Diagnostic Medical Sonography
A GUIDE TO CLINICAL PRACTICE

VOLUME I
Obstetrics and Gynecology

VOLUME I   **Obstetrics and Gynecology**

Edited by
MIMI C. BERMAN, PH.D., R.D.M.S.
Associate Professor, Diagnostic Medical Imaging Program
College of Health Related Professions
State University of New York
Health Science Center at Brooklyn
Brooklyn, New York

VOLUME II   **Echocardiography**

Edited by
MARVEEN CRAIG, R.D.M.S.
Founder
International Ultrasound Institute
Dallas, Texas

VOLUME III   **Abdomen**

Edited by
DIANE M. KAWAMURA, M.ED., R.T.(R), R.D.M.S.
Professor, Radiological Sciences
Weber State College
Ogden, Utah

Diagnostic Medical Sonography

A GUIDE TO CLINICAL PRACTICE

VOLUME I **Obstetrics and Gynecology**

Edited by
MIMI C. BERMAN, PH.D., R.D.M.S.

J.B. Lippincott Company

PHILADELPHIA   NEW YORK   ST. LOUIS
LONDON   SYDNEY   TOKYO

Acquisitions Editor: Charles McCormick
Developmental Editor: Kimberley Cox
Production Manager: Janet Greenwood
Production: Editorial Services of New England
Compositor: University Graphics, Inc.
Printer/Binder: Halliday Lithograph

5 6 4

Library of Congress Cataloging-in-Publication Data

Obstetrics and gynecology / edited by Mimi C. Berman.
    p.   cm.—(Diagnostic medical sonography; v.   1)
  Includes bibliographical references.
  Includes index.
  1. Ultrasonic in obstetrics.   2. Generative organs, Female-
Ultrasonic imaging.   I. Berman, Mimi C.   II. Series.
  [DNLM: 1. Gynecology.   2. Obstetrics.   WB 289 D5355 v.   1}
RC78.7.U4D48   vol.   1
{RG527.5.U48}
616.07′543 s—dc20
[618.1′07543}
DLC
for Library of Congress   90-6249
                                                                     CIP

ISBN 0-397-50952-9
ISBN 0-397-50954-5 (set)

The authors and publisher have exerted every effort to ensure that drug selection and dosage
set forth in this text are in accord with current recommendations and practice at the time of
publication. However, in view of ongoing research, changes in government regulations, and
the constant flow of information relating to drug therapy and drug reactions, the reader is
urged to check the package insert for each drug for any change in indications and dosage and
for added warnings and precautions. This is particularly important when the recommended
agent is a new or infrequently employed drug.

To Marvin, my parents, and my students, who have taught me the qualities necessary to produce this book—love, knowledge, patience, perseverance, and awe.

And to those who will use this book:

"The bees plunder the flowers here and there, but afterward they make of them honey, which is all theirs; it is no longer thyme or marjoram. Even so with the pieces borrowed from others; he will transform and blend them to make a work that is all his own, to wit, his judgment. His education, work and study aim only at forming this." *Michel de Montaigne—Of the Education of Children*

Contributors

Dunstan Abraham, M.P.H., R.D.M.S.
Clinical Instructor,
New York University Medical Center, School of
Diagnostic Medical Sonography,
New York, New York;
Supervisor of Ultrasound,
Bronx Municipal Hospital Center,
Bronx, New York

Birgit Bader-Armstrong, R.D.M.S.
Assistant in Obstetrics and Gynecology,
University of Rochester School of Medicine and
Dentistry;
Administrator,
Strong Memorial Hospital,
Rochester, New York

Raymond Atwood, B.S., R.D.M.S.
Clinical Instructor, Diagnostic Medical Imaging
Program,
College of Health Related Professions,
State University of New York, Health Science
Center at Brooklyn;
Staff Sonographer,
Kings County Hospital,
Brooklyn, New York

Carol B. Benson, M.D.
Associate Director of Ultrasound,
Brigham and Women's Hospital;
Assistant Professor of Radiology,

Harvard Medical School,
Boston, Massachusetts

Mimi C. Berman, Ph.D., R.D.M.S.
Associate Professor, Diagnostic Medical Imaging
Program,
College of Health Related Professions,
State University of New York, Health Science
Center at Brooklyn,
Brooklyn, New York

Paul D. Cayea, M.D.
Assistant Professor of Clinical Radiology,
University Hospital at Stony Brook,
Stony Brook, New York;
Director of Ultrasound,
Winthrop-University Hospital,
Mineola, New York

Frank Cervantes, B.A., R.T., R.D.M.S.
Associate Director, Department of Radiology;
Supervisor, Division of Ultrasound,
State University of New York, Health Science
Center at Brooklyn,
Brooklyn, New York

Linda M. Chase, B.A., B.S., R.D.M.S.
Clinical Assistant Professor, Diagnostic Medical
Imaging Program,
College of Health Related Professions,
State University of New York, Health Science
Center at Brooklyn,
Brooklyn, New York

Frank A. Chervenak, M.D.
Director of Ultrasound and Ethics,
Department of Obstetrics and Gynecology,
New York Hospital,
Cornell University Medical Center,
New York, New York

Harris L. Cohen, M.D.
Associate Professor of Radiology,
Cornell University Medical College;
Associate Director, Division of Ultrasound,
Chief, Section of Pediatric Ultrasound,
North Shore University Hospital,
Manhasset, New York

Marveen Craig, R.D.M.S.
Founder, International Ultrasound Institute,
Dallas, Texas

Reva A. Curry, M.Ed., R.T. (R), R.D.M.S.
Program Coordinator,
Diagnostic Medical Sonography,
Department of Diagnostic Imaging,
College of Allied Health Science,
Thomas Jefferson University,
Philadelphia, Pennsylvania

Dale R. Cyr, B.S., R.D.M.S.
Chief Sonographer,
Division of Diagnostic Ultrasound,
Department of Radiology,
University of Washington,
Seattle, Washington

Sharon DalCompo, R.T., R.D.M.S.
Supervisor, Diagnostic Ultrasound Center,
Prentice Women's Pavilion,
Northwestern Memorial Hospital,
Chicago, Illinois

Marie DeLange, B.S., R.D.M.S.
Program Director and Chief Sonographer,
Section of Diagnostic Ultrasound,
Department of Radiation Sciences,
Loma Linda University Medical Center,
Loma Linda, Calfornia

Mark A. Dennis, M.D.
Chief Radiologist, Division of Diagnostic
Ultrasound,
Rose Medical Center;
Clinical Faculty, Department of Radiology,
University of Colorado Health Sciences Center,
Denver, Colorado

Julia A. Drose, B.A., R.T., R.D.M.S.
Chief Diagnostic Medical Sonographer,
Division of Diagnostic Ultrasound;
Instructor, Department of Radiology,
University of Colorado Health Sciences Center,
Denver, Colorado

Terry J. DuBose, B.B.A., A.S., R.R.T., R.D.M.S.
Senior Sonographer,
Austin Radiological Association;
Director, Diagnostic Medical Sonography,
Austin Community College,
Austin, Texas

Mary Beth Geagan, B.S., R.T., R.D.M.S.
Assistant Supervisor, Division of Ultrasound,
State University of New York, Health Science
Center at Brooklyn,
Brooklyn, New York

Steven R. Goldstein, M.D.
Assistant Professor of Clinical Obstetrics and
Gynecology,
New York University School of Medicine,
New York, New York

William Greenhut, B.A., R.D.M.S.
Instructor, School of Diagnostic Medical
Sonography,
New York University Medical Center,
New York, New York;
Diagnostic Medical Imaging Program,
State University of New York, Health Science
Center at Brooklyn,
Brooklyn, New York;
Diagnostic Medical Ultrasonography Program,
University of Medicine and Dentistry of New
Jersey,
Newark, New Jersey;
Staff Technologist,
Bronx Muncipal Hospital Center,
Bronx, New York

Gerald L. Grube, M.D.
Director of Diagnostic Ultrasound,
Section of Diagnostic Ultrasound,
Department of Radiation Sciences,
Loma Linda University Medical Center,
Loma Linda, California

Warren G. Guntheroth, M.D.
Professor of Pediatrics (Cardiology),
Attending Pediatric Cardiologist,
University of Washington,
Seattle, Washington

Rebecca Hall, M.S., R.D.M.S.
Lecturer, Program Director,
Diagnostic Medical Sonography Program,
Allied Health Sciences, School of Medicine,
University of New Mexico,
Albuquerque, New Mexico

Jack O. Haller, M.D.
Professor and Vice Chairman,
Department of Radiology,
State University of New York, Health Science
Center at Brooklyn,
Brooklyn, New York

Kathleen S. Howe, M.A., R.D.M.S.
Sonographic Support Services,
Albuquerque, New Mexico

Glenn Isaacson, M.D.
Assistant Professor of Otolaryngology,
Section of Pediatric Otolaryngology,
St. Christoper's Hospital for Children,
Philadelphia, Pennsylvania

Diana Kawai, B.S., R.D.M.S.
Program Director,
Maryland Institute of Ultrasound Technology,
Greater Baltimore Medical Center,
Baltimore, Maryland

Diane M. Kawamura, M.Ed., R.T.(R), R.D.M.S.
Professor, Radiological Sciences,
Weber State College,
Ogden, Utah

H. J. Khamis, Ph.D.
Associate Director, Statistical Consulting Center,
Associate Professor, Department of Mathematics
& Statistics and Department of Community
Health,
School of Medicine,
Wright State University,
Dayton, Ohio

Mordecai Koenigsberg, M.D.
Associate Professor of Radiology,
Albert Einstein College of Medicine;
Director of Ultrasound,
Weiler Hospital of the Albert Einstein College of
Medicine,
Bronx, New York

Michelle Lanigan, M.D.
Radiologist,
Staten Island University Hospital,
Staten Island, New York

Ji-Bin Liu, M.D.
Research Fellow,
Division of Diagnostic Ultrasound, Department
of Radiology,
Thomas Jefferson University Hospital,
Philadelphia, Pennsylvania

Laurence A. Mack, M.D.
Professor of Radiology,
University of Washington,
Seattle, Washington

Laurence B. McCullough, Ph.D.
Professor of Medicine and Community Medicine,
Center for Ethics, Medicine, and Public Issues,
Baylor College of Medicine,
Houston, Texas

Joyce A. Miller, M.A., R.D.M.S.
Assistant Professor,
Diagnostic Medical Imaging Program,
College of Health Related Professions,
State University of New York, Health Science
Center at Brooklyn,
Brooklyn, New York

Susan E. Nealer, B.S., R.D.M.S.
Chief Sonographer,
Department of Radiology,
State University of New York, Health Science
Center at Syracuse,
Syracuse, New York

Martha Newelt, B.S., R.D.M.S.
Adjunct Lecturer,
Diagnostic Medical Imaging Program,
College of Health Related Professions,
State University of New York, Health Science
Center at Brooklyn;
Coordinating Manager, Kings County Hospital,
Brooklyn, New York

Lawrence D. Platt, M.D.
Professor,
University of California;
Chairman,
Department of Obstetrics and Gynecology,
Cedars Sinai Medical Center,
Los Angeles, California

Regina Rodrick, R.T., R.D.M.S.
Staff Sonographer,
Maryland Institute of Ultrasound Technology,
Greater Baltimore Medical Center,
Baltimore, Maryland

Joanne Rosenberg, B.S., R.D.M.S.
Chief Sonographer,
Division of Maternal-Fetal Medicine,
University of Medicine and Dentistry of
New Jersey,
Robert Wood Johnson Medical School,
New Brunswick, New Jersey

Ruth Rosenblatt, M.D.
Associate Professor of Radiology,
Albert Einstein College of Medicine;
Attending Radiologist,
Montefiore Hospital and Radiology,
Bronx, New York

Rudy E. Sabbagha, M.D.
Professor of Obstetrics and Gynecology,
Northwestern University;
Director,
Diagnostic Ultrasound Center,
Prentice Women's Pavilion,
Northwestern Memorial Hospital,
Chicago, Illinois

Roger C. Sanders, M.D.
Medical Director,
Ultrasound Institute of Baltimore,
Baltimore, Maryland

Sathyanarayana, M.D.
Assistant Professor of Radiology,
Chief, Section of Diagnostic Ultrasound;
Medical Director,
Diagnostic Medical Sonography Program,
Medical College of Georgia,
Augusta, Georgia

George I. Solish, M.D., M.S., Ph.D.
Professor of Obstetrics and Gynecology,
State University of New York, Health Science
Center at Brooklyn;
Director of Medical Genetic Services,
Maimonides Hospital,
Brooklyn, New York

Beverly A. Spirt, M.D.
Professor of Radiology,
Chief of Ultrasound,
Department of Radiology,
State University of New York,
Health Science Center at Syracuse,
Syracuse, New York

Jean Lea Spitz, M.Ph., R.D.M.S.
Professor and Program Director of Sonography,
University of Oklahoma,
College of Allied Health,
Oklahoma City, Oklahoma

Katharine Steurer, R.D.M.S.
Sonographer,
The Johns Hopkins Medical Institutions,
Baltimore, Maryland

Jane Streltzoff, B.S., R.D.M.S.
Chief Sonographer,
Obstetrical Ultrasound,
New York Hospital, Cornell University Medical
Center,
New York, New York

Phil-Ann Tan-Sinn, R.T., R.D.M.S.
Clinical Staff Sonographer,
Section of Diagnostic Ultrasound, Department of
Radiation Sciences,
Loma Linda University Medical Center,
Loma Linda, California

Linda J. Wadsworth, R.T., R.D.M.S.
Staff Sonographer,
Department of Radiology,
State University of New York, Health Science
Center at Syracuse,
Syracuse, New York

Larry Waldroup, B.S., R.D.M.S.
Technical Manager,
Division of Diagnostic Ultrasound, Department
of Radiology,
Thomas Jefferson University Hospital,
Philadelphia, Pennsylvania

Catherine A. Walla, R.N., M.A., M.N.
Assistant Clinical Professor,
University of California, Los Angeles;
Clinical Research Specialist,
Los Angeles County and University of Southern
California Medical Center,
Los Angeles, California

Lisa A. Warneke, R.D.M.S.
Assistant Chief Technologist,

Brigham and Women's Hospital,
Harvard Medical School,
Boston, Massachusetts

Roger W. Warner, M.S., R.D.M.S.
Senior Consultant and Manager of Physician
Services,
Administrative Health Management Group,
Dayton, Ohio

Paula S. Woletz, B.A., R.D.M.S., R.D.C.S.
Adjunct Faculty Member,
School of Graduate Medical Education,
Seton Hall University,
South Orange, New Jersey;
Perinatal Testing Coordinator,
St. Joseph's Hospital and Medical Center,
Paterson, New Jersey

John Yaghoobian, M.D.
Director,
Radiology Department,
Victory Memorial Hospital
Brooklyn, New York

Preface

One of the most dynamic specialties in the field of diagnostic ultrasound is obstetrics and gynecology, not only because constantly improving technology is expanding diagnostic capabilities, but because it matches the continuously changing treatment of gynecologic and obstetric problems. In vitro fertilization, selective infanticide, intrauterine transfusion, and chorionic villus sampling are some new treatment options that are enhanced by or depend on sonographic imaging. Although progress in gynecology has not been as dramatic, the increasing use of Doppler investigation of uterine and ovarian blood flow and the exquisite resolution of pelvic organs afforded by transvaginal transducers show early promise in providing answers to infertility problems and to the early detection of lethal gynecologic malignancies.

This volume has been designed to include the most current and reliable information available to date. To ensure a permanent value to its content, the text includes at least equal coverage of the normal gynecologic and obstetric applications of sonography. Clinical principles, sonographic techniques, and the interpretive criteria that form the theoretical base of obstetric and gynecologic sonography have been emphasized and they will apply to most of the innovations that will inevitably occur. Chapters on ethics, embryology, and maternal-fetal emotional interactions, statistics, and computers will likewise be of lasting interest.

Each chapter has been written and critiqued by practitioners with recognized expertise in the topic. To make the content clear, concise, and easy to use in daily practice, summary tables, schematics, and diagrams have been included in addition to the sonographic illustrations. Every effort has been made to offer sonographers and physicians a book that is accurate, comprehensive, and useful.

We would like to acknowledge the contributors to this volume for their willingness to share their experience, knowledge, and dedication to our profession.

MIMI C. BERMAN, PH.D., R.D.M.S.
MARVEEN CRAIG, R.D.M.S.
DIANE M. KAWAMURA, M.ED., R.T.(R), R.D.M.S.

Contents

PART III   Obstetric Sonography

PART IV **Technical and Psychosocial Topics in Gynecologic and Obstetric Sonography**

List of Tables

PART ONE

Basic Principles of Scanning Techniques

CHAPTER 1

Principles of Scanning Technique in Obstetric and Gynecologic Ultrasound

MIMI C. BERMAN

Using proper technique to examine gynecologic and obstetric patients will result in diagnostic-quality sonograms, minimal ultrasound exposure for the patient, cost containment, and minimal patient discomfort. Much of the art of scanning has disappeared, as most articulated-arm machines have been put into mothballs, but the importance of a scientific approach to the examination has increased with the advent of real-time scanning. Articulated-arm scanners allowed complete sections of the body to be imaged. When they were applied with the proper art to a sonographically "photogenic" patient, the images were often comparable to those produced by computed tomography (CT) and magnetic resonance imaging (MRI). Ironically, although manipulating the equipment has become easier, producing diagnostic-quality images now requires better knowledge of anatomy, disease processes, and sonographic data. Real-time imaging demands that the sonographer develop a systematic approach to scanning, to avoid missing any section of the body. However, today's sonographer, unlike early clinicians, has the benefit of a large body of research and experience in ultrasound, which provides guidelines on technique and criteria.

In this chapter I describe the basic techniques and protocols of scanning in obstetrics and gynecology. Routines specific to the topics discussed are explained in subsequent chapters.

Parity and Last Menstrual Period

Knowing the patient's reproductive history gives the sonographer important information with which to design and interpret the sonographic examination. There are variations to the coding system used, but the following method is generally applicable: *Gravidity* (G) refers to the number of pregnancies the patient has had and includes the current one. A pregnant woman who had an ectopic pregnancy and gave birth to twins would be G3. *Parity* (P) refers to the number of pregnancies the patient has carried to term; thus, an ectopic pregnancy would be recorded as P0 and a twin gestation would be P1. The numbers used after P refer, in the order presented, to the number of term pregnancies, premature deliveries, abortions, and living children. Thus G3P1012 would mean the woman has had 3 pregnancies, 1 full-term pregnancy, no premature deliveries, 1 abortion (the ectopic pregnancy in this case), and two full-term births, in this case, a set of twins.[7]

It is generally accepted that the first day of the last menstrual period (LMP) is used to date pregnancies. The LMP usually occurs about 2 weeks before conception, but it is chosen because women can document this date. Still, some 20 to 40% of pregnant women are uncertain of their LMP, so this date may be unreliable for dating a pregnancy. Ultrasound can narrow the estimated date of deliv-

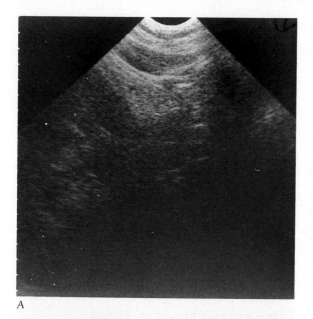

A

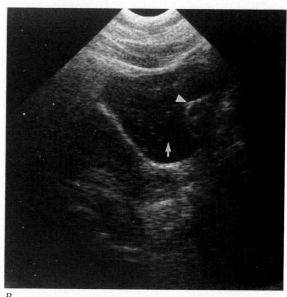

B

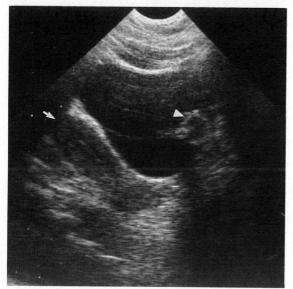

C

Figure 1-1. (A) This sagittal transabdominal scan through an empty bladder does not visualize the uterus and adnexa. (B) The bladder has been partially filled with saline. Although the uterus is visualized better, the bladder is not filled enough to allow complete evaluation of the fundal region. The balloon (*arrowhead*) from the Foley catheter can be seen, as can echoes (*arrow*) produced by the air that entered the bladder with the fluid. (C) With the bladder adequately filled, the fundus (*arrow*) can be evaluated, as can the echogenicity of the myometrium and endometrium (*arrowhead*, balloon from the catheter).

ery to as little as ±2.7 days by using at least three crown-rump length (CRL) measurements.[8]

Patient Preparation
Gynecologic Ultrasound Examinations
Anyone remotely involved with general ultrasound knows that a full bladder is required for performing gynecologic exams (Fig. 1-1). The use of this window has become almost the hallmark of obstetric and gynecologic scanning, but over the years its use has been modified or refined to suit particular examinations, problems, and transducers.

Instructions to a patient on how to prepare for an examination should be tailored to the patient,

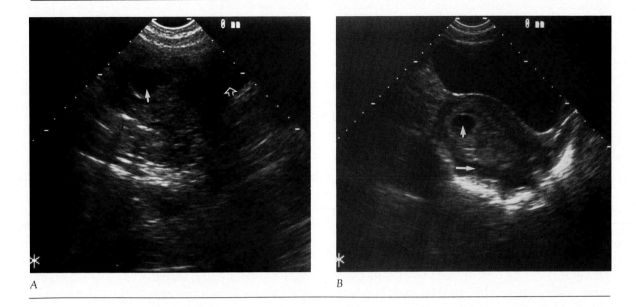

FIGURE 1-2. (A) The urinary bladder *(open arrow)* has a small amount of urine in it, but not enough to determine whether the fluid-filled structure *(short arrow)* is a gestational sac and whether it is within or outside the uterus. (B) The uterus with the fundal gestational sac *(arrow)* can now be clearly delineated because the bladder is full. A cul-de-sac fluid collection *(long arrow)* is also apparent.

the examination objectives, and the transducer that will be used. A young woman who is to be examined for a possible ovarian cyst can be instructed to eat normally, drink four 8-ounce glasses of water, and not void for 2 hours prior to the exam. These directions should ensure that she will be properly prepared for the study. On the other hand, a postmenopausal woman in her 60s or 70s who is being scheduled because of uterine bleeding may have decreased bladder capacity or may suffer from incontinence.[24] The directions to her could be to eat normally, drink three 8-ounce glasses of water, and not void for 1 hour before the examination. If a patient is scheduled for a transvaginal examination, no urinary bladder filling is required; however, if transabdominal scanning is to be performed prior to the transvaginal examination, it is still advisable to instruct the patient to come prepared with a full bladder.

If the patient's bladder is so distended that it compresses and displaces the pelvic viscera, or the patient cannot tolerate the examination, it may be wise to instruct her to pass some urine. Patients usually respond, "I can't control the flow. I'll empty everything." If given a cup and told to empty as many cups as the sonographer thinks is necessary, patients usually are able to comply.

Obstetric Examinations

The degree of bladder filling required depends on the stage of the gestation. In the first trimester, a full bladder is needed for transabdominal scanning because the intestines have not been pushed out of the false pelvis by the uterus and therefore cast obliterating echoes over it (Fig. 1-2). From the second trimester on, it is usually not necessary for the patient to have a full bladder. In normal pregnancies there is sufficient amniotic fluid to provide a window to the fetus, and the expanded uterus fills the pelvic cavity and pushes the intestines out of the way.[22]

There are particular situations, however, when some filling of the bladder enhances visualization of the cervical portion of the uterus—the internal os, to be specific. When examining for an incompetent os, the bladder affords an unobstructed view of that area.[21] Postvoiding scans are necessary on the os, to demonstrate the extent of dilation without the mechanical pressure exerted by a full bladder. When identifying the location of a suspiciously low-lying placenta, a moderately full bladder enhances imaging in the area. Also, when the fetal head lies very deep in the pelvis, a partially filled bladder may displace the head upward into a position where the biparietal diameter (BPD) can be measured. A rule of thumb for estimating whether the bladder is full enough has been that it should extend slightly beyond the uterine fundus. This can be applied in gynecologic scanning when the uterus is normal in size or retroverted, but it is not a hard and fast rule. Once again, the sonographer must use common sense: If the uterus and adnexa are clearly delineated, the bladder is full enough; if not, the patient should be instructed to drink more water. This may or may not help. Other bladder manipulation techniques that should be kept in mind involve asking the patient to lie in a left or right posterior oblique (LPO, RPO) position, so that the bladder drapes over a structure being scanned, such as the lateral section of the uterus, the adnexa, or a mass.

Performing the Gynecologic Examination

When the patient arrives for her gynecologic examination, the sonographer assists her onto the examination table. The patient should be informed about the examination procedure—how long it will take, what sensations she will feel, how the transducer will be moved over her pelvis. At the same time, the sonographer should confirm the patient's identity and record all pertinent clinical information on the examination report. This information should include the patient's age, last menstrual period, parity, history of surgical procedures, and other pertinent medical history. The sonographer is required to obtain this information from the patient if it is not already on the examination request. Then the examination can begin. Mineral oil was often used with articulated-arm scanners, but today a variety of gels are on the market that are more viscous and more suitable for real-time transducers. The gel should be applied liberally to the pelvis to provide an effective medium for sound transmission. It makes the exami-

nation more pleasant if the gel is warmed to body temperature. If a laboratory is not equipped with a gel warmer, the container can be placed in hot water for a few minutes to remove the chill. Cold gel and a full bladder is a bad combination.

In many laboratories, the sonographer and the sonologist develop scanning protocols for each type of examination. In some laboratories, these are printed in a reference manual. Suggested protocols have been developed for obstetric scanning by the American Institute of Ultrasound in Medicine (AIUM; Display 1-1) and the Society of Diagnostic Medical Sonographers (SDMS; Table 1-1). Less standardization has been achieved in gynecologic scanning, but the SDMS does recommend following certain procedures (see Table 1-1). A sonographer developing his or her own protocols should keep in mind that the sonographic examination must demonstrate clearly through a series of images that the findings are normal or abnormal. For gynecologic examinations this requires that each pertinent section of the pelvis be scanned thoroughly and that representative scans be recorded that demonstrate the normal or abnormal findings.

Regardless of the indications for it, a gynecologic examination should include the following images: sagittal: midline of uterus including the cervix and vagina, right and left lateral views of the uterus, right and left ovaries; transverse: fundus with cornua of uterus, corpus, cervix, vagina, right and left ovaries. If the sonographic examination is being done to rule out pathology of any kind, these views should be recorded along with clear documentation of the characteristics of the pathology. The sonographic record should include several sagittal and transverse views, including measurements, gain studies of the echogenicity and transsonicity of the lesion, and clear delineation of the relationship of the mass or abnormality to other organs and structures. If results of the sonographic examination are negative, the area of interest should be imaged to show that no pathology was seen.

The sonographer must also be aware of the findings that often are associated with particular diseases. For instance, upon finding a solid ovarian mass the sonographer should carefully examine the cul-de-sac, Morison's pouch, the liver edge, and the flanks for ascites. In addition, the liver, kidneys, and perivascular areas should be examined for ev-

Table 1-1. SDMS suggested scanning protocols for obstetrics and female pelvis

Obstetrics (preparation, full bladder)
A. First trimester
  1. Real-time (essential)
    a. Document
      1. Uterus
      2. Gestational sac
      3. Fetal pole
      4. Yolk sac
      5. Fetal heart movement (FHM)
      6. Ovaries
    b. Measure
      1. Gestational sac
      2. Crown-rump (CRL)
      3. Biparietal diameter (BPD) and femur length (FL) (11-12 weeks)
  2. Static scan (optional)
    a. Sagittal and transverse
    b. 1-cm increments
B. Second and third trimester
  1. Real-time (essential)
    a. Document
      1. Fetal position
      2. Internal os
      3. Placental position and grade
      4. Fetal anatomy
        *Stomach
        Liver
        Spleen
        *FHM
        *Kidneys
        *Bladder
        *Spine
        *Cranial anatomy
        Lungs
        Extremities
        Umbilical cord
        Genitalia
        Amniotic fluid
    b. Measure
      *1. BPD at thalamus
      *2. Head circumference (HC)
      *3. FL

      *4. Abdominal circumference (AC) at umbilical vein
      5. Binocular measurements
  2. Static scan by 1- or 2-cm increments, sagittal and transverse
  3. For twins
    a. Document both heads in one image if possible
    b. Document septum if applicable
  4. To rule out placenta previa
    a. Scan internal os before and after voiding
    b. Head-sacrum measurement
  5. For growth retardation
    a. Use ratios FL/AC HC/AC
    b. Total intrauterine volume (TIUV)
    c. Fetal weight
  6. To rule out ectopic
    a. Routine pelvic
    b. If fluid seen in cul-de-sac, scan Morison's pouch
Pelvic
A. General
  1. Note LMP
  2. Full bladder
  3. Static and transverse by 1-cm increments (to tilt of uterus)
  4. Document
    a. Uterus
    b. Ovaries
    c. Adnexa
    d. Vaginal canal
    e. Bowel peristalsis
  5. Pelvic with adnexal masses
    a. Document kidneys
  6. If free fluid seen
    a. Document Morison's pouch
  7. Equivocal masses
    a. Use H_2O enema
B. To rule out ectopic
  1. Routine pelvic
  2. If fluid seen in cul-de-sac, scan Morison's pouch

*Essential anatomy and measurements
(Adapted from Bell BT, Nowers C. SDMS suggested scanning protocols. J Diagn Med Sonogr. 1986; 2:343–347.)

idence of metastases. Every examination must be performed thoroughly; the added time it takes is minimal when using real-time scanners and the findings may be critical to the patient's well-being. Although sonographic images of gynecologic masses often are frustratingly nonspecific, with optimal technique, characteristics related to particular masses can be visualized sonographically. In the following chapters specific techniques are described. Table 1-2 summarizes general approaches the sonographer can use to enhance visualization of particular aspects of masses.

A good understanding of the physical principles of ultrasound gives the sonographer a valuable tool for solving diagnostic scanning problems. Many excellent textbooks explain these principles.[9,10,12,16]

Display 1-1.   Antepartum Obstetrical Ultrasound Examination Guidelines

These guidelines have been developed for use by practitioners performing obstetrical ultrasound studies. In some cases, additional and/or specialized examination may be necessary. While it is not possible to detect all structural congenital anomalies with diagnostic ultrasound, adherence to the following guidelines will maximize the possibility of detecting many fetal abnormalities.

Equipment

These studies should be conducted with real-time or a combination of real-time and static scanners, but never solely with a static scanner. A transducer of appropriate frequency (3 to 5 MHz) should be used.

Comment. Real-time is necessary to reliably confirm the presence of fetal life through observation of cardiac activity, respiration, and active movement. Real-time studies simplify evaluation of fetal anatomy as well as the task of obtaining fetal measurements.

The choice of frequency is a trade-off between beam penetration and resolution. With modern equipment 3- to 5-MHz transducers allow sufficient penetration in nearly all patients, while providing adequate resolution. During early pregnancy, a 5-MHz transducer may provide adequate penetration and produce superior resolution.

Documentation

Adequate documentation of the study is essential for high-quality patient care. This should include a permanent record of the ultrasound images, incorporating whenever possible the measurement parameters and anatomical findings proposed in the following sections of this document. Images should be appropriately labeled with the examination date, patient identification, and image orientation. A written report of the ultrasound findings should be included in the patient's medical record regardless of where the study is performed.

Guidelines for First Trimester Sonography

1. The location of the gestational sac should be documented. The embryo should be identified and the crown-rump length recorded.

Comment. The crown-rump length is an accurate indicator of fetal age. Comparison should be made to standard tables. During the late first trimester, biparietal diameter and other fetal measurements may also be used to establish fetal age.

2. Presence or absence of fetal life should be reported.

Comment: Real-time observation is critical in this diagnosis. It should be noted that fetal cardiac activity may not be visible prior to seven weeks as determined by crown-rump length. Thus, confirmation of fetal life may require follow-up evaluation.

3. Fetal number should be documented.

Comment. Multiple pregnancy should be reported only in those instances where multiple embryos are seen. Due to variability in fusion between the amnion and chorion, the appearance of more than one sac-like structure in early pregnancy is often noted and may be confused with multiple gestation or amniotic bands.

4. Evaluation of the uterus (including cervix) and adnexal structures should be performed.

Comment. This will allow recognition of incidental findings of potential clinical significance. The presence, location, and size of myomas and adnexal masses should be recorded.

Guidelines for Second and Third Trimester Sonography

1. Fetal life, number, and presentation should be documented.

Comment. Abnormal heart rate and/or rhythm should be reported. Multiple pregnancies require the reporting of additional information: placental number, sac number, and comparison of fetal size.

2. An estimate of the amount of amniotic fluid (increased, decreased, normal) should be reported.

Comment. While this evaluation is subjective, there is little difficulty in recognizing the extremes of amniotic fluid volume. Physiologic variation with stage of pregnancy must be taken into account.

3. The placental location should be recorded and its relationship to the internal cervical os determined.

Comment. It is recognized that placental position early in pregnancy may not correlate well with its location at the time of delivery.

4. Assessment of gestational age in the second and third trimester should be accomplished using a combination of biparietal diameter (or head circumference) and femur length. Fetal growth assessment (as opposed to age) requires the addition of abdominal circumferences. If previous studies have been done, an estimate of the appropriateness of interval change should be given.

Comment. Third trimester measurements may not accurately reflect gestational age. Initial determination of gestational age should be performed prior to 26 weeks whenever possible.

4A. Biparietal diameter at a standard reference level (which should include the cavum septi pellucidi, the thalamus, or the cerebral peduncles) should be measured and recorded.

Comment. If the fetal head is dolichocephalic or brachycephalic, the biparietal diameter alone may be misleading. In such situations, the head circumference is required.

4B. Head circumference is measured at the same level as the biparietal diameter.
4C. Femur length should be measured routinely and recorded after the 14th week of gestation.

Comment. As with biparietal diameter, considerable biological variation is present late in pregnancy.

4D. Abdominal circumference should be determined at the level of the junction of the umbilical vein and portal sinus.

Comment. Abdominal circumference measurement may allow detection of asymmetric growth retardation—a condition of the late second and third trimester. Comparison of the abdominal circumference with the head circumference should be made. If the abdominal measurement is below that expected for a stated gestation, it is recommended that circumferences of the head and body be measured and the head circumference/abdominal circumference ratio be reported. The use of circumferences is also suggested in those instances where the shape of either the head or body is different from that normally encountered.

5. Evaluation of the uterus and adnexal structures should be performed.

Comment. This will allow recognition of incidental findings of potential clinical significance. The presence, location, and size of myomas and adnexal masses should be recorded.

6. The study should include, but not necessarily be limited to, the following fetal anatomy: cerebral ventricles, spine, stomach, urinary bladder, umbilical cord insertion site on the anterior abdominal wall, and renal region.

Comment. It is recognized that not all malformations of the above-mentioned organ systems (such as the spine) can be detected using ultrasonography. Nevertheless, a careful anatomical survey may allow diagnosis of certain birth defects which would otherwise go unrecognized. Suspected abnormalities may require a specialized evaluation.

(Leopold GR. Antepartum obstetrical ultrasound examination guidelines. J Ultrasound Med. 1986; 5:241–242.)

Chapter 37 describes the artifacts sonographers should be aware of when scanning. The sonographer should make every effort to minimize them. Certain basic scanning principles should be utilized to achieve the best, most informative images:

1. The sonographic beam should be perpendicular to the area of interest.
2. The best resolution occurs within the focal zone of the transducer.
3. Higher-megahertz transducers display more detail in the area through which the focal portion of the beam passes.
4. Signals from lower-megahertz transducers penetrate farther than those from higher-megahertz ones.
5. Fluid-filled structures enhance the transmission of sound.
6. Solid structures usually attenuate the sound to varying degrees, depending on the nature of the tissue.

Performing the Obstetric Examination

Scanning a pregnant patient before the 15th week of gestation requires basically the same technique

TABLE 1-2. General principles of gynecologic scanning techniques

CHARACTERISTICS OF MASS	SCANNING TECHNIQUE
Size	Measure three longest dimensions: length, height, width
Mobility	Turn patient, empty bladder, apply transducer pressure
Tissue composition	Change transducer: high- to low-frequency Compare to urine, which is fluid and anechoic Raise gain settings to see septations, lower gain to see shadows from calcifications Look for edge shadowing and anterior reverberation artifacts in fluid-filled structures Check for peristalsis in mass to determine whether it is bowel
Extension	Examine bladder wall, which should appear as clean, echogenic line measuring 3 to 6 mm Examine cul-de-sac, flanks, Morison's pouch for ascites Examine liver for metastases Examine kidneys for hydronephrosis and metastases Examine perivascular area for enlarged nodes

as a gynecologic examination. The protocol detailing the number of exams and measurements that need to be taken is summarized in Table 1-1 and is described more fully in subsequent chapters.

Later in pregnancy, from about 20 weeks,[8] some women suffer from caval compression syndrome and cannot lie on their back for long periods. The sonographer can accommodate such patients by elevating their back or performing as much of the scan as possible with patients lying on the left side. Also, scanning in the most efficient manner possible reduces the time the patient lies on the table. The sonographer should establish an organized routine for scanning, for example, beginning the scan at the fetal head and carefully examining each organ and limb while moving toward the femurs. Images that demonstrate the findings can be recorded as the thorough survey is completed. Consistency in performing each scan saves the sonographer from having to design a new approach for each patient, makes doing complete examinations habitual, and alerts the sonographer very quickly when something is abnormal.

Safety of Ultrasound

The patient undoubtedly will ask questions about the findings of the examinations and about the safety to the fetus and herself of exposure to diagnostic ultrasound. The sonographer must answer these questions accurately and clearly. Extensive research has been done on the potential deleterious effects of diagnostic ultrasound. The AIUM, the

SDMS, the National Institutes of Health (NIH), and the United States Food and Drug Administration (FDA) carefully monitor results of epidemiologic and biologic studies. In 1984 the NIH and the FDA convened a Consensus Development Conference on Diagnostic Ultrasound Imaging in Pregnancy. The report generated by the proceedings of that meeting included the following statements: "It is the consensus of the panel that ultrasound examination in pregnancy should be performed for a specific medical indication. The data on clinical efficacy and safety do not allow a recommendation for routine screening at this time." In this same vein, the AIUM published a Bioeffects Report[1] in which the following safety statement and two conclusions appeared:

American Institute of Ultrasound in Medicine Official Statement on Clinical Safety. Approved October 1982; revised and approved March 1988.
Diagnostic ultrasound has been in use since the late 1950s. Given its known benefits and recognized efficacy for medical diagnosis, including use during human pregnancy, the AIUM herein addresses the clinical safety of such use:

No confirmed biological effects on patients or instrument operators caused by exposure at intensities typical of present diagnostic ultrasound instruments have ever been reported. Although the possibility exists that such biological effects may be identified in the future, current data indicate that the benefits to patients of the prudent use of diagnostic ultrasound outweigh the risks, if any, that may be present.

Conclusions Regarding Epidemiology. Approved October 1987.

1. Widespread clinical use over 25 years has not established any adverse effect arising from exposure to diagnostic ultrasound.
2. Randomized clinical studies are the most rigorous method for assessing potential adverse effects of diagnostic ultrasound. Studies using this methodology show no evidence of an effect on birthweight in humans.[a]
3. Other epidemiologic studies have shown no causal association of diagnostic ultrasound with any of the adverse fetal outcomes studied.[a]

[a](The acoustic exposure levels in these studies may not be representative of the full range of current fetal exposures.)

Conclusions Regarding In Vivo *Mammalian Bioeffects. Approved October 1987.*

A review of bioeffects data supports the following statement as an update of the AIUM Statement on *In Vivo* Mammalian Bioeffects:

In the low megahertz frequency range there have been (as of this date) no independently confirmed significant biological effects in mammalian tissues exposed in vivo to unfocused ultrasound with intensities[a] below 100 mW/cm², or to focused[b] ultrasound with intensities below 1 W/cm². Furthermore, for exposure times[c] greater than 1 second and less than 500 seconds for unfocused ultrasound or 50 seconds for focused ultrasound, such effects have not been demonstrated even at higher intensities, when the product of intensity and exposure time is less than 50 joules/cm².

[a]Free-field spatial peak, temporal average (SPTA) for continuous wave exposures, and for pulsed-mode exposures with pulses repeated at a frequency greater than 100 hz.
[b]Quarter-power (-db) beam width smaller than 4 wavelengths or 4 mm, whichever is less at the exposure frequency.
[c]Total time including off-time as well as on-time for repeated pulse exposures.

These conclusions and statements apply equally to the use of Doppler ultrasound, although presently the FDA has established guidelines that restrict the power levels used in fetal scanning below those used prior to 1976. If higher levels are used, with no clinical indication, the clinician or investigator must submit an Investigational Device Exemption to the FDA. These guidelines are likely to change in the near future, as the AIUM Bioeffects Committee is working with the FDA to develop guidelines that reflect the bioeffects research, as summarized in the above conclusions.[18] The AIUM's position statement on the use of Doppler ultrasound is this:

AIUM feels that there is currently sufficient information to justify clinical use of continuous wave, pulsed and color flow Doppler ultrasound to evaluate blood flow in urine, umbilical and fetal vessels, the fetal cardiovascular system and to image flow in these structures using color flow imaging technology. (AIUM Newsletter, Oct. 1988)

If the patient asks, the sonographer should convey the gist of these statements to allay any immediate fears but should also indicate that examinations should not be performed indiscriminately.

Sharing the results of the examination with the patient depends on many factors, most of them involving the use of common sense. The physician who ordered the sonographic examination is the best person to explain and discuss the findings with the patient. Whether patients are given immediate reassurance and are allowed to view the images, especially in a normal pregnancy, depends on the philosophy of the ultrasound laboratory. The impact on the patient of seeing the images should be the primary consideration. The bonding that occurs when the mother and father view the sonograms is discussed in Chapter 34 and the ethical considerations in Chapter 38. The sonographer should be aware of all aspects of the ultrasound examination before deciding how much information to share with the patient.

Transducer Selection

The choice of a transducer for gynecologic and obstetric scanning depends on several factors, including patient habitus, stage of pregnancy, and examination objectives. In addition to real-time models, of which there are many varieties, Doppler, color-coded Doppler, and transvaginal transducers are used in obstetrics and gynecology. Each laboratory should have a selection to choose from, to accommodate routine situations. Sector scanners, because they have small scanning surfaces, are more maneuverable, and therefore more effective in most gynecologic and early gestation examinations. Linear transducers, which come in a variety of sizes, are best suited to wider fields of view and to survey scanning. They tend to be more effective later in pregnancy. Frequency and focal point considerations depend on the patient: 2.5 MHz is about the lowest frequency available and should be used on larger patients, whereas 7.5 MHz provides excellent resolution on children and smaller women. Transvaginal transducers range from 3.0 to 7.5 MHz.[23] Choice of focal point (most transducers offer near, mid- and far) also depends on patient size and the organs of interest. If more than one transducer is available, the sonographer must become accustomed to changing them during the examination. Some transducers offer variable focusing that can be programmed from the machine console.

At this time transvaginal imaging is proving to be superior to transabdominal scanning for some gynecologic and obstetric conditions and complementary in many others (Table 1-3),[4–6,11,13,15,17,25,27] so transvaginal transducers are becoming part of the standard equipment of most labs. At least 14 manufacturers offer transvaginal transducers, which incorporate a variety of shapes and features.[23]

Transvaginal Scanning

Techniques of transvaginal scanning are currently being developed, as are image presentations. At this time, transvaginal scans are often performed after a transabdominal scan. Since the transvaginal transducer depicts anatomy best within a focal range of 2 to 7 cm and is confined to the area of the fornices (Fig. 1-3), it is limited to visualizing the uterus and adnexa. In most clinical situations when ultrasound examination is required, a more extensive view of the pelvis and abdomen is required than can be provided by the transvaginal probe alone (Fig. 1-4).

The procedure should be explained carefully to the patient. In some institutions, the patient is asked to sign an informed consent form prior to the examination.[19]

TECHNIQUE
1. Patients are usually scanned with an empty bladder. Timor-Tritsch recommends that patients being examined for low-lying placenta have a half-full bladder to help outline the internal os and anterior portion of the cervix.[27]

TABLE 1-3. Indications and applications of transvaginal ultrasound

1. Patients who are suboptimal for transabdominal scanning due to obesity, bowel gas, adhesions, and inability to distend bladder
2. Infertility management
     Follicular monitoring—size and internal features of follicles
     Oocyte harvesting
     Cyclic endometrial changes
3. Ectopic *v* early intrauterine pregnancy (IUP)
     Documentation of IUP (7–10 d earlier than transabdominally)
     Visualization of extrauterine gestation
4. Ovarian and adnexal abnormalities
     Better echoarchitectural characterization
     Transvaginal sonography possible as screening technique
     For carcinoma in postmenopausal women
     Determine organ of origin—uterus *v* adnexa
5. Uterus
     Retroversion—better visualization
     Anomalies
     Fibroids—definition and localization
     Endometrial abnormalities and normal cyclic changes
6. Cervical abnormality—incompetence
7. Fallopian tubal pathology
8. First trimester IUP
     Documentation
     Sac morphology
     Assessment of decidual reaction
     Yolk sac, cardiac activity, embryo
     Early detection of placental localization, helpful with chorionic villi sampling
     Embryonic development and detection of anomalies
9. Mid- to late pregnancy—evaluation of presenting fetal part (probably contraindicated in third trimester bleeding)
10. Sonographically guided biopsies of pelvic lesions
11. Nongynecologic pathology
     Pelvic abscesses
     Tumors such as bladder carcinoma
12. Free fluid *v* fluid-filled bowel

(Mendelson EB, Böhm-Vélez M, Neiman HL, et al. Transvaginal sonography in gynecologic imaging. Semin Ultrasound LT MR. 1988; 9:102–121.)

2. The lithotomy position is used, or a pillow may be placed under the supine patient's buttocks. Timor-Tritsch suggests that the patient's upper body be positioned higher than the pelvis, to permit pooling of any fluid in the cul-de-sac.[27]

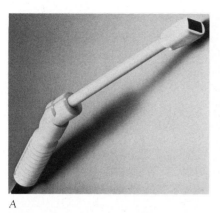
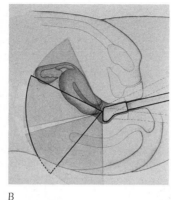
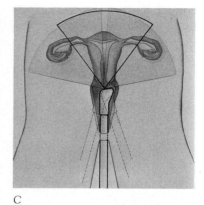

A   B   C

FIGURE 1-3. (A) A transducer designed for transvaginal scanning. (B) Moving the transducer within the fornix produces sagittal sectors of the cervical to the fundal portions of the normal uterus. (C) Rotating the transducer 90 degrees results in coronal images, which often appear as transverse sections because the uterus and adnexa are anteflexed when the bladder is empty. (Images courtesy of General Electric Company.)

Also, he has found that higher structures may be imaged better if the patient lifts her knees toward her chest.

3. The transducer is covered with a condom or a digit of a surgical glove into which gel has been placed. All air bubbles must be removed from the condom or glove.

4. A lubricant usually is not necessary on the outside of the condom. If it is, scanning gel or K-Y jelly can be placed on the condom-covered probe. If the patient is being treated for infertility, no gel should be used because of its spermicidal effect[26]; instead, the probe can be lubricated with saline.

5. Depending on institutional policy, either patient, physician, or sonographer can insert the transducer into the vagina. In some settings, a female chaperone is present in the examination room when a male sonographer or physician performs the transvaginal examination.[19]

6. The sonographer manipulates the transducer to image sagittal, coronal, transverse sections of the uterus and adnexa. Enlarging the image enhances visualization.

7. Because the orientation of the images differs from transabdominal scans, it is important to indicate the location and directions on each scan. Orientation and labelling have not been standardized, but referencing images by using anatomic landmarks is recommended (e.g., demonstrating the ovaries in relationship to the iliac vessels). A minimal amount of urine in the bladder may assist in locating the other pelvic organs.

8. At the completion of the examination, the condom should be removed carefully and the transducer disinfected by soaking it in Cidex, Sporiciden, or another recommended disinfectant.

Professional Responsibilities of the Sonographer

Persons who choose diagnostic ultrasound as a profession should take the certifying examination given by the American Registry of Diagnostic Medical Sonographers and should become members of the professional society that represents sonographers, the Society of Diagnostic Medical Sonographers. While in most hospitals it is not mandatory to be registered, passing the registry examination

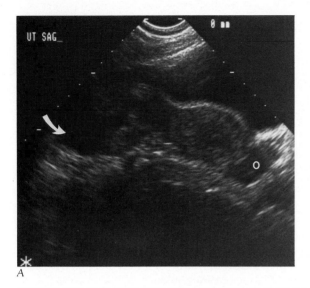

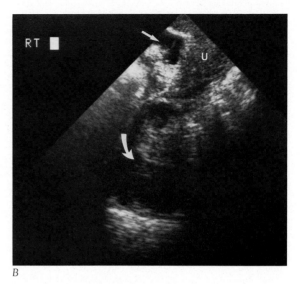

FIGURE 1-4. (A) A transabdominal scan demonstrates a large complex mass (*curved arrow*) located superior to and to the right of the uterus (O, ovary). The mass was thought to represent a chronic ectopic pregnancy. On a follow-up exam 1 week later, the size of the mass had decreased slightly. (B) The endovaginal scan in the area of the right adnexa provided a vague outline of the mass (*curved arrow*) that did not contribute additional diagnostic information (U, uterus; *straight arrow*, bowel).

attests that the sonographer has a practicing level of knowledge in the specialties in which he or she is registered. The registered sonographer can use the designation RDMS (registered diagnostic medical sonographer) after his or her name and to maintain this status must compile 30 hours of continuing education credits every 3 years. In a field as dynamic as diagnostic ultrasound, keeping informed of its innovations is imperative.

Membership in the SDMS brings with it the benefits of being part of a professional organization whose goals are to keep its members informed and competent. Among the resources the SDMS provides are educational guidelines, profiles of sonographer characteristics (including salary levels), a peer-reviewed journal (*The Journal of Diagnostic Medical Sonography*), and annual national and regional scientific meetings. It also keeps its membership informed of legislation and current societal trends that can affect the practice of ultrasound.

References

1. AIUM Bioeffects Reports Sub-Committee. Bioeffects considerations for the study of diagnostic ultrasound. J Ultrasound Med. 1988; 7:S4.
2. AIUM presents position statement on fetal Doppler. AIUM Newsletter. October 1988; 3.
3. Bell BB, Nowers CN. SDMS suggested scanning protocols. J Diagn Med Sonogr. 1986; 2:343–347.
4. Coleman BG, Arger PH, Grumbach K, et al. Transvaginal and transabdominal sonography: Prospective comparison. Radiology. 1988; 168:639–643.
5. Dashefsky SM, Lyons EA, Levi SC, et al. Suspected ectopic pregnancy: Endovaginal and transvesical US. Radiology. 1988; 169:181–184.
6. Goldstein SR. Endovaginal technique and efficacy. Presented at Thirteenth Annual Spring Symposium in Diagnostic Ultrasound, Department of Radiology, State University of New York, Health Science Center at Brooklyn, April 29, 1989.
7. Hacker NF, Moore JG. Essentials of Obstetrics and Gynecology. Philadelphia: WB Saunders; 1986.
8. Hansmann M, Hackeloer B-J, Staudach A. Ultra-

sound Diagnosis in Obstetrics and Gynecology. Berlin: Springer-Verlag; 1985.

9. Hussey M. Basic Physics and Technology of Medical Diagnostic Ultrasound. New York: Elsevier; 1985.

10. Hykes D, Hedrick WR, Starchman DE. Ultrasound Physics & Instrumentation. New York: Churchill Livingstone; 1985.

11. Jain KA, Hamper UM, Sanders RC. Comparison of transvaginal and transabdominal sonography in the detection of early pregnancy and its complications. AJR. 1988; 151:1139–1143.

12. Kremkau F. Diagnostic Ultrasound: Principles, Instruments and Exercises. 3rd ed. Philadelphia: WB Saunders; 1988.

13. Leibman AJ, Kruse B, McSweeney MB. Transvaginal sonography: Comparison with transabdominal sonography in the diagnosis of pelvic masses. AJR. 1988; 151:89–92.

14. Leopold GR. Antepartum obstetrical ultrasound examination guidelines. J Ultrasound Med. 1986; 5:241–242. Editorial.

15. Lyons EA. Early pregnancy loss. Presented at Thirteenth Annual Spring Symposium in Diagnostic Ultrasound, Department of Radiology, State University of New York, Health Science Center at Brooklyn, April 29, 1989.

16. McDicken WN. Diagnostic Ultrasonics: Principles and Use of Instruments. 2nd ed. New York: John Wiley; 1981.

17. Mendelson EB, Bohm-Velez M, Neiman HL, Russo J. Transvaginal sonography in gynecologic imaging. Semin Ultrasound. 1988; 9:102–121.

18. Meyer RA. Doppler in fetal investigation. August 1, 1986. Letter to AIUM members.

19. Midwest region conducts survey on endocavitary ultrasound. SDMS Newsletter. March/April 1989; 10:1.

20. NICHD consensus report: Diagnostic ultrasound imaging in pregnancy. US Dept of Health and Human Services, PHS, NIH Publication No. 84-667. Washington, DC: 1984.

21. Parulekar SG, Kiwi R. Dynamic incompetent cervix uteri. J Ultrasound Med. 1988; 7:481–485.

22. Persutte WG, Lenke RR. Maternal urinary bladder filling for middle- and late-trimester ultrasound. Is it really necessary? J Ultrasound Med. 1988; 7:207–209.

23. Platt LD. New look in ultrasound: The vaginal probe. Technology 1988. Contemp Ob/Gyn. Special Issue. 1987; 99–105.

24. Raz S. Female Urology. Philadelphia: WB Saunders; 1983.

25. Rempen A. Vaginal sonography in ectopic pregnancy—A prospective evaluation. J Ultrasound Med. 1988; 7:381–387.

26. Schwimer SR, Rothman CR, Lebovic J, et al. The effect of ultrasound coupling gels on sperm motility in vitro. Fertil Steril. 1984; 42:946.

27. Timor-Tritsch IE. How to do vaginal sonography. Presented at The First International Conference on Transvaginal Sonography: Clinical Applications. Columbia University College of Physicians and Surgeons and Sloane Hospital for Women; March 17–18, 1988; New York, NY.

Gynecologic Sonography

CHAPTER **2**

Embryonic Development of the Female Genital System

JOYCE A. MILLER

Knowledge of the embryogenesis of any internal organ is essential to understanding its anatomy. This is especially true in the female pelvis, where developmental anomalies may distort the normal sonographic appearance of the uterus and present diagnostic dilemmas. An understanding of the close developmental relationship between the primitive urinary system and the reproductive system can guide the sonographer to examine both when an anomaly exists in either one. The urogenital system can be demonstrated in utero and in later life, permitting diagnosis of morphologic anomalies when they are large enough for sonographic resolution or when they produce sonographic or clinical symptoms. Sonographers may discover evidence of pelvic anomalies in three different periods of life.

Fetal Period

Most congenital anomalies discovered in fetuses in utero have occurred in the genitourinary system.[12] In a large epidemiologic study of approximately 12,000 pregnant women, the overall prevalence of fetal malformations was found to be 0.5%; urinary tract abnormalities represent about 50% of the total number.[8] These anomalies presented in a wide range from complete agenesis of the kidney and ureter to partial malformations, duplications, and obstructions with concomitant cyst formation. Prenatal ultrasound may also detect congenital anomalies in the ovaries, uterus, and vagina, especially when they enlarge and produce a pelvic mass. Hydrometrocolpos of the vagina and uterus, which presents as a hypoechoic mass posterior to the bladder, is the most common genital anomaly detected in utero.[5] In some fetuses with this condition, the hydrometrocolpos also compresses the urinary tract and causes hydronephrosis or hydroureter.

Neonatal Period

As in the fetal period, the most common mass lesions in neonates are of renal origin[12]; however, hydrometrocolpos secondary to an atretic vagina is a well-known cause of abdominal masses in newborn girls.[3] Sonographic survey of a newborn girl should include identification of normal urinary bladder, uterus, vagina, and (whenever possible) ovaries, to rule out masses and obstructions.

Premenarche Through Adulthood

It is in this age group that the sonographer most frequently finds genital anomalies. Presentation of genital anomalies often occurs at the onset of puberty, when menstrual irregularities are apparent. For example, in the patient with a duplicated uterus with one septated vagina, obstruction to menstrual flow from one side can present as unilateral hematocolpos.[2] Some patients, however, have no symptoms and their congenital anomalies may first be discovered while scanning to rule out other conditions.

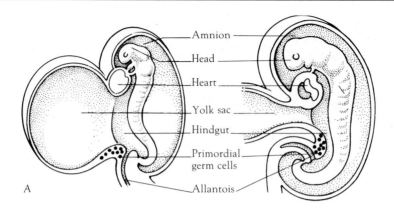

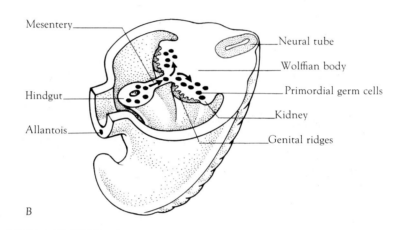

FIGURE 2-1. (A) Primordial germ cells in wall of yolk sac. (B) Migration path of primordial germ cells.

A review of the embryonic development of the female genitalia elucidates how such conditions arise.

Expression of Gender in an Embryo

THE PRIMORDIAL GERM CELLS

The gender or sex of an embryo is determined at fertilization. If the male gamete (the spermatozoon) contributes an X chromosome to its union with the female gamete (the ovum), which always contains an X, a female embryo (XX) results. If the male gamete contributes a Y chromosome, a male embryo (XY) results. The *primordial germ cells* that express or produce this femaleness or maleness are first dis-cernible in the embryo about 21 days after conception. They differentiate from cells in the caudal part of the yolk sac, close to the allantois, a small diverticulum of the yolk sac that extends into the connecting stalk (Fig. 2-1A). Simultaneously, the *genital* or *gonadal ridges* are formed. They are the precursors to the ovaries in females and to the testes in males. These ridges are located on the anteromedial sides of the wolffian bodies, the embryonic regions where the kidneys develop (Fig. 2-1B).[15] The urinary system and the reproductive system are intimately associated in origin, development, and certain final relations. Both arise from mesoderm that initially takes the form of a com-

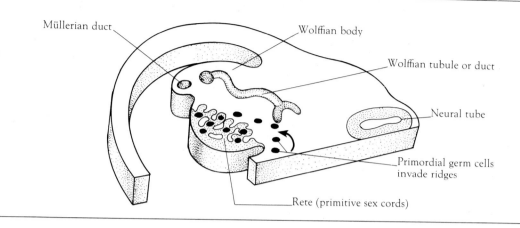

FIGURE 2-2. Development of embryo on one side. Indifferent gonad stage; formation of primitive sex cords.

mon ridge (wolffian body) located on both sides of the median plane. Both systems continue to develop in close proximity; they drain into a common cloaca, and slightly later into a urogenital sinus, which is a subdivision of the cloaca. Some parts of the urogenital system disappear after a transitory existence.[1] For example, by the fifth developmental week, the first-stage kidney (pronephros) has differentiated and has already disappeared.[11] Certain common primordia transform differently in males and females.

Inducer Germ Cells

During the fifth week of development, the primordial germ cells migrate by ameboid movement from their origin in the yolk sac along the dorsal mesentery. In the sixth week they invade the gonadal ridges (see Fig. 2-1B). If by chance they do not reach the ridges, the gonads cease to develop. Thus these primordial germ cells act as *inducers* of the gonads. Note that at this time in development (the sixth week), the mesonephros, or second-stage kidney, and its wolffian duct have developed lateral to the gonadal ridges.[9,13]

As the primordial cells are invading the ridges, an outer layer of fetal tissue called coelomic epithelium grows into the underlying mesenchymal tissue, or embryonic connective tissue. Active tissue growth here forms a network, or rete, called the primitive sex cords (Fig. 2-2). This rete forms anas-

tomoses with a portion of the wolffian duct, thus establishing the first urogenital connections in the embryo. After the degeneration of the second-stage kidney, the mesonephros, the male embryo appropriates its wolffian duct and converts it into genital canals. This stage of development is often termed the *indifferent gonad stage*, since it is still not possible to distinguish morphologic sex differences.[9,13,15]

In the seventh week, if the embryo is a genetic male the primitive sex cords continue to proliferate and eventually give rise to the rete testis. If the embryo is a genetic female the primitive sex cords break up into irregularly shaped cell clusters, which eventually disappear. They are replaced by a vascular stroma, a supporting tissue, that will later form the ovarian medulla.[15]

In a female gonad (the ovary) the outer layer of epithelium continues to proliferate, giving rise to a second group of cords, which eventually occupy the cortex of the ovary. These are the *cortical cords*, or *Pluger's tubules* (Fig. 2-3).[15]

In the fourth month, the cortical cords split into isolated cell clusters, each surrounding one or more primitive germ cells. Now the primitive germ cells will differentiate into *oogonia*, which divide repeatedly by mitosis to reach a maximum number of 7 million by the 5th month of prenatal life. Many oogonia subsequently degenerate, so at birth their number is approximately 1 million (Fig. 2-4).[7]

The surviving oogonia differentiate into *primary*

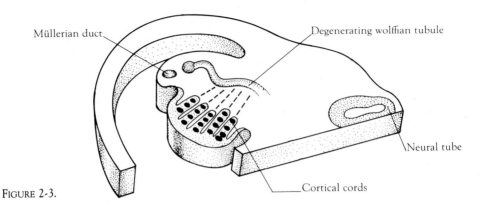

FIGURE 2-3.

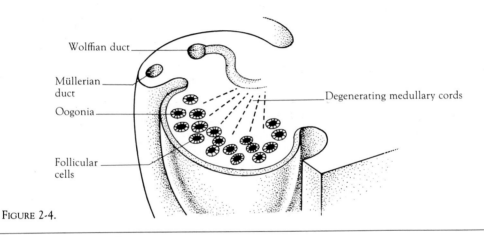

FIGURE 2-4.

FIGURE 2-3. Formation of the cortical cords.

FIGURE 2-4. Differentiation of primitive germ cells into oogonia in the 4th month.

oocytes during prenatal life and are surrounded by a single layer of granulosa cells derived from the cortical cords. The primary oocyte with its surrounding granulosa cells is called a *primordial follicle.* Many undergo degeneration during childhood and adolescence so that by puberty approximately 500,000 remain. Between puberty and menopause approximately 300 to 400 fertile ova are produced.[7]

Genital Ducts

We need to backtrack in time to trace the development of the ductal system that occurs simultaneously with the development of the gonads (ova-

ries or testes). In the *indifferent gonad stage* (until the 7th week) the genital tracts of both male and female embryos have the same appearance and are comprised of two pairs of ducts. The wolffian ducts arise from the second-stage kidney, the mesonephros. The müllerian ducts arise from an invagination or pocket of coelomic epithelium lateral to the cranial end of each wolffian duct. Growth progresses caudad, eventually hollowing out to form an open duct.[9] Development of the embryonic ductal system and external genitalia occurs under the influence of circulating hormones in the fetus. In males, fetal testes produce an *inducer* substance that causes differentiation and growth of the wolffian

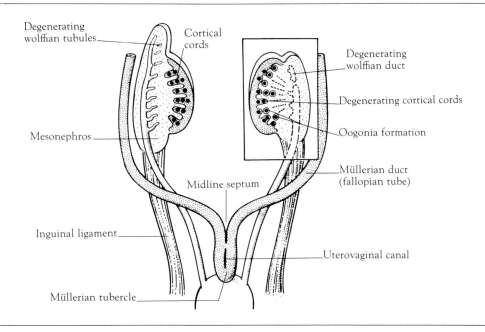

FIGURE 2-5. Formation of uterovaginal canal, 8th week. Inset: ovary at 4th month, forming the oogonia.

ducts and inhibition of the müllerian ducts. In females, because the male inducer substance is absent, the wolffian ducts regress while the müllerian ductal system, influenced by maternal and placental estrogens, develops into the fallopian tubes and uterus.[9]

The müllerian ducts first extend downward parallel to the wolffian ducts then turn mediad in the lower abdomen, crossing anterior to the wolffian ducts and fusing together in the midline to form a single duct, the *uterovaginal canal* (Fig. 2-5). This fusion begins caudally and progresses up to the site of the future fallopian tubes. In normal development, the midline septum disappears by the end of the 3rd month and the uterine corpus and cervix are formed. They are surrounded by a layer of mesenchyme, which will eventually form the muscular coat of the uterus (the myometrium) and its peritoneal covering (the perimetrium).[9,13]

Formation of the Fallopian Tubes
After the formation of the *uterovaginal canal,* the segment of each müllerian duct positioned above

the junction of the inguinal ligament becomes a fallopian tube. The craniad orifice of the müllerian duct, which stays open to the peritoneal cavity, becomes the fimbriae of the fallopian tube. Initially, the fallopian tube lies in a vertical position. As development proceeds, it moves to the interior of the abdominal cavity to lie horizontally. This causes the ovary, which is attached to the fallopian tube by the mesovarium, to descend and finally to assume a position dorsal to the fallopian tube (Table 2-1, Fig. 2-6).[7,9,13]

Formation of the Broad Ligament
As the müllerian duct fuses medially and the ovary is successfully located cranial and finally dorsal to the fallopian tubes, the mesenteries follow these positional changes.[13] This movement causes the folds of the peritoneum to be elevated from the posterolateral wall, thus creating a large transverse pelvic fold called the *broad ligament,* which extends from the lateral sides of the fused müllerian ducts toward the wall of the pelvis. The fallopian tube will be located on its superior surface and on its

Table 2-1. Embryonic development chart for female urogenital system

	Urinary System	Gonads	Ducts	Mesenteries
3rd Week	Pronephros differentiates	Primordial cells seen in allantois		
4th Week	Pronephros disappears and mesonephros differentiates	Formation of genital ridges		
5th Week	Metanephros starts to differentiate	Migration of primordial germ cells		
6th Week		Primitive germ cells invade gonadal ridges Formation of primitive sex cords "indifferent stage"	Two sets of ducts exist wolffian (kidney) müllerian (genital ridge)	
7th Week		Primitive sex cords disappear Cortical cords arise		
8th Week	Mesonephros disappears, only its duct (wolffian) remains			
8th Week ↓	Wolffian duct regresses almost completely		Müllerian ducts fuse to form uterovaginal canal and fallopian tubes	
12th Week		Ovary descends	Median septum disappears	
12th Week ↓ 5th Month	Metanephros-3rd stage kidney	Cortical cords split up and surround primitive germ cells to produce 7,000,000 oogonia		Formation of mesosalpinx, mesovarium, broad ligament, proper ovarian ligament, and suspensory ligament

posterior surface, the ovary (Fig. 2-6). The ovary is suspended by several structures: (1) The *mesovarium* is a double-layered fold of peritoneum that is continuous with the posterosuperior layer of the broad ligament. (2) The *proper ligament of the ovary* is a band of connective tissue that lies between the two layers of the broad ligament and connects the lower pole of the ovary with the lateral uterine wall. (3) The *suspensory ligament* is a triangular fold of peritoneum that actually forms the upper lateral corner of the broad ligament. This ligament suspends both the ovary and the fallopian tube by its confluence with the parietal peritoneum at the pelvic brim.[6]

Formation of the Vagina

The vagina has a dual origin: Its upper region is derived from the mesodermal tissue of the müllerian ducts and its lower region, from the urogenital sinus. The urogenital sinus is the ventral half of the primitive cloaca (hindgut) after it has been divided by the urorectal septum. The upper portion of the urogenital sinus will become the urinary bladder and the lower portion is divided into two portions—the pars pelvina, involved in formation of the vagina, and the pars phallica, which is related to the primordia (developing organs) of the external genitalia. This can best be understood by following the development of the vagina step by step. First, the distal end of the uterovaginal canal makes contact with the posterior wall of the urogenital sinus (Fig. 2-7A). As these structures fuse, a solid group of cells called the *vaginal plate* is formed (Fig. 2-7B). From the vaginal plate two outgrowths (*sinovaginal bulbs*) surround the uterovaginal canal and fuse on opposite sides (Fig. 2-7C). If the sinovaginal bulbs do not fuse normally, a vagina with two outlets, or a vagina with one normal outlet and one atretic one may result.[9,13]

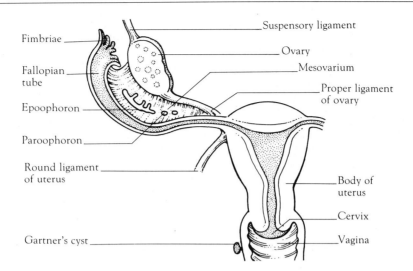

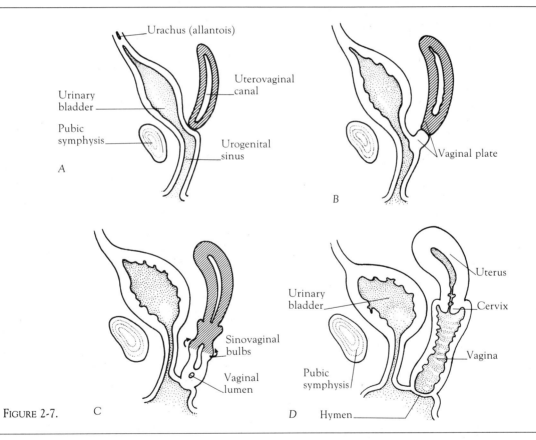

Figure 2-6. Fully developed female reproductive organs.

Figure 2-7. Formation of the vagina: (A) Uterovaginal canal makes contact with wall of urogenital sinus. (B) Formation of vaginal plate. (C) Sinovaginal bulbs encircle the vaginal plate and elongate. (D) Canalization of vaginal plate to form the vagina; separation of vagina and urogenital sinus by the hymen.

Following normal development, the center core of cells hollows out to form a lumen in the vagina. The vagina is now separated from the urogenital sinus only by a thin tissue plate, the *hymen* (Fig. 2-7D). The vaginal fornices, which surround the ends of the uterus (cervix), are thought to be of müllerian duct origin.

In the majority of female fetuses these developmental steps proceed uneventfully to culminate in normal pelvic viscera, which can be examined with ultrasound. Chapter 4 discusses ultrasound's role in diagnosing congenital abnormalities.

References

1. Arey L. Developmental Anatomy. 7th ed. Philadelphia: WB Saunders Co; 1974.
2. Benson R. Obstetric and Gynecologic Diagnosis and Treatment. 2nd ed. Los Altos, CA: Lange; 1978.
3. Burbige KA, Hensle T. Uterus didelphis and vaginal duplication with unilateral obstruction presenting as a newborn abdominal mass. J Urol. 1984; 132:1195–1198.
4. Cormack DH. Introduction to Histology. Philadelphia: JB Lippincott; 1984.
5. Crade M, Gilloley L, Taylor K. Ovarian cystic mass in utero. J Clin Ultrasound 1980; 8:251.
6. Crafts RC, Krieger HP. Gross anatomy of the female reproductive tract, pituitary, and hypothalamus. In: Danforth DN, Scott JR, eds. Obstetrics and Gynecology. 5th ed. Philadelphia: JB Lippincott; 1986.
7. Crowley LV. Introduction to Clinical Embryology. Chicago: Year Book Medical Publishers; 1974.
8. Helin I, Persson P. Prenatal diagnosis of urinary tract abnormalities by ultrasound. Pediatrics. 1986; 78: 879–883.
9. Langeman J. Medical Embryology. 4th ed. Baltimore: Williams & Wilkins, 1981; 234–267.
10. Pritchard JA, McDonald PC, Gant NF. The anatomy of the reproductive tract of women. In: Williams Obstetrics. 17th ed. New York: Appleton-Century Crofts; 1971; 11–14.
11. Ramsey EM. Embryology and developmental defects of the reproductive tract. In: Danforth DN, ed. Obstetrics and Gynecology. 5th ed. Philadelphia: JB Lippincott; 1986.
12. Schulman CC, Elkhazen N, Picard C. Diagnostic chez le foetus des malformations urinaires par l'echographie. J Urologie. 1981; 87:431.
13. Tuchmann-Duplessis H, Haegel P. Illustrated Human Embryology. Berlin: Springer-Verlag; 1972; 2.
14. Wiersma A. Uterine anomalies associated with unilateral renal agenesis. Obstet Gynecol. 1976; 47:654.
15. Zuckerman L, Weir B. The Ovary. 2nd ed. New York: Academic Press; 1977; 1:42–52.

C H A P T E R 3

Sonographic Anatomy of the Female Pelvis

LARRY WALDROUP, JI-BIN LIU

A thorough knowledge of the gross and cross-sectional anatomy of the female pelvis is essential for the sonographer who must seek pathology in this area. This anatomy can more easily be assimilated and understood by building up a mental picture of the layers of the pelvis, beginning with the bony framework.

The Pelvic Skeleton

In adults, the osseous pelvis is essentially a ring composed of four bones: the *sacrum,* the *coccyx,* and the two large *innominate bones,* which result from fusion of the ilium, ischium, and pubis (Fig. 3-1).[6] The sacrum and coccyx form the posterior wall of the pelvis, and the innominate bones form the lateral and anterior walls (Fig. 3-2). The innominate bones are joined together posteriorly through the sacrum and anteriorly in the midline at the pubic symphysis. The outer surface of the innominate bone forms the acetabulum, the socket for the femoral head (see Fig. 3-2).

The sacrum and coccyx are modified segments of the vertebral column. The sacrum results from fusion of the five sacral vertebrae, and the coccyx (our vestigial tail) consists of four fused coccygeal vertebrae (see Fig. 3-3). Between the sacrum and coccyx is an articulation that permits little or no motion.

The female pelvis serves three principal functions. First, it provides a weight-bearing bridge between the spinal column and the bones of the lower limbs via the sacrum and the innominate bones. Second, it directs the pathway of the fetal head during childbirth (parturition). Third, it protects the organs of reproduction.

The bones of the pelvis define two distinct spaces, the true pelvis and the false pelvis, which are separated by an imaginary line (the *linea terminalis*) extending from the sacral prominence along the inner surface of the innominate bone down to the symphysis pubis anteriorly (Figs. 3-4 to 3-6).[6] The true pelvis lies below the linea terminalis and has a horizontally oriented inlet but a vertically oriented outlet (Fig. 3-7). The inlet of the true pelvis is entirely walled by bone, but the outlet is only partially so (see Figs. 3-2, 3-5, and 3-6). It is apparent that other structures are needed to fill in the gaps, and these include the membranes, ligaments, and muscles of the pelvic floor.

The Pelvic Muscles

Forming much of the abdominal body wall and lining the osseous framework of the pelvis are muscles that can be demonstrated by ultrasound. Most are paired structures that are bilaterally symmetric. Table 3-1 lists the pelvic muscles by region and pelvic location. The pelvic skeletal muscles, along with the osseous pelvis, define the limits of the space that must be investigated by pelvic sonography. The sonographer should be able to recognize these pelvic muscles in order to avoid confusing them with a mass. Skeletal muscle appears less

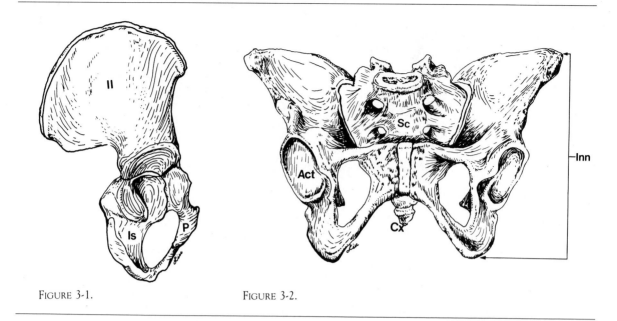

FIGURE 3-1.   FIGURE 3-2.

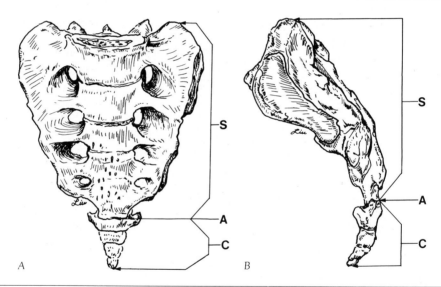

FIGURE 3-3.   A   B

FIGURE 3-1. Three bones fuse to form the innominate bone. (Il, ilium; Is, ischium; P, pubis).

FIGURE 3-2. The female pelvis viewed from the front. The pelvis has been tilted up to better show the acetabula and pubic rami. See Figure 3-5 for the correct angle of the pelvis in life. (Act, acetabulum; Inn, innominate bone; Sc, sacrum; Cx, coccyx.)

FIGURE 3-3. (A) Ventral and (B) lateral surfaces of the adult sacrum (S) and coccyx (C). Note the five fused vertebral bodies forming the sacrum, the four fused bodies that form the coccyx, and the shallow S-shaped curve that these bones establish in the posterior wall of the pelvis. (A, articulation between sacrum and coccyx.)

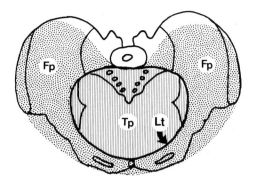

FIGURE 3-4.

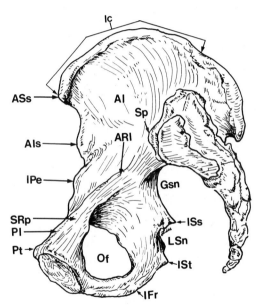

FIGURE 3-5.

FIGURE 3-4. The true and false pelvic cavities. The wide but shallow false pelvis (Fp) surrounds the deep central true pelvis (Tp.) The dividing line between the two spaces is the linea terminalis (Lt).

FIGURE 3-5. Pelvis viewed from the side with the left innominate bone removed. The linea terminalis (innnominate line) is made up of the pectineal line and the arcuate line. (Sp, sacral prominence; Al, ala (wing) of the ilium bone forming iliac fossa; Ic, iliac crest; ASs, anterior superior iliac spine; AIs, anterior inferior iliac spine; Pt, pubic tubercle; ISt, ischial tuberosity; ISs, ischial spine; Gsn, greater sciatic notch; LSn, lesser sciatic notch; IFr, inferior ramus of pubis; Of, obturator foramen; SRp, superior ramis of pubis; IPe, iliopubic eminence; Pl, pectineal line; ARl, arcuate line.)

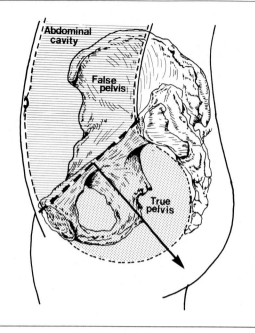

FIGURE 3-6. Relationship of the abdominal cavity to the true and false pelvic cavities. The false pelvis forms the walls of the most inferior part of the abdominal cavity. The true pelvis extends farther posterior than the false pelvis. When viewed from the side, the axis of the true pelvic cavity is directed posterior and inferior at about 45 degrees. The inlet is steeply tilted (about 60 degrees from horizontal) while the outlet is almost horizontal. The curve of the sacrum provides the transition between these two angles, and serves to direct the fetal head downward and then forward during parturition.

TABLE 3-1. The pelvic muscles

Region	Muscle	Location
Abdominopelvic	Rectus abdominis	Anterior wall
	Psoas major	Posterior wall
False pelvis	Iliacus	Iliac fossa
True pelvis	Obturator internus	Lateral wall
	Piriformis	Posterior wall
	Coccygeus	Posterior floor
	Levator ani	Middle and anterior floor

echoic than fat or smooth muscle and exhibits linear internal echoes outlining the muscle bundles (see Fig. 3-11). The borders of the muscle are outlined by the echogenic fascia and retroperitoneal fat.

Two of the muscles commonly demonstrated on transverse pelvic scans (rectus abdominis and psoas) are not exclusively pelvic muscles because they also extend through the abdominal region. The *rectus abdominis* muscles form much of the anterior body wall. They extend from the pubic symphysis and pubic crest to the costal cartilages of the fifth, sixth, and seventh ribs and the xiphoid process (Fig. 3-8).[5] On cross section each rectus muscle is ovoid or lens-shaped (lenticular), most strikingly so in the lower abdomen.

The *psoas major* muscle originates from the lower thoracic and the lumbar vertebrae.[5] This cylindri-

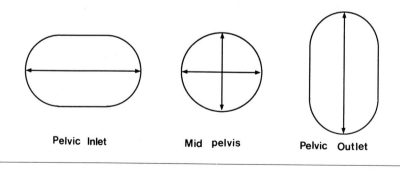

Pelvic Inlet   Mid pelvis   Pelvic Outlet

FIGURE 3-7. Shape of the true pelvis at its inlet, midpelvis, and outlet. Although the inlet and outlet are similar in shape, their axes differ by 90 degrees. Consider how these shapes affect the orientation of the fetal head during parturition.

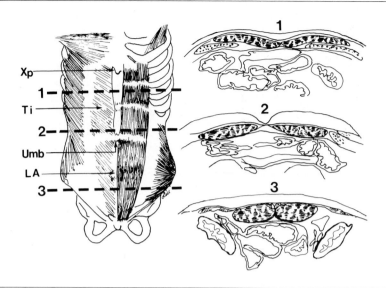

FIGURE 3-8. The rectus abdominis muscles seen from the front with representative cross sections (*dashed lines.*) The left and right columns of muscle are separated by the midline linea alba (LA) and are interrupted by transverse tendinous intersections (Ti) at the level of the umbilicus, between the umbilicus (Umb) and the xiphoid, and at the xiphoid process (Xp).

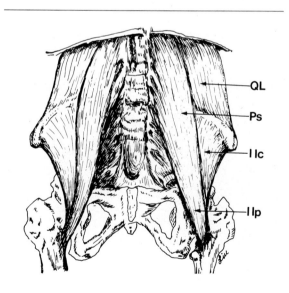

FIGURE 3-9. Muscles of the posterior body wall and the false pelvis, viewed from the front. (Ps, psoas major; QL, quadratus lumborum; Ilc, iliacus; Ilp, iliopsoas.)

cal muscle then courses laterad and anterior as it descends through the lower abdomen (Fig. 3-9). Above the level of the fourth lumbar vertebra (L4) the psoas is closely attached to the lateral margins of the vertebral column. At about the fifth lumbar vertebra it separates from the spine and begins to move more laterad, creating a space between the psoas and spine through which the common iliac vessels run. Below the level of the iliac crest, fibers of the psoas major lie adjacent to or begin to interdigitate with fibers from the medial aspect of the *iliacus muscle,* thus creating the *iliopsoas.* This composite muscle continues its lateral and anterior course through the false pelvis, passing over the pelvic brim to insert on the lesser trochanter of the femur.

Through most of the false pelvis, the cross-sectional shape of the psoas-iliopsoas is that of an oddly shaped hook with a bulbous medial limb (Fig. 3-10, section 4). On sagittal ultrasound scans, these muscles appear as a long, dark strip whose posterior margin courses upward toward the anterior body wall as the muscle complex descends

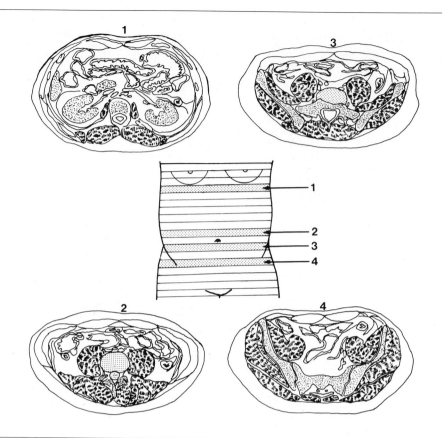

FIGURE 3-10. Shape of the psoas-iliacus-iliopsoas muscles on cross section at various levels in the abdomen and pelvis.

through the pelvis (Fig. 3-11). The iliopsoas never enters the true pelvis. In the false pelvis, its medial margin coincides with the linea terminalis and thus marks the border between the true and false pelvis (Fig. 3-12).

Within the true pelvic space is the *obturator internus* (Fig. 3-13). This triangular sheet of muscle originates as bands of fibers anchored along the brim of the true pelvis and from the inner surface of the obturator membrane, which closes the obturator foramen.[5] The muscle extends posteriorly and medial along the side wall of the true pelvis, passing beneath the levator ani muscles to exit from the pelvic space through the lesser sciatic foramen. Because it lies parallel and adjacent to the lateral pel-

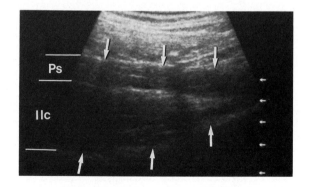

FIGURE 3-11. Sagittal scan of the psoas major (Ps) and iliac muscles (Ilc) in the false pelvis. Faint lines within the muscle arise from the fiber bundles and fascial planes. Note the upward slant of the posterior wall of the muscle group and how the image ends at the bone of the ilium.

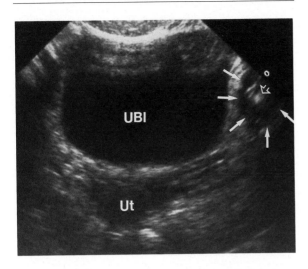

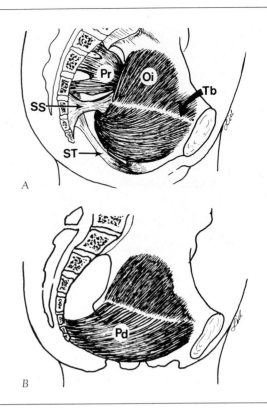

FIGURE 3-12. Transverse scan of the midpelvis. The iliopsoas muscle complex is almost always seen on transverse pelvic scans. The bright echo (*open arrow*) within the muscle arises from the femoral nerve, the iliopsoas tendon, and fat filling in a groove formed by the line of fusion between the two contributor muscles. Although the anatomic location of this bright echo complex is not actually central to the iliopsoas composite muscle, it usually appears central on the sonogram because the lateral region of the iliacus is rarely seen well owing to overlying bowel gas. (UBl, urinary bladder; Ut, uterus.)

FIGURE 3-13. (A) Lateral view of pelvis with the deep pelvic sidewall muscles shown. The piriformis muscle (Pr) exits the true pelvic space through the greater sciatic foramen; the obturator internus (Oi) exits the true pelvis through the lesser sciatic foramen. These foramina are defined by the sacrospinous (SS) and the sacrotuberous (ST) ligaments. (Tb, tendinous band.) (B) The obturator internus muscle exhibits a tendinous band (Tb) that runs anterior to posterior across the muscle. This band is the point of attachment for the pelvic diaphragm (Pd), which is in part suspended from the surface of the obturator internus muscle.

vic wall, the obturator internus is difficult to identify on a sagittal ultrasound image. At normal gain levels it is often obscured on transverse scans as well; however, when it is visible the obturator appears as a thin, hypoechoic, vertical strip lining the wall of the pelvis (Fig. 3-14).

Deeply posterior in the true pelvis is another roughly triangular muscle, the *piriformis*, which takes origin from the sacrum and then courses laterally through the greater sciatic foramen to insert on the greater trochanter of the femur (Fig. 3-15).[5] Unless the urinary bladder is very full, the piriformis is usually obscured by overlying bowel gas in the sigmoid colon.

The floor of the true pelvis is made up of a complex group of similar muscles that collectively form a two-layered pelvic diaphragm. The outermost layer is composed of the muscles of the *perineum*, which are rarely identifiable in transabdominal ultrasound images. In contrast, the innermost layer of the pelvic diaphragm is commonly visualized in transverse ultrasound scans. The named muscles of the innermost group include (from posterior to an-

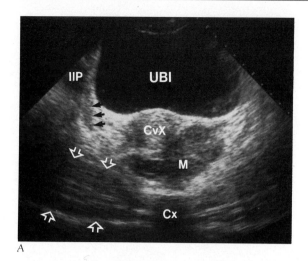
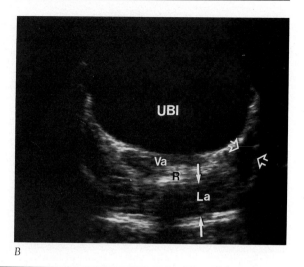

FIGURE 3-14. (A) Transverse scan of the pelvis demonstrates the obturator internus muscle as a thin, hypoechoic strip *(black arrows)* adjacent to the lateral pelvic wall. The upper margin of the muscle is just below the brim of the pelvis. The levator ani muscle group is also well seen *(open arrows)*. (UBl, urinary bladder; CvX, cervix; Cx, coccyx; M, mass adjacent to cervix; Ilp, iliopsoas muscle.) (B) Forming the floor of the true pelvic space is the levator ani muscle group *(arrows)*, which attaches to the medial surface of the obturator internus muscle *(open arrows)*. (UBl, urinary bladder; La, levator ani muscle; R, rectum; Va, vagina.)

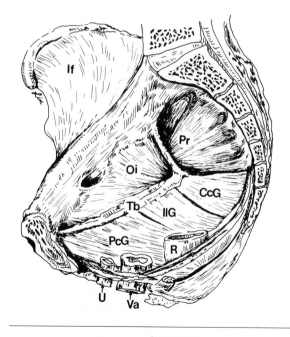

FIGURE 3-15. A more detailed view of the pelvic muscles with the pelvic diaphragm in place. The ragged edges along the tendinous band of the obturator internus are the cut edges of the fascial membrane that covers these muscles. The major orifices that pass through the pelvic diaphragm are also shown. (Oi, obturator internus muscle; Pr, piriformis muscle; Tb, tendinous band; CcG, coccygeus muscle; IlG, iliococcygeus; PcG, pubococcygeus; U, urethra; Va, vagina; R, rectum; If, iliac fossa.)

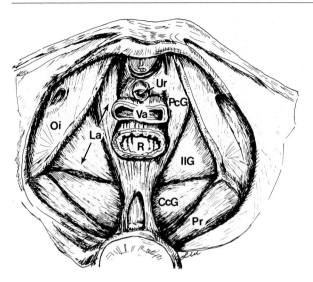

FIGURE 3-16. A view from above and posterior looking down into the true pelvis. Relate the position of the muscles in this view to the view shown in Figure 3-15. (Oi, obturator internus muscle; Pr, piriformis muscle; CcG, coccygeus muscle; IlG, iliococcygeus; PcG, pubococcygeus; La, levator ani muscle group; R, rectum; Ur, urethra; Va, vagina.)

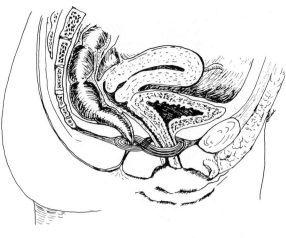

FIGURE 3-17. Relationship of the pubococcygeus muscle of the levator ani to the orifices that pass through the pelvic diaphragm.

terior) the coccygeus, the iliococcygeus, and the pubococcygeus (part of which is classified as the puborectalis; Figs. 3-15, 3-16).[5] The iliococcygeus, pubococcygeus, and puborectalis are more correctly described as the *levator ani* muscles. Most authorities include the coccygeus as part of the levator ani, some do not because, unlike other muscles, it functions only to support the sacrum.

The levator ani is like a hammock stretched between the pubis and the coccyx. Its lateral margins attach to a thickened band of the tough membrane (obturator fascia) that covers the obturator internus muscle, thus anchoring the levator ani to the lateral pelvic walls.[5] In the midline, fibers from the levator ani insert on the walls of the rectum, vagina, and urethra as they pass through the pelvic diaphragm.

The levator ani functions to resist increased intraabdominal pressure (as from coughing or strain-ing) and to resist gravity, holding the pelvic organs in place (Fig. 3-17).[5] If these muscles fail to function properly, one of the results is "prolapse" of the pelvic organs through the pelvic diaphragm.

The Pelvic Organs

The pelvic organs include three hollow muscular viscera and one parenchymatous organ. These are (1) the urinary bladder and urethra; (2) the uterus, fallopian tubes, and vagina; (3) the pelvic colon and rectum; (4) and the ovaries.

Before beginning a detailed examination of the organs of the female pelvis, the reader should take a moment to conceptualize the various layers of the pelvic walls formed by the bones, muscles, and tendons. Like the walls of a house, this organic wall provides a relatively rigid framework that supports a layer of fascia composed of loose connective tissue, through which run the plumbing (arteries, veins, and lymphatics) and the electrical and communication lines (nerves). Almost everywhere in the pelvis, the fascia is covered by a layer of insulation (the retroperitoneal fat, which lies between the peritoneum and the endopelvic fascia). The "wallpaper" over the surface of the walls is the peritoneum. Inside the "room" defined by these

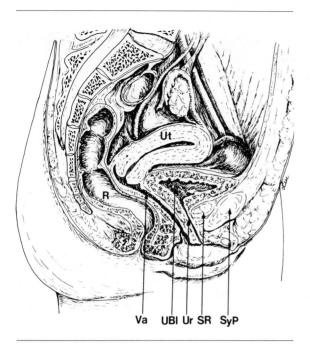

FIGURE 3-18. Organs of the pelvis. (Ut, uterus; R, rectum; Va, vagina; UBl, urinary bladder; Ur, urethra.) Also noted are certain non-organ structures, including the space of Retzius (SR) and the symphysis pubis (SyP).

walls will be found the organs. The analogy breaks down a bit here, because most of the organs of the female pelvis (urinary bladder, uterus, rectum) technically are not inside the room but push into it from the walls or floor without ever breaking through the wallpaper (peritoneum). From a practical standpoint, however, the pelvic organs must be conceptualized as being inside the room of the pelvic space because these organs constantly change dimensions. The urinary bladder and the rectum must expand and contract over relatively brief periods of time. Over a longer time frame the uterus must expand during pregnancy and contract after expulsion of the fetus.

The arrangement of the organs within the pelvic space (Fig. 3-18) facilitates dimensional changes, but it also means that the position and contour of each organ will vary in response to the degree of filling of the other organs that share the same space. These variations dramatically affect the ultrasound image as we will see later in this chapter.

URINARY BLADDER AND URETHRA

The *urinary bladder* is a thick-walled, highly distensible muscular sac that lies between the symphysis pubis and the vagina. When empty, its shape on a sagittal section is an inverted triangle whose apex is formed by the orifice of the urethra.

The anterior surface of the bladder is loosely anchored to the pubic arch by fibrous connective tissue (the pubovesical ligament) but is separated

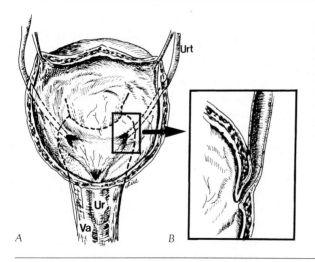

FIGURE 3-19. (A) Cutaway view of the posterior wall of the urinary bladder. Deeper structures including the cervix and the upper region of the vagina are indicated by dotted lines. (B) The ureters enter the bladder at the level of the cervix and on the posterior and inferior wall of the bladder. Their passage through the bladder wall is oblique, forming a passive valve system that resists urine reflex. (Ur, urethra; Va, vagina; Urt, ureter.)

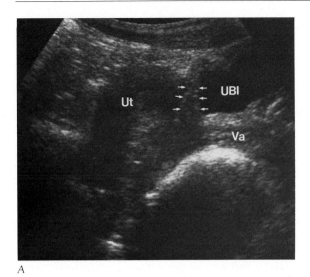
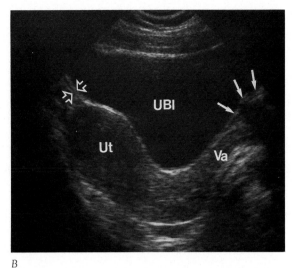

A

B

FIGURE 3-20. (A) Sagittal scan in midline. When the urinary bladder contains only a small amount of urine, the bladder walls (arrows) are thick and easily demonstrated. (Ut, uterus; UBl, urinary bladder; Va, vagina.) (B) Sagittal scan in midline. When fully distended, the bladder walls (open arrows) nearly disappear from the image. The "urethral hump" formed by the internal sphincter is clearly visible in this scan (solid arrows). (UBl, urinary bladder; Ut, uterus; Va, vagina.)

from the symphysis pubis by an interposed pad of extraperitoneal fat in the space of Retzius, or retropubic space.[12] The posterior wall is composed largely of the *trigone* region, which is defined by the orifices of the two ureters and the urethra (Fig. 3-19). The trigone region is thicker and more rigid than the rest of the bladder wall and is separated from the anterior vaginal wall only by a thin layer of fat and loose connective tissue. The superior wall (the *dome* of the bladder) is covered by the coelomic peritoneum and usually is in contact with the anterior wall of the uterus, which folds forward to rest on the dome of the bladder (see Fig. 3-18).

The walls of the urinary bladder are composed of three layers, but only two are visible on sonography. The thick middle layer (the muscularis or detrusor muscle) is composed predominantly of smooth muscle fibers, which give the bladder its contractility. The outer epithelial layer is not visible in ultrasound scans because it is thin and in intimate contact with adjacent layers of fascia and fatty tissues that cover most of the anterior and posterior walls. The inner layer of the bladder is the mucosa, which is very echogenic, but sonographic demonstration of the muscularis and mucosa depends on the degree of bladder filling. When empty, the bladder mucosa is quite thick and easily demonstrated (Fig. 3-20A). When the bladder is distended, the stretched mucosa becomes so thin that it can no longer be recognized as a discrete layer of the bladder wall.

Extending from the urinary bladder are three tubular structures: the two *ureters*, which carry urine from the kidneys to the bladder, and the *urethra*, which conducts urine from the bladder to the urethral orifice, which lies between the labia minora of the external female genitalia. At its exit from the bladder the urethra is surrounded by a thickened region of bladder wall known as the internal sphincter. This thickening may be observed on the sagittal sonogram, marking the urethral exit (Fig. 3-20B).

Urine is transported through the ureters by peristaltic contraction of the walls. As the contraction

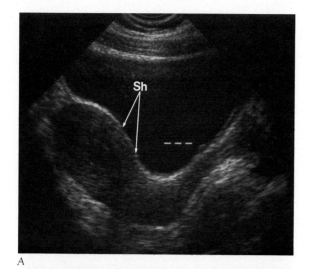

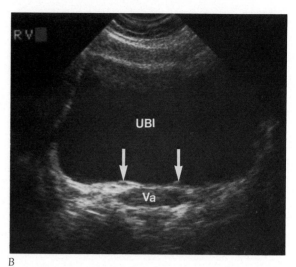

A

B

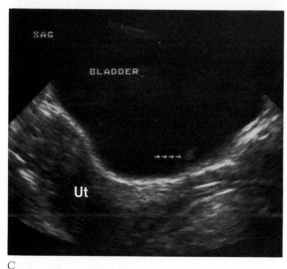

C

Figure 3-21. (A) Sagittal scan slightly to the left of midline. The ureteric valve is visible occasionally as a small projection (*dashed line*). When the valve structure is normal, this projection appears only briefly as the valve pops open. If persistent, it may represent a ureterocele. This image is also a good example of the typical reflection shadow (Sh), which occurs as a result of the relationship between the curve of the anterior uterine wall and the angle of incidence of the acoustic beam. This shadow is artifactual but normal. (B) A slightly oblique transverse scan shows the right ureter (*left arrow*) anterior to the vagina (Va) and just beneath the urinary bladder (UBl) wall. The left ureteric valve (*right arrow*) is in the process of opening. (C) A ureteric jet (*arrows*). This echo pattern lasts only a second or two (Ut, uterus).

reaches the bladder, back-pressure from the bladder must be overcome; the ureteral valve pops open and a bolus of urine enters the bladder in a brief jet (Fig. 3-21). Urine jets can be observed routinely on sonography with high gain, but the jet is transient and the echoes disappear quickly. The cause of these echoes is the subject of debate, but it is probable that the pressure differential between the jet and the surrounding urine is sufficient explanation. Urine in the renal pelvis, ureters, and urinary bladder is normally sterile and completely anechoic.

The contour of the urinary bladder does not change uniformly as it expands with filling. The dome is the most distensible region of the bladder, so we might expect it to expand uniformly upward in the pelvis as it fills, but two factors dictate nonuniform expansion of the bladder walls. First, the trigone is thicker and more rigid; second, the bladder must accommodate the space requirements of the other organs in the pelvis, chiefly the uterus. Since the uterus normally folds forward to rest on the posterior and midregions of the dome, the part of the bladder wall that experiences least resistance

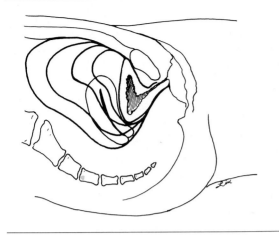

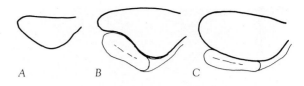

FIGURE 3-22. Contours of the urinary bladder with progressive filling. The uterus is shown in its initial position, folded forward over the dome of the empty urinary bladder. For clarity, the corresponding positions of the uterus are not shown, although the indentation of the posterior bladder wall by the uterus is indicated for each stage of filling.

FIGURE 3-23. The urinary bladder contour is directly influenced by the presence of the uterus within the fixed space of the pelvis. When the uterus has been surgically removed or is congenitally absent, the bladder contour is distinctly deltoid (A). The normal anteflexed uterus creates a gentle indentation of the moderately distended bladder (B). The degree of indentation is influenced by the size of the uterus and the degree of bladder filling. If overdistended, the bladder can compress the uterus excessively, altering the uterine shape and echo pattern (C). The ideal degree of filling results in extension of the bladder 1 to 2 cm above the fundus of the uterus, while preserving the normal uterine contour.

to expansion is the extreme anterior portion. This region needs displace only highly mobile loops of small bowel, which normally fill any unoccupied space in the true pelvis. So the anterior part of the urinary bladder expands upward more rapidly, resulting in the typical asymmetric shape of the distended bladder on sagittal section (Fig. 3-22).

Because the bladder contour reflects the presence of both normal and abnormal structures with which it is in contact, the examiner should look carefully at the urinary bladder before trying to determine the identity and relationship of other structures in the pelvis. The urinary bladder contours provide a "reverse map" of the pelvis (Figs. 3-23, 3-24). In addition, urine in the bladder provides both a window and a reference standard. Like water, urine attenuates ultrasound frequencies only slightly, permitting transmission deep into the pelvis with minimal energy loss. If there are echoes in the urine (with the exception of the normal anterior wall artifact seen on transabdominal sonography), then either the gain setting is too high or the urine is abnormal.

Cell casts from the renal tubules and uric acid crystals can cause punctate echoes in the urine, but

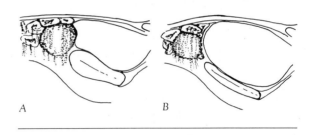

FIGURE 3-24. The cephalad margin of the urinary bladder can provide an important clue to the presence of a mass superior to the urinary bladder and uterine fundus (A). If the bladder is only moderately distended, it can respond to the weight of a mass by forming a gentle curve around the mass (B). As the bladder becomes tense with overdistention, the weight of a cephalad mass may be insufficient to alter the bladder contour. As masses cephalad to the urinary bladder and uterine fundus may be surrounded by loops of small bowel, the bladder contour may be the only indication of the presence of the mass.

sonographers encounter these only rarely. More often, echoes in the urine represent "noise" associated with a gain or output level that is too high. If such false echoes are appearing in the urine, they will also appear in soft tissues, where they may not

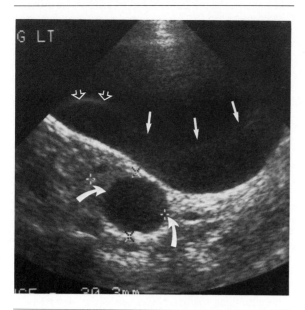

Figure 3-25. Excessive gain is evidenced by false echoes (*straight arrows*) in the bladder. These false echoes also appear in the follicular cyst in the ovary (*curved arrows*). Also noted on this scan is a typical "thumbnail" artifact within the bladder (*open arrows*) caused by rough handling of the film used to record the scan.

be recognized as false. The most common technical error in gynecologic sonography is excessive gain obscuring subtle details within the soft tissues. A good rule of thumb is to use the minimum output and gain level consistent with adequate demonstration of tissue echo patterns. The second way in which urine serves as a reference standard is for comparison with other echo patterns in pelvic structures. If the gain is set so that no echoes appear in the normally anechoic urine, then no echoes should appear within cysts (such as follicles), which are wider than the ultrasound beam and which contain homogeneous fluid (Fig. 3-25).

By comparing the echogenicity of the urine with the echogenicity of the unknown structure at various gain levels, one can qualitatively assess the structural similarity or dissimilarity of the two. A word of caution is in order here: Too often, the assumption is made that anechoic content always represents fluid; this is not so. Echogenicity alone

cannot be used as a definitive criterion for the presence of fluid. Homogeneous solids (e.g., myoma) can be anechoic at normal gain levels and fluids (blood, pus) can be echogenic. Both echogenicity and through-transmission must be used as criteria for distinguishing fluids from solids.

The Vagina

The *vagina* is a relatively thin-walled, 7- to 10-cm-long muscular tube that extends from the cervix of the uterus to the vestibule of the external genitalia and lies between the urinary bladder and the rectum.[7] Its wall is composed of smooth muscle and elastic connective tissue and is lined with stratified squamous epithelium, very similar to skin (hence its name; the vagina is essentially an invagination of the skin). The outer surface of the vagina (the adventitial coat) is a thin, fibrous layer that is continuous with the surrounding endopelvic fascia (Fig. 3-26). Normally the vaginal canal is a potential space, because the anterior and posterior walls are in apposition. When collapsed, the vagina assumes a rounded **H** shape on cross section, and the inner mucosal surface of the wall wrinkles up to form transverse ridges (rugae), which largely disappear when the vaginal wall is stretched (Fig. 3-27).

The posterior wall of the vagina is longer than the anterior wall. The upper end of the vagina attaches to the cervix of the uterus along an oblique line about halfway up the length of the cervix.[12] This form of attachment creates a ring-shaped, blind pocket (the *fornix*) between the outer wall of the cervix and the inner surface of the vaginal wall. By convention, this continuous ring-shaped space is divided into anterior, lateral, and posterior fornices (Fig. 3-28). Because of the oblique attachment of the vagina to the cervix, the posterior fornix is deeper than the anterior, and its posterior location causes it to be the site of pooling of urine, pus, blood, or other fluid that originates in the vagina or escapes into it.

The length and wall thickness of the vagina vary in response to filling of the urinary bladder. The vagina is attached to the uterus, which is displaced upward and backward by bladder filling, thus stretching and reducing the thickness of the vaginal wall as the bladder expands. The combined thickness of the normal anterior and posterior va-

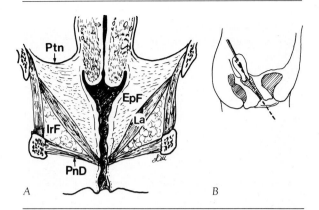

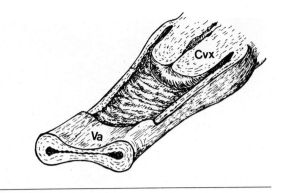

FIGURE 3-26. (*A*) Oblique section through lower uterus and vagina. The plane of section is indicated in (*B*). The uterus has been elevated to stretch the vagina and align it with the plane of section. Note the relationship between the perineal diaphragm and the levator ani muscle group. (PnD, perineal diaphragm; La, levator ani; EpF, endopelvic fascia; Ptn, peritoneum; IrF, ischiorectal fossa.)

FIGURE 3-27. Cutaway view of vagina. Note cross section when collapsed and relationship of uterine cervix (Cvx) to vaginal (Va) walls.

ginal walls should not exceed 1 cm[17] when measured from a transvesical scan made with the urinary bladder distended.

On sonograms, the muscular walls of the vagina produce a moderately hypoechoic pattern typical of smooth muscle (Fig. 3-29). The mucosa of the vagina is highly echogenic, but it may be difficult to differentiate if the vaginal walls are stretched by a distended bladder (Fig. 3-30). Although the vagina can move laterally in response to pressure from a distended rectum, it is most commonly found at or near the sagittal midline of the pelvis. Its anteroposterior position, however, varies substantially in response to the degree of filling of the urinary bladder and the rectum. In addition, the upper part of the vagina will follow the cervix if the uterus is displaced laterally by a pelvic mass or a distended rectum or sigmoid colon.

The introduction of transvaginal ultrasound imaging has placed new emphasis on the importance of a complete understanding of the anatomy of the vagina and its relationship to the surrounding organs. The typical transvaginal scan is performed with the urinary bladder empty or containing only

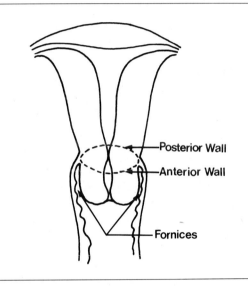

FIGURE 3-28. Relationship between uterus and vagina. The posterior vaginal wall attaches higher on the cervix than the anterior wall. The fornices are the blind pockets formed by the inner surface of the vaginal walls and the outer surface of the cervix. These spaces are normally collapsed or contain only a small amount of mucus.

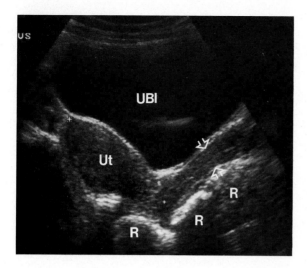

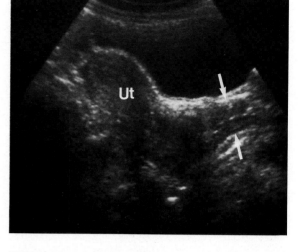

Figure 3-29. Median sagittal scan with the bladder only moderately filled. Note the thickness (*arrows*) and cephalocaudad length of the vaginal walls. The vaginal canal is indicated by the interrupted bright line separating the anterior and posterior walls. (Ut, uterus.)

Figure 3-30. Echo pattern of the vagina when the bladder is fully distended. The vaginal walls can be identified readily (*open arrows*). The linear echo in the bladder is an artifact. (Ut, uterus; UBl, urinary bladder; R, rectum.)

a little urine (Fig. 3-31). A specially designed transducer is inserted into the vagina so that the active face of the transducer is positioned at the tip of the cervix or in the fornix. The ultrasound beam may then be directed anteriorly and cephalad to image the uterus, fallopian tubes, and ovaries, or the transducer can be rotated to view the lateral pelvic walls.[19]

While the remarkable flexibility of the vagina affords substantial latitude in positioning the ultrasound probe, the shape of the pelvic cavity imposes some limitations. In addition, the probe must be manipulated judiciously. The patient may have limited tolerance for probe movement, particularly in the case of pelvic inflammation or adhesions. The examiner also must be aware of the differences in anatomic position and mobility of the pelvic organs when the urinary bladder is empty. For example, the uterus is much lower and more anterior in the pelvic cavity when the bladder is empty, and the ovaries are usually in the posterolateral region of the pelvis and may lie at some distance from the uterus. This is in contrast with transabdominal pelvic scans, on which the ovaries are usually deeper

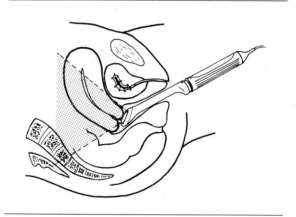

Figure 3-31. Transvaginal sonography permits the specially adapted transducer to be placed close to the organs of interest. These transducers usually generate higher acoustic frequencies than those used for transvesical imaging.

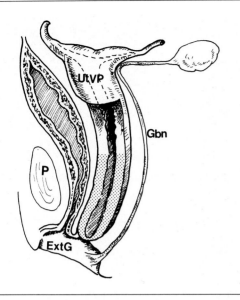

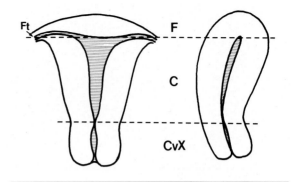

FIGURE 3-33. Schematic diagram of uterine regions. (F, fundus; C, corpus; CvX, cervix; Ft, fallopian tube.)

FIGURE 3-32. The embryonic uterus and fallopian tubes arise from the paired paramesonephric ducts. The upper (cranial) regions of these ducts remain separate and form the fallopian tubes. The caudal regions fuse to form the uterovaginal primordium, which later differentiates into the uterus and the vagina. The shaded area on the figure indicates the area that will differentiate into the vagina. (P, pubis; Gbn, gubernaculum; UtVP, uterovaginal primordium; ExtG, external genitalia.)

in the true pelvic space and are pressed against the lateral or superior margins of the uterus.

THE UTERUS

In nulliparous women the *uterus* is a small, pear-shaped muscular viscus suspended in the midpelvis. In one sense, the uterus is only a prominent bulge in the middle section of a continuous muscular canal that begins with the fallopian tubes and ends with the external orifice of the vagina (Fig. 3-32), but, because its structure and size differentiate it so dramatically from the fallopian tubes and the vagina, the uterus is usually considered as a separate organ. Its sole function is reproductive; that is, to receive the fertilized egg, to nourish the developing conceptus, and ultimately to expel the fetus.

Regions of the Uterus. The uterus is described as having four parts or regions—fundus, corpus, isthmus, and cervix. The regions are arbitrarily defined on the basis of the uterine contour and structure (Fig. 3-33).

Fundus. The uppermost region of the uterus is the fundus ("bottom"), which begins at the point where the fallopian tubes arise from the uterine walls. (The "bottom" of the uterus is its uppermost region because the uterine regions are named for the Greek wine bottle, the amphora, which it resembles. In this case, the wine bottle is upside down with its neck pushed into the vaginal canal.) The fundus is the least distinctive region of the uterus. It is a rounded or dome-shaped area characterized only by its location above the level of the uterine cavity. It narrows at its outer and lateral margins to form the cornu (horn) of the uterus,[13] through which passes the interstitial portion of the fallopian tube (see Fig. 3-33).

Corpus and Isthmus. The corpus (body) is the largest uterine region and houses the uterine cavity. On cross section the corpus appears rounded or ovoid (Fig. 3-34). In both sagittal and coronal sections the corpus usually appears cylindrical or slightly tapered, narrowing as it approaches the isthmus, or waist, of the uterus. The isthmus marks the transition from the corpus to the cervix, or neck. The isthmus is important in that it is the point at which the uterus is most flexible. With the urinary bladder empty, the uterus folds or bends at the isthmus, so that the axis of the corpus and the axis of the cervix form a shallow angle.

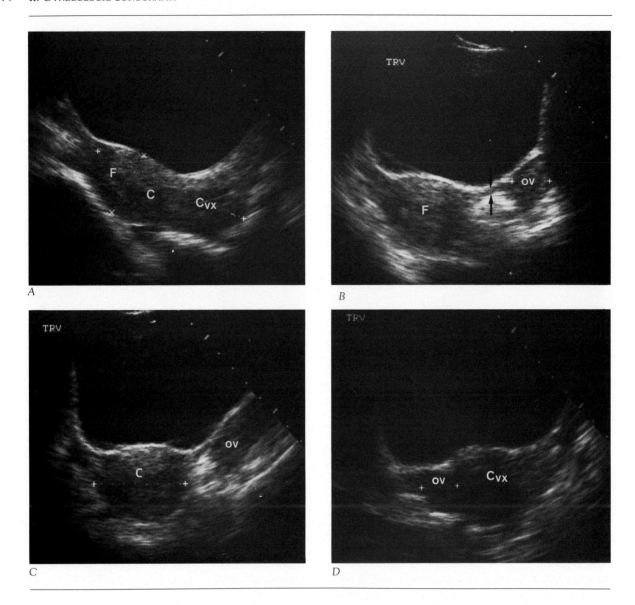

FIGURE 3-34. (A) Median sagittal scan of normal uterus and vagina. (F, fundus; C, corpus; Cvx, cervix). (B) Transverse scan at the level of the fundus. The left ovary (OV) is demonstrated. The broad ligament and/or fallopian tube (arrows) bridges the space between the uterine fundus and the ovary. (C) Transverse scan at the level of the corpus. (D) Transverse scan at the level of the cervix. The right ovary (OV) is seen adjacent to the cervix. In this position, it occupies most of the posterior cul-de-sac.

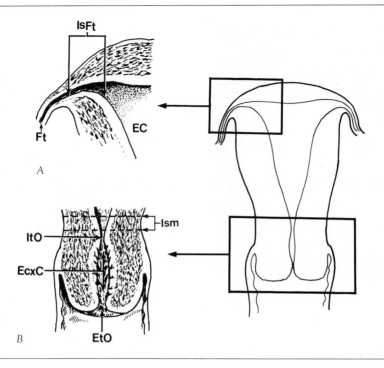

FIGURE 3-35. Structure of the cornual (*A*) and cervical (*B*) regions of the uterus. (EC, endometrial cavity; Ft, fallopian tube; ItO, internal os; EtO, external os; EcxC, endocervical canal; IsFt, interstitial portion of the fallopian tube; Ism, isthmus.)

Cervix. The cervix is the cylindrical neck of the uterus (Fig. 3-35). It is different from the rest of the uterine tissue in being more fibrous and less muscular, and by having a distinctive endothelium. It may be described as a barrel-shaped cylinder, slightly wider in the middle and 2 to 3 cm long in nulliparous females.[13] It is penetrated by the spindle-shaped endocervical canal, which extends from the internal to the external os (small opening). The canal is lined with a mucosa whose anterior and posterior surfaces are characterized by oblique ridges or palmate folds that slant downward toward the external os.[13] The endocervical mucosa is richly supplied with mucous glands (Fig. 3-36). The mucus serves to impede upward migration of bacteria. In pregnancy, the mucosa of the endocervical canal under goes hypertrophy and the glands produce a dense, sticky mucous plug (the mucous plug of pregnancy).

The Uterine Cavity. The uterine cavity is shaped like an inverted triangle with its basal angles defined by the ostia of the fallopian tubes and its apex defined by the internal os of the cervix. The cavity is widest at the fundus and narrowest at the isthmus and is flattened front to back, so that the anterior and posterior endometrial surfaces are normally separated only by a thin layer of mucus.

Layers of the Uterus. The walls of the uterus are composed of three tissue layers (Fig. 3-37). The outermost layer is quite thin and not visible on sonography. It consists of a layer of fascia that is continuous with the pelvic fascia and forms a serosa that invests the uterine walls. The thick middle layer (the myometrium) is composed of smooth muscle cells and interspersed connective tissue fibers. Lining the inner surface of the uterus is a mucosa known as the endometrium, which forms the walls of the uterine cavity.

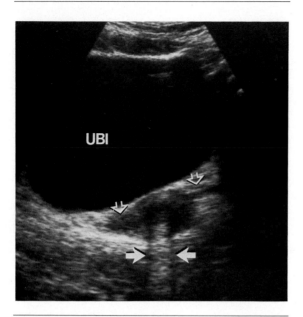

FIGURE 3-36. Transverse scan of a cervix that is shifted to the left side of the pelvic cavity. Note the lateral extensions of the cervical echo pattern *(open arrows)*. These ill-defined "wings" are the transverse cervical ligaments. Also note the edge shadows *(solid arrows)*, which bracket a central zone of enhanced echoes. This pattern is characteristic of the cervix. (UBl, urinary bladder.)

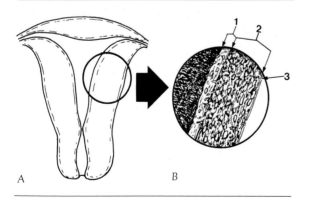

FIGURE 3-37. (A) Frontal plane schematic of the uterus. (B) Enlarged view of tissues that form the uterine wall. (1, endometrium; 2, myometrium; 3, serosa.)

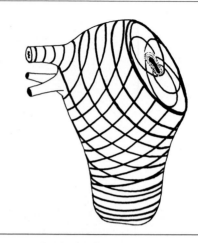

FIGURE 3-38. Schematic diagram of spiral smooth muscle fibers of the uterus. Contraction of these fibers tends to increase pressure in the uterine lumen.

Myometrium. The thick, muscular middle layer of the uterus (the myometrium) forms most of the bulk of the uterine body. Within this layer, the major muscle fibers are arranged in a complex spiral pattern (Fig. 3-38). The myometrium may be further subdivided into three rather indistinct layers: an outer layer characterized by longitudinal muscle fibers, a thick middle layer that is richly vascular, and a denser inner layer whose muscle fibers are arranged both longitudinally and obliquely.[13] Throughout the reproductive years, the muscular tissues of the uterus participate in low-amplitude contractile activity, which serves to maintain the muscle tone of the uterus. Just before and during the menstrual flow, this contractile activity becomes more focused and results in slow, subsensate, ripple-like contractions, which originate in the fundus and sweep down the length of the uterus to the internal os. These contractions are of very low amplitude and quite slow, requiring several seconds to progress from fundus to isthmus. They can be recognized during transvaginal imaging of the uterus as a progressive focal rippling distortion of the endometrial echo pattern. In contrast with these menstrual contractions, one group of investigators[15] reported observing reverse contractions, which sweep upward from the internal os to the fundus. These contractions were observed during transvaginal sonography and were found to be most frequent at the time of ovulation. The inves-

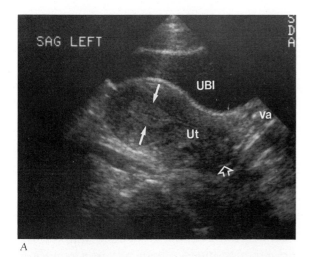

A

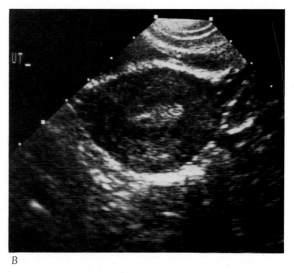

B

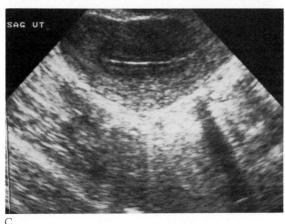

C

FIGURE 3-39. (A) Sagittal scan of uterus (Ut) and vagina (Va). This immediately premenstrual (day 27) endometrium (*arrows*) is producing abundant mucus, which has outlined the uterine cavity. Four distinct echo layers can be identified. The outermost dark layer is myometrium and should not be included in measurement of the endometrium. This layer abuts on the thick, echogenic glandular layer that forms the bulk of the endometrium. A hypoechoic inner layer separates the echogenic glandular layer from a thin, highly echogenic line formed by mucus and the surfaces of the endometrium. Mucus has also outlined the posterior fornix (*open arrow*). (UBl, urinary bladder.) (B) In this transverse transvesical scan of a midsecretory-phase endometrium, the layers are more difficult to identify precisely, and the echo pattern in the glandular layer is patchy. (C) The distinct layers are more easily appreciated in this transvaginal sagittal scan of the uterine corpus during the late proliferative stage.

tigators speculate that these contractions assist migration of sperm upward through the uterus to the fallopian tubes.[15]

Endometrium. The endometrium is a specialized mucosa that varies in thickness and composition through the menstrual cycle. Covering the surface are ciliated cells interrupted at intervals by the orifices of mucous glands.[14] The hairlike cilia flex in synchronized waves that tend to force surface mucus toward the cervix. This steady downward flow of a sticky tide of mucus prevents bacteria from migrating upward into the uterine cavity. Although the vagina is richly colonized by bacteria, the endometrium and the endocervical canal are normally free of foreign organisms. The amount of mucus present at any given time is highly variable, but typically is greatest just before the menstrual flow begins or at the onset of pregnancy.

Following menstruation the thickness of a single layer of endometrium is about 0.5 to 1 mm[12]; it increases to a maximum 5 to 7 mm at the onset of the next menstrual flow. Sonographic measurements of the endometrium are usually made across the long axis of the uterus, including layers of endometrium on the anterior and posterior walls. When measured this way, endometrial thickness ranges from approximately 1 mm immediately following menstruation to about 14 mm immediately before menstruation (Fig. 3-39A). When measuring the endo-

TABLE 3-2. The endometrium

PHASE	DAYS OF CYCLE	THICKNESS (MM)	ENDOMETRIAL ECHO PATTERN
Menstrual	1–5	<0.5	Thin echogenic line
Postmenstrual	6–9	1–2	Mostly anechoic
Proliferative	10–13	2–4	Slightly echogenic
Secretory	14–28	5–7	Highly echogenic

metrium, the outermost, hypoechoic layer should be excluded, because it is myometrial in origin. This layer is most likely the result of the extensive vascular channels in the muscle layer closest to the endometrium.[4] Within the endometrium proper, two or even three layers may be identified (Fig. 3-39A). Their exact clinical significance is a matter of debate, but Hackeloer[9] and others[3] have noted that a thin hypoechoic layer can sometimes be seen lining the innermost surface of the endometrial cavity at the time of ovulation or immediately afterward (Fig. 3-39B). This "inner ring" sign may be useful as a confirmation of ovulation, but it has not been identified consistently in studies by other investigators.[3]

Attempts have been made to precisely correlate the echo pattern or thickness of the endometrium with the stage of the menstrual cycle. Although the variations during the menstrual cycle for an individual are relatively consistent from cycle to cycle, the range of variation from individual to individual is great, and only generalizations may safely be made. The average menstrual cycle of 28 days may be regarded as having four phases associated with histomorphologic changes in the endometrium. These phases, their duration, endometrial thickness, and echo pattern are shown in Table 3-2.

Although transvaginal scanning has greatly improved our ability to delineate the endometrium with ultrasound (Fig. 3-39C), it is doubtful that endometrial thickness or echo pattern will prove to be reliable clinical indicators, except when either is grossly abnormal.

Uterine Size and Shape. The size and shape of the uterus vary markedly with age and obstetric history (Fig. 3-40A). In the fetus, the uterus grows at a rate consistent with the rest of the body until early in the third trimester. For the remainder of the gestational period, growth of the uterine corpus is ac-

celerated because of the high level of maternal estrogen produced as term approaches. As a result, the uterus is larger and has a more "adult" contour in newborns than in children.[11] Immediately after birth, withdrawal of the influence of maternal estrogen causes the uterine corpus to shrink, and significant growth will not occur again until the ovaries begin to produce hormones as a prelude to puberty. In infants, the uterus rides high in the pelvis, is cylindrical, and lies along the same axis as the vagina. In young girls the uterus remains nearly cylindrical (Fig. 3-40B), but the body (corpus and fundus) of the uterus becomes more globular as it matures. By puberty, the uterus has assumed the characteristic inverted pear shape. With each pregnancy the corpus and fundus grow thicker, increasing the globularity of the multiparous uterus (Fig. 3-40C). After menopause the corpus and fundus shrink and regress to the prepubertal state (Fig. 3-40D) and in elderly women, they may appear as little more than a cap above the cervix. Throughout life, changes in uterine size are mostly the result of changes in the muscularis layer, predominantly in the corpus. Because of its smaller proportion of muscle to connective tissue, the cervix varies least in size and is least flexible of all the uterine regions.

A Caveat About Uterine Dimensions. The range of individual variation in organ size increases steadily from the fetal period through adulthood. Additionally, the linear dimensions of the uterus are influenced by many factors, including pressure from surrounding organs, stage of the menstrual cycle, and obstetric history. Normal dimensions given for the uterus must be regarded only as arbitrarily defined points on the continuum of uterine development, growth, and regression (Fig. 3-40). The uterus of a child typically is 2.5 cm long and has an anteroposterior diameter of about 1 cm.[18] The length of the adult nulliparous uterus typically is 8 cm or less, the width 5.5 cm, and the anteriorpos-

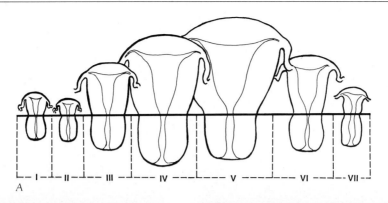

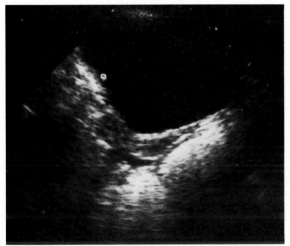

B

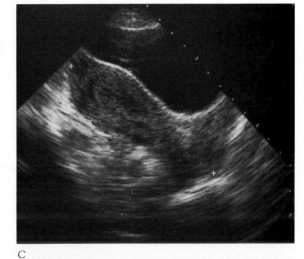

C

Figure 3-40. (A) Relationship between cervical length and the length of the combined corpus and fundus at various stages of a woman's life. In childhood, the cervix may constitute two-thirds and the corpus and fundus one-third of the total uterine length. By puberty, the ratio has become 1 to 1 and continues to shift steadily until the adult nulliparous ratio is two-thirds corpus and fundus to one-third cervix. (I, birth; II, childhood; III, at puberty; IV, adult nuliparous; V, adult parous; VI, at menopause; VII, elderly.) (B) Sagittal scan of the uterus in a child, aged 8 years. The uterus is mostly cylindrical with only slight rounding of the corpus and fundus. (C) Sagittal scan of the uterus of a multiparous woman. (D) Sagittal scan of the uterus of a postmenopausal 58-year-old woman.

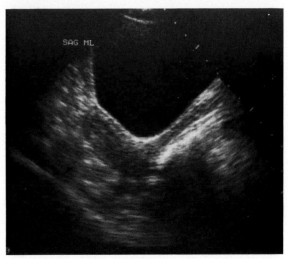

D

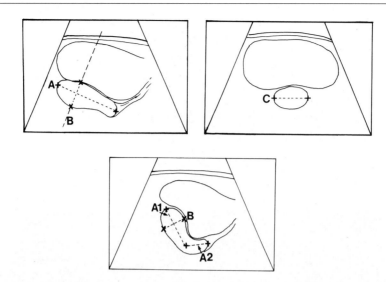

FIGURE 3-41. Measurement technique for the uterus. The long axis of the uterus should be measured from the fundus to the tip of the cervix (line A). When making this measurement, carefully identify the true long axis of the uterus, since it is seldom parallel to the pelvic midline. Gain and scan plane are then adjusted to optimally demonstrate the tip of the cervix. The posterior wall of the vagina serves as a guide; its curve can be followed around the posterior lip of the cervix to more precisely identify where the cervix ends and the vaginal wall begins. On the same image, the greatest AP diameter of the uterus should be measured along a line perpendicular to line A at a point where the uterus appears widest in the AP plane. Then the midpoint of the field of view is centered on the same line used to measure the AP diameter, and the transducer is rotated 90 degrees, maintaining a constant tilt. This assures that the transverse diameter (line C) is measured in the same plane as the AP diameter (line B), which results in more consistent and accurate measurements of the uterus. If the uterus is strongly anteflexed, two measurements of the long axis (Lines A1 and A2) should be made and added together to obtain the true length.

terior dimension 3 cm.[11] The sonographer should use a consistent method to measure the uterus. One such method is shown in Figure 3-41. Small variations of uterine size are not clinically significant.

The Uterine Ligaments. Unlike the urinary bladder and rectum, which are relatively closely attached to the walls of the pelvic space, the uterus is loosely suspended in the center of the pelvic cavity.

The *cardinal ligaments* (also called transverse cervical ligaments) consist of ill-defined, wide bands of condensed fibromuscular tissue that originate from the lateral region of the cervix and along the lateral margin of the uterine corpus. These bands

insert over a broad region of the lateral pelvic wall and extend posteriorly to the margins of the sacrum.[12] The posterior edge of the cardinal ligaments is more condensed than other regions and is identified as the uterosacral ligaments (Fig. 3-42). These extend from the posterolateral margin of the cervix to the sacrum. Together, the cardinal and uterosacral ligaments anchor the cervix and orient its axis so that it is roughly parallel to the central axis of the body.

The *round ligaments* (Fig. 3-42) are fibromuscular bands originating from the uterine cornua and extending across the pelvic space from posterior to anterior. They cross over the pelvic brim, pass

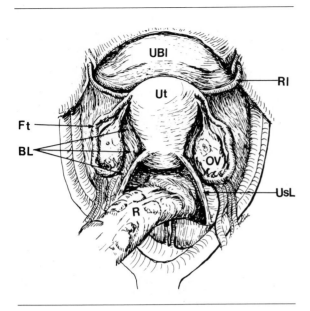

FIGURE 3-42. View looking down into the pelvic cavity from behind, with the organs in place: Ut, uterus; OV, ovary; Ft, fallopian tube; Rl, round ligament; UsL, uterosacral ligament; R, rectum; UBl, urinary bladder; Bl, broad ligament.

through the inguinal ring, and then disperse as fibers anchored in the labia majora of the external genitalia.[12] They serve to loosely tether the uterine fundus and tilt it forward in the pelvis, aiding in the normal anteflexion of the uterus at the isthmus.

Of all the ligaments of the pelvis, the *broad ligament* is the most difficult to describe because it is not a true ligament but simply a double fold of *peritoneum*. The peritoneum is a thin, glistening serous membrane that forms a sac that lines the abdominopelvic cavity. Its function is to permit organs to slide over each other with minimal friction, and this is aided by a thin layer of serous fluid produced by the peritoneum.

To understand the relationship of the peritoneum to the organs in the pelvis, the reader might imagine a container that will represent the abdominopelvic cavity. Put into it a pear to represent the uterus. Now stuff a sac into the container so that it covers the pear, folding back on itself, and extending down in front and back. At the sides of the pear, the sac will form a double layer, which is analogous to the broad ligament. The broad ligament

is simply the double layer of peritoneum, with fat, vessels, and nerves between the two layers. This arrangement probably has only minimal function in suspension of the uterus, but the broad ligament is important because it incompletely divides the true pelvis into anterior and posterior pelvic compartments. The ovaries are attached to the posterior surface of the broad ligament, thus limiting their movements to the posterior pelvic compartment.

Spaces Adjacent to the Uterus. In addition to its anatomic function of isolating and lubricating the surfaces of organs, the peritoneum is also responsible for formation of certain spaces in relationship to the uterus and other organs of the pelvis (Figs. 3-42, 3-43). The peritoneum reflects, or folds back, from the anterior wall of the pelvic cavity to cover the dome of the bladder and then folds more sharply to cover the anterior surface of the uterus. This fold forms the relatively shallow *anterior cul de sac* (vesicouterine pouch), which lies between the anterior wall of the uterus and the urinary bladder.[12] This space virtually disappears as the urinary bladder fills; normally it is not significant to the sonographer. In contrast, the similar pocket formed by reflection of the peritoneum from the posterior wall of the pelvis (covering the rectum) to the posterior wall of the uterus is very important. The *posterior cul de sac* (pouch of Douglas or rectouterine pouch) is the most posterior and dependent portion of the peritoneal sac lining the abdominopelvic cavity.[8] Fluid originating anywhere in the peritoneal sac tends to drain into the posterior cul de sac. This space is relatively complex in its configuration. Its most inferior extent consists of a deep, narrow pocket that extends down between the rectum and the cervix and is defined at its upper margins by the uterosacral ligaments. Above these ligaments the cul de sac widens out and is continuous with the broad, shallow spaces to the side of the uterus. These shallow *adnexal* spaces are lined by the peritoneum, forming the broad ligament.

Variants of Uterine Position. In some women the uterus does not maintain the anteflexed position, instead bending backward so that the fundus of the uterus comes to rest in the posterior cul-de-sac (Fig. 3-44).[14] This retroflexion of the uterus is relatively

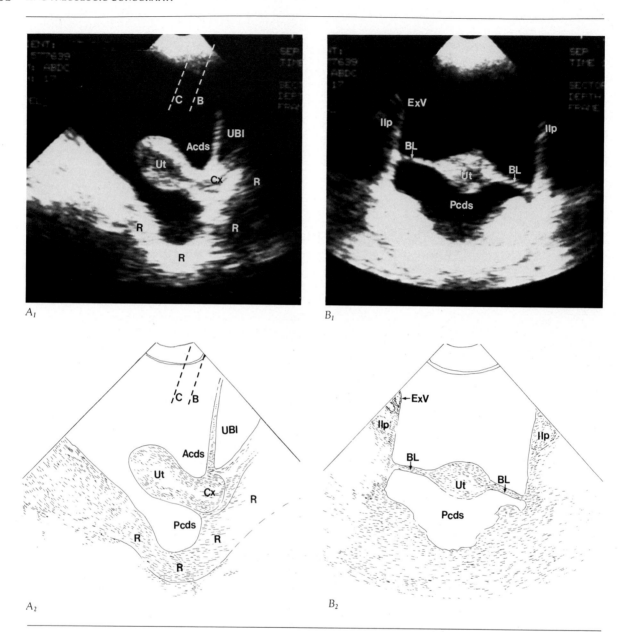

A_1

B_1

A_2

B_2

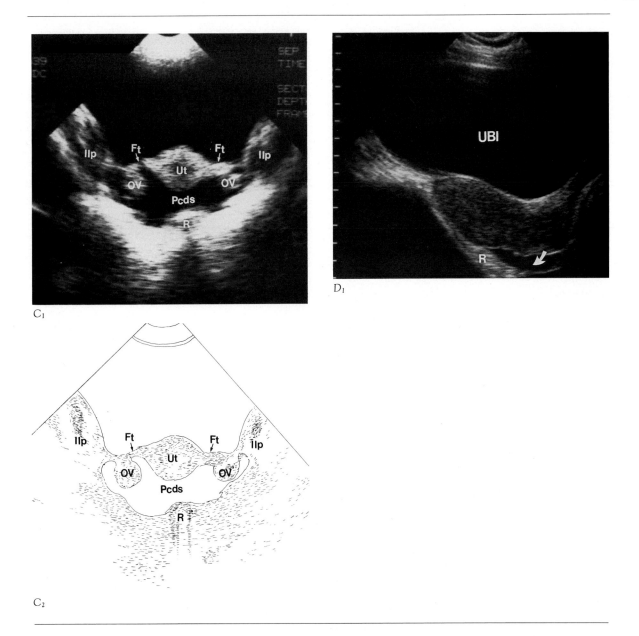

FIGURE 3-43. (A₁) Sagittal scan of the pelvis of a patient with massive ascites. Fluid fills the pelvic cavity, outlining the uterus. Note how the shape of the posterior cul-de-sac compares with the shape of the anterior cul-de-sac. The dashed lines indicate the plane of scan for images B and C. (A₂) UBl, urinary bladder; Acds, anterior cul-de-sac; Ut, uterus; Cx, cervix; Pcds, posterior cul-de-sac; R, rectum. (B₁) Transverse scan at the level of the uterine isthmus demonstrates the broad ligaments and posterior cul-de-sac. (B₂) ExV, external iliac artery and vein; llp, iliopsoas muscle; BL, broad ligament; Ut, uterus; Pcds, posterior cul-de-sac. (C₁) Transverse scan at the level of the uterine fundus demonstrates the uterus, ovaries, fallopian tubes, and rectum. (C₂) llp, iliopsoas muscle; Ft, fallopian tube; Ut, uterus; OV, ovary; Pcds, posterior cul-de-sac; R, rectum. (D₁) Typical pattern of a moderate amount of fluid in the posterior cul-de-sac (curved arrow). Compare with image A to appreciate the shape of the posterior cul-de-sac with varying amounts of fluid in it.

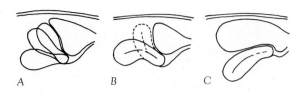

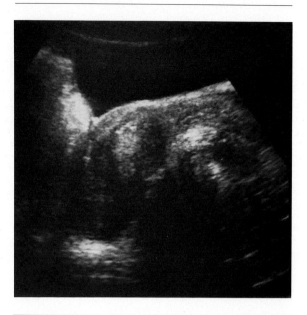

FIGURE 3-44. Variants of uterine position within the pelvis. (A) Normal physiologic retroversion of the uterus by filling of the urinary bladder. (B) Retroflexion of the uterus. The cervix maintains a normal position but the corpus and fundus flex backward into the posterior pelvic compartment. Note that the point of flexion is at the isthmus. (C) Retroflexion and retroversion. All regions of the uterus are abnormal in position. Positions B and C are commonly lumped together in the category of "retroversion."

FIGURE 3-45. Sagittal scan of a retroflexed multiparous uterus. The ill-defined fundus mimics a mass in the posterior cul-de-sac. Note the abnormal contour of the posterior wall of the urinary bladder.

common, rarely has clinical significance, and may be transient or persistent in a given woman.

Retroflexion of the uterus is responsible for significant alterations in the uterus echo pattern produced by transabdominal scanning. Normally, the uterus lies in a plane roughly perpendicular to an ultrasound beam entering through the full urinary bladder. Most of the uterus lies at a relatively constant depth from the transducer, so the echo pattern is uniform throughout the myometrium. In contrast, the corpus and fundus of a retroflexed uterus are tilted back into the pelvic cavity, and the acoustic beam must traverse the muscle tissue of the corpus to reach the fundus. As a result, the fundus of a retroflexed uterus often appears echo poor when compared with the corpus (Fig. 3-45).[11] This difference is due to absorption of the ultrasound beam by the muscle of the corpus. In extreme cases, the hypoechoic fundus may be misidentified as a mass in the cul-de-sac.

THE FALLOPIAN TUBES

The *fallopian tubes* (*oviducts* or *salpinges* [singular: *salpinx*]) are paired musculomembranous tubes that extend from the fundus of the uterus to the ovary and lateral pelvic wall. Most of the length of the fallopian tube lies within the free edge of the fold of peritoneum that forms the broad ligament. Like the uterine wall, the wall of the fallopian tube

consists of three layers: an outer serosal coat (which is continuous with the overlying peritoneum over the isthmic portion of the tube), a middle muscular layer, and an inner mucosa. By convention the tube is divided into the intramural, isthmic, and ampullary portions (Fig. 3-46). The total tubal length in an adult (7 to 14 cm)[12] is usually greater than the distance from the uterus to the lateral pelvic wall, so in its normal state the tube is more tortuous than its wall structure alone would impose. The tubal lumen widens as it moves away from the uterus. The intramural portion is the narrowest (< 1 mm), and the third portion or ampulla is the widest (about 6 mm).[13] The ampullary portion terminates in the trumpet-shaped infundibulum, which is open to the inside of the peritoneal sac that lines the abdominopelvic cavity. This trumpet-shaped opening is about 1 cm wide and is fringed by delicate fingerlike projections called fimbriae. Usually one of these, the *fimbria ovarica*, is attached to the ovary and serves to maintain a close relationship between the opening of the tube and the ovarian surface.[12]

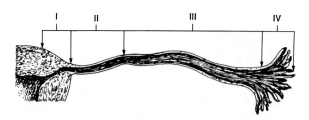

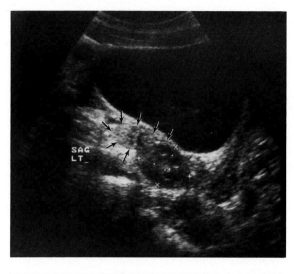

FIGURE 3-46. Regions of the fallopian tube. For this illustration, the tube has been stretched horizontally. The intramural (interstitial) portion (I) is relatively straight and is located within the uterine wall. The isthmic portion (II) is longer and slightly wavy in its course. The ampullary portion (III) is the longest section of the tube and is quite tortuous in vivo. It terminates in the trumpet-shaped infundibulum (IV), which is fringed with fingerlike projections, the fimbriae.

FIGURE 3-47. Sagittal scan of the left ovary (outlined by the measurement markers). The fallopian tube *(small arrows)* is seen over the upper pole of the ovary in this transvesical scan. Without the small amount of fluid that defines the crescentic lumen, it would not be possible to positively identify these echoes as representing the tube.

Because the echo pattern of the fallopian tube is similar to that of the surrounding structures, it is commonly demonstrated but rarely recognized in transabdominal ultrasound images, except when distended with fluid. Occasionally, a typical pattern is seen at the lateral pole of the ovary where the infundibulum is usually located (Fig. 3-47). Because of the relative thinness of its wall, the characteristic echo pattern of the fallopian tube is that of the hyperechoic mucosa bordered by a thin layer of hypoechoic muscle tissue surrounding a crescentic or cylindrical lumen.

THE OVARIES

The *ovary* is unlike the other organs of the female pelvis in many respects. It is a solid (parenchymatous) structure; it secretes hormones; it is not covered by peritoneum; and it is the only organ that is entirely "inside" the peritoneal sac.

In a term infant, the ovary is an elongated structure shaped like a round-edged prism and located in the posterior segment of the false pelvis, directly adjacent to the posterior uterine surface. Its size is approximately $25 \times 15 \times 5$ mm.[10] By menarche, the ovary has moved into the true pelvic space and has assumed its almond-shaped adult contour and location.

The normal dimensions for the adult ovary are length, 2.5 to 5.0 cm; width, 1.5 to 3.0 cm; and anteroposterior thickness, 0.6 to 2.2 cm.[10] Individual variation for a single linear dimension of the ovary is greater than either the average of the three linear dimensions or the volume. In other words, short ovaries tend to be thicker, and thin ovaries tend to be longer. For this reason, a single linear dimension of the ovary should not be used to assess normalcy of size. Instead, a volume calculation should be used (length $\times$ width $\times$ height $/2$ = volume in cm^3). With this approach, the upper normal value for the prepubertal ovary is 1 cm^3. During the reproductive years, ovarian volume should not exceed 6 cm^3.[11]

The anterior margin of the ovary is relatively thin and is attached to the posterior surface of the broad ligament by the mesovarium (Fig. 3-48). The posterior or free edge of the ovary is thicker and bows outward, giving the ovary its characteristic asymmetric almond shape.

The ovary is suspended in the pelvic space by

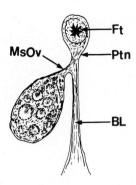

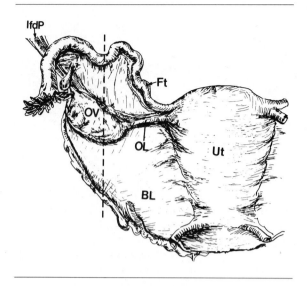

FIGURE 3-48. The peritoneum which forms the broad ligament covers the fallopian tube and forms a short suspensory ligament, the mesovarium, which supports and anchors the ovary to the posterior surface of the broad ligament. The plane of this figure is shown on Figure 3-49 as a dotted line. (Ft, fallopian tube; Ptn, peritoneum; MsOv, mesovarium; BL, broad ligament.)

FIGURE 3-49. The ovary and its suspensory structures. This view of the posterior surface of the broad ligament shows the relationship of the ovary to the broad ligament, fallopian tube, infundibulopelvic ligament, and ovarian ligament. The fallopian tube has been lifted up to expose the ovary and its ligaments. (Ft, fallopian tube; OL, ovarian ligament; lfdP, infundibulopelvic ligament; OV, ovary; Ut, uterus; BL, broad ligament.)

three anchoring structures (Fig. 3-49). The *ovarian ligament* is a flattened fibromuscular band extending from the uterine cornu, where the fallopian tube exits the uterine wall, to the inferior (medial or uterine) pole of the ovary. The *infundibulopelvic ligament* consists of fibromuscular strands intertwined with the ovarian vessels and lymphatics as they pass from the brim of the pelvis to the lateral pole of the ovary. These vessels and their supporting fibers form a ridge in the overlying peritoneum, which is thicker in this region and contributes to the suspensory effect. The infundibulopelvic ligament suspends the superior (lateral or pelvic brim) pole of the ovary from the posterolateral pelvic wall at the brim of the true pelvic space. The *mesovarium* is a short double layer of peritoneum extending from the posterior surface of the broad ligament. The mesovarium provides only a minimal suspensory effect in comparison with the fibromuscular ovarian ligament, but it does provide the primary route of access for vessels traveling into and out of the ovarian hilus.

The outer layer of the ovary is composed of so-called *germinal epithelium*, which is neither germinal nor a true epithelium. (The early anatomists made some incorrect assumptions.) It is actually a modified form of the peritoneum but sufficiently differ-

ent to result in the ovary's being considered "nude," that is, not covered by the coelomic peritoneum.[12] Immediately beneath the germinal epithelium is a thin layer of fibrous tissue, which forms the *tunica albuginea (white coat),* or capsule, of the ovary.

The bulk of the ovarian substance consists of a thick layer of ovarian parenchyma (the cortex) containing a large number of primordial follicles (Fig. 3-50). In the center of the ovary is the medulla, which contains blood vessels and connective tissue but no follicles.[12] Along the margins of the ovarian hilus, the ovarian germinal epithelium is continuous with the peritoneum that forms the broad ligament. Occasionally the hilus also contains vestigial remnants of the primitive mesonephros, which persist in the adult ovary as a cluster of tubules known as the epoöphoron.[12] These are of some interest to the sonographer because they occasionally give rise to benign simple cysts (parovar-

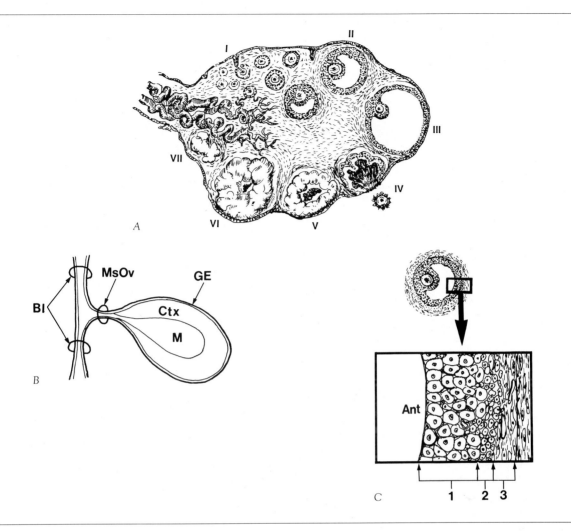

FIGURE 3-50. (A) Diagrammatic representation of the ovary in cross section. The stages of development of a follicle are shown clockwise from upper left: I, primitive oocytes and early developmental stages of the follicle; II, graafian follicle; III, mature follicle; IV, rupture of the follicle (ovulation); V, early stages of corpus luteum formation; VI, mature corpus luteum; VII, corpus albicans. (B) Ovarian suspension and regions. (Bl, broad ligament; MsOv, mesovarium; GE, germinal epithelium; Ctx, cortex of ovary; M, medulla of ovary.) (C) Cellular construction of a developing follicle: 1, granulosa; 2, theca interna; 3, theca externa; Ant, antrum.

ian cysts), which, when very large, can be mistaken for the urinary bladder.

Each ovary of a newborn infant contains about a million or more primordial follicles, but this number is substantially reduced through spontaneous follicular regression as the infant matures. Only 300 to 400 of the many thousands of follicles that persist into adult life will actually progress through development and ovulation over the 30 or more reproductive years.[10] It is interesting to contemplate that ovulation occurring when a woman is 40 years old will release an egg that is approximately 40 years and 8 months old, containing DNA-encoded patterns that extend back through time to the primordial organism with which life began on this planet.

Follicular Development

The stages of follicular development (Fig. 3-50) have been of particular interest to sonographers since the advent of fertility therapy using ultrasound monitoring of follicular growth. These stages are controlled by a complex cycle of chemical interchanges between the brain, the anterior hypophysis of the pituitary gland, and the ovary. (For more information on pituitary-gonadal axis relationships, see Fig. 12-1.) The early developing follicle is a solid mass consisting of granulosa cells surrounding the central ovum. External to the granulosa layer are two thinner layers of theca cells, the theca interna, which is richly vascularized, and the theca externa, which is primarily connective tissue. With further development, a fluid-filled crescentic cavity forms eccentrically within the granulosa layer. As this cavity (the antrum) enlarges, the ovum contained within a surrounding mound of granulosa cells projects into the cavity, forming a structure known as the cumulus oöphorus (also called discus proligerus).[10] As the follicle continues to develop, it enlarges and becomes a follicular cyst, eventually impinging on the tunica albuginea of the ovarian surface. Typically, a mature follicle reaches 20 mm in size before rupturing.

The ripening follicle is referred to as a graafian follicle. Each month during the reproductive years, five to seven or more of these follicles in each ovary are triggered into rapid growth by follicle-stimulating hormone (FSH) produced by the pituitary gland (Fig. 3-51A). In a normal ovulatory cycle, only one of these follicles becomes dominant and ruptures through the tunica albuginea, releasing its contained egg; this is known as ovulation (Fig. 3-51B). The other follicles undergo atresia,[10] rapidly shrinking to eventually become an amorphous mass of hyalin scar tissue known as the corpus albicans. Artificial stimulation of follicular development (i.e., fertility therapy) can result in simultaneous development of multiple follicles (Fig. 3-51C).

At ovulation, the combination of the discharged liquor folliculi and hemorrhage associated with follicular rupture results in accumulation of 5 to 10 ml of fluid in the posterior cul-de-sac, where it can be observed as a crescentic anechoic collection behind the cervix (Fig. 3-51D).[1] The process of ovulation may be associated with midcycle pain (mittelschmerz). The ruptured follicle cavity within the ovary becomes the corpus luteum (yellow or golden body). In this process, there is hemorrhage into the theca interna, extending to fill the vacant cavity of the follicle. The stigma (the opening through which the egg was discharged) is sealed by a blood clot, thus reestablishing a closed cystic structure filled with clotted blood. In the normal development of the corpus luteum, the blood clot is gradually resorbed as the theca interna layer undergoes rapid proliferation and luteinization through deposit within the cells of golden or reddish brown pigment and fat.[10] The resolving clot often forms bizarre stands of fibrin in the center of the corpus luteum.[19]

If the discharged egg is fertilized, the corpus luteum is maintained and enlarges to become the corpus luteum cyst of pregnancy. This cystic structure can become quite large (5 to 6 cm is not unusual) and persists through the early stages of pregnancy. If fertilization does not occur, the corpus luteum undergoes regression, involuting to become the corpus albicans. The surface of the ovary where rupture of the follicle occurred becomes puckered inward as a scar forms, giving the aging ovary a quilted or cobbled surface. At menopause, the remaining follicles undergo atresia over the subsequent 4 or 5 years, although occasionally a postmenopausal follicle may undergo development, ovulation, and corpus luteum formation.[10] This, however, is rare, and any persistent cyst in the postmenopausal ovary must be regarded with suspicion. After menopause the ovary shrinks steadily until it is less than one third of its mature size.[10] Occasionally, dilated veins can mimic follicles in postmenopausal women, and the sonographer may misinterpret the persistent fluid-filled structure as a persistent follicle. Doppler ultrasound can easily distinguish a true cyst from a dilated vessel.

Ultrasound measurements of the follicle are most often performed using an average of the follicular diameter in three planes, but when precise measurements are required, the follicle can be measured in the same manner as the ovary. A volume can be calculated using (length × width × height)

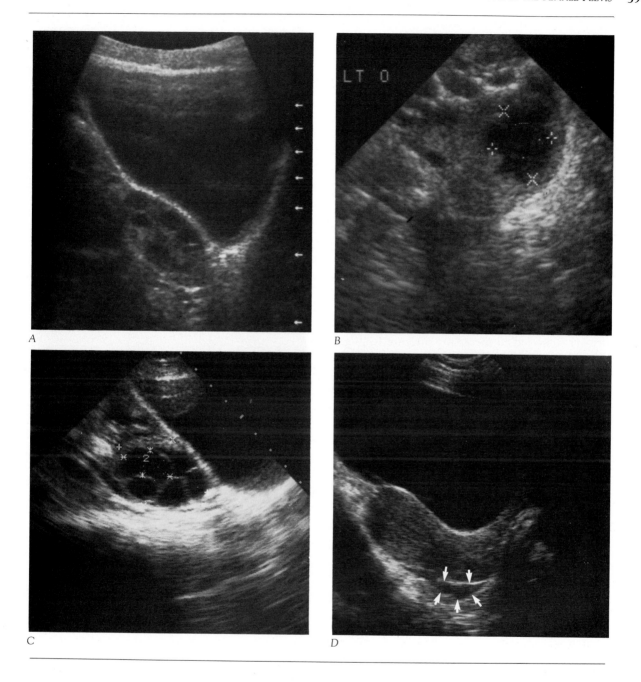

FIGURE 3-51. (A) Transvesical sagittal scan of a normal adult ovary on day 7 of the menstrual cycle. Several small follicles are seen within the ovarian substance. (B) Transvaginal sagittal scan of a dominant follicle immediately after its rupture at ovulation. Note the partially collapsed walls resulting from loss of most of the liquor folliculi. (C) Transvesical scan of an ovary that has been artificially stimulated during fertility therapy. Five follicles are seen in this scan plane. (D) Transvesical sagittal scan of the uterus immediately after ovulation, showing a small amount of echogenic fluid in the posterior cul-de-sac (arrows). This fluid most likely represents blood and serous fluid from the follicle.

/ 2 = volume in cm³. If only two diameters are available the formula is (diameter A × diameter B × diameter B) / 2.

Location and Acoustic Patterns of the Ovary

When the bladder is empty, the ovary rests in the ovarian fossa, a shallow depression on the posterolateral pelvic wall just beneath the brim of the pelvis and formed by the external iliac vessels and the ureter. In this position, with the uterine fundus in its normal position resting on the dome of the urinary bladder, the ovary is substantially superior and posterior to the fundus of the uterus. As the bladder fills, the uterus is physiologically retroverted and pushed upward toward the sacral prominence. As filling progresses, the ovaries tend to remain stationary in their ovarian fossae and come to lie at the sides of the uterine fundus. (The uterus moves upward while the ovaries stay in place, Fig. 3-52.) With further filling of the bladder, the ovaries are subjected to increasing pressure from the bladder and are usually forced downward in the adnexal space. Frequently one of them slips farther down into the posterior cul-de-sac. With excessive filling of the bladder, the ovaries are often forced out of the lower regions of the posterior pelvic compartment and come to rest above (cephalad to) the fundus of the uterus in what is often called the axial position.

The ovary may be found in any of three regions of the posterior pelvic compartment: the posterior cul-de-sac, the adnexal space to the side of the uterus, or above (cephalad to) or behind the fundus of the uterus. The normal ovary is not found anterior to the broad ligament (in front of the uterus, between the uterus and the urinary bladder, or in the anterior cul-de-sac) because of its attachment via the mesovarium to the posterior surface of the broad ligament (see Fig. 3-49).

Movements of the ovaries are governed by the complex relationship of the configuration of the true pelvic space, the degree of filling of the rectum, ovarian and uterine size, and the degree of filling of the urinary bladder. When meticulous scanning with gain variations does not reveal the ovary, the sonographer should consider having the patient void partially, especially if the bladder is too distended. This usually causes the ovaries to as-

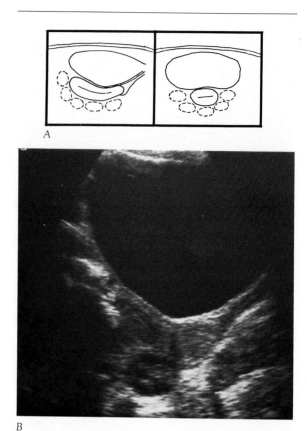

FIGURE 3-52. (A) Positions of the ovary. Because of its attachment to the posterior surface of the broad ligament, the ovary may be found in the posterior pelvic compartment or above the fundus of the uterus, in the adnexal spaces or in the posterior cul-de-sac, but not in the anterior cul-de-sac or between the urinary bladder and the uterus. (B) Parasagittal scan slightly to the right of midline shows a normal ovary located in the posterior cul-de-sac. Part of the fundus of the uterus is not visualized in this plane of scan. Note the excellent acoustic penetration deep to the ovary.

sume a new position, most commonly adjacent to the uterine fundus, where they may be visualized more easily.

Transvaginal ultrasound imaging is the method of choice when the primary interest is detailed visualization of the ovaries; however, the advantages of transvaginal imaging must be balanced against the limitations of less depth of penetration and a

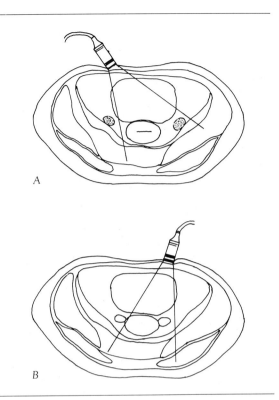

FIGURE 3-53. (A) The ovary can be differentiated from the obturator internus muscle by scanning in a transverse plane and angling the beam in from the side of the pelvis opposite the ovary to be demonstrated. This steep angle brings the ultrasound beam more perpendicular to the surface of the obturator internus muscle and usually demonstrates the thin layer of fat overlying the muscle, thus separating the dark echo pattern of the ovary from the similar dark pattern of the muscle. (B) A more difficult task is to separate the ovary from the myometrium when the two are in apposition. Scanning in a transverse plane with the transducer positioned on the same side of the pelvis as the ovary of interest and angled slightly back toward the midline often permits demonstration of a thin line between the ovary and the uterus, which confirms that the structure is an ovary and not a small subserosal fibroid. Careful attention to matching ovarian position with the focal zone of the ultrasound beam also helps. Placing the patient in a decubitus position may make it easier to obtain certain steeply angled scan planes.

limited range of transducer positions. For the initial evaluation of the pelvic organs, especially when a pelvic mass is suspected, transabdominal imaging is the method of choice. This examination may then be supplemented by transvaginal imaging to obtain more detailed images of specific structures. Transvaginal imaging alone can be used for follow-up examinations and in cases in which only the ovaries are to be evaluated (e.g., in fertility therapy) and for the few cases in which the patient is unable to maintain a distended urinary bladder.

The adult ovary normal echo pattern consists of a background of low-amplitude echoes (compared with the uterine myometrium) through which is scattered a coarse pattern of punctate bright reflectors and the distinctive anechoic spaces of the developing follicles. The bright reflections are most likely caused by corpora albicantia in the ovarian cortex and small vessels in the ovarian medulla. On both transvesical and transvaginal ultrasound, the ovary can be identified by its characteristic "Swiss cheese" pattern of anechoic follicles against the low-amplitude gray of the ovarian cortex.

Infants' ovaries may be difficult or impossible to locate, and in postmenopausal women the ovaries become increasingly difficult to detect as they becomes isoechoic with the surrounding parametrial tissues. With transabdominal scanning of patients in the reproductive years of life the ovary may be difficult to separate from the adjacent myometrium or obturator internus muscle (Fig. 3-53). Since the echo patterns of the uterus and the ovary are subtly different, placing the focal zone at a level where both structures are intersected permits optimal differentiation. Many instruments today permit selective positioning of the focal zone, greatly facilitating demonstration of the ovary as separate from the adjacent uterus.

In especially difficult cases, an acoustic property of the ovary may provide the only clue to its location. The ovary exhibits nearly as much acoustic transmission as a serous cyst of the same size. To locate a difficult ovary, the examiner should reduce gain levels so that most of the echoes from the uterus and the parametrium disappear. The ovary will be revealed by the burst of acoustic enhancement (increased through-transmission) seen beneath it as a column of brighter echoes (Fig. 3-54).

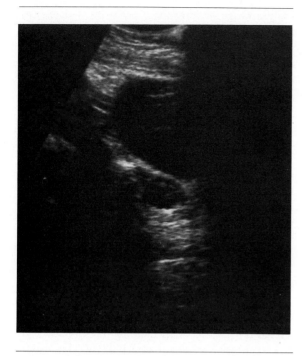

FIGURE 3-54. Sagittal scan of the right ovary at very low gain setting. Note the burst of bright echoes that "mark" the position of the overlying ovary.

The Pelvic Bowel

The bowel is a much neglected component of the pelvic viscera. Most sonographers fail to recognize the bowel when it is evident in the image, and so fail to fully appreciate its influence on other organs in the pelvis. To a large extent, the position of the uterus and ovaries is influenced by the degree of filling of the rectum, and bowel may be easily mistaken for a pelvic mass, especially when peristalsis is not readily evident in the real-time image. The *descending colon* becomes the *sigmoid colon* and enters the pelvic space through the left iliac fossa. The sigmoid typically forms one or more S curves, which loop back and forth along the curve of the sacrum (Fig. 3-55).

Whereas the descending colon is partially buried in the retroperitoneal fat of the colic gutter, the sigmoid emerges to become completely covered by peritoneum, which forms a short suspensory membrane known as the *mesocolon*. It is the flexibility of this mesocolon that permits the sigmoid colon to

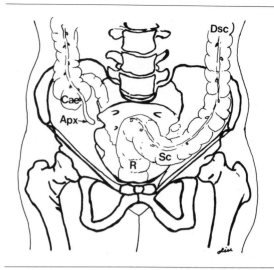

FIGURE 3-55. Schematic diagram of the large bowel and its relationship to the false pelvis. The false pelvis is usually filled with loops of small bowel. The cecum and appendix are found on the right side of the false pelvis, and the pelvic portion of the descending colon and the proximal (upper) part of the sigmoid colon are found on the left. The location of the appendix is highly variable, and it may be found virtually anywhere in the right false pelvis, or even in the true pelvis. (Cae, caecum; Apx, appendix; Dsc, descending colon; Sc, sigmoid colon; R, rectum.)

move about over a relatively wide area of the posterior pelvic compartment. When the urinary bladder is empty, the sigmoid (along with loops of small bowel) occupies the posterior cul-de-sac. This location of the sigmoid can create some difficulty during transvaginal sonography. If the transducer is placed in the posterior fornix, curves of the sigmoid colon may lie between the transducer and the ovaries. In such cases, transfer of the probe to the lateral fornix may permit better visualization. This is not a problem in transvesical scanning because the distended urinary bladder forces the sigmoid and loops of small bowel upward so that they move above and behind the fundus of the uterus.

When filled with fecal material, the sigmoid colon usually can be followed from its entry at the left posterolateral brim of the pelvis, down into the cul-de-sac. At about the midpoint of the sacral

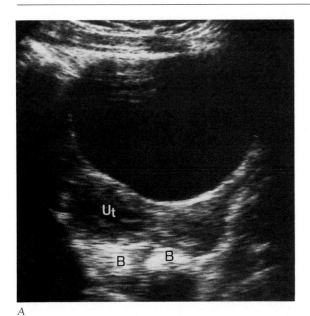

A

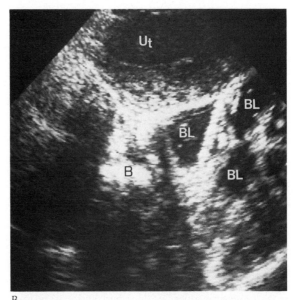

B

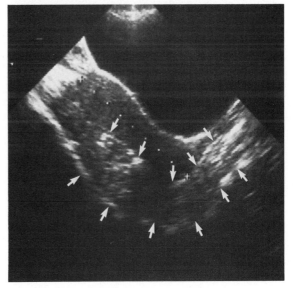

C

FIGURE 3-56. (A) Parasagittal scan of the pelvis demonstrating boluses of fecal material (B) with typical "dirty" shadows (*arrows*). (Ut, uterus.) (B) Transvaginal scan of the uterus. Fluid-filled loops of bowel (BL) are seen posterior to the uterus. (C) Sagittal view of the pelvis. The space between the posterior uterine wall and the curve of the sacrum is occupied by the rectum (*arrows*). In this person the fecal material contains little gas, permitting good visualization of the curve of the sacrum, as indicated by the abrupt cut-off of the ultrasound image.

curve, the sigmoid moves posterior to the peritoneum and, like the descending colon, becomes partially buried, so that only its anterior surface and part of its lateral surfaces are covered by peritoneum. From this point to its terminus at the anus, the large bowel is the *rectum*, which is characterized by thicker and more muscular walls.

In the ultrasound image, the rectum is commonly recognized by deduction. That is, the rectum walls usually are not visible, but the content of the rectum is easily demonstrated. Boluses of fecal material in the rectum cause irregular ("dirty") shadows and produce a pattern of very dense, bright echoes typical of material containing many small bubbles of gas (Fig. 3-56A). Fluid in the rectum or fecal material containing little gas

TABLE 3-3. Echo pattern of bowel

	ECHO PATTERN	SHADOWS
Small bowel	Variably echogenic content with thin, anechoic ring representing the muscular wall	Shifts with movement of bowel and content
Caecum	Variably echogenic content with thin, anechoic ring representing the muscular wall	Constant except when peristalsis occurs
Sigmoid	Echogenic content with thin, anechoic ring representing the muscular wall	Constant except when peristalsis occurs
Rectum	Echogenic content with thin, anechoic ring representing the muscular wall	Constant and nearly complete; only top surface of fecal boluses can be seen

permits visualization of the anterior surface of the sacrum lying deep to the rectum (Fig. 3-56C). On real-time observation, the upper parts of the pelvic bowel and any intruding loops of small bowel are actively peristaltic and can be easily differentiated as bowel, particularly if filled with fluid (Fig. 3-56B). In contrast, rectal peristalsis is infrequent and the rectum must be identified by location and echo pattern rather than by its motion.

The *caecum* and *appendix* can usually be identified in the right iliac fossa. The appendix is one of the most variable structures in the human body, and although technically it is an abdominal structure, it may be found in the pelvis.[2]

Bowel is relatively easy to differentiate from other pelvic organs and from muscle in most cases. If there appears to be a mass in the posterior cul-de-sac but it is not possible to determine whether it is bowel, a water enema may be administered while the suspect area is simultaneously observed with real-time ultrasound imaging. Movement of water through the rectum and sigmoid should permit positive identification of these structures. Table 3-3 lists some of the salient features of the echo pattern and shadowing for each of the pelvic bowel segments.

The Pelvic Vascular System

Until recently, information about the pelvic vascular system had little direct value for sonographers. Occasionally, they encountered dilated pelvic veins mimicking a complex mass, but these were rare. Today, Doppler examination of the pelvic vessels is becoming an increasingly important tool in obstetric ultrasound, and it shows promise of having applications in gynecologic sonography as well.

The pelvic vascular system consists of three distinct components: the arteries, the veins, and the lymphatics. The lymphatic channels usually have no significance in pelvic sonography.

The spatial relationship of the great vessels (aorta and vena cava) changes as they descend through the abdomen. In the upper abdomen, the vena cava is more anterior than the aorta. Just above the level of the umbilicus, these two vessels come to lie side by side, and then at their bifurcation the veins come to lie posterior to the arteries.[16] From the bifurcation through the pelvic region, the arteries are more anterior than the veins. A simple way to remember this is with the phrase "*arteries before veins.*"

ARTERIAL SYSTEM OF THE PELVIS

The *aorta* usually bifurcates at a point slightly higher than the inferior vena cava, giving rise to the *common iliac arteries,* which are quite short, extending only for a few centimeters until they branch into the large *external iliac artery* and the smaller *internal iliac (hypogastric) artery* (Fig. 3-57). The external iliac artery runs along the medial border of the iliopsoas muscle at the brim of the true pelvic space. When it reaches the lower margin of the pelvis, the external iliac artery passes beneath the inguinal ligament to enter the thigh.

The hypogastric or internal iliac artery is smaller than the external iliac artery, and it courses from the bifurcation at the upper and posterior margin of the true pelvic space down into the pelvic cavity along the lateral wall for a distance of only 1 or 2 cm. It then gives rise to the relatively large and posteriorly directed *superior gluteal artery.* The hypogastric artery continues downward along the pelvic wall, giving rise to four small branches that course

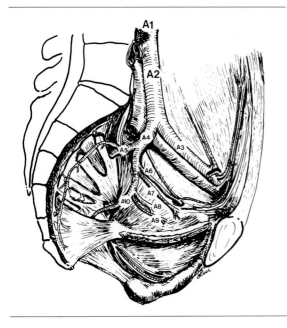

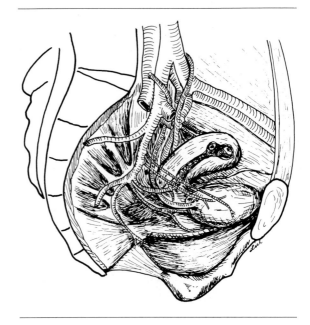

FIGURE 3-57. The pelvic vascular system. Although only the arteries are shown in detail, the veins follow the same pattern but lie posterior to the arteries. The one exception to the pattern of naming the vessels is the hypogastric artery, whose companion vein is named the internal iliac vein rather than the hypogastric. Note the triangular space defined by the vessels at the bifurcation of the common iliac vessels. This open-based triangle is the ovarian fossa (Waldeyer's fossa). (A1, aorta; A2, common iliac artery; A3, external iliac artery; A4, hypogastric artery; A5, superior gluteal artery; A6, obturator artery; A7, umbilical artery; A8, uterine artery; A9, superior vesical artery; A10, internal pudendal and inferior gluteal arteries.)

FIGURE 3-58. Arterial supply to the uterus. The broad ligament has been removed to expose the uterine artery as it courses upward from the level of the cervix to the cornu of the uterus, where it makes a sharp turn to run along the underside of the fallopian tube. The uterine artery forms an anastomosis with the ovarian artery beneath the fallopian tube. Thus, although the uterine artery is the principal supplier of blood to the uterus, it is not the sole supplier. Anastomotic connections are not limited to the uterine-ovarian arteries. They are found throughout the pelvis, providing an elaborate fail-safe network of alternate channels to each of the organs.

anterior along the pelvic wall: the *obturator artery,* the *umbilical artery,* the *uterine-vaginal artery,* and the *superior vesical artery.* Finally, the hypogastric terminates in two posteriorly directed branches: the *internal pudendal* and the *inferior gluteal arteries.* Except for these last two posteriorly directed branches, the branches of the hypogastric artery and their many subdivisions fan out along the lateral wall of the pelvis, descending to the pelvic floor to pass over the pelvic diaphragm to reach their target organs or muscles.[16] The hypogastric artery is the primary blood supply for the uterus, vagina, urinary bladder, and most of the muscles of the pelvic floor. It should be kept in mind that branching patterns of blood vessels are highly variable.

Most of the smaller branches of the hypogastric artery are not individually identifiable in the ultrasound image, but one branch, the uterine artery, is important to sonographers. The uterine artery extends across the pelvic floor to reach the uterus at approximately the level of the tip of the cervix (Fig. 3-58). At this point, it bifurcates into a uterine branch and a descending vaginal branch. Its uterine component turns upward to run along the lateral margin of the uterus to the fallopian tube, where it again makes a sharp turn to run along the length of the fallopian tube. Just past the cervical

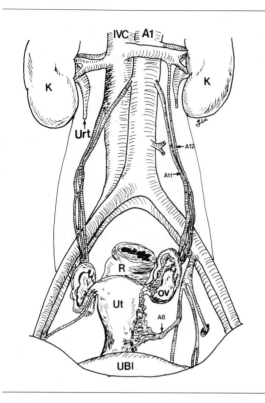

FIGURE 3-59. The blood supply of the ovaries (OV). The uterine artery (A8) and the ovarian artery (A11) form anastomoses in the region of the ovarian hilus. Note the difference in the pattern of ovarian artery origin versus ovarian vein (A12) termination. Since lymphatics follow the gonadal (ovarian) vessels, tumor spread from the pelvis to the paraaortic nodes at the level of the renal pelvis is common. (Urt, ureter; K, kidney; Ut, uterus; UBl, urinary bladder; IVC, inferior vena cava; R, rectum.)

"right angle" turn, the uterine artery is relatively straight as it ascends alongside the cervix. It is at this point that the artery is most accessible for Doppler evaluation with transvaginal probe. As it courses upward along the lateral border of the uterus, the uterine artery becomes very tortuous.

On the basis of the description thus far, one might reasonably conclude that the uterine artery is the exclusive supplier of arterial blood to the uterus; however, the organs of reproduction, like the brain, are provided with an elaborate fail-safe blood supply. In addition to terminating in capillaries embedded in the target organ, the internal pudendal artery, vaginal artery, and uterine artery all have anastomotic branches that form a complex network of interconnected channels around the vagina and most of the uterus. This anastomotic network ensures that compromised flow through any one of these arteries will not result in tissue damage in the target organ. Other feeder vessels of the network will provide an immediate compensatory flow, thus preserving tissue function. An even more elaborate system exists to supply the ovary.

The embryonic ovaries originate in the abdominal region from a common mesenchymal tissue, which also gives rise to the adrenal glands. This explains why tumors in the region of the adrenal may produce sex hormones and why tumors that have adrenal characteristics may be found in the pelvis. In the later stages of embryonic life, the ovaries descend into the pelvis, guided by a ligamentous band called the *gubernaculum*. As the embryonic ovaries descend, they bring with them their original blood supply derived from the aorta and draining into the vena cava. These vessels persist in adult life as the *ovarian artery* and *vein*. In women, the ovarian arteries originate as lateral branches of the aorta at about the level of the lower margin of the renal pelvis (Fig. 3-59). These arteries course downward over the psoas muscles and along the same path followed by the ureters, crossing over the common iliac artery just superior to its bifurcation into the external and internal iliac arteries. The ovarian artery then bridges across from the upper margin of the pelvis to the ovary through the infundibulopelvic ligament. From the infundibulopelvic ligament it passes through the mesovarium to reach the ovarian hilus, where it supplies the ovarian parenchyma. In addition, the ovarian artery forms anastomoses with the ovarian branches of the uterine artery, thus providing a closed loop or fail-safe blood supply originating from two widely divergent points in the arterial system.

VENOUS SYSTEM OF THE PELVIS
The venous system of the pelvis follows a pattern virtually identical to that of the arterial system. The *inferior vena cava* bifurcates slightly below the level of the aortic bifurcation, giving rise to the *common iliac veins,* which run beneath the *common iliac arteries.* These short vessels in turn give rise to

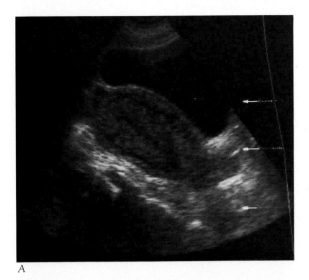

A

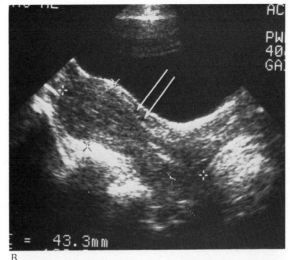

B

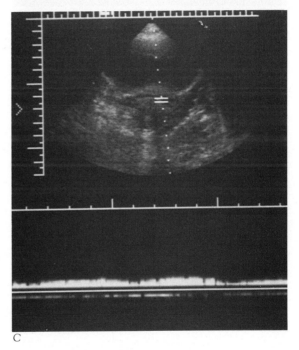

C

FIGURE 3-60. (A) Dilated venous channels in the superficial regions of the myometrium cause this uterus to appear to have separate layers within the myometrium. Such a pronounced degree of dilatation is unusual. (Note: the small arrows along the right margin of the image indicate focal zones, not structures.) (B) More typical vascular channels (*arrows*) in the uterine myometrium. These appear as small, often irregular or serpiginous anechoic spaces within the myometrium. They are most commonly seen within the superficial layers. (C) Doppler can be used to determine whether flow is present in the suspected vascular channel. Since the dilated vessels are veins, the Doppler signal will typically be low in amplitude and the flow nearly constant.

the large external *iliac veins*, which drain the legs, and the smaller *internal iliac veins*, which drain the pelvic organs and muscles. The ovarian veins follow the same course as the ovarian arteries until they reach the midabdomen, where the *right ovarian vein* drains directly into the vena cava and the *left ovarian vein* drains into the left renal vein.

Because the veins are thin walled, they are highly distensible and vary in size with certain conditions, most notably pregnancy. After parturition, the venous channels usually shrink, but rarely to the prepregnant state, and they may remain prominent and easily visible. If venous congestion occurs, the veins may form pelvic varices, which are readily

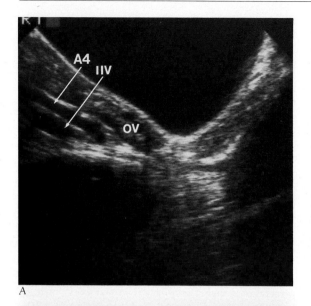

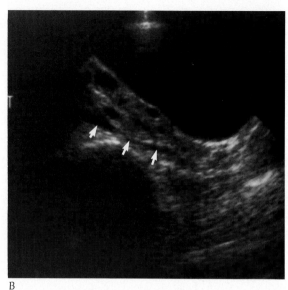

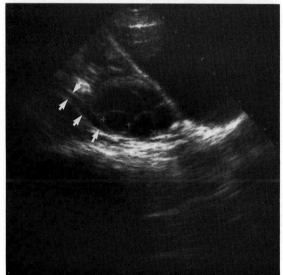

FIGURE 3-61. Sagittal scans of the ovary (OV) and surrounding vessels. (*A*) The most lateral scan plane will demonstrate the hypogastric artery (A4), internal iliac vein (Ilv), and a small part of the lateral aspect of the ovary. (*B*) A more medial scan plane will demonstrate mostly ovarian tissue, with the ureter (*arrows*) running beneath the ovary. (*C*) The ureter (*arrows*) is more clearly seen superior to and deep to a hormonally stimulated ovary.

identifiable in the ultrasound image. In some women, particularly after parturition, the venous channels in the outer regions of the myometrium may appear to separate the muscle layer into two regions (Fig. 3-60).

The Ureter

The *ureter* is commonly observed as it courses along the lateral pelvic wall posterior to the ovary. These musculomembranous tubes move urine via peristalsis, and enter the pelvis at a point just caudad to the bifurcation of the common iliac vessels. This results in the ureter being the most anterior and lateral of the three tubular structures seen deep to the ovary in its most common position lateral to the uterus (Fig. 3-61). As the ureter descends into the pelvic space, it moves mediad, to reach the trigone of the urinary bladder, therefore oblique scan planes are usually required to demonstrate long segments of the ureter in the pelvis. Ureteral contractions are readily observed with real-time ultrasound, and the ureter can be identified most clearly with vaginal scanning.

References

1. Athey PA. Sonographic appearance of the normal female pelvis. In: Athey PA, Hadlock FP. Ultrasound in Obstetrics and Gynecology. St. Louis: CV Mosby; 1981.
2. Blount RF. The digestive system. In: Schaeffer JP, ed. Morris' Human Anatomy. 11th ed. New York: McGraw-Hill; 1953.
3. Fleischer AC, Kalemeris GC, Entman SS. Sonographic depiction of the endometrium during normal cycles. Ultrasound Med. Biol. 1986; 12:271–277.
4. Fleischer AC, Kalemeris GC, Machin JE, et al. Sonographic depiction of normal and abnormal endometrium with histopathologic correlation. J Ultrasound Med. 1986; 5:445–452.
5. Grant JCB, Smith CG. The musculature. In: Schaeffer JP, ed. Morris' Human Anatomy. 11th ed. New York: McGraw-Hill; 1953.
6. Gray H. Osteology. In: Goss CM, ed. Gray's Anatomy. 28th ed. Philadelphia: Lea & Febiger; 1966.
7. Gray H. The urogenital system. In: Goss CM, ed. Gray's Anatomy, 28th ed. Philadelphia: Lea & Febiger; 1966.
8. Green JH, Silver PHS. An Introduction to Human Anatomy. New York: Oxford University Press; 1981.
9. Hackeloer B. The role of ultrasound in female infertility management. Ultrasound Med Biol. 1984; 10:44.
10. Kistner RW. Gynecology, Principles and Practice. 3rd ed. Chicago: Year Book Medical Publishers; 1980.
11. Kurtz AB, Rifkin MD. Normal anatomy of the female pelvis. In: Sanders RC, James AE, eds. The Principles and Practice of Ultrasonography in Obstetrics and Gynecology. 3rd ed. New York: Appleton-Century-Crofts; 1985.
12. Markee JE. The urogenital system. In: Schaeffer JP, ed. Morris' Human Anatomy. 11th ed. New York: McGraw-Hill; 1953.
13. Muckle CW. Clinical anatomy of the uterus, fallopian tubes, and ovaries. In: Droegemueller W, Sciarra J, eds. Gynecology and Obstetrics. Philadelphia: JB Lippincott; 1988; 1.
14. Netter FH, Oppenheimer E, eds. The CIBA Collection of Medical Illustrations. Reproductive System. West Caldwell, NJ: Ciba Pharmaceutical Company; 1965.
15. Oike K, Obata S, Takagi K, et al. Observation of endometrial movement with transvaginal ultrasonography. (Abst #1524). J Ultrasound Med. 1988; 7:S99.
16. Patten BM. The cardiovascular system. In: Schaeffer JP, ed. Morris' Human Anatomy. 11th ed. New York: McGraw-Hill; 1953.
17. Sample WF. Gray scale ultrasonography of the normal female pelvis. In: Sanders RC, James AE, eds. The Principles and Practice of Ultrasonography in Obstetrics and Gynecology. 2nd ed. New York: Appleton-Century-Crofts; 1980.
18. Sample WF, Lippe BM, Gyepes MT. Gray-scale ultrasonography of the normal female pelvis. Radiology 1977; 125:477–483.
19. Timor-Tritsch IE, Rottem S, Elgali S. How transvaginal sonography is done. In: Timor-Tritsch IE, Rottem S, eds. Transvaginal Sonography. New York: Elsevier; 1988.

CHAPTER 4

Congenital Anomalies of the Female Genital System

MIMI C. BERMAN, JOYCE A. MILLER

Congenital anomalies of the female reproductive tract are an uncommon occurrence. The reported incidence is between 0.1 and 0.5%.[1,2,23] Because these anomalies are rare and usually present with no clinical symptoms,[13] sonographers seldom image them. Congenital malformations can, however, mimic other pelvic pathology, such as myoma, adnexal mass, ectopic pregnancy, and twin gestation, so it is important for practitioners to be familiar with the appearance of the different anomalies. Usually patients are sent for a sonogram at puberty or during a pregnancy when suspicion arises that there may be some irregularity in the configuration of the uterus. Also, because uterine anomalies occur in at least 50%[14,19] of patients with developmental urinary tract disorders, such as renal agenesis and ectopic kidney, sonographers should make it a practice to examine both systems whenever an anomaly exists in either one.

In nonpregnant patients, congenital anomalies are suspected when at puberty a mass is palpated in the pelvis or the patient experiences dysmenorrhea, dyspareunia, or pelvic pain. These symptoms are often caused by obstruction at some level of the uterus, cervix, or vagina, resulting in an accumulation of mucus or menstrual blood. Obstruction can be caused by an intact hymen or by congenital absence of the vagina. Ultrasound can contribute essential information when no vagina is found on physical exam and when a mass is palpated.

Nonpregnant postpubertal patients may present with clinical symptoms other than those usually ex-perienced by pubertal girls. These include infertility, habitual abortion, unsuccessful dilation and curettage (because only one uterus was treated), cervical incompetence, and failure of an intrauterine device (IUD). Although uterine anomalies that allow passage of the ovum and sperm and implantation do not affect fertility, they are associated with increased rates of abortion and premature delivery, possibly owing to the weakness of the cervical muscles and the decreased vascularity in some implantation sites, such as the septum.[1,11,12] In septate or bicornuate uteri, the conceptus may implant on the septum, often resulting in an early abortion,[11,25] An 8- to 12% incidence of congenital anomalies has been reported in women who experience habitual abortion and infertility.[23]

Once the patient becomes pregnant, it is important to be aware of any unsual configurations that could interfere with a normal pregnancy. Higher incidences of premature deliveries, abnormal fetal presentations, premature labor, prolonged labor, low birth weight, and fetal malformations have been reported.[12,16,23] A sonogram is the first imaging modality to use to examine pregnant patients for anomalies.

Anatomy of Congenital Anomalies

The vagina and uterus are formed by the müllerian ducts fusing together in the midline to form a single duct, the *uterovaginal canal.* At first, there is a midline septum in this canal that normally disappears by the end of the third month of prenatal development (see Fig. 2-5). Most types of malformations in this region may be attributed to total or partial atresia of the müllerian ducts, failure of the müllerian ducts to fuse properly, or failure of the uterovaginal septum to be resorbed.

VAGINA

The vagina, which is the connection between the interior and exterior portions of the genitalia, is a frequent site of maldevelopment of the müllerian system. The lumen of the vagina remains separated from the urogenital sinus by a thin tissue plate, the *hymen*. This tissue usually ruptures during prenatal life; however, if it doesn't, an *imperforate hymen* results (see Fig. 2-7). This diagnosis is usually made at menarche, when a physician observes a tense, bulging membrane, which may represent hematocolpos (retention of menstrual blood in the vagina), hematometra (retention of menstrual blood in the uterus), or hematometrocolpos.[10] Sonography can be very helpful in establishing this diagnosis.

Vaginal Agenesis or Atresia. Vaginal agenesis or atresia may occur if the sinovaginal bulbs do not develop or develop improperly. Transverse septa, or partitions, can also form during embryonic development of the vagina; when they do, they are usually located on the upper third of the vagina. These septa, like an imperforate hymen, may close off the vagina to the exterior and result in similar clinical and sonographic findings.[10]

UTERUS

Fusion Failure. Vaginal abnormalities are often associated with concomitant cervical and uterine anomalies, as virtually all are caused by failure of some stage of development in the müllerian duct system. Partial or total failure of fusion of the müllerian ducts may cause any degree of duplication of the system from the minor anomaly seen in uterus arcuatus, which has a slighly indented fundus, to a completely duplicated uterus, *uterus didelphys*, including duplicate cervix and vagina (Fig. 4-1A–I).[18] One of the most common anomalies encountered in the uterus is *uterus bicornis*, either *bicervical* or *unicervical* (Figs. 4-1D, 4-1F) which has two horns entering a common vagina.[28]

Müllerian Duct Atresia. Another cause of uterine and cervical anomalies occurs when there is partial or complete atresia of one of the müllerian ducts. *Aplasia* or *hypoplasia* of the entire uterus or cervix may occur, or only one side may be atretic and may not communicate with the vagina. A rudimentary or hypoplastic uterus usually is not functional, but if menstrual bleeding does occur in a horn that has no communication with the vagina, hydrometrocolpos can result (Fig. 4-1H).[28]

Failure of the Urogenital Septum to Disappear. The septum can persist to any degree, causing any degree of separation of the uterine corpus from slight (Fig. 4-1D,F) to complete.[28] In *uterus subseptus* the septum is only partially resorbed (Fig. 4-1C).

Diethylstilbestrol Syndrome. From the late 1940s to the early 1970s many women were exposed in utero to diethylstilbestrol (DES) administered to their mothers primarily for the treatment of threatened abortion. Women exposed to DES in utero are able to conceive, but many have poor pregnancy outcomes. Thirty-five percent of them have been found to have vaginal epithelial changes (adenosis), and 42% have an abnormally shaped uterine cavity. The most significant DES stigmata are a T-shaped uterus, constricting bands in the uterus, and intrauterine wall defects.[10,27]

FALLOPIAN TUBES

Very rarely, both fallopian tubes are absent. Unilateral absence is associated with absence of the uterus on that side. Rare doubling of the tube can also occur on one side. The most common problem encountered here is *atresia* of a portion of a tube. This may cause infertility or tubal pregnancy.[10] With transvaginal scanning, documenting the absence of fallopian tubes might become more feasible.

OVARIES

Congenital agenesis or atresia of the ovaries is very rare.[10] When it does occur, the fallopian tubes usually are also absent (Fig. 4-1E). *Supernumerary* (extra) ovaries are found occasionally at a site remote from the normal ovary. They probably result from development of separate primordia in an ectopic portion of the gonadal ridge. Benign terato-

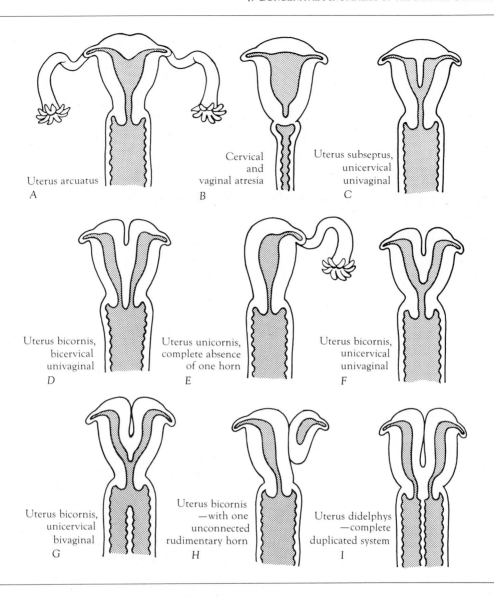

FIGURE 4-1. Drawings of congenital anomalies of the uterus.

mas and dermoid cysts of these supernumerary ovaries have been found in the omentum and in the retroperitoneum.[10]

Occasionally, an ovary may be split into separate portions. *Accessory ovarian tissue*, usually less than 1 cm in diameter, can be found in the broad ligament near the normal ovary or near the cornua of the uterus.[10] Ectopic ovarian tissue may also be found near the kidney or in the retroperitoneal space.

Parovarian cysts arising from the Rosenmüller's organ, a vestigial portion of the wolffian duct system, may be found. The outer extremity of this "duct" can become dilated and form a cystic, pedunculated structure known as the *hydatid cyst of Morgagni*. These may become infarcted and cause pain when they twist on their pedicles. Gartner's duct, remnants of the wolffian duct in the broad ligament, has a propensity to cystic dilatation and infection with the attendant symptoms.[10,24]

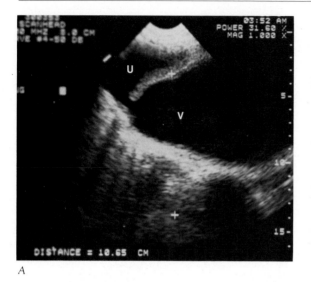

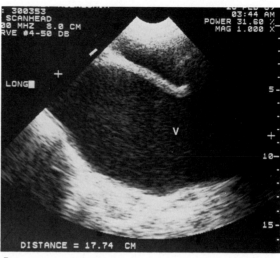

A   B

FIGURE 4-2. A 12-year-old girl with hematometrocolpos. Sagittal sonogram demonstrates the fluid-filled dilated vagina (V). Superior to the vagina is a smaller blood-filled structure representing the dilated uterus (U). (B) This sagittal section of the hematometrocolpos has the characteristic low-level echoes representing clotted blood. The lack of convergence of the inferior borders of the dilated vagina is characteristic of hematocolpos.

Sonographic Scanning Technique and Appearance

VAGINAL ANOMALIES

Most vaginal anomalies, such as transverse and longitudinal septa and duplicated vagina, cannot be imaged by transabdominal or transvaginal ultrasound.[20] Likewise, an intact hymen cannot be seen directly, but sequelae, such as accumulations of mucus or blood in the vagina (colpos) or endometrial canal (metra), can be visualized (Fig. 4-2A,B). As in all ultrasound imaging, gross changes in the normal appearance of the vagina can be seen. Thus a Gartner's duct cyst, a remnant of the wolffian duct, appears as a small anechoic mass in the anterolateral portion of the vagina (Fig. 4-3). Complete absence of the vagina will be apparent by the missing normal vaginal echoes (Fig. 4-4). This condition occurs in about 1 in 5000 patients[4] and may affect part of the vagina. When there is agenesis of a small inferior section, ultrasound can be useful in identifying the atretic area[26] by mapping out the section where no normal echoes are visualized.

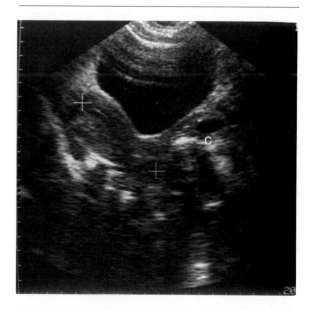

FIGURE 4-3. A cyst (C) in the vagina, a Gartner's duct cyst.

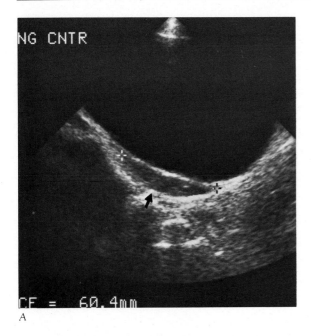

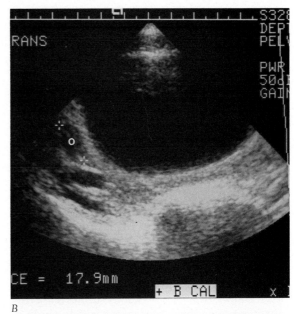

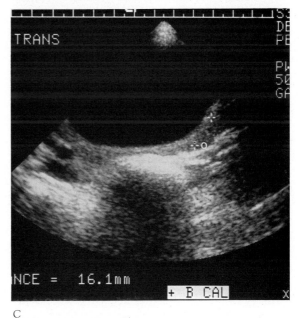

Figure 4-4. (A) Sagittal scan through the rudimentary uterus (*arrow*) of a 16-year-old girl with primary amenorrhea. Reconstructive surgery was performed to create a vagina. (B,C) Transverse scans of the right and left ovaries (O). (Courtesy Dr. Ruth Rosenblatt, Montefiore Hospital, Bronx, NY.)

The importance of ultrasound in detecting the cause of pelvic masses in females with asymmetric duplication of the uterus resulting in one imperforate vagina has been reported.[6,17,21] Although the shape of the masses varied because each duplication above the vagina was somewhat different, the basic sonographic appearance was of a mass adjacent to a uterus and filled with either clear fluid (anechoic) or with low-level echoes (hypoechoic) from blood or mucus. The ultrasound findings spared several of these patients from having hysterectomies and exploratory surgery. Subsequently

Table 4-1. Sonographic appearance of congenital vaginal anomalies

Anomaly	Sonographic Appearance
Hydrocolpos or hematocolpos	Anechoic to hypoechoic pear-shaped mass with no normal vaginal echoes located adjacent and posterior to the bladder (Fig. 4-2)
Vaginal septa	Normal vaginal echoes
Double vagina	Either no significant change in appearance of normal vagina or enlarged vagina; transvaginal scanning may demonstrate second vagina
Absent vagina	Absence of normal vaginal echoes (Fig. 4-4)
Duplicated uterus with unilateral imperforate vagina	Vagina appears normal; lateral to normal uterus, an anechoic or echo-filled mass might be seen. Kidney ipsilateral to mass is usually absent.
Intact hymen	In postmenarchal symptomatic patient, hematocolpos or hematometrocolpos might be found (Fig. 4-2).
Gartner's duct cyst	Anechoic small mass in anterolateral vagina (Fig. 4-3)

they had corrective surgery that involved incision and drainage of the fluid followed by reconstruction of a vagina or excision of a septum if it was causing the obstruction.[8] The kidney on the side of the asymmetric duplication almost always is absent; only one case has been reported in which a kidney was found on the ipsilateral side.[4] It follows that if a sonographer suspects that a parauterine mass is a duplication of part of the uterus, the kidneys should be examined.

Technique. A full bladder is necessary for sonographic examination for vaginal anomalies, to permit sound transmission posterior to the pubic symphysis. A sector scanner provides more maneuverability in this area. Beginning with a sagittal plane of the pelvis and lowering the gain until the transvaginal canal is clearly seen is the first step. The canal with the surrounding vaginal muscles should appear continuous with the cervix. Absence of this continuity could indicate atresia and should be further documented with transverse scans at the region of no vaginal echoes and inferior and superior to this area.

In cases of hydrocolpos or hematocolpos no vagina is visible separate from the fluid-filled mass. The typical appearances of vaginal anomalies are summarized in Table 4-1.

Uterine Anomalies

Since uterine anomalies run the gamut from absence of uterus and vagina (Rokitansky-Küster-Hauser syndrome) to complete duplication of uterus, cervix, and vagina (uterus didelphys), there

are a wide variety of sonographic appearances (Table 4-2).[5] However, in the nonpregnant patient without symptoms, unless the anomaly manifests in gross changes in the morphology of the uterus (Figs. 4-4 through 4-7), ultrasound cannot make the diagnosis.

When examining a patient for a uterine anomaly, the sonographer must keep in mind the various combinations of uterine, cervical, and vaginal malformations. As in every gynecologic ultrasound exam, a transabdominal scan requires a full bladder. Sagittal plane scans should be used to outline the vagina. Then, to best visualize duplications of the cervix and uterus, transverse images are more revealing. The transverse scan through a duplicated cervix will appear as two echogenic connected or contiguous cervices (Figs. 4-5, 4-6). The uterus likewise presents as two connected or adjacent uteri. Depending on the extent of the cleft in a bicornuate uterus, the fundal portion will appear enlarged or separated. Septae in the uterine corpus, either subseptate or total septation, usually are not visualizable in nonpregnant women, but duplicated endometrial echoes may be followed to where they fuse into one common endometrial cavity (Fig. 4-7). The sonographer must systematically scan through the cervix, looking carefully for two endocervical canals and measuring the width of the cervix. If the width of the cervix or uterus is much more than the normal 5 cm, the possibility of duplication must be explored.

Then the examination should continue through the uterine corpus, varying the gain settings to visualize the endometrial and myometrial echoes. A

Table 4-2. Sonographic appearance of uterine anomalies

Anomaly	Sonographic Appearance	
	Nonpregnant Uterus	Pregnant Uterus*
Cervical atresia	No cervical echoes but corpus of uterus appears as echogenic mass[19]	
Uterine agenesis	Absence of echoes in area of uterus or small remnant of apparently fibrous tissue[19]	
Unicornuate uterus	Normal to slightly asymmetric uterus,[7] loss of pear shape,[19] lateral displacement	In advanced pregnancy, no abnormalities
Didelphic uterus	Double cervix, uterine corpora, enlarged uterus, two endometrial canal echoes visualized (Figs. 4-5, 4-6)	Pregnancy in one uterus; decidual reaction and enlarged other
Bicornuate uterus	Dependent on degree of cleft between horns: broad uterine fundus, two distinct cornua, two endometrial cavity echoes, or normal-looking uterus are all possible[19]	Eccentric implantation of gestational sac (Figs. 4-9, 4-10)
Subseptate uterus	Depends on extent of septum (partial or complete). Two endometrial echoes might be seen until fusion of endometrium (Fig. 4-7).	Thick septum might be seen in early pregnancy. Sac might extend across septum (see Fig. 12-10).
		Differentials include large ovarian cyst, degenerated cystic fibroid, ectopic gestation (see Fig. 21-5)

*After 22 weeks' gestation, most anomalies cannot be visualized.

widened uterus with two endometrial echoes is characteristic of duplication. Finally, the fundus must be carefully examined, concentrating on the midsagittal line, looking for an indentation, and the cornua should be examined to look for symmetry in their configuration. An indentation could indicate a uterus didelphys (see Figs. 4-5, 4-6), bicornuate, or arcuate uterus. Transvaginal scanning can help differentiate between these by tracing the endometrial cavity echoes from the fundus to the vagina (see Fig. 4-6). Asymmetry in the cornua could represent a unicornuate uterus. Once transverse scans raise a suspicion of an anomaly, the structures of interest should be studied further and documented in sagittal views.

Because aplasia and hypoplasia of the uterus are other possibilities, the size of the uterus relative to the patient's age and parity should be accounted for. If the uterus is absent or small, it is particularly important to examine for a vagina, since it is frequently absent in these cases (Mayer-Rokitansky-Hauser syndrome) (see Fig. 4-4).[2]

Potential Pitfalls. Pedunculated and subserosal myomas located in the cervical or fundal areas can present as enlargements of these structures that are suggestive of duplication (Fig. 4-8).[3] Myomas will not have endocervical echoes and usually will not have the same degree of echogenicity as endometrial tissue. Most important, on sagittal scans there will not be continuity with the rest of the uterus.

UTERINE ANOMALIES IN PREGNANT PATIENTS
After 22 weeks' gestation, pregnancy tends to obliterate some anatomic variants, so if there is clinical suspicion of an anomaly, the patient should be examined before this juncture. It is important for the physician to know whether an anomaly exists, because anomalies tend to be associated with premature delivery, low birth weights, and complicated delivery, often requiring cesarean section.

Pregnancy can occur in one or both duplicated uteri, in arcuate, unicornuate, and septate uteri; therefore, the sonographic appearance will vary with the individual anomaly and pregnancy. Pregnant women with a uterine corpus not connected to a vagina may present with a pelvic mass representing the nonpregnant uterus which is enlarged in response to hormonal stimulation or which is filled with blood or mucus. Early in pregnancy the

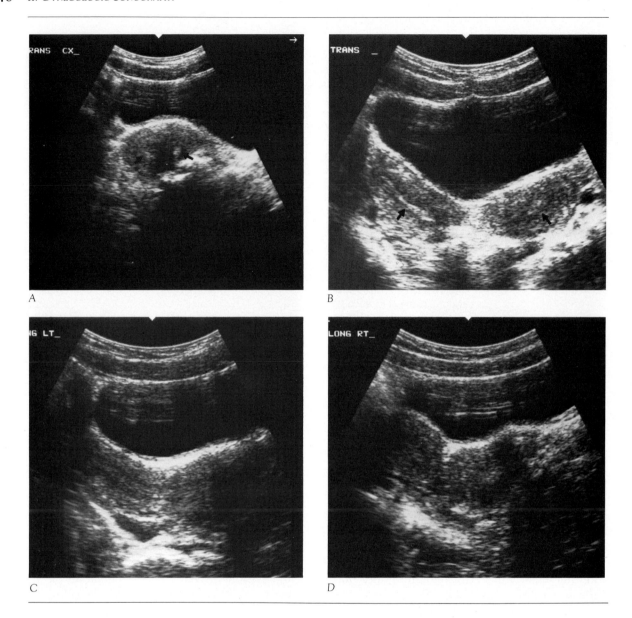

FIGURE 4-5. (A) Transverse scan through the cervix of a patient with uterus didelphys. Two separate endocervical echoes *(arrows)*. (B) Transverse scan through a more superior section of the uterus demonstrates separate uterine bodies with their endometrial canal echoes *(arrows)*. (C,D) Sagittal scans through the left (C) and right (D) uteri. With anomalous uteri, it may be difficult to clearly outline each individual uterus. (Courtesy Birgit Bader-Armstrong, University of Rochester Medical Center, Rochester, NY.)

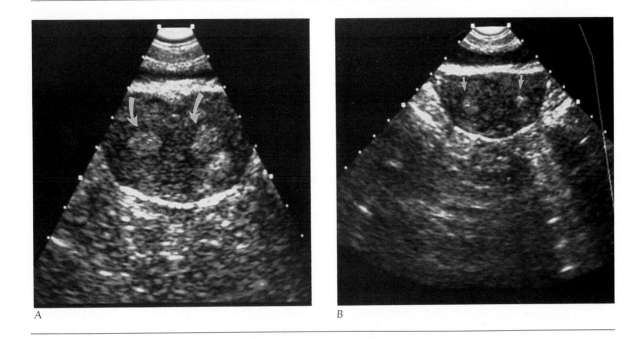

FIGURE 4-6. (A) Transvaginal coronal view of uterine fundus in a uterus didelphys showing two endometrial echoes (*curved arrows*). (B) More caudad coronal transvaginal view of uterus at level of cervix again shows two groups of echoes (*arrows*) continuous with the duplicated endometria. (Mendelson EB, Bohm-Velez M, Neiman HL, Russo J. Transvaginal sonography in gynecologic imaging. Ultrasound CT MR. 1988; 9:102-121.)

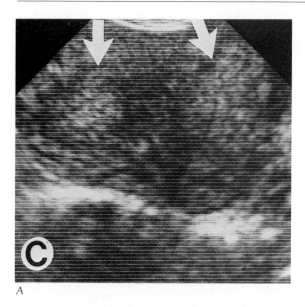

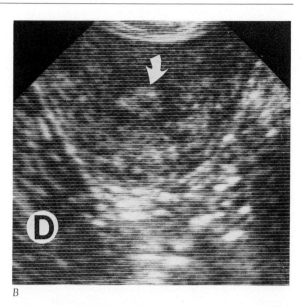

A

B

FIGURE 4-7. (A) Uterus subseptus. Endovaginal coronal scan at level of fundus demonstrates two sets of endometrial echoes *(arrows)*. (B) On a caudal section, inferior to the septum, only one endometrial echo is visualized *(arrow)*. (Mendelson EB, Bohm-Velez M, Neiman HL, Russo J. Transvaginal sonography in gynecologic imaging. Ultrasound CT MR. 1988; 9:102-121.)

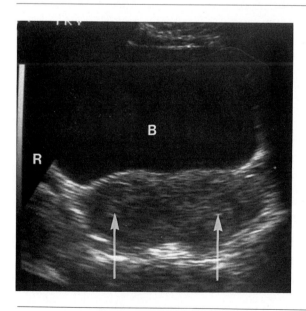

FIGURE 4-8. Transverse sonogram of a young woman with a history of several first-trimester miscarriages who was thought to have a bicornuate uterus. Uterus has a symmetric bilobed appearance. Echoes from two apparent canals *(arrows)* are seen, although entire right side is slightly more hypoechoic. Hysterosalpingography revealed a normal central cavity and outlined a mass consistent with a fibroid on the right side (R), confirmed on a follow-up sonogram. (B, bladder.) (Baltarowich OH, Kurtz AB, Pennell RG, et al. Pitfalls in the sonographic diagnosis of uterine fibroids. AJR. 1988; 151:725-728.)

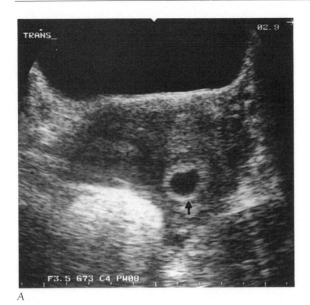

A

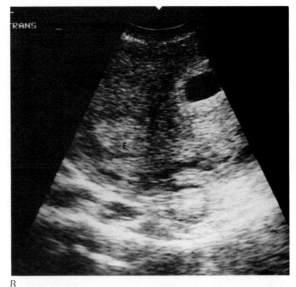

B

FIGURE 4-9. (A) Transabdominal transverse scan of a duplicated uterus with a gestational sac *(arrow)* in the left uterus. The prominent echoes (E) in the right uterus represent the decidual reaction. A transvaginal scan (B) more clearly defines the decidual reaction (E) in the right uterus and (C) the embryo *(arrow)* in the left uterus. (Courtesy Birgit Bader-Armstrong, University of Rochester Medical Center, Rochester, NY.)

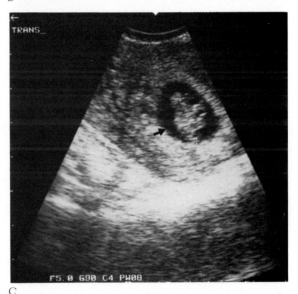

C

gravid uterus is located eccentrically, and the non-gravid uterus often demonstrates a decidual reaction and enlargement (Figs. 4-9, 4-10). The decidual reaction may look like a gestational sac but will have neither an embryo nor the double sac sign of a true pregnancy. Transvaginal scanning can clearly differentiate between a true gestation and the endometrial reaction.

The septum in a septate uterus can be seen when it is surrounded by amniotic fluid. A subseptate uterus can also be imaged and appears as a broad uterine septum (see Fig. 20-10). The septum often causes the fetus to lie in an abnormal position.

Potential Pitfalls. Sonographic findings that can simulate one of the many variations of anomalies are:

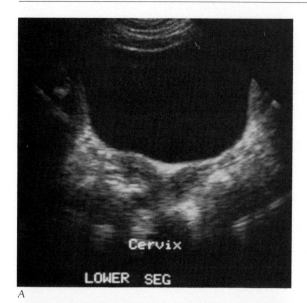

A

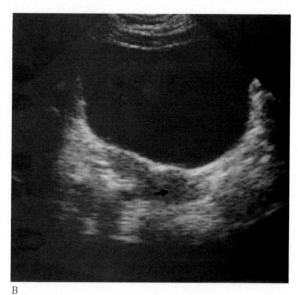

B

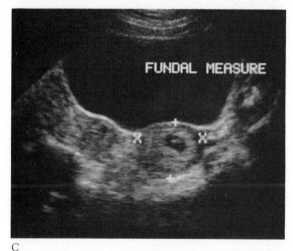

C

FIGURE 4-10. Example of clearly separated fundi in a pregnant patient with uterus didelphys. (A) Sonogram through the cervices, which are joined. (B) More cephalad section through the uterine bodies demonstrates that they are still joined, but the left (pregnant) uterus (arrow) is enlarged. (C) A sonogram through the fundal area shows two separate fundi with a gestational sac in the uterus. (Courtesy Ultrasound Lab, Raritan Bay Medical Center, Raritan, NJ.)

a gestational sac in a fallopian tube may look like a pregnancy in a uterine horn; a cornual uterine fibroid may look like a nonpregnant horn (Fig. 4-8); the decidual reaction in the nonpregnant uterus may suggest a twin gestation; the amniotic membrane may be confused for the septum in a septate uterus. Being alert to the patient's symptoms and the sonograpic characteristics of each entity will help to differentiate between these. Pennes suggests that the amniotic membrane is not as thick as a uterine septation and tends to move in the amniotic fluid whereas the septum is rigid.[3,23]

Treatment

When anomalies such as absent vagina or cervix prohibit normal impregnation or cause symptoms because they prevent menstrual blood and fluid from escaping, modern surgical techniques and more potent antibiotics allow these sections of the reproductive tract to be reconstructed.[9] Septa in the vagina can be removed; connections between duplicated uteri can be made to allow the flow of blood between them; and metroplasty, the joining of two uteri, can be performed, to increase the success of future pregnancies.[25]

Other Imaging Modalities

Although ultrasound is the first imaging technique to be used, in equivocal cases magnetic resonance imaging has been used to identify a small gap in the vagina. Hansmann feels that ultrasound is limited to imaging a bicornuate uterus in patients who are pregnant and that in other cases hysteroscopy and hysterosalpingography are superior to ultrasound.[4,15]

With a good knowledge of the characteristics of congenital anomalies and the use of transvaginal scanning, sonography's ability to identify these developmental variations should improve dramatically.

References

1. Akhtar AZ. Congenital abnormalities of genital tract-uterine malformation. JPMA. 1986; 36:261–266.
2. Alper MM, Garner PR, Spence JEH. Coexistence of gonadal dysgenesis and uterine aplasia. Reproduct Med. 1985; 30:232–234.
3. Baltarowich OH, Kurtz AB, Pennell RG, et al. Pitfalls in the sonographic diagnosis of uterine fibroids. AJR. 1988; 151:725–728.
4. Barach B, Falces E, Benzian SR. Magnetic resonance imaging for diagnosis and preoperative planning in agenesis of the distal vagina. Ann Plast Surg. 1987; 19:192–194.
5. Baramki TA. Treatment of congenital anomalies in girls and women. Reproduct Med. 1984; 29:376–384.
6. Berman L, Stringer DA, St Onge O, et al. Case report: Unilateral haematocolpos in uterine duplication associated with renal agenesis. Clin Radiol. 1987; 38:545–547.
7. Bowie JD. Sonography of the uterus. In: Sabbagha RE, ed. Diagnostic Ultrasound. Philadelphia: J.B. Lippincott; 1987.
8. Cohen RC, Davey RB, LeQuesne GW. Ultrasonography in the diagnosis and management of unilateral hematometracolpos and associated renal agenesis. Austral Paediatr J. 1982; 18:287–290.
9. Cukier J, Batzofin JH, Conner JS, et al. Genital tract reconstruction in a patient with congenital absence of the vagina and hypoplasia of the cervix. Obstet Gynecol. 1986; 68:32S–36S.
10. Durfee RB. Congenital anomalies in female genital tract. In: Benson R, ed. Current Obstetric and Gynecology: Diagnosis and Treatment, 2nd ed. Los Altos, CA: Lange; 1978.
11. Fedele L, Dorta, M, Brioschi D, et al. Pregnancies in septate uteri: Outcome in relation to site of uterine implantation as determined by sonography. AJR. 1989; 52:781–784.
12. Fedele L, Zamberletti D, d'Alberton A, et al. Gestational aspects of uterus didelphys. J Reproduct Med. 1988; 33:353–355.
13. Fliegner JRH. Uncommon problems of the double uterus. Med J Austral 1986; 145:510–512.
14. Hacker NF, Moore, JG. Essentials of Obstetrics and Gynecology. Philadelphia: WB Saunders; 1986.
15. Hansmann M, Hackeloer B-J, Staudach A. Ultrasound Diagnosis in Obstetrics and Gynecology. Berlin: Springer-Verlag, 1985.
16. Hochner-Celnikier D, Hurwitz A, Beller U, et al. Ultrasound diagnosis in the case of an adnexal mass as a presenting symptom in early pregnancy. Eur J Obstet Gynecol Reprod Biol. 1984; 16:339–342.
17. Johnson J, Hillman BJ. Uterine duplication, unilateral imperforate vagina and normal kidneys. AJR. 1986; 147:1197–1198.
18. Langman J. Medical Embryology, 4th ed. Baltimore: Williams and Wilkins; 1981.
19. Malini S, Valdes C, Malinak R. Sonographic diagnosis and classification of anomalies of the female genital tract. J Ultrasound Med 1984; 3:397–404.
20. Mendelson EB, Bohm-Velez M, Neiman HL, et al. Transvaginal sonography in gynecologic imaging. Semin Ultrasound CT MR. 1988; 9:102–121.
21. Miyazaki Y, Ebisuno S, Uekado Y, et al. Uterus didelphys with unilateral imperforate vagina and ipsilateral renal agenesis. J Urol. 1986; 135:107–109.
22. Novak ER, Jones GS, Jones HW. Novak's Textbook of Gynecology. 8th ed. Baltimore: Williams & Wilkins; 1970.
23. Pennes DR, Bowerman RA, Silver TM. Congenital uterine anomalies and associated pregnancies. J Ultrasound Med. 1985; 4:531–538.
24. Ramsey D. Embryology and developmental defects of the female reproductive tract. In: Danforth D, Scott Jr, eds. Obstetrics and Gynecology. 5th ed. Philadelphia: JB Lippincott; 1986.
25. Rock JA, Zacur HA. The clinical management of repeated early pregnancy wastage. Fertil Steril. 1983; 39:123–140.

26. Rulin MC, Yoder DA, Hayashi TT. Congenital atresia of the lower vagina with regular menses through a fistula: A therapeutic approach. Obstet Gynecol 1985; 65:88S–90S.

27. Sharp H. Reproductive tract disorders. In: Danforth D, Scott R, eds. Obstetrics and Gynecology. 5th ed. Philadelphia: JB Lippincott; 1986.

28. Tuchman-Duplessis H, Hagel P. Organogenesis. In: Illustrated Human Embryology. New York: Springer-Verlag; 1974; 2.

CHAPTER **5**

Pediatric Gynecologic Ultrasound

MARY BETH GEAGAN, JACK O. HALLER, HARRIS L. COHEN

Major indications for gynecologic ultrasound examination of young girls include vaginal bleeding or discharge, ambiguous genitalia, and abdominal mass. Although pregnancy is often found to be the cause of an abdominal mass in older adolescents, because this chapter deals with premenarchal patients, pregnancy is not discussed here.

Because internal pelvic examination of young girls generally is not desirable or possible, ultrasound assumes a role of great importance as a relatively simple and painless method of viewing the internal anatomy. With the exception of transvaginal ultrasound, which is also contraindicated in children, sonography has opened new horizons in the field of pediatric gynecologic imaging. Much information about the nature and extent of the abnormality can be collected with little trauma to the child. More invasive procedures, such as examination under anesthesia, diagnostic laparoscopy, or exploratory laparotomy, may be avoided or postponed.

Anatomy and Physiology

The uterus is approximately 3.5 cm long for the first 6 to 8 weeks of life and, owing to maternal hormonal stimulation, it has the adult configuration. After the immediate postnatal period, the uterus gradually decreases in length to 2.5 cm and regresses to premenarchal shape, in which the cervix predominates (Fig. 5-1). The ratio of cervix to corpus length in premenarchal girls is 2:1.[18] Hansmann and co-workers report the prepubertal length to be 1.5 to 3 cm and corpus width, 0.5 to 1 cm; the cervix width is 1.5 to 3 cm.[17] The size of the uterus does not change appreciably until age 7 years. At this point, it begins to increase in size, with a proportionally greater increase in the corpus than in the cervix.[23] The mean total uterine length increases from 2.5 cm at 7 years, to 3.5 cm at 10 years, to 6.2 cm at 13 years (Fig. 5-2).[19]

At birth, the ovaries usually have descended to their normal position in the pelvis. As in adults, the adnexa(e) may be found in the posterior cul-de-sac, at the lateral pelvic wall, or rarely, above the pelvic brim. Identifying the iliac vessels and pelvic musculature may aid in locating the ovaries. The ovaries' shape may vary, but usually they are elongated and symmetric, as in adults. The pediatric ovary measures 15 mm long, 2.5 mm thick, and 3 mm wide and grows gradually until the onset of puberty, when it has adult proportions—24 to 41 mm long, 8.5 to 19.4 mm thick, and 15 to 24 mm wide. Ovarian volume increases from 1 cm^3 before puberty to the reported adult value of 6 cm^3.[16] Our ovarian volume measurements for both children and adults are somewhat larger.

A cyst in a child's ovary is usually no cause for concern. Many follicles in all stages of development are present constantly in girls' ovaries, and a

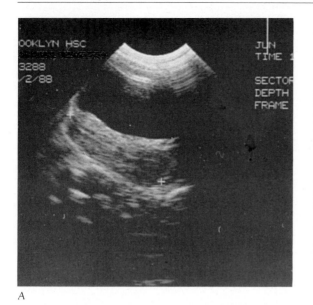

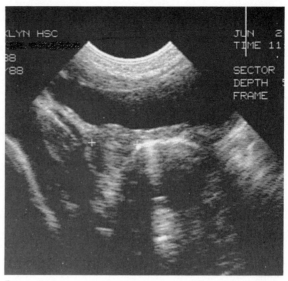

A

B

FIGURE 5-1. Normal infantile uterus. A 5-day-old infant had vaginal bleeding; no hematocolpos was found. Enlargement is due to maternal hormonal situation. (A) Sagittal scan through the uterus. (B) Transverse scan through uterine fundus.

greater portion of these follicles generally are in earlier stages of development than in women.

Usually, follicular regression in fetal or postnatal life begins before the follicle attains any appreciable size, but follicles can measure several millimeters. Up to 5% of neonatal ovaries contain cysts, which range in size from 0.5 to 7 mm. These may occur at any time before menarche, and they differ from true follicles in that they contain no ova.[18] Stanhope and colleagues found that a maximum follicular diameter of 7 mm was normal in early childhood.[28]

Vascularization increases slowly in infants and young children to approximately the adult level by age 6 or 8 years, at which time the medullary zone of the ovary becomes identifiable histologically. By age 11 or 12 years, primordial follicles are seen in the cortical zone. Under normal conditions, these primordial follicles regress as follicles containing ova develop.[16]

Sonographic Examination Technique and Protocols

Before beginning a sonographic examination of a pediatric patient, it is wise to spend a few minutes explaining "the test" and the equipment, at least to older girls. The explanation and demonstration should be tailored to the age of the patient. For example, the child should be allowed to touch the transducer, feel the "jelly," and locate the "TV" where she will "see her belly." Allowing one or both parents to stay with the child during the examination may reduce the anxiety level of all concerned. Bottle, pacifier, and a key ring for an infant and perhaps a favorite toy for an older child may also alleviate the patient's anxiety. Nursery rhymes, songs, and riddles can also be employed to distract the child's attention from "the test." Often a child will cry at the start of the examination despite the examiner's explanations and endeavors; invariably she will stop once she realizes the ex-

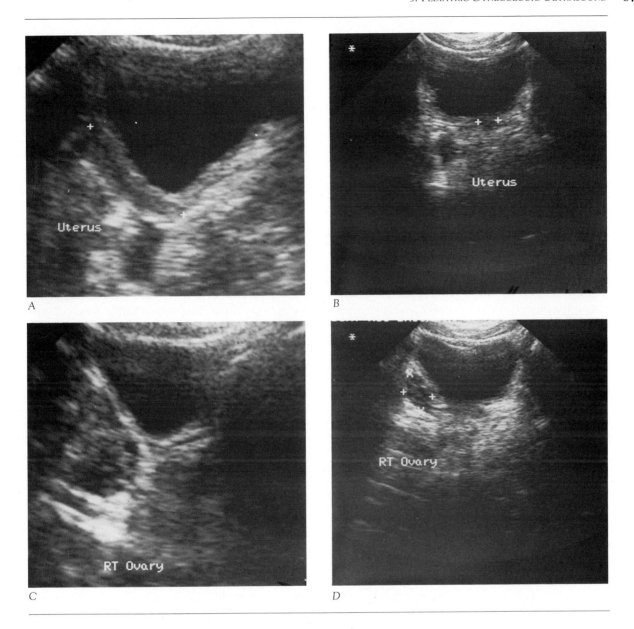

FIGURE 5-2. Normal prepubertal uterus and ovaries of 10-year-old. Sagittal (A) and transverse (B) scans of uterus. (C,D) Sagittal and transverse scans of ovary.

amination is not painful and that her parents are not going to leave her. At the termination of the ultrasound procedure, the examiner might give the patient a "happy face" or some similar sticker as a reward.

As for adults, pelvic sonography of a pediatric patient requires a full urinary bladder. The older child should drink 24 ounces of noncarbonated fluid 45 minutes to 1 hour before the study and can usually maintain a full bladder for the time required to complete the examination. A bottle 30 minutes prior to the study may provide adequate bladder filling in a patient who is not toilet trained, but catheterization may be necessary to ensure proper filling for optimal pelvic evaluation. An 8 French feeding tube is generally an adequate catheter substitute for an infant; age and size determine the catheter of choice for older children. Sedation is rarely necessary, but it may be indicated when repeated attempts fail to calm the child enough to permit a diagnostically adequate examination. Speed and accuracy are of prime importance in scanning pediatric patients, as bladder control is limited and the patient, especially a very young child, may void at any time.

The scanning planes used and the images obtained are the same as for adults. Considerable patience and fortitude may be required to obtain these views, however, if the child presents a squirming, moving target. Transducer frequency generally ranges from 5 to 7.5 MHz; the higher-frequency transducer is preferred for younger children. The prepubertal uterus and ovaries are usually small in comparison to the filled urinary bladder. Therefore, the gain must be set low enough to allow these structures to be distinguished from surrounding muscle and bowel.

As in adults, if an abnormality is found in the pelvis, the appropriate upper abdominal organs should be examined to preclude related findings, such as hydronephrosis or metastatic lesions in the lymph nodes or liver.

Pathology

Genital tumors are quite rare in children and young adolescents but approximately 50% of those found are malignant or potentially malignant. Almost every tumor that occurs in an adult has also been described in a child.[11] Here, we emphasize the more common pathologic lesions of children, which will be grouped into benign and malignant categories.

VAGINA, UTERUS, AND FALLOPIAN TUBES

Primary tumors are rare in children. Malignant tumors are more common, and the vagina is involved more often than the uterus.[25]

Benign Lesions. Gartner's duct cysts and pelvic inflammatory disease occur most often. Gartner's duct cysts are the most common cystic lesions of the vagina. These benign mesonephric duct remnants are rare in children and are found as single or multiple lesions along the anteromedial aspect of the vaginal wall.[6,20]

It is possible for hydrosalpinx or pyosalpinx to occur, often in a sexually abused child. Inflammatory debris may be present, which together with the fusiform shape and thickened tubal walls, help differentiate this entity from an ovarian cyst. Tuboovarian abscess occurs when the infection extends to involve the ovary.[2]

Malignant Lesions. Sarcoma botryoides is the most common malignant vaginal and uterine lesion of young girls. It is a polypoid form of embryonal rhabdomyosarcoma, which usually originates in the vagina and spreads to the uterus, although the reverse may occur. The mass is soft and may fill the entire abdomen without being palpable. Symptoms include a bloody vaginal discharge and a grapelike mass in the vagina or protruding from it.[9,10,15,25]

On sonography, a large, poorly circumscribed mass with a mixed echogenic pattern and areas of cystic degeneration is usually demonstrated. Invasion of the bladder and surrounding pelvic structures often makes it impossible to determine the organ of origin.[15] Radiation and chemotherapy are used to shrink the mass to a size suitable for conservative excision. Ultrasound, MRI, and computed tomography (CT) may be used for serial follow-up examinations.

Primary adenocarcinoma of the uterus and vagina has been reported, some in daughters of mothers exposed to diethylstilbestrol (DES). Approximately one-third occur in children less than 1 year of age. Almost all cases occur before age 11.[15] It presents with vaginal bleeding and a rapidly growing tumor not associated with sexual precocity. Sonography usually reveals a solid tumor with no distinguishing characteristics.

Endodermal sinus tumor, a soft, often cystic and highly malignant tumor of the vagina and cervix, usually occurs by age 3 years and simulates sarcoma botryoides clinically.[11]

OVARY

The ovary is the most common site of tumors in the female genital tract in childhood. Ovarian tumors often present with pain, abdominal swelling, or a palpable abdominal mass. Ultrasound is often useful in determining the organ of origin, narrowing the possible differential diagnoses, and directing further diagnostic work-up.

Benign Masses. Single or multiple cysts, usually nonneoplastic, account for more than 70% of ovarian masses and are the most common pelvic tumors of childhood and adolescence. These are usually follicular retention cysts, corpus luteum cysts, or hemorrhagic cysts. Hormone secretion by the lining cells of some cysts may lead to precocious puberty. Fetal ovarian cysts have been reported, which may cause dystocia if they are large. Parovarian cysts, located in the mesosalpinx between the tube and ovary, are generally indistinguishable from simple ovarian cysts.[16] With the exception of hemorrhagic cysts, which may contain internal debris, these masses are usually purely cystic and often asymptomatic. Polycystic ovaries may have a sonographic appearance identical to that of multiple primordial follicles. The cysts may be too small to distinguish and simply appear as enlarged ovaries. All of these masses are subject to torsion when they attain sufficient size.[25]

The benign cystic teratoma (BCT, dermoid cyst) is the most common tumor during the reproductive years, but it is relatively uncommon before puberty. It occurs more often on the right side and often presents with abdominal pain secondary to torsion, which may easily be confused with appendicitis.[2] In children, the mass is predominantly cystic, with small foci of fat, hair, and calcification, the latter being less than in adults.[11] The appearance of a cyst-within-a-cyst has been described by Haller and colleagues. Fifteen to 20% of BCTs are reported to be bilateral.[16]

There have been reports of serous and mucinous cystadenomas in prepubertal girls. These tumors of epithelial origin are almost exclusively unilateral in children, and although rare, they are more common than their malignant counterparts.[11] The diagnosis can be suspected by demonstrating septa, a frequent finding in these masses. Ovarian fibroma, which may be associated with Meig's syndrome, is a rare benign solid connective tissue tumor occasionally found in children. It also is subject to torsion.[8]

Malignant Masses. As a group, germ cell tumors are the most common malignant tumors involving the pediatric genital tract. Dysgerminoma is the most common pediatric ovarian mass and is thought to be the counterpart of the testicular seminoma. Fortunately, this tumor has low-grade malignancy and is very radiosensitive, so it is potentially curable. The sonogram usually demonstrates a solid mass ranging in size from a small nodule to one of pelvoabdominal proportions. Hemorrhagic necrosis may lead to a complex appearance. Ascites, retroperitoneal adenopathy, and hepatic metastases may be seen in advanced cases.[16] Dysgerminoma is bilateral in 10 to 15% of cases and may contain foci of calcification. Levels of human chorionic gonadotropin (HCG), lactic dehydrogenase (LDH), and α_1-fetoprotein (AFP) may all be elevated.[11] The image is nonspecific and the differential diagnosis requires appropriate clinical and laboratory correlation. Ovarian torsion and appendiceal abscess have a similar sonographic appearance and must be ruled out.

Treatment is somewhat controversial. When the tumor is localized to one ovary, some advocate unilateral oophorectomy, with or without postoperative radiation; others recommend total abdominal hysterectomy with postoperative radiation. The more aggressive surgery is always indicated if the tumor is bilateral or locally extensive or if ascites or adenopathy is present.[24]

The other germ cell tumors are endodermal sinus tumor, malignant teratoma, primary choriocarcinoma of the ovary, and embryonal carcinoma. Endodermal sinus tumor, the second most common of the germ cell tumors, grows rapidly and is unilateral.[11] Malignant teratoma may be indistinguishable from BCT, but generally it contains more solid components. The peak incidence is at age 3 years, and 60% of teratomas show calcification on x-ray examination.[21] Embryonal carcinoma is highly malignant, unilateral, and may lead to precocious puberty. Nongestational choriocarcinoma, though rarer, likewise may lead to precocious puberty.[11] The appearance of these tumors ranges from almost purely cystic to purely solid and highly echogenic. Cul-de-sac fluid is found in 50% of these patients. Nodal metastases, abdominal ascites, and liver metastases are not uncommon.[25]

Tumors of gonadal (sex cord) origin such as the

granulosa-theca cell and arrhenoblastoma (Sertoli-Leydig cell) are generally less malignant and exert hormonal influences. Granulosa-theca cell tumors are feminizing tumors that lead to precocious puberty. Approximately 5% occur prepubertally, and less than 5% are bilateral. They are prone to late recurrence, which requires lifelong postoperative follow-up of the patient. Arrhenoblastomas are masculinizing tumors. When they recur in children it is usually during the first 3 years after operation.[11]

Serous and mucinous cystadenocarcinomas are malignant tumors of epithelial origin. In children, they are even rarer than their benign counterparts. The serous type is twice as common as the mucinous type. These tumors are often multilocular with thick septa and solid elements.[11,21]

The ovary may be involved by tumor metastases. Neuroblastoma, rhabdomyosarcoma, Krukenberg's tumor, lymphoma, and leukemia have all been reported to involve the ovary.[7,14,16] The genital involvement of acute lymphocytic leukemia at autopsy is 11.5 to 80% in females. The sonographic appearance has been described as solid, hypoechoic ovarian masses. Gonadal involvement often coincides with marrow remission.[3] Tumor recurrence is likely if the sequestered tumor is not treated adequately.[10]

Genital Anomalies, Gonadal Dysgenesis, Ambiguous Genitalia

Congenital uterine anomalies are difficult to detect in infants and young children. Often the sonogram is obtained as a precaution in the presence of other anomalies such as absence of the vagina, imperforate anus, or urinary tract anomalies. In DES-exposed infant girls, a T-shaped uterus (one that is relatively short and wide) has been described. Ultrasound may be of some use in identifying this anomaly,[10] though it is usually diagnosed after menarche. Vaginal anomalies are even more difficult to detect than uterine ones, and often it is possible to establish only that a vagina is indeed present. Occasionally, an increased anteroposterior vaginal diameter may suggest an abnormality when compared to a child of the same age. In the case of vaginal atresia, stenosis, or hypoplasia, sonography can provide useful information on the presence or absence of the upper one-third of the vagina, the uterus, and the ovaries prior to corrective surgery.[15]

Ovarian agenesis is extremely rare and is thought to be an acquired condition secondary to torsion and necrosis in utero. Hypoplasia is often associated with endocrine disorders, intersex disorders, and gonadal dysgenesis.[15]

Gonadal dysgenesis is marked by rudimentary gonads. In the most familiar type, Turner's syndrome, the ovaries are deficient. They may reach varying stages of development, ranging from absent to infantile to adult. Turner's patients have a 45,XO karyotype (chromosome pattern). Anomalies include dwarfism, webbed neck, shield-shaped chest, infantile sexual development, and amenorrhea. The ovary has no primordial follicles and is often represented only as a fibrous streak.[29] Sonographic study of these patients prior to the commencement of hormonal therapy rarely demonstrates the ovaries (volume less than 1 cm^3) and reveals a uterus with a prepubertal size and configuration, even in older adolescents. Ultrasound is useful to follow and document the changes in size and shape that occur in response to hormone therapy.[16]

In androgen insensitivity (testicular feminization) the karyotype is 46,XY and the patient often has uterine or vaginal defects, normal breast development, little or no pubic or axillary hair, and abdominal or inguinal testes. The testosterone level is close to normal, but the end organs are insensitive.[18] Patients with gonadal dysgenesis may have "streak" gonads. These resemble ovaries but contain no germ cells or follicular apparatus. The presence of a Y chromosome in such a child is cause for concern, as the child's risk of developing a tumor such as a dysgerminoma or a gonadoblastoma is greater than 30%. Gonadectomy is recommended for these patients.[1,5]

Ambiguous genitalia is one of the main indications for sonography of neonates. Early diagnosis is important to avoid serious psychologic disturbances. The presence of vaginal atresia, fused labia, clitoromegaly, or cryptorchidism should prompt an effort to define the internal anatomy with sonography and to locate a uterus, vagina, ovaries, or testes. Images of the adrenal glands and kidneys should be obtained to exclude congenital adrenal hyperplasia and renal anomalies.[18] The sonogram can easily be obtained while awaiting results of hormonal and chromosomal studies and may afford the parents some peace of mind.

Intersex occurs as an isolated entity in 1 birth in 1000 and is more common in association with other anomalies.[15] By defining the internal anatomy, ultrasound helps speed diagnosis and sex assignment of such infants.[15,25] A true hermaphrodite has both ovarian and testicular tissue. The structures may be joined, as an ovitestis, or separate ovaries and testes may be seen on each side of the pelvis. A uterus may or may not be present. A female pseudohermaphrodite is a chromosomal female (46,XX) with ovaries but with masculinized external genitalia, including an enlarged clitoris and prominent fused labia. This condition may be due to congenital adrenal hyperplasia, in which case a uterus is always present, or to increased androgen production caused by a virilizing maternal condition, in which case a uterus may not be present.

A male pseudohermaphrodite is a chromosomal male (46,XY) with feminized external genitalia due to decreased androgens, poor target organs, or an enzyme defect. Sonography is difficult and usually fails to locate undescended testicles unless they lie in the inguinal canal or high in the scrotum, but it can exclude the presence of a uterus and ovaries. These patients may have two testes or one testicle and one streak gonad.

Precocious Puberty

True isosexual precocious puberty is idiopathic in the majority of cases, secondary to activation of the hypothalamic-pituitary-gonadal axis. It can be defined as the onset of the normal physiologic and endocrine processes of puberty in girls before age 8 years. It usually follows the developmental sequence seen in normal children, that is, breast development followed by pubic and axillary hair development, followed by the onset of menstruation. The ovaries reach postpubertal size and volume and the uterus assumes the adult configuration, with a corpus-to-cervix ratio of 1:1.[18] True precocious puberty may occasionally be related to a central nervous system lesion that affects the hypo-thalamus.[10] Isolated premature development of the breasts (thelarche) or pubic hair (adrenarche) is not considered true precocious puberty.

Pseudoprecocious or incomplete precocious puberty results from adrenal or ovarian dysfunction. The accompanying clinical signs may be identical to those of the true type, although the menses are usually more irregular. Granulosa-theca cell tumors account for 60% of the cases with an ovarian cause.[25] Rarely, dysgerminoma, choriocarcinoma, arrhenoblastoma, and follicular retention cysts have been demonstrated as the cause of pseudoprecocious puberty. Adrenal causes include congenital hyperplasia, adenoma, and carcinoma. Hypothyroidism has occasionally been reported as a cause of breast development but has not produced menses.[10,25]

McCune-Albright syndrome, characterized by fibrous dysplasia of bone associated with café-au-lait skin pigmentation and possible endocrine hyperfunction has also been associated with precocious puberty. These patients tend to have the largest ovarian cysts and the largest size discrepancy between the two ovaries.[26]

Prior to the development of ultrasound, surgical exploration was required to search for ovarian or adrenal masses in patients with precocious puberty. Sonography has virtually eliminated this. The size of the uterus and ovaries can be assessed accurately. Findings of a large uterus and symmetric ovarian enlargement lead to a diagnosis of pituitary axis stimulation (true precocious puberty; Fig. 5-3). Unilateral ovarian enlargement and a prepubertal-sized uterus suggest ovarian tumor; however, primordial cysts may be a normal cause of ovarian enlargement. An infantile uterus and ovaries suggest premature thelarche or adrenarche rather than true precocious puberty (Fig. 5-4).[7] Therefore, careful study of the adrenal and hypothalamic regions must also be undertaken before precocious puberty can be attributed to an ovarian cyst.[16] Both areas are better studied by CT or magnetic resonance imaging (MRI) than by sonography.

When true precocious puberty is treated by hormone replacement therapy (luteinizing hormone-releasing factor [LHRF] analog therapy to decrease the pituitary response to gonadotropin-releasing hormone [GRH]), sonography is part of the pro-

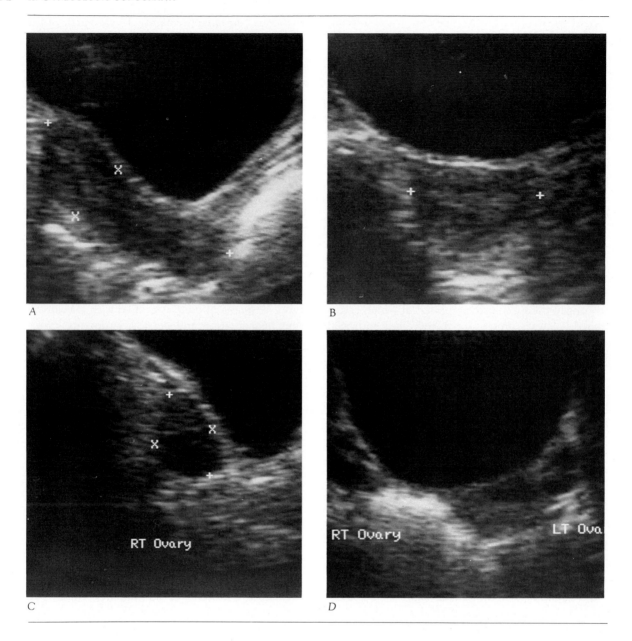

FIGURE 5-3. Precocious puberty. Note adult size and configuration of the uterus and ovaries of an 8-year-old girl with true precocious puberty. (A) Sagittal scan through uterus. (B) Transverse scan through uterine fundus. (C) On sagittal scan of right ovary, note follicles. (D) Transverse scan of ovaries and uterus.

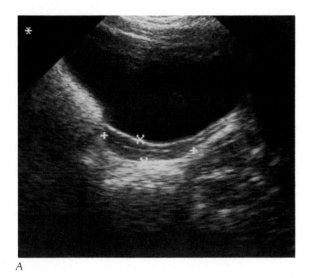
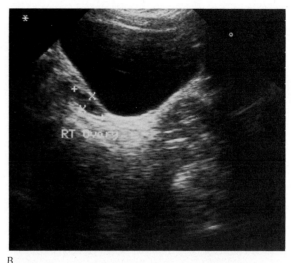

A

B

FIGURE 5-4. Pseudoprecocious puberty. Normal prepubertal uterus and ovaries in a 7½-year-old with precocious breast development (thelarche). (A) Sagittal scan through uterus. (B) Sagittal scan through right ovary; note small follicles.

tocol, to monitor the size and volume changes of the uterus and ovaries.[13,28] Serial sonograms document regression in response to therapy.

Hydrocolpos

Fluid or blood may accumulate in the vagina (hydrocolpos, hematocolpos), the uterus (hydrometra, hematometra), or both (hydrometrocolpos, hematometrocolpos). The cause is most often related to imperforate hymen, vaginal septum, duplication anomaly with unilateral obstruction, or acquired obstructing lesion.[2,9,10,15,21,25] Although these conditions often go undetected until menarche, they may present in a neonate as an abdominal mass or bulging hymen. Indeed, they account for 15% of abdominal masses in newborn girls; the incidence is slightly greater than that of ovarian cysts.[18] Maternal hormones prompt increased uterine secretions in newborns. This leads to distension of the uterus and/or vagina proximal to the point of obstruction (Fig. 5-5).

Sonography reveals a hypoechoic, transonic, pear-shaped mass in the midline arising from the pelvis between the bladder and rectum (Fig. 5-6).

As they both may present with internal echoes resulting from cellular debris or blood, pyometria and hematometria may not be differentiated.[32] A normal uterus and vagina cannot be identified.[2,25] It is important for the urinary bladder to be distended in order to prove that this mass is not the bladder.

Severe distension can lead to hydronephrosis and obstruction of the venous and lymphatic channels of the lower extremity.[27] If the condition presents in utero, urinary tract obstruction associated with fetal anuria, oligohydramnios, and pulmonary hypoplasia may result.[21]

Except for pure imperforate hymen, hydrocolpos is often accompanied by other severe congenital malformations, such as imperforate anus and urinary tract anomalies as well as genital, cardiac, and skeletal anomalies. Therefore, an attempt should be made to identify associated anomalies such as unilateral renal agenesis or hypoplasia. Uterine anomalies occur in only 0.1 to 0.5% of all females, but the incidence is 48 to 70% in females with renal abnormalities. Accordingly, discovery of a major renal anomaly should prompt evaluation of the uterus for potential anomalies.[4] In cases

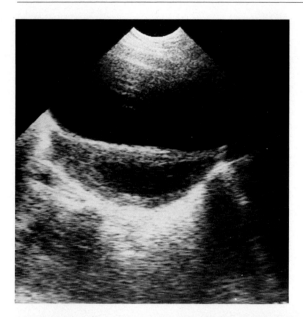

FIGURE 5-5. Hydrocolpos. Sagittal scan through an infant uterus. Note hypoechoic material distending the cervix and vagina.

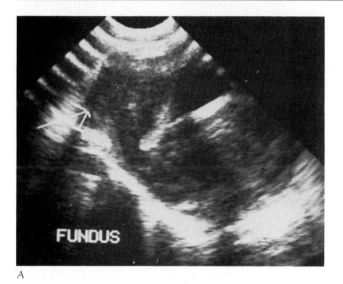

A

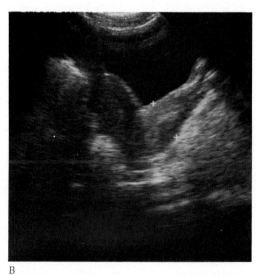

B

FIGURE 5-6. Hematometrocolpos. Abdominal mass in a 13-year-old. (A) Sagittal scan shows distended vagina and uterus; arrow indicates fundus. (B) Postoperative scan after surgery for vaginal web shows normal uterus.

TABLE 5-1. Differential diagnoses of the complex pediatric ovarian mass

MASS	HISTORY	PHYSICAL FINDINGS	LABORATORY STUDIES	SONOGRAPHIC FINDINGS
Hemorrhagic ovarian cyst	Lower abdominal pain, occasional nausea	None, or palpable mass; fever with torsion	↑ WBC if torsion	Variable: thick-walled cyst; septated cyst; homogeneous low-level echoes with poor sound attenuation; cyst containing solid components, fluid in cul-de-sac; change in appearance in follow-up study
Benign cystic teratoma	Lower abdominal pain, nausea, vomiting; pain increase with torsion	Lower abdominal or pelvic mass; torsion in 25% cases, w/ associated fever and acute abdomen	↑ WBC if torsion	Complex mass with hyperechoic zones with acoustic shadowing; "tip-of-the-iceberg sign"; solid mass with cystic components with or without scattered internal echoes; fat-fluid level; pelvic radiograph with calcium in 47 to 54%
Torsion of normal uterine adnexa	Acute abdominal pain; 50% have had similar episodes with spontaneous recovery in past; nausea, vomiting	Small, tender adnexal mass or lower abdominal mass, possible rebound tenderness, fever	↑ WBC	Predominantly solid ovarian mass with good through-transmission; fluid in cul-de-sac
Appendiceal abscess	Right lower-quadrant pain, nausea, vomiting .	Tender right, lower abdominal mass; may have rebound tenderness; fever	↑ WBC	Nonspecific complex adnexal mass; fecalith with shadowing fluid in cul-de-sac
Tuboovarian abscess	Lower abdominal pain, vaginal discharge, history of PID	Tender lower abdominal or adnexal mass; fever; purulent cervical drainage	↑ WBC	Nonspecific complex mass; fluid in cul-de-sac
Malignant neoplasm	May have lower abdominal pain which is acute, subacute, or chronic; nausea, vomiting	Lower abdominal mass; fever with torsion; ascites, lymphadenopathy, metastases	↑ WBC if torsion	Nonspecific complex ovarian mass; central cystic area of necrosis; uterus may not be identifiable; fluid in cul-de-sac in 50%; ascites, liver and peritoneal metastases, lymphadenopathy

(Adapted from Haller JO, et al. Pelvic masses in girls: An 8-year retrospective analysis stressing ultrasound as the prime imaging modality. Ped. Rad.; Springer-Verlag; 1984; 14:367.)

where corrective surgery is performed, serial sono-grams may be obtained to follow the postoperative course.

Ovarian Torsion

Torsion of a normal or an abnormal ovary is an infrequent but important cause of abdominal pain. There is an unexplained right-sided predominance ratio of 3:2.[30] Torsion of the normal adnexa usually occurs in the first decade of life and is less common than torsion of an ovary containing a mass (i.e., BCT or dysgerminoma). It is thought to be related to the particular mobility of the pediatric adnexa, which allows twisting at the mesosalpinx as a result of changes in intra-abdominal pressure or in body position. The torsion may involve the tube, the ovary, or both. If the ovary is to be salvaged, sur-gical treatment must be carried out promptly.[16]

Clinical symptoms include lower abdominal pain, usually of more than 48 hours' duration, fever, anorexia, nausea, and vomiting. The pain is often acute in onset, sharp, and radiates to the groin or flank. The presence of fever and leukocy-tosis usually indicates that necrosis and/or abscess formation has begun. Fifty percent of patients have a history of pain with spontaneous recovery[6,31] Di-agnostic confusion may result, especially in the case of pediatric patients, whose symptoms are often attributed to such entities as appendicitis, gastroenteritis, pyelonephritis, intussusception, or Meckel's diverticulitis.[16]

Sonographic signs are often nonspecific and in-clude a markedly enlarged ovary (mean volume may be 28 times normal), cul-de-sac fluid, periph-eral structures most likely representing follicles, and other adnexal pathology such as a cyst or tumor.[12,31] Vascular congestion in the mass leads to good sound transmission and numerous internal echoes. Incomplete torsion, with its associated ab-normal venous and lymphatic drainage, can lead to marked ovarian enlargement over several days and the appearance of a solid mass. When torsion is as-sociated with an intraovarian mass, a complex pelvo-abdominal mass is usually identified.[10]

The sonographic differential diagnosis includes ovarian neoplasm, ectopic pregnancy, hemorrhagic cyst, pelvic inflammatory disease (PID), and periap-pendiceal abscess. A proper index of suspicion in

TABLE 5-2. Differential diagnoses of cystic and solid gynecologic masses in children

CYSTIC	SOLID
Anterior meningocele	Chordoma
Neurenteric cysts	Neuroblastoma
Retrorectal cysts	Ganglioneuroma
Ectopic kidney (hydronephrotic)	Neurofibroma
Massive hydroureter	Sacral bone tumors
Bladder diverticulum	Retroperitoneal sarcomas
Hydrosalpinx	Lymphosarcoma
Ovarian cyst	Rhabdomyosarcoma
Hydrometrocolpos	Yolk sac carcinoma

the face of a clinical history that is atypical for these entities may lead to early diagnosis of torsion and salvage of the ovary.[6]

Diagnostic Criteria

The diagnostic criteria are essentially the same for pediatric as for adult gynecologic disorders. Masses can be described as cystic, solid, or complex. Ex-amination techniques such as gain studies should be performed to ensure that hypoechoic homoge-neously solid masses, such as lymphoma, are not mistaken for cystic masses. The presence of ascites, irregular borders, or papillary projections with thickened septa in a mass favors, but is not diag-nostic of, malignancy. Identification of the abnor-mality in relation to normal landmarks often re-veals the organ of origin even in confusing cases.

It must be remembered that sonography is a method to describe and characterize, not make a specific diagnosis. The final diagnosis in most cases requires clinical, radiographic, and laboratory input to narrow the differential possibilities and ar-rive at the diagnosis. Sonography is of prime im-portance in directing further work-up.

Differential Diagnosis

The differential diagnosis of a pediatric gynecologic disorder is extensive and varied. Cystic masses may be of gynecologic origin (ovarian cyst, hy-drosalpinx, hydrocolpos) or of urinary tract origin (bladder diverticulum, hydroureter). In addition, mesenteric cyst, gastrointestinal duplication cyst, pseudocyst, and presacral meningocele must be considered.

Complex masses may be secondary to abscesses, including appendiceal abscess, hematoma (depends on stage of clot), torsion of a mass, or ectopic pregnancy.

Solid masses may represent torsiverted tumors, gynecologic tumors, presacral neural tumors, lymph nodes, and sarcomas of bone origin. Tables 5-1 and 5-2 describe some of the pediatric gynecologic masses and their differential diagnoses.

The sonographic information, clinical history, laboratory values, and hormone assays must all be used in conjunction to narrow the possibilities and arrive at the most likely diagnosis.

References

1. Baramki TA. Treatment of congenital anomalies in girls and women. J Reprod Med. 1984; 29:376–384.
2. Bass IS, Haller JO, Friedman A, et al. Sonography of cystic masses of the pelvis in children. Part 2. Masses originating in female genitalia. Appl Radiol. 1984; 13:144–149.
3. Bicker GH, Siebert JJ, Anderson JC, et al. Sonography of ovarian involvement in childhood acute lymphocytic leukemia. AJR. 1981; 137:399–401.
4. Bowie JD. Sonography of the uterus. In: Sabbagha RE, ed. Diagnostic Ultrasound Applied to Obstetrics and Gynecology. 2nd ed. Philadelphia: JB Lippincott; 1987.
5. Cabrol S, Haseltine FP, Taylor KJ, et al. Ultrasound examination of pubertal girls and of patients with gonadal dysgenesis. J Adolesc Health Care 1981; 1:185–192.
6. Farrell TP, Boal DK, Teele RL, et al. Acute torsion of normal uterine adnexa in children: Sonographic demonstration. AJR. 1982; 139:1223–1225.
7. Fleischer AC, Entmann SS. Sonographic evaluation of the ovary and related disorders. In: Sabbagha RE, ed. Diagnostic Ultrasound Applied to Obstetrics and Gynecology. 2nd ed. Philadelphia; JB Lippincott; 1987.
8. Fleischer AC, Entmann SS, Burnett LS, et al. Principles of differential diagnosis of pelvic masses by sonography. In: Sanders RC, James AE, eds. The Principles and Practice of Ultrasonography in Obstetrics and Gynecology. 3rd ed. Norwalk, CT: Appleton-Century-Crofts; 1985.
9. Fleischer AC, Entmann SS, Porrath SA, et al. Sonographic evaluation of uterine malformations and disorders. In: Sanders RC, James AE, eds. The Princi-
ples and Practice of Ultrasonography in Obstetrics and Gynecology, 3rd ed. Norwalk, CT: Appleton-Century-Crofts; 1985.
10. Fleischer AC, Shawker TH. The role of sonography in pediatric gynecology. Clin Obstet Gynecol. 1987; 30:735–746.
11. Foster CM, Feuillan R, Padmanabhan V, et al. Ovarian function in girls with McCune-Albright syndrome. Pediatr Res 1986; 20:859–863.
12. Gallup D, Talledo OE. Benign and malignant tumors. Clin Obstet Gynecol. 1987; 30:662–670.
13. Graif M, Shaler J, Strauss S, et al. Torsion of the ovary: Sonographic features. Am J Radiol. 1984; 143:1331.
14. Hall DA, Crowley WF, Wierman ME, et al. Sonographic monitoring of LHRH analogue therapy in idiopathic precocious puberty in young girls. J Clin Ultrasound. 1986; 14:331–338.
15. Haller JO, Bass IS, Friedman AP. Pelvic masses in girls: An 8-year retrospective analysis stressing ultrasound as the prime imaging modality. Pediatr Radiol. 1984; 14:363–368.
16. Haller JO, Fellows RA. The pelvis. In: Haller JO, Shkolnik A, eds. Ultrasound in Pediatrics. New York: Churchill Livingstone; 1981.
17. Haller JO, Friedman AP, Schaffer R, et al. The normal and abnormal ovary in childhood and adolescence. Semin Ultrasound. 1983; 4:206–225.
18. Haller JO, Schneider M. The reproductive system. In: Haller JO, Schneider M, eds. Pediatric Ultrasound. Chicago: Year Book Medical Publishers; 1980.
19. Hansmann M, Hackeloer B-J, Staudach A. Examination of the female pelvis. In: Hansmann M, Hackeloer B-J, Staudach A, eds. Ultrasound Diagnosis in Obstetrics and Gynecology. Berlin: Springer-Verlag; 1985.
20. Ivarsson SA, Nilsson KO, Persson PH. Ultrasonography of the pelvic organs in prepubertal and postpubertal girls. Arch Dis Child. 1983; 58:352–354.
21. McCarthy S, Taylor KJW. Sonography of vaginal masses. Am J Radiol. 1983; 140:1005.
22. Merten DF, Kirks DR. Diagnostic imaging of pediatric abdominal masses. Pediatr Clin North Am. 1985; 32:1397–1425.
23. Morely P, Barnett E. The ovarian mass. In: Sanders RC, James AE, eds. The Principles and Practice of Ultrasonography in Obstetrics and Gynecology. 3rd ed. Norwalk, CT: Appleton-Century-Crofts; 1985.
24. Salardi S, Orsini LF, Cacciari E, et al. Pelvic ultrasonography in premenarchal girls: Relation to puberty and sex hormone concentrations. Arch Dis Child. 1985; 60(2):120–125.
25. Schaffer RM, Haller JO, Friedman AP, et al. Sono-

graphic diagnosis of ovarian dysgerminoma in children. Med Ultrasound. 1982; 6:118–119.

26. Schneider M, Grossman H. Sonography of the female child's reproductive system. Ped Ann. 1980; 9:180–186.

27. Shawker T, Comite F, Rieth KG, et al. Ultrasound evaluation of female isosexual precocious puberty. J Ultrasound Med. 1984; 3:309.

28. Shkolnik A. Applications of ultrasound in the neonatal abdomen. Radiol Clin North Am. 1985; 23:361–365.

29. Stanhope R, Adams J, Jacobs HS, et al. Ovarian ultrasound assessment in normal children, idiopathic precocious puberty, and during low-dose pulsatile gonadotrophin-releasing hormone treatment of hypogonadotrophic hypogonadism. Arch Dis Child. 1985; 60:116–119.

30. Stedman TL. Stedman's Medical Dictionary Illustrated. 23rd ed. Baltimore: Williams & Wilkins; 1976:1391.

31. Warner M, Fleischer A, et al. Torsion of the adnexa. Sonographic findings. Radiology. 1985; 154:773.

32. Worthington-Kirsch RL, Raptopoulos V, Cohen IT. Sequential bilateral torsion of normal ovaries in a child. J Ultrasound Med. 1986; 5:663–664.

33. Yaghoobian J, Yankelevitz DF, Pinck RL, et al. Pyometrium in a three-year-old girl: Sonographic findings. J Ultrasound Med. 1984; 3:87–88.

CHAPTER 6

Benign Diseases of the Vagina, Cervix, and Uterus

SATHYANARAYANA, REVA A. CURRY

Ultrasonography of the female pelvis has enabled physicians to assess benign pathologic conditions in detail. A well-trained sonographer can identify the size, shape, internal texture, and location of pathologic lesions, thus narrowing the differential diagnosis and improving patient management.

Ultrasound is noninvasive and presents little discomfort to the patient other than that of a full bladder. The advent of transvaginal sonography eliminates the full-bladder technique and enables better visualization of pelvic structures that lie in the field of view. Closer structures, such as the vagina and cervix, may be visualized better than more distant structures, especially if disease has distorted normal anatomy. Myomas in the fundus of a grossly enlarged uterus, for example, may be too distant to be visualized effectively with the transvaginal technique.

In this chapter we present benign conditions of the vagina, cervix, and uterus. The cause, symptoms, and ultrasound appearance of each lesion are described.

Benign Diseases of the Vagina

GARTNER'S DUCT CYST

Gartner's duct cysts arise from the caudal remnants of the mesonephric duct and usually occur on the anterolateral wall of the vagina.[8,17] The cysts may be single or multiple and are the common cystic lesion of the vagina. They rarely cause symptoms, but if large, they may cause pain and dyspareunia.

Sonography is helpful in delineating the location of the cyst in the anterolateral vaginal wall. The lesion appears as an anechoic mass, with well-defined margins and good sound transmission (see Fig. 4-3).[23]

PRESENCE OF A TAMPON

Care should be taken to avoid mistaking a tampon for an abnormality. The sonographer can avoid this error by asking the patient whether she is wearing a tampon. A tampon in the vaginal canal can be easily identified as an irregularly shaped echogenic focus (Fig 6-1).[22] As the tampon absorbs menstrual blood, it enlarges to fill the vaginal cavity and may appear to distort the vaginal wall. Several risks are associated with the use of tampons. These include vaginal ulcers, toxic shock syndrome, and the "forgotten" tampon.[4]

Occasionally, when a vaginal mass is detected, a thorough patient history may reveal the presence of a tampon. A lost or forgotten tampon appears high in the vagina and may be associated with an unpleasant odor.[4] Vaginal contraceptive sponges are another device that may lie in the vaginal canal. The sponge produces a curvilinear echo in the vagina and casts an acoustic shadow.[19]

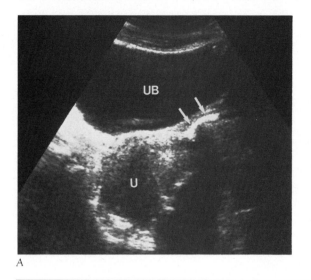
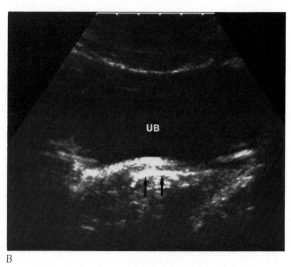

A   B

FIGURE 6-1. A curvilinear, brightly echogenic structure (*arrows*) is present in the vagina in longitudinal (A) and transverse (B) views. This represents a tampon. (U, uterus, UB, urinary bladder.)

Benign Diseases of the Cervix

Benign conditions that produce an enlarged cervix include cervical myoma, nabothian cysts, and cervical polyps.

CERVICAL MYOMA

Cervical myomas are similar histologically to myomas of the uterine corpus and may be confused with myomas from the uterine isthmus. Three to eight percent of myomas are classified as cervical, and most are small and cause no symptoms. Like corpus myomas, asymptomatic masses are observed for growth. Symptoms may include dyspareunia, dysuria, urgency, genitourinary obstruction, cervical obstruction, and prolapse. Symptomatic lesions may be resected, or a hysterectomy may be indicated, depending on the age and reproductive plans of the patient.[4]

Sonographically, cervical myomas may distort the cervix and appear hyper- to hypoechoic, depending on the degree of degeneration (Fig. 6-2).

NABOTHIAN CYSTS

Nabothian cysts are retention cysts of endocervical columnar cells that frequently are seen on vaginal speculum examination as an incidental finding. Nabothian cysts may range from 3 mm to 3 cm in size.[4] They are formed in response to inflammation or squamous epithelial proliferation that blocks the endocervical gland.[4] Mucous secretions accumulate and form retention cysts (nabothian cysts).[4]

Although nabothian cysts are incidental findings on vaginal speculum examinations, sonography is helpful in detecting cysts located high in the cervical canal (Fig. 6-3).[6] Nabothian cysts present as anechoic masses with smooth geometric borders and enhanced sound transmission on ultrasound.

POLYPS

Cervical polyps are common benign neoplasms of the cervix that most often occur in multiparous women in the 40-to 50-year age group,[4] and rarely in postmenopausal women.[10] Polyps are usually attached to the cervical wall by pedicles and may reach a size of several centimeters.[4,17]

Although it is easier to identify small polyps with a transvaginal approach than transabdominally,[30] they are difficult to identify sonographically because of their size. Polyps can appear sonographically as small echogenic foci in the cervix.

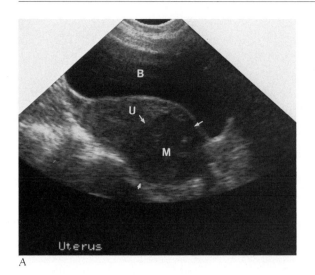

A

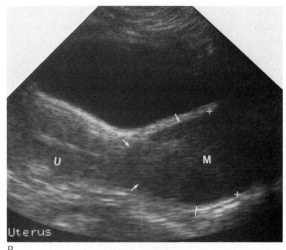

B

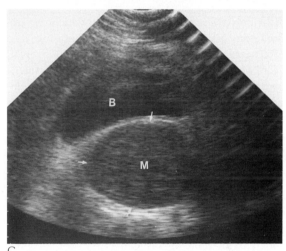

C

FIGURE 6-2. (A) Longitudinal sonogram of the uterus (U) shows large cervical leiomyoma (M) with a mixed, predominantly echopenic echo pattern causing extrinsic compression on the urinary bladder (B). Arrows define the borders of the myoma. (B) Longitudinal and (C) transverse sonograms of the uterus (U) and vaginal canal of a different patient show a large hypoechoic solid mass (M) in the vaginal canal representing a prolapsed cervical leiomyoma. Arrows define the borders of the myoma.

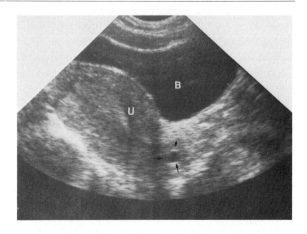

FIGURE 6-3. Longitudinal sonogram of the uterus (U) shows a 1-cm, well-defined, cystic mass in the cervical region (arrows) representing a nabothian cyst. (B, urinary bladder.)

Condylomata Acuminata (Venereal Warts)

Condylomata acuminata, also known as vulvar condylomata acuminata or genital, venereal, or anogenital warts,[4] are transmitted sexually. The incidence of the disease has increased 500% in the last 15 years.[4] The appearance ranges from small papillary growths to large cauliflowerlike masses.[4,10] Condylomata acuminata most often appear in the vulvar area, but they can be found in the vagina and on the cervix.[4,10] The lesions tend to grow during pregnancy and can obstruct the birth canal.[10] A large lesion can appear on ultrasound as an irregular hyperechoic mass and may distort cervical and vaginal contours.

Benign Diseases of the Uterus

Adenomyosis

Adenomyosis is a benign disease in which the endometrial glands and stroma grow deep into the myometrium. Frequently seen in women over 50 years of age, the common symptoms are dysmenorrhea and abnormal bleeding. The cause of adenomyosis is not clear, but it may be secondary to abnormally high levels of estrogen.[4] Adenomyosis is frequently a diffuse process involving the entire uterine wall and resulting in uterine enlargement. The enlargement of the uterus is not usually as prominent as that seen with leiomyoma, but leiomyoma can often coexist with adenomyosis. A focal form of adenomysis can occur with discrete nodules presenting in the myometrium. This is called an adenomyoma (Fig. 6-4).[4,17]

Adenomyosis can be classified into three categories[10]: grade I, restricted to the immediate basal layer; grade II, present in the inner half of the myometrium; and grade III, present in the outer half of the myometrium. Although adenomyosis is considered distinct from endometriosis, the two are associated in 13% of women studied.[33]

Sonographic Findings. Sonographic findings for adenomyosis include an enlarged uterus with normal contours.[2,24] Uterine echogenicity may range from normal[24] to slightly hypoechoic.[2] Areas of decreased echogenicity may represent menstrual engorgement of the endometrial glands (Fig. 6-5).[33]

Sonographers must pay careful attention to technique to accurately assess uterine size, contour, and

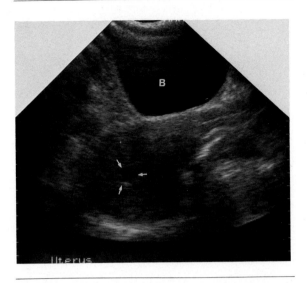

FIGURE 6-4. Longitudinal sonogram of the uterus shows 1-cm cystic lesion (*arrows*) in the myometrium of a retroverted uterus. Although the lesion appeared similar to cystic degeneration of a small leiomyoma, it was found to be a focal adenomyoma. (B, urinary bladder.)

texture. The urinary bladder must cover the fundal area in order that accurate uterine measurements may be obtained. If proper bladder distension is not possible or the uterus is too large, the transducer should be placed at the pubis and angled sharply cephalad. This may help identify the fundal area by enlarging the bladder window.

Leiomyoma

Uterine leiomyomas (also called fibroids) are benign muscle tumors.[4,10,16,17,22] While the term "fibroid tumor" denotes the fibrous tissue components present in some myomas, the proper term is leiomyoma. Other acceptable descriptive terms are fibroma, fibromyoma, and myoma.[4,10]

Leiomyomas are the most common female pelvic tumors and are usually multiple.[8] It has been estimated that up to 20% of women past 35 years of age have leiomyomas.[10,17] The occurrence is markedly greater in blacks than in whites.[4,10] Leiomyomas are usually found in the uterine corpus, but they may also be found in the cervix[4,10,17] and broad ligament.[17] They vary in size from microscopic to

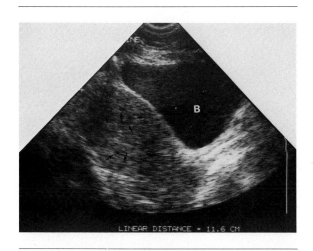

FIGURE 6-5. Longitudinal sonogram of the uterus shows generalized enlargement of the uterus with multiple small 3- to 4-mm cystic areas in the myometrium (*arrows*). Upon histologic examination, this was found to be generalized adenomyosis. (B, urinary bladder.)

large; there is one report of a fibroid weighing over 100 pounds.[10,17]

Pathophysiology. Leiomyomas develop from immature smooth muscle cells of the uterine myometrium. Small myomas are composed entirely of smooth muscle. As they grow, fibrous tissue strands appear between the bundles of smooth muscle.[17] Myomas are described by their location in relation to the uterine wall. The submucous forms lie beneath the endometrium and often project into the endometrial cavity. Large submucous myomas may distort the cavity. Intramural leiomyomas develop interstitially within the myometrium; subserous myomas lie close to the peritoneal surface of the uterus.[4,10,17]

Myomas cause the uterus to contract, and as a result the myomas are compressed and displaced either toward the endometrial cavity (submucous leiomyoma) or toward the peritoneal surface (subserous myoma).[25] Myomas may grow away from myometrium and become pedunculated.[10] Torsion to the pedicle can occur with subsequent infarction, degeneration, and necrosis. Occasionally, pendunculated subserous leiomyomas can detach from the uterus and become parasitic or wandering myomas, deriving their blood supply from the omentum or intestine.[4] Myomas can also grow between the layers of the broad ligaments; such ones are called intraligamentous leiomyomas.[4]

The cause of leiomyomas is unknown. It appears that leiomyoma development may be related to estrogen stimulation.[4,10] This is supported by the fact that myomas are not commonly seen before menarche and usually do not grow after menopause. It is also reported that myomas grow rapidly in women with anovulatory menstrual cycles, where there seems to be unopposed estrogen action.[25]

Degenerative Changes. Leiomyomas have no true capsules. Surrounding uterine muscles often compress the tumor and form a pseudocapsule from which they derive their blood supply.[4] When the myoma outgrows its blood supply, degeneration occurs. The extent of degeneration depends on the severity of the discrepancy between the myoma's growth and its blood supply.[8] Two-thirds of all myomas show some form of degeneration. Various types of degeneration can occur, including hyaline, myxomatous, cystic, calcific, fatty, red degeneration, and necrosis.[17]

The most common types are hyaline degeneration (65%), myxomatous degeneration (15%), and calcific degeneration (10%).[4] In hyaline degeneration, smooth muscle cells are replaced by fibrous tissue. In cystic degeneration, degeneration of hyaline tissue occurs as a result of decreased blood supply, which leads to liquefaction necrosis.

Calcific degeneration occurs most often after menopause.[17] Carnous, or red, degeneration is an acute form resulting from muscle infarction that may occur during pregnancy and can cause acute pain that may require medical treatment. Sarcomatous degeneration is very rare.[4,17] Many types of degeneration are without symptoms. Secondary infection may occur in myomas with advanced degeneration.[4]

Signs and Symptoms. The majority of myomas produce no symptoms. When they do, the most common symptom is alteration in menstrual bleeding—heavy or prolonged flow (or both) with very little change in cycle.[4,10] The submucous and intramural myomas that distort the endometrial cavity

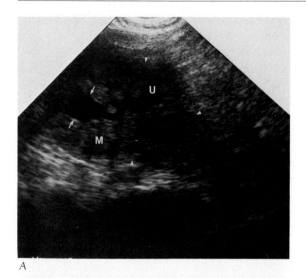

A

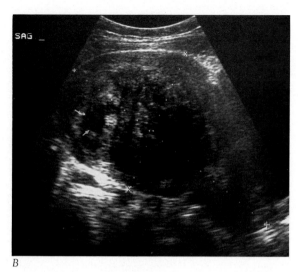

B

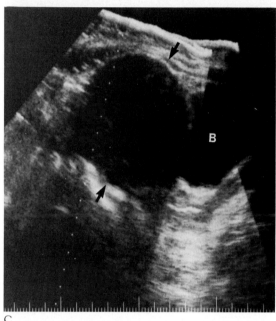

C

FIGURE 6-6. (A) Longitudinal sonogram of the uterus (U) shows anechoic areas (*arrowheads*) with good through-transmission representing cystic degeneration in an echogenic myoma (M). This fundal myoma is intramural (*arrows*). (B) An area of cystic degeneration (*arrows*) is present in this uterus enlarged by leiomyomas. (C) Longitudinal static sonogram of an enlarged uterus depicts a large anechoic mass with poor sound transmission replacing the uterine fundus (*arrows*). This was found to be a large intramural myoma with hyaline degeneration. (B, urinary bladder.)

cause abnormal bleeding. Dysmenorrhea is not a common symptom; however, it can occur with pedunculated submucous myomas.[4]

The signs and symptoms of degeneration depend on the size and location of the myoma. Pain may indicate some form of a degenerative process, or it may be the result of torsion of the pedunculated myoma, an infection, or large tumors pressing on pelvic nerve roots.

Leiomyomas may produce pressure symptoms on bladder or rectum in the form of frequent urination or difficult evacuation.[4] Infertility can result if the tumor is close to the isthmic area and if it causes distortion of the fallopian tubes. Leiomyomas can also cause uterine inertia and can obstruct normal vaginal delivery. Spontaneous abortion may occur if implantation is on or near a submucous leiomyoma.

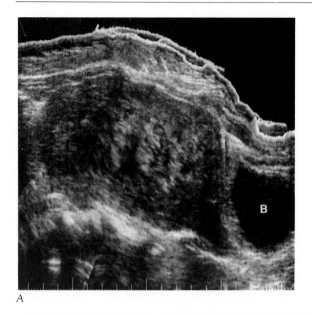 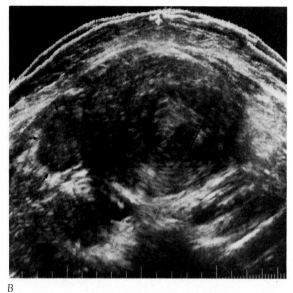

A   B

FIGURE 6-7. (A) Longitudinal and (B) transverse static sonograms show an enlarged uterus with lobulated margins. Also depicted is a large intramural fibroid with a whorled internal architecture. A small pedunculated fibroid is also seen on the right side of the fundus on a transverse scan *(arrows)*. (B, urinary bladder.)

Sonographic Appearance. A wide range of sonographic findings are associated with myomas.[1,9] The sonographic appearance of myomas depends on the degree and type of degeneration present and can range from hypoechoic to echogenic. Cystic degeneration can cause hypoechoic areas within the myoma (Fig. 6-6). A whorled internal architecture can form when bundles of smooth muscle and fibrous tissue are arranged concentrically within a myoma (Fig. 6-7). Calcific degeneration may cause shadowing (Fig. 6-8). A whorled, calcific myoma can even resemble a fetal head (Fig. 6-9). Red degeneration can present as medium echoes with good sound transmission.[11]

The sonographic appearance of myomas also depends on their number, size, and location. Large myomas disrupt uterine contour much more than smaller ones (Fig. 6-10). Multiple large subserous myomas may cause an enlarged uterus with a lobulated contour (Fig. 6-11); large intramural and submucous myomas can distend the uterine cavity and distort the endometrial echoes (Figs. 6-12, 6-13). Large myomas in the anterior and posterior uterine walls can cause extrinsic compression on the urinary bladder and rectum that appears sonographically to indent the usually smooth uterus-bladder interface (Fig. 6-10A).

Because leiomyomas can enlarge the uterus considerably and may present outside the uterus in a pedunculated form, care must be taken to demonstrate the entire pelvic area to document both uterine and extrauterine myomas (see Fig. 6-7B). A pedunculated fibroid can be mistaken for a number of conditions, including bicornuate uterus (Fig. 6-14), ovarian mass, hydatidiform mole, and ectopic pregnancy.[1]

Accurate gain settings are important for proper assessment of the extent of degeneration. The cervix can be used as a reference point for normal uterine texture when severe degeneration has occurred or when multiple myomas distort normal uterine echo patterns. When the uterus is grossly enlarged, it is likely that the bladder will not be able to cover the fundus. Cephalad transducer an-

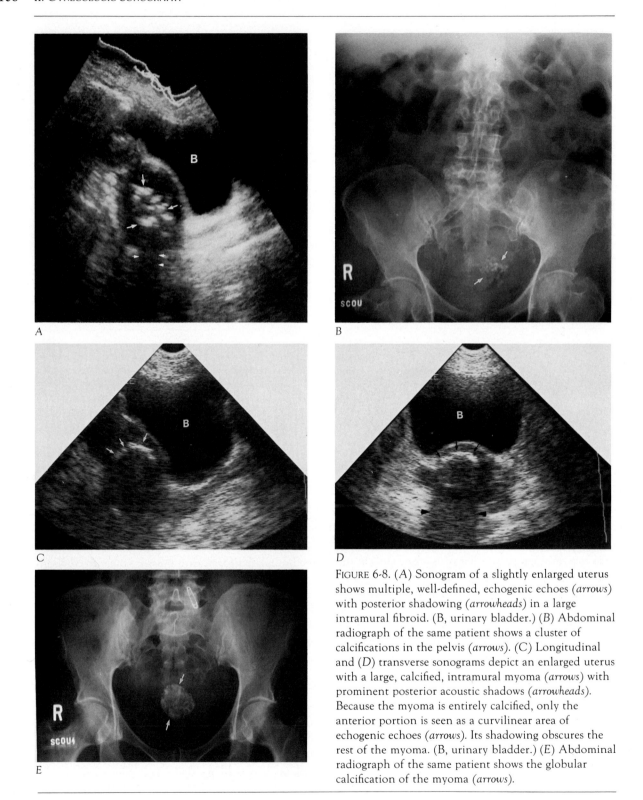

FIGURE 6-8. (A) Sonogram of a slightly enlarged uterus shows multiple, well-defined, echogenic echoes (*arrows*) with posterior shadowing (*arrowheads*) in a large intramural fibroid. (B, urinary bladder.) (B) Abdominal radiograph of the same patient shows a cluster of calcifications in the pelvis (*arrows*). (C) Longitudinal and (D) transverse sonograms depict an enlarged uterus with a large, calcified, intramural myoma (*arrows*) with prominent posterior acoustic shadows (*arrowheads*). Because the myoma is entirely calcified, only the anterior portion is seen as a curvilinear area of echogenic echoes (*arrows*). Its shadowing obscures the rest of the myoma. (B, urinary bladder.) (E) Abdominal radiograph of the same patient shows the globular calcification of the myoma (*arrows*).

FIGURE 6-9. Sector image, sagittal plane, depicts fetal skull *(arrows)* and calcified myoma *(arrowheads)*.

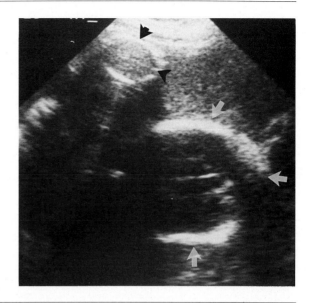

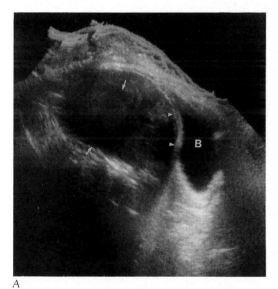

A

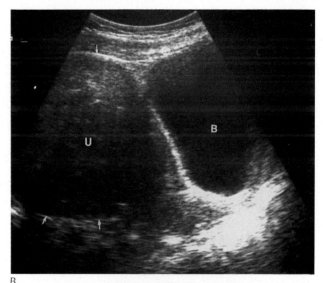

B

FIGURE 6-10. (A) Longitudinal static sonogram shows an enlarged uterus with a large hypoechoic fundal myoma *(arrows)*. There is extrinsic compression *(arrowheads)* on the urinary bladder (B). (B) A uterus (U) enlarged by leiomyomas may be difficult to visualize in its entirety on one sonogram. Arrows define the border of the uterus. (B, urinary bladder.) (C) Longitudinal sonogram shows an enlarged uterus with a somewhat lobulated contour depicting multiple small intramural and subserous myomas, which are predominantly hypoechoic *(arrows)*. (B, urinary bladder.)

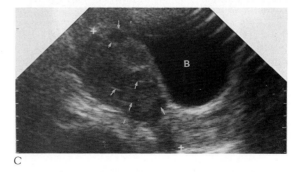

C

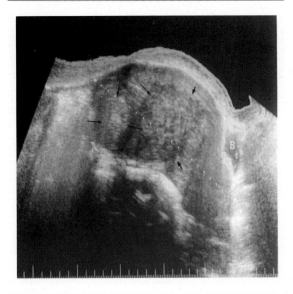

FIGURE 6-11. Longitudinal static sonogram of a grossly enlarged uterus shows a lobulated contour from multiple subserous and intramural myomas (arrows). An intramural myoma was found to protrude into the uterine cavity. (B, urinary bladder.)

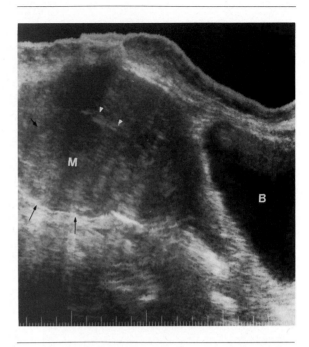

FIGURE 6-12. Longitudinal static sonogram of the uterus depicts a large intramural myoma (M) in the posterior uterine wall (arrows) displacing the endometrial cavity anteriorly (arrowheads). (B, urinary bladder.)

gulation avoids overlying bowel. Increased gain settings may be needed to assess myomas in enlarged uteri in lieu of a bladder window.

Anteroposterior measurements generally are not difficult to obtain because, as the uterus enlarges, it moves farther anterior and, therefore, closer to the body wall. Proper focal depth settings and transducer selection will be important. A 3.0- or 3.5-MHz transducer should be used, depending on the size of the uterus. Pertinent uterine dimensions include the length and the anteroposterior diameter, both of which are measured in the sagittal plane, and the width, which is measured in the transverse plane. If possible, measurements should be obtained of the myomas as well. Sonographers should bear in mind that general uterine enlargement is normal for a multiparous uterus. Accurate uterine measurements help the clinician monitor myoma growth and can be useful in planning surgical removal of the myomas.

Transvaginal imaging of leiomyomas. Transvaginal sonography has improved the diagnostic capability of ultrasound examinations of the pelvis. Several studies have shown transvaginal sonography to be superior to transabdominal imaging in the detection of pelvic masses, including leiomyomas (Figs. 6-15, 6-16).[3,13,29,31] Transvaginal sonography can provide improved visualization and additional information of pelvic structures and conditions.[3,13,29,31]

The advantages of the transvaginal technique include improved tissue characterization (Fig. 6-17), higher resolution, and shorter examination time (a full bladder is not necessary).[13] Disadvantages include a decreased field of view (grossly enlarged uteri and very large myomas may not be seen in their entirety) and the challenge of viewing anatomic structures in a new orientation.[13] Improved visualization of leiomyomas with the transvaginal technique can provide better assessment of texture, number, and location of myomas.

Magnetic resonance imaging of leiomyomas. Recent

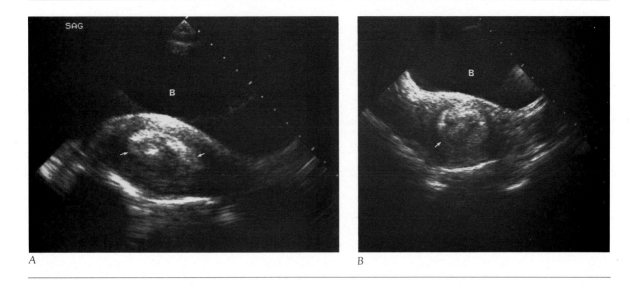

FIGURE 6-13. Longitudinal (A) and transverse (B) sonograms depict a brightly echogenic, curvilinear structure (arrows) in the area of the endometrial cavity. This finding is consistent with a submucosal myoma. (B, urinary bladder.)

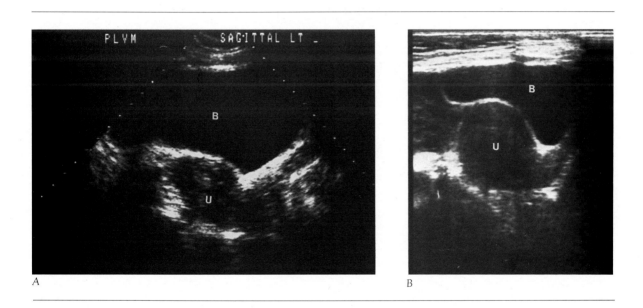

FIGURE 6-14. (A) Sector image, sagittal plane, of the left horn of a bicornuate uterus (U). (B, urinary bladder.) (B) Same patient. Linear array image, sagittal plane of the right horn of the bicornuate uterus (U), enlarged by leiomyomas. (B, urinary bladder.)

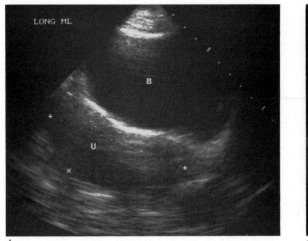

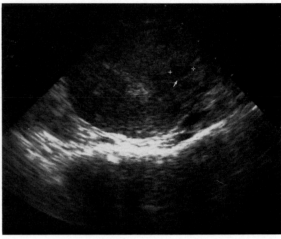

A

B

FIGURE 6-15. (A) Transabdominal image of uterus (U) enlarged with myomas. (B, urinary bladder.) The echo pattern of the uterus is not well seen. (B) Same patient. Transvaginal scan of the uterine fundus depicts the heterogeneous echo pattern of the uterus, including areas of cystic degeneration (*arrow*).

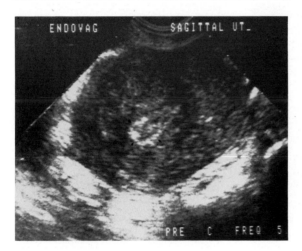

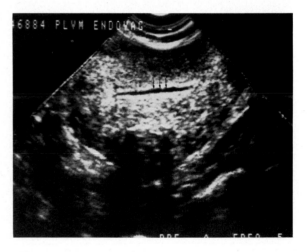

FIGURE 6-16. Sagittal transvaginal view of the uterus depicts a heterogeneous echo pattern with areas of cystic degeneration. Also present is an area of intense echogenicity (*arrows*). Findings are consistent with leiomyoma.

FIGURE 6-17. Transvaginal scan of a myomatous uterus with a fluid collection in the endometrial cavity (*arrows*). As this patient was postmenopausal and presented with vaginal bleeding, endometrial carcinoma was suspected.

studies indicate that magnetic resonance imaging (MRI) may improve visualization of leiomyomas.[5,34] MRI examinations were able to detect the number, location, and size of myomas better than transabdominal ultrasound.[5,34] MRI evaluation is recommended to locate myomas prior to surgery.[5]

DIETHYLSTILBESTROL

The drug diethylstilbestrol (DES) was given to pregnant women between the 1940s and the 1950s[20] to prevent premature labor and reduce pregnancy complications[26] in pregnancies complicated by toxemia, diabetes, premature labor, or threatened abortion. It was later discovered that DES provided no benefit to the women who received the drug and actually increased the incidence of abortions, premature births, and neonatal deaths.[26] It is estimated that 2 to 3 million male and female offspring were exposed to the drug in utero; they are at increased risk for anatomic and reproductive malformations.[26]

Approximately 50 to 75% of female offspring of mothers who took DES are affected by vaginal adenosis,[26] a condition characterized by the atypical presence of glandular structures in the vagina, which have a tendency to undergo squamous metaplasia.[7,20] It had been suggested that adenosis may precede the development of clear cell carcinoma.[7,20] DES-exposed female offspring are at a greater risk, especially before age 19, of developing clear cell carcinoma; however, the overall prevalence is low compared to the total number of females exposed to DES.[26] Other anomalies include cervical and vaginal malformations.[7,20]

DES-exposed females are at increased risk of pregnancy complications such as ectopic pregnancy, first-trimester abortion, and premature labor.[12] Premature labor may be caused in part by an incompetent cervix,[14,15] another side effect of DES exposure. Serial sonograms have been recommended to assess the cervix for incompetency during pregnancy.[14,15]

Documented uterine anomalies include a small uterus and T-shaped uterus.[18,21,32] Uterine texture is normal in both entities. The T-shaped uterus is best demonstrated in the transverse view.[20,21] Uterine tissue resembling a T can be seen in the fundal area. Careful technique and attention to detail are necessary, as the uterus may be smaller than normal.

TABLE 6-1. Sonographic appearance of benign lesions of the vagina, cervix, and uterus

CONDITION	ULTRASOUND APPEARANCE
Gartner's duct cyst	Anechoic mass with well-defined margins and good sound transmission located in the anterolateral wall of the vagina
Tampon	Echogenic mass producing acoustic shadowing posteriorly, within the vaginal canal
Nabothian cyst	Anechoic mass (3 mm–3 cm) with good sound transmission located in the cervical canal
Cervical polyp	Often very small and difficult to identify sonographically
Condylomata acuminata	Large lesion involving the cervix, can appear as irregular solid mass distorting cervix; sonography cannot demonstrate small lesions
Adenomyosis	Enlarged uterus with smooth contour
Leiomyoma	Varies in echogenicity and appears as hypoechoic or echogenic nodules. Hyaline degeneration within a myoma appears as an anechoic mass with poor sound transmission. Cystic degeneration within a myoma appears as an anechoic mass with good sound transmission. Calcification within a myoma produces focal echogenic areas with acoustic shadowing.
DES exposure in utero	Nonpregnant uterus small and T-shaped, possible incompetent cervix in pregnancy

Male offspring exposed to DES have been found to have less motile sperm, lower sperm count, and a higher incidence of testicular anomalies and epididymal cysts.[26] Ultrasound may be useful in documenting testicular size and texture and in locating epididymal cysts.

References

1. Baltarowich OH, Kurtz AB, Pennell RG, et al. Pitfalls in the sonographic diagnosis of uterine fibroids. AJR. 1988; 151:725–728.

2. Bohlman ME, Ensor RE, Sanders RC. Sonographic findings in adenomyosis of the uterus. AJR. 1987; 148:765–766.

3. Coleman BG, Arger PH, Grumback K, et al. Transvaginal and transabdominal sonography: Prospective comparison. Radiology. 1988; 168:639–643.

4. Droegemueller W, Herbst AL, Mishell DR, et al. Comprehensive Gynecology. St. Louis: CV Mosby; 1987.

5. Dudiak CM, Turner DA, Patel SK, et al. Uterine leiomyomas in the infertile patient: Preoperative localization with MR imaging versus US and hysterosalpingography. Radiology. 1988; 176:627–630.

6. Fogel SR, Slaskey BS. Sonography of nabothian cysts. AJR. 1982; 138:927.

7. Fox H, Buckley CH. Pathology for Gynecologists. Baltimore: University Park Press; 1983.

8. Gompel C, Silverberg SG. Pathology in Gynecology and Obstetrics. 3rd ed. Philadelphia: JB Lippincott Co; 1985.

9. Gross BH, Siver TM, Jaffe MH. Sonographic features of uterine leiomyomas: Analysis of 41 proven cases. Ultrasound Med. 1983; 2:401–406.

10. Hale RW, Krieger J, eds. Gynecology: A Concise Textbook. Garden City, NY: Medical Examination Publishing Co: 1983.

11. Lev-Toaff AS, Coleman BG, Arger PH, et al. Leiomyomas in pregnancy: Sonographic study. Radiology. 1987; 164:375–380.

12. Mangan CE, Borrow L, Burtnett-Rubin MM, et al. Pregnancy outcome in 98 women exposed to diethylstilbestrol in utero, their mothers, and unexposed siblings. Obstet Gynecol. 1982; 59:315–319.

13. Mendelson EB, Bohm-Velez M, Joseph N, et al. Gynecologic imaging: Comparison of transabdominal and transvaginal sonography. Radiology. 1988; 166:321–324.

14. Michaels WH, Montgomery C, Karo J, et al. Ultrasound differentiation of the competent from the incompetent cervix: Prevention of preterm delivery. Am J Obstet Gynecol. 1986; 154:537–546.

15. Michaels WH, Thompson HO, Schreiber FR, et al. Ultrasound surveillance of the cervix during pregnancy in diethylstilbestrol-exposed offspring. Obstet Gynecol. 1989; 79:230–238.

16. Novak ER, Jones GS, Jones HW Jr. Novak's Textbook of Gynecology. 9th ed. Baltimore: Williams & Wilkins; 1975.

17. Novak ER, Woodruff JD, eds. Novak's Gynecologic and Obstetric Pathology. 8th ed. Philadelphia: WB Saunders Co; 1979.

18. Nunley WC, Pope TL. Upper reproductive tract radiography findings. AJR. 1984; 142:337–339.

19. Odwin C. Sonographic appearance of a vaginal contraceptive sponge. Diagn Med Sonog. 1985; 1:65–67.

20. Peckham B, Shapiro S. Signs and Symptoms in Gynecology. Philadelphia: JB Lippincott; 1983.

21. Sabbagha R, ed. Diagnostic Ultrasound Applied to Obstetrics and Gynecology. 2nd ed. Philadelphia: JB Lippincott, 480–482.

22. Sanders R, James AE, eds. Principles and Practice of Ultrasonography in Obstetrics and Gynecology. 3rd ed. New York: Appleton-Century-Crofts; 1985.

23. Scheible FW. Ultrasonic features of Gartner's duct cysts. J Clin Ultrasound. 1978; 6:438.

24. Siedler D, Laing FC, Jeffrey RB Jr, Wing VW. Uterine adenomyosis—A difficult sonographic diagnosis. Ultrasound Med. 1987; 6:345–349.

25. Smith JP, Weiser EB, Karnei RF, et al. Sonography of rapidly growing uterine leiomyomata associated with anovulatory cycles. Radiology. 1980; 134:713–716.

26. Stillman RJ. In utero exposure to diethylstilbestrol: Adverse effects on the reproductive tract and reproductive performance in male and female offspring. Am J Obstet Gynecol. 1982; 142:905–920.

29. Tessler Fn, Schiller VL, Perrella RR, et al. Transabdominal versus endovaginal pelvic sonography: Prospective study. Radiology. 1988; 170:553–556.

30. Timor-Tritsch IE, Rottem S. Transvaginal Sonography. New York: Elsevier; 1988.

31. Vilaro MM, Rifkin MD, Pennell RG, et al. Endovaginal ultrasound—A technique for evaluation of nonfollicular pelvic masses. J Ultrasound Med. 1987; 6:697–701.

32. Viscomi GN, Gonzalez R, Taylor KJW. Ultrasound detection of uterine anomalies. Radiology. 1980; 136:733.

33. Walsh JW, Taylor KJW, Rosenfield AT. Gray scale ultrasonography in the diagnosis of endometriosis and adenomyosis. AJR. 1979; 132:87–90.

34. Weinreb JC, Brown CE, Lowe TW, et al. Pelvic masses in pregnant patients: MR and US imaging. Radiology. 1986; 159:717–724.

CHAPTER 7

Malignant Diseases
of the Uterus and Cervix

RUTH ROSENBLATT

The uterus is the most common site of pelvic malignancy, accounting for 10% of cancers diagnosed in women.[1] A number of pathologically and clinically distinct lesions are encountered. Three of these are discussed here: endometrial carcinoma, carcinoma of the cervix, and malignant gestational trophoblastic diseases.

A reversal in the incidence of carcinoma of the endometrium and cervix has been observed in the past several decades. Carcinoma of the endometrium has become statistically more significant, being twice as common now as carcinoma of the cervix. This is due in part to better control of carcinoma of the cervix as a result of early diagnosis by means of the Papanicolaou (Pap) smear. Furthermore, endometrial carcinoma occurs later in life than carcinoma of the cervix, and the increased life span in recent years undoubtedly has a bearing on the reversed incidence of endometrial carcinoma.

Mortality from carcinoma of the cervix is more than twice that of carcinoma of the endometrium.[1] This is probably due to the fact that carcinoma of the cervix is a more virulent disease when allowed to progress beyond the early stages; in addition, this malignancy is more commonly seen among the low socioeconomic strata, where the availability of routine examination may be limited.

Morphologic changes produced by endometrial carcinoma may be observed with ultrasound. Intracavitary transducers (transvaginal and endorectal)

further improve visualization of the regional anatomy in many cases, providing information that can aid in staging of endometrial and cervical malignancies. Therefore, the role of ultrasound in the diagnosis and management of carcinoma of the uterus and cervix has been expanding.

Endometrial Carcinoma

CLINICAL INFORMATION

Epidemiology and Risk Factors. In the United States endometrial carcinoma is the most commonly encountered malignancy of the female genital tract. About three-quarters of the patients are diagnosed and treated at a relatively early stage, and an overall 5-year cure rate of close to 75% may be attained.[3] Carcinoma of the endometrium is seen frequently in the clinical setting of obesity, hypertension, diabetes, and, it is claimed, short stature. It is also more common among Jewish women, suggesting some genetic predisposition.[16]

There is evidence to suggest a relationship between elevated estrogen levels in perimenopausal and postmenopausal patients and the development of endometrial carcinoma.[12] Estrogen has a proliferative effect on the endometrium. A number of premenopausal conditions, probably related to estrogen imbalance, place some women at higher risk for developing carcinoma of the endometrium later—dysfunctional uterine bleeding with failure of ovulation, adenomatous hyperplasia of the

Table 7-1. Uterine carcinoma: Relationship of FIGO stage to 5-year survival

FIGO	Staging of Carcinoma of the Uterus	5-Year Survival (%)
Stage I	Lesion confined to body of uterus	76
I A	Uterus not larger than 8 cm	
I B	Uterus larger than 8 cm	
Stage II	Lesion extends to involve the cervix	50
Stage III	Extension beyond uterus but within the pelvis	30
Stage IV	Involvement of bladder, rectum, or distant metastases	9

(Adapted from Thigpen JT. Approaches to the evaluation and management of endometrial carcinoma. In: Forastiere AA, ed. Gynecologic Cancer. New York: Churchill Livingstone; 1984: 219.)

endometrium, and polycystic ovaries (Stein-Leventhal syndrome). In the perimenopausal and postmenopausal age group, the presence of a functioning theca-granulosa cell tumor of the ovary (usually estrogen-producing) is associated with an increased incidence of endometrial carcinoma. Prolonged intake of therapeutic estrogen after menopause, which some women take to alleviate postmenopausal symptoms including osteoporosis, has been implicated as a risk factor.[16]

Pathophysiology. On gross examination, endometrial carcinoma may be exophytic and polypoid, sometimes filling the uterine cavity. Growth toward the myometrium produces first superficial, then deep, myometrial infiltration. Uterine enlargement is often, but not always, present. Myometrial infiltration is more apt to occur with poorly differentiated tumors and is associated with an increased incidence of lymph node metastases and poorer prognosis. Spread to the cervix is an important criterion for tumor staging. In late stages, transmural spread of tumor to the adnexa occurs. Another route for pelvic extension is retrograde, toward the fallopian tubes and ovaries. Distant metastases occur via the pelvic lymphatics, eventually involving retroperitoneal lymph nodes. Histologically, endometrial carcinoma is classified into grades I through III, depending on the degree of tumor differentiation. This histologic classification is distinct from staging of disease, which is based on extent of tumor spread (Table 7-1). Both tumor grade and stage are diagnostic parameters that influence treatment.

Clinical Diagnosis. Carcinoma of the endometrium is usually diagnosed in the sixth or seventh decade and the principal presenting symptom is abnormal bleeding or discharge. Pain may also occur because of uterine distension resulting from intracavity bleeding associated with cervical blockage. Dilation and curettage and endometrial biopsy provide the tissue necessary to confirm the diagnosis of endometrial carcinoma. Important diagnostic features in staging the disease include depth of myometrial invasion; involvement of the cervix; spread to the tubes, ovaries, or pelvic lymph nodes; and distant metastases (see Table 7-1). Prognosis depends also on pathologic grade.

Treatment. Carcinoma of the endometrium is treated by total hysterectomy and bilateral salpingo-oophorectomy. Depending on tumor grade and stage, radiation therapy is frequently added before or after surgery. In more advanced cases, preoperative intrauterine radium therapy is sometimes used. Treatment of stage IV disease is individualized and may include chemotherapy. The 5-year survival statistics range from 9 to 76%, depending on the stage of disease at the time of diagnosis.[21]

Sonographic Imaging

Diagnostic Features. For patients with abnormal uterine bleeding pelvic ultrasound (US) is often the initial study. The uterus may appear entirely normal sonographically in the early stage of endometrial carcinoma.[18] In most cases, however, some change in the size, shape, and acoustic texture of the uterus will be observed. A common finding is increased uterine size, either length or anteroposterior diameter. In the absence of fibroids, a postmenopausal uterus should not exceed 7 cm in length and 2 cm in anteroposterior dimension. A bulbous or lobulated uterine contour may also be present.[4,18] When seen in a postmenopausal

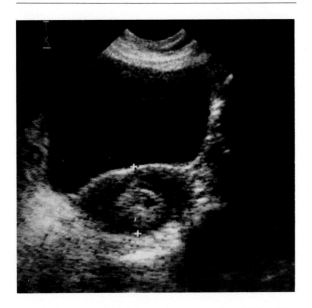

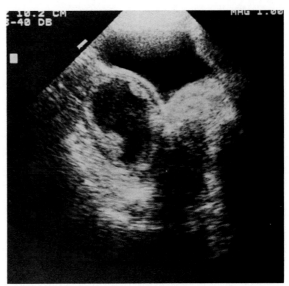

FIGURE 7-1. Stage I endometrial carcinoma. The 60-year-old patient experienced postmenopausal bleeding. A transverse view of the enlarged uterus demonstrates irregular thickening of the endometrium and fluid collections in the endometrial cavity representing blood and tissue necrosis.

FIGURE 7-2. Stage I endometrial carcinoma with cervical stenosis. The 91-year-old patient had abdominal pain. The sagittal scan of the pelvis shows hematometra. Note the echogenic fluid and nodular endometrial surface. (Courtesy Janet Hoffman and Flora Mincer, Albert Einstein College of Medicine.)

woman, a more suspicious finding is thickening of the endometrial reflection (exceeding 3 mm; Fig. 7-1).[4] The prominent endometrial pattern, together with fluid in the cavity representing blood or secretions, may resemble a distorted gestational sac (Fig. 7-2).

Recently, attention has been focused on the role of sonographic imaging in staging of endometrial carcinoma and determining myometrial extension after the diagnosis has been made histologically. Accurate staging is an important guide to successful management of the disease. For example, if an imaging test suggests myometrial extension (which increases the likelihood of lymphatic involvement) the patient may receive preoperative radiation therapy.

Detailed analysis of the endometrial reflection and the subendometrial sonolucent halo (which corresponds in location to the compact vascular inner myometrial segment) may provide a clue to the presence or extent of myometrial invasion (Fig. 7-3). In a recent study of 20 cases of endometrial carcinoma, sonographic analysis of myometrial involvement was accurate within 10% in 14 of 20 cases.[6] It has been suggested that preservation of the subendometrial halo in the presence of endometrial carcinoma would imply superficial involvement only. In many cases, transvaginal scanning facilitates the detailed study of endometrial and myometrial texture (Fig. 7-4). Recently, intrauterine scanning has also been advocated as an accurate means of determining extent of myometrial invasion by tumor.[14] This procedure, which requires dilation of the cervix and insertion of a probe into the uterus, is, of course, more invasive, requiring anesthesia and it is not likely to be used routinely. Myometrial tumor invasion may be hypoechoic or hyperechoic. The increased echogenicity may be related to a more differentiated mucin-producing lesion, whereas the hypoechoic areas may indicate zones of necrosis or an anaplastic lesion that does not form glandular elements.[6]

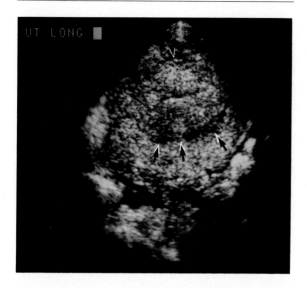

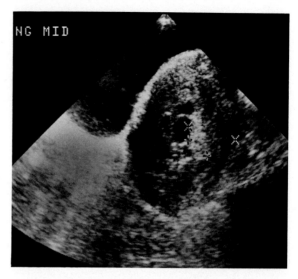

FIGURE 7-3. Stage I endometrial carcinoma. The 80-year-old patient reported vaginal bleeding. The longitudinal view of the uterus using the transvaginal probe shows marked thickening of endometrium (to 50% of the total uterine thickness). Note the partially visualized sonolucent subendometrial halo (arrows).

FIGURE 7-4. Stage I endometrial carcinoma with myometrial invasion. A 79-year-old woman had vaginal bleeding and a history of breast carcinoma. The sagittal transvaginal view of the uterus demonstrated an irregularly thickened endometrial reflection measuring 11 mm (between cursors), suggesting myometrial extension of tumor.

US has a useful role in helping to distinguish carcinoma confined to the uterus (stage I or II) from carcinoma extending beyond the uterus (stage III or IV). Presence of a mass adjacent to the uterus may represent direct extension, metastases to the ovary, lymph node enlargement, or a coincidental ovarian mass. Attention to the uterine cervix, especially to expansion greater than 2 or 3 cm, and heterogeneous sonographic pattern may also separate stage I from stage II disease (Table 7-1). If the urinary bladder is involved with tumor, ureteral obstruction is likely to be present. The kidneys should be scanned for evidence of hydronephrosis.

The major role of US in treatment planning is the delineation and assessment of endometrial length.[9] When intracavitary radiotherapy is contemplated this information is valuable in facilitating the selection of an appropriate applicator (Fig. 7-5). Proper placement of the applicator can be monitored with US, and the scan also provides spatial relationships that allow calculation of the ra-

diation dose to the surrounding tissue and bladder wall (see Fig. 7-5).

Although pelvic US may be used to monitor treated patients for recurrent disease, computed tomography (CT) is more commonly employed because it affords better definition of pelvic side walls and retroperitoneal anatomy.

Technique and Protocol. A systematic sonographic examination of the pelvis with special attention to the uterus should include a number of anatomic structures. The uterus should be depicted in its long axis (which is not necessarily paralled to the long axis of the patient). The dimension from the fundus to and including the cervix should be measured. Insertion of a tampon or Foley catheter (with balloon inflated) into the vagina prior to scanning helps to identify the cervix. The sonographer should observe the cervix for changes in size and echogenicity if endometrial carcinoma is sus-

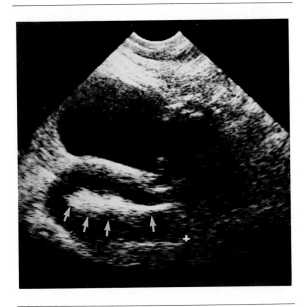

FIGURE 7-5. Stage II endometrial carcinoma with involvement of the cervix. The 61-year-old patient presented with bleeding. Patient had preoperative radiotherapy with intracavitary tandem. Sagittal scan of the uterus demonstrates a high-amplitude reflection from the endometrium representing the tandem and the endometrial thickening (arrows). Study was done to monitor position of the tandem prior to insertion of radioactive sources.

pected. Overall thickness of the uterus is measured in the anteroposterior axis.

It is important to identify the endometrial reflection, which represents the endometrial canal. Endometrial thickening, if present, may be expressed as a percentage of total myometrial thickness by dividing the thickness of the thickest portion of the endometrium (from the lumen to the margin) by the myometrial wall thickness and multiplying by 100 (Fig. 7-3). The sonographer should note whether the myometrial echoes are homogeneous or heterogeneous.

Attention should then be focused on the adnexal region, to identify the ovaries and any adnexal masses. Pelvic and abdominal ascites should be noted.

Whenever sonographic findings in the pelvis suggest a neoplasm, the examination should be ex-

tended to the liver to search for possible metastases. In addition, the paraaortic and paracaval areas should be scanned to search for adenopathy. Finally the kidneys should be imaged to document the presence or absence of hydronephrosis.

OTHER IMAGING MODALITIES

CT is most useful for determining the extent of tumor inside and outside the pelvis of patients who have stage III or IV disease. Enlarged retroperitoneal lymph nodes, urinary tract obstruction, and liver metastases are readily visualized.

The advantage of magnetic resonance imaging (MRI) of the pelvis is the ability to provide sagittal, coronal, and transverse images and to display intrinsic tissue contrast of fat, bowel gas, bone, and blood vessels. These factors contribute to good anatomic resolution in the pelvis. Furthermore, obesity is not an impediment to MRI. (Patients with endometrial carcinoma frequently are obese.) The origin of a mass can be assigned to the appropriate organ with reasonable accuracy. The ability of MRI to resolve different layers of the uterus (e.g., endometrium and myometrium separated by the junctional zone) has made it a valuable tool for assessing the presence and degree of myometrial invasion by tumor.[11]

DIFFERENTIAL DIAGNOSIS

Prominence and thickening of the endometrial layer seen on ultrasound are not specific signs of endometrial carcinoma. The differential diagnosis includes endometrial hyperplasia, which may be a precursor to carcinoma in some cases. Endometrial polyps may also increase echogenicity, as may secretions or blood in the endometrial cavity. In postmenopausal women all of these conditions are likely to be accompanied by abnormal bleeding and would, in most cases, call for curettage. The most common cause of uterine enlargement is leiomyoma; so an enlarged bulbous or lobulated uterus associated with abnormal bleeding does not necessarily imply endometrial carcinoma but could be due to fibroids, either alone or associated with endometrial carcinoma. Fibroids could also distort the endometrial reflection, making it difficult to appreciate any endometrial thickening. Hematometra and pyometra may also be secondary to cervical carcinoma or cervical stenosis. When endometrial carcinoma extends to the cervix it may resemble primary cervical carcinoma sonographically.

LEIOMYOSARCOMA

Leiomyosarcoma is a rare malignancy, accounting for only 3% of uterine tumors. This lesion is derived from smooth muscle in the wall of the uterus. It is believed to arise from preexisting leiomyoma or fibroid. The diagnosis of leiomyosarcoma may be suspected when a fibroid undergoes a growth spurt (rather than regression) in a perimenopausal or postmenopausal patient. The lesion is rarely diagnosed preoperatively. Sonographically, leiomyosarcoma may be indistinguishable from the myoma, especially when cystic degeneration is present.

Carcinoma of the Cervix

CLINICAL INFORMATION

Epidemiology and Risk Factors. Carcinoma of the cervix accounts for 6% of malignancies of women. Its incidence is about half that of carcinoma of the endometrium. In the past few decades, a decrease in the incidence of invasive carcinoma of the cervix has been observed, a trend that is due largely to the increasing availability of the Pap test. Unlike the ovary, which by virtue of its location deep in the pelvis often is not amenable to early diagnosis of malignancy, the cervix is easily accessible to visual inspection and palpation in the course of a gynecologic examination. As a result, there has been an increase in the diagnosis of early carcinoma (carcinoma in situ). The availability of cytologic screening has led to a reduction in mortality.

Epidemiologic studies suggest a number of individual risk factors for carcinoma of the cervix, of which the most consistent are early sexual activity, multiple sex partners, and herpes virus type 2 infection.[12] Cancer of the cervix develops at an earlier age in India, where early marriage has been customary. Conversely, the disease is virtually unknown among celibate women. In the United States, the disease is more prevalent among the Puerto Rican and black populations and least common among Jewish women. This ethnic variation has led some authors to speculate on the possible significance of coitus with uncircumcised men. It has been suggested that secretions contained in the smegma of uncircumcised men constitute an irritant to the cervical mucosa and promote cancer in susceptible women.[12]

The incidence of adenocarcinoma of the cervix and vagina is increased among women who were exposed to diethylstilbestrol (DES) in utero. This drug was used during the 1940s and 1950s to support pregnancy for habitual aborters.

Pathophysiology. Two types of cells form the lining of the cervix. The mucosal covering of the lower cervix is squamous epithelium, which gives rise to squamous carcinoma and accounts for 90 to 95% of lesions. The cervical canal (endocervix) is lined with columnar epithelium, which may give rise to adenocarcinoma. The junction between the two types of epithelium is the site of active mitotic activity, or metaplasia. The transition from columnar to squamous epithelium occurs most actively during menarche and pregnancy with eversion of the cervix. Cervical cancer invariably arises at this junction, initially as carcinoma in situ. The concept that has been proposed is that this site of physiologic mitotic activity (metaplasia) is subject to transformation into neoplastic growth by exposure to external carcinogens.

Initially the carcinoma is confined to the cervix and may form a superficial ulcerating mass with bulky expansion of the cervix. The lesion spreads locally to involve the vagina, upper cervix, and parametria, and may spread to neighboring structures such as bladder and rectum. A clinical staging system proposed by the International Federation of Gynecology and Obstetrics (FIGO) provides criteria for staging of the disease (Table 7-2). Stage of disease determines the type of therapy. The cervix has a rich plexus of lymphatics that drain to the hypogastric and presacral area, and lymph node metastases occur early: Nodes are involved in 15% of women with stage I disease, 28% with stage II, and 47% with stage III disease.[17]

Clinical Diagnosis. Cervical cancer occurs at a younger age than carcinoma of the endometrium (mean age 45). Carcinoma in situ is often diagnosed between ages 25 and 40.[12] Abnormal vaginal discharge and bleeding, especially after intercourse, are typical presenting symptoms. Delay in seeking medical attention after the onset of symptoms is

TABLE 7-2. Invasive cervical carcinoma: Relationship of stage to 5-year survival

FIGO	STAGING SYSTEM FOR INVASIVE CARCINOMA OF THE CERVIX	5-YEAR SURVIVAL %
Stage I	Carcinoma confined to the cervix	92
Stage II	Carcinoma extends beyond the cervix but not to pelvic wall; upper one-third of vagina may be involved	
II A	Involvement of medial parametrium	84
II B	Involvement of lateral parametrium	67
Stage III	Carcinoma extends to pelvic wall. Lower one-third of vagina may be involved. Ureteral obstruction may be present.	40
Stage IV	Carcinoma extends beyond the true pelvis; bladder or rectal involvement present. Distant metastases to liver, bone, or lungs may be present.	14

(Adapted from Fletcher GH. Cancer of the uterine cervix. AJR. 1971; 111:225–242.© The American Roentgen Ray Society.)

common. In more advanced stages, symptoms of bladder irritability, low back pain from lumbosacral root involvement, and parametrial involvement may be seen. Unilateral or bilateral ureteral obstruction is invariably present in advanced disease, and uremia has been the most common cause of death from carcinoma of the cervix. The diagnosis is often suspected from the Pap smear and can be established with cervical biopsy. Colposcopy has considerable value. Physical examination helps determine the initial clinical stage. Additional methods used for staging include cystoscopy, intravenous pyelography, barium enema, lymphangiography, and chest examination. In the past decade CT, US, and MRI have been added to the diagnostic work-up.

Treatment. The type of treatment, whether primarily surgical or radiation therapy, is determined by the stage of disease. Limited surgery—excision of a cone of tissue around the cervical os—is sometimes performed in early cancers when fertility preservation is desired. A radical hysterectomy is usually performed when parametria are free of tumor (stage II or earlier).

Radiation therapy is given to patients whose disease involves the parametria and when nodal extension is likely. Ultrasound can play an important role in enhancing the precision of radiation therapy, especially with intracavitary treatment. Intracavitary radiation therapy consists of placing radioactive sources in the uterus and the vaginal

fornices, usually for 24 to 48 hours, in order to deliver high-intensity local radiation. Distances from the radiation source to sensitive adjacent organs such as bladder are crucial. Radiation dose is calculated on the basis of these distances. A metal tandem (a hollow tube) is placed into the uterine cavity while the patient is in the operating room and anesthetized. Later the radioactive material is loaded into the tube. A sonographic survey of the uterus with the intracavitary tandem in place demonstrates the spatial relationship of the radioactive material to the urinary bladder and to the lesion (see Fig. 7-5).[5]

SONOGRAPHIC IMAGING

In stage I and II of carcinoma of the cervix US offers little diagnostic information because the cervix is usually of normal size and echogenicity. Occasionally, expansion of the cervix is observed (Fig. 7-6). Changes in the echogenicity of an enlarged cervix may also be observed with carcinoma. In the presence of cervical stenosis, hematometra may be noted.

Sonographic identification of the cervix may be difficult. Some authors have suggested placing a fluid-soaked tampon in the vagina to facilitate visualization of the cervix.[7] Placing an inflated Foley catheter balloon in the upper vagina is another method that has been used to aid in the identification of the cervix.[5] It is likely that a few milliliters of sterile saline will serve the same purpose and in addition may define the vaginal fornices.

Involvement of the bladder in stage IV disease may be readily appreciated with ultrasound because of the natural contrast provided by fluid in the bladder (Fig. 7-7A, B). Rectal involvement and parametrial infiltration are more difficult to demonstrate unless a bulky adnexal mass is present. Obstruction and dilatation of the distal ureter may mimic an ovarian cyst, but ipsilateral hydronephrosis would usually clarify such a finding. The kidneys should be scanned routinely to exclude obstructive hydronephrosis, which would indicate stage III disease. Survey of the retroperitoneal nodal areas may disclose adenopathy (Fig. 7-7C), and, as with any pelvic malignancy, the liver should be surveyed for possible metastases.

Reports on the use of transrectal and transvaginal sonography in staging of cervical cancer have suggested that this type of examination may facilitate staging of early lesions.[2] With endosonography, high-frequency transducers scanning at close range through a balloon water path provide sufficient anatomic resolution to distinguish between stage I and stage II and to determine depth of tumor infiltration. Although it is not possible to differentiate between a malignant and a benign mass, US can be used to guide an accurate biopsy. Transrectal and transvesical scanning have also been reported to have benefits in treatment planning during intracavitary irradiation.[2]

Conventional real-time US is used as a guide to interventional procedures in the management of patients with pelvic malignancy. For example, in the presence of bilateral ureteral obstruction, percutaneous nephrostomy is often performed using ultrasound guidance.

OTHER IMAGING MODALITIES
Lymphangiography and CT. Since lymph node involvement is an important parameter in establishing the extent of disease, both lymphangiography and CT scanning have been used for this purpose. Although lymphangiography has a high specificity when positive, it has a high false negative rate. Lymphangiography has a wide range of sensitivity and specificity for lymph node disease.[13] CT has become the method of choice for staging cervical carcinoma. Parametrial extension is manifested by a nodularity and mass extending laterally from the cervix and obliteration of fat planes and loss of

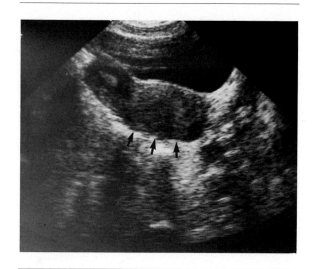

FIGURE 7-6. Stage II carcinoma of the cervix with a mass extending to the upper third of the vagina. The 28-year-old patient's Pap smear was abnormal. A sagittal scan of the pelvis shows marked expansion of the cervix (*arrows*).

periureteral fat. CT has been shown to be more accurate in the diagnosis and staging of lesions beyond stage III but is less accurate in differentiating stage I from stage II disease.[13]

Magnetic Resonance Imaging. Cervical carcinomatous masses are consistently demonstrated well on MRI and appear as tumors of high signal intensity. Parametrial invasion with tumor may be visualized as well, but advantages of MRI over CT in this regard are not as yet clear-cut.[22] MRI may have an advantage over CT in distinguishing enlarged pelvic lymph nodes from adjacent blood vessels. This is because flowing blood produces a low-intensity signal and therefore creates a contrast between the vasculature and lymph nodes.

DIFFERENTIAL DIAGNOSIS
The main consideration in the differential diagnosis when a bulky cervix is present is leiomyoma involving the lower uterine segment. Benign endometrial polyps may prolapse into the cervical canal, causing expansion in the cervix and changes in acoustic texture. Occasionally cancer of the endo-

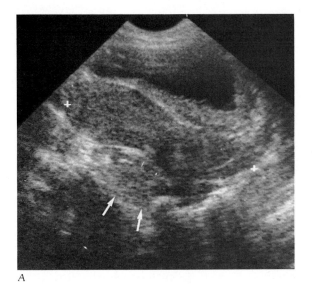

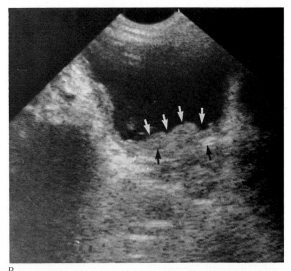

A

B

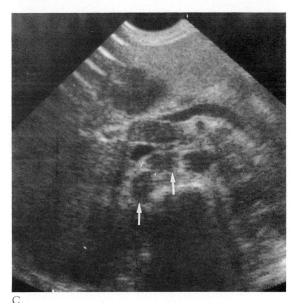

C

FIGURE 7-7. Stage IV carcinoma of the cervix. The 32-year-old patient presented with intermenstrual bleeding. (*A*) Sagittal scan of the pelvis demonstrates enlargement of the cervix and an ill-defined mass in the cul-de-sac (*arrows*). (*B*) Transverse view shows nodularity and thickening of the posterior wall of the bladder (*arrows*). (*C*) Transverse view of the upper abdomen at the level of the splenic vein demonstrates retroperitoneal adenopathy (*arrows*).

metrium may involve the cervix, causing bulky expansion.

Gestational Trophoblastic Disease

CLINICAL INFORMATION

Epidemiology. Gestational trophoblastic disease is a group of rare neoplasms of the uterus that occur as a complication of pregnancy or conception. These lesions include benign hydatidiform mole, invasive (but not metastasizing) mole, and choriocarcinoma, a highly malignant lesion. The reader is referred to Chapter 22 for a complete discussion of the spectrum of gestational trophoblastic disease. The present discussion focuses on invasive mole and choriocarcinoma. In approximately 20% of cases, hydatidiform mole may develop into an invasive mole. Rarely (in 3 to 5% of patients) choriocarcinoma may result. The highest incidence of invasive mole and choriocarcinoma is seen in Southeast Asia and the tropics, where hydatidiform mole is more common.[15]

Pathophysiology of Invasive Mole and Choriocarcinoma. The *invasive mole* is characterized by extensive proliferation of trophoblastic tissue and swollen chorionic villi. These tissue components invade the myometrium, forming hemorrhagic masses. In the case of hydatidiform mole they distend the endometrial cavity. The focal invasion of myometrium and blood vessels may cause uterine rupture and intraperitoneal hemorrhage. Because the growth is primarily into the myometrium, diagnostic curettage may not yield tumor tissue, whereas significant abnormalities are likely to be present on ultrasound and MR images.[10]

Choriocarcinoma is also characterized by extensive proliferation of trophoblastic tissue, but in contrast to invasive mole, no villi are present. It is possible that the absence of villi is due to their rapid destruction by the malignant tissue. Choriocarcinoma is more aggressive than invasive mole, and extension to the cervix and vagina sometimes occurs. A typical feature of the malignant behavior of choriocarcinoma is invasion of blood vessels and embolization of trophoblastic tissue to the lungs, where it may obstruct the pulmonary venous circulation, causing right-sided heart failure or spread to the pulmonary arterial system. Embolization to the systemic circulation is not uncommon, accounting for tumor implants in brain, liver, and soft tissues.

Theca lutein cysts involving one or both ovaries are frequently observed with gestational trophoblastic disease (Fig. 7-8B; see Fig. 22-2). It has been suggested that these cysts may be the result of the high levels of beta subunit of human chorionic gonadotropin (β-HCG) a hormone similar to luteinizing hormone (LH) produced by the pituitary.[12] Theca lutein cysts may be seen in 20% of cases of trophoblastic disease. When they are present, they constitute an additional risk factor for the presence or development of invasive disease.

Clinical Diagnosis. Invasive mole is usually diagnosed in the setting of previous evacuation of a hydatidiform mole and persistent bleeding and elevation of β-HCG titer. Choriocarcinoma may be preceded by a hydatidiform mole in 50% of cases, by a normal pregnancy in 30%, and by a spontaneous abortion in 20%.[12]

Abnormal vaginal bleeding in conjunction with a pregnancy is a common presenting symptom. Often incomplete or impending abortion is suspected. Should intrauterine hemorrhage or perforation occur, the patient is likely to present in shock. The presenting symptoms (cough, hemoptysis, or neurologic disturbances) may be related to metastatic disease.

Malignant trophoblastic disease is divided into two groups: nonmetastatic and metastatic. The former includes invasive mole or choriocarcinoma that is confined to the uterus. Patients with metastatic disease are classified in low-, intermediate-, or high-risk categories, depending on the duration of disease, the β-HCG titer, and the site of metastases.

SONOGRAPHIC IMAGING

US examination of invasive mole or choriocarcinoma may be indistinguishable from complete mole. The uterus is usually enlarged in both conditions. When the invasive mole is focal, echogenic foci may be noted within the myometrium (see Fig. 7-8A). Hypoechoic areas may be seen within the masses, representing hemorrhage or vascular lakes with arteriovenous shunting (Fig. 7-8B).[19]

Doppler ultrasound has provided additional data, demonstrating the significant increase of tissue perfusion that is associated with gestational trophoblastic disease.[20] Initial reports on the use of Doppler interrogation of the uterine wall and ovarian artery have demonstrated high-amplitude systolic and diastolic frequency shifts, indicating increased perfusion with low impedance to blood flow. Such increase in blood flow is also seen in normal pregnancy during the late second and early third trimester but not in the first trimester, during which period the diagnosis of trophoblastic disease is usually made. A study reporting the use of color Doppler in the investigation of invasive trophoblastic mole has also confirmed that the rapid blood flow in this condition can be demonstrated. The Doppler studies were repeated after treatment, and resolution of the hypervascularity generally paralleled the positive response to chemotherapy.[19]

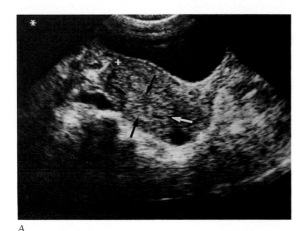

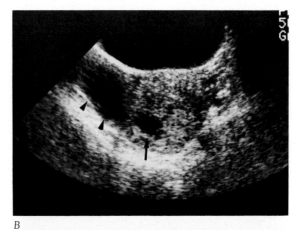

A

B

FIGURE 7-8. Choriocarcinoma in a 21-year-old woman with persistent elevation of β-HCG titer following an abortion. (A) Sagittal view of the pelvis shows a slightly enlarged uterus with an eccentrically situated echogenic mass (*arrows*) representing tumor tissue in the myometrium. (B) Transverse view of the pelvis shows a fluid collection within the uterine outline (*arrows*) and a right-sided adnexal corpus luteum cyst (*arrowheads*). (C) A Doppler tracing of the sonolucent zone within the uterus demonstrates pulsatile flow, suggesting the presence of arteriovenous lakes.

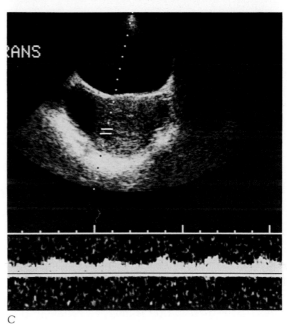

C

Although further studies are needed to establish the specificity and sensitivity of Doppler studies in these patients, this preliminary information suggests that Doppler ultrasound is a promising tool in diagnosis and management of this disease.

Associated adnexal multicystic masses representing theca lutein cysts may be unilateral or bilateral and range in size from 4 to 10 cm (Fig. 7-8B; see Fig. 22-2). These cysts occur in association with the classic mole, invasive mole, and choriocarcinoma. The liver is a common site of metastases in choriocar-cinoma, and it should be included in the sono-graphic evaluation.

OTHER IMAGING MODALITIES

Chest radiography is an important part of the evaluation and follow-up of patients diagnosed with choriocarcinoma (Fig. 7-9). CT of the chest may be necessary to find small pulmonary lesions. CT of the brain has been an important modality in determining the presence of cerebral metastases.

The excellent resolution of MRI of the central

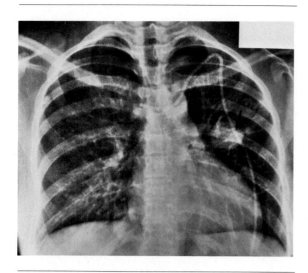

FIGURE 7-9. Choriocarcinoma in a 16-year-old girl with a history of previous evaluation for hydatidiform mole who presented with hemoptysis. Frontal view of the chest shows a metastatic lung mass *(arrows)*.

nervous system as well as the pelvis and the sensitivity of MRI in detecting hemorrhage suggest that it may also become the modality of choice in evaluating the brain and the uterus.[10]

DIFFERENTIAL DIAGNOSIS

An early failed pregnancy with incomplete abortion and hydropic degeneration of the placenta may be confused with trophoblastic disease and therefore should be included in the differential diagnosis. The β-HCG titer is likely to be low in this condition because, not only is there an absence of trophoblastic proliferation, but function of this tissue is decreased or diminished. Retained products of conception or a degenerating uterine fibroid with areas of hemorrhage may also produce an appearance of numerous small cysts within an expanded uterine outline. Intramural fibroids may resemble invasive molar tissue, especially when they are undergoing degeneration. Some ovarian tumors such as cystic papillary adenoma or dermoids may have a morphologic similarity to molar tissue. This source of confusion can be minimized if every attempt is made to search for and identify the uterus. In this regard, one of the strengths of transvaginal

scanning is its ability to separate uterine from adnexal structures, thereby enhancing the potential value of the ultrasound examination.

References

1. American Cancer Society. Cancer Statistics 1988. Cancer J Clinic. 1988; 38:1:5–22.
2. Bernaschek G, Dertinger J, Bartl W, et al. Endosonographic staging of carcinoma of the uterine cervix. Arch Gynecol. 1986; 239:21–36.
3. Boronow RC, Morrow CP, Creasmon WT, et al. Surgical staging in endometrial CA: Clinicopathologic findings of a prospective study. Obstet Gynecol. 1984; 63:825–832.
4. Chambers CB, Unis JS. Ultrasonographic evidence of uterine malignancy in the postmenopausal uterus. Am J Obstet Gynecol. 1986; 154:1194–1199.
5. De Wit JJ, Smit BJ. The role of ultrasound in the management of cervical carcinoma, a preliminary report. SA Med J. 1983; 64:381–383.
6. Fleischer AC, Dudley BS, Entmann SS, et al. Myometrial invasion by endometrial carcinoma: Sonographic assessment. Radiology. 1987; 162:307–310.
7. Fleischer AC, Entmin SS, Parroth SA, et al. Sonographic evaluation of uterine malformations and disorders. In: Sanders RC, James AE, eds. The Principles and Practice of Ultrasonography in Obstetrics and Gynecology. 3rd ed. Norwalk, CT: Appleton-Century-Crofts; 1985.
8. Fletcher GH. Cancer of the uterine cervix. AJR. 1971; 111:225–242.
9. Girinski T, Leclere J, Pejovic MH, et al. Prospective comparison of US and CT in evaluation of the size of the uterus: Can these methods be used for intracavitary treatment planning of cancer of the uterus. Int J Radiation Oncol Biol Physiol. 1987; 13:789–793.
10. Hricak H, Demas BE, Braga CA, et al. Gestational trophoblastic neoplasm of the uterus: MR assessment. Radiology. 1986; 161:11–16.
11. Hricak H, Stern JL, Fisher MR, et al. Endometrial cancer staging by MR imaging. Radiology. 1987; 162:297–307.
12. Jones HW, Jones GS. Novak's Textbook of Gynecology. 11th ed. Baltimore: Williams & Wilkins; 1988.
13. Lewis E. The use and abuse of imaging in gynecologic cancer. Cancer. 1987; 60:1993-2009.
14. Obata A, Akamatsu N, Sekiba K. Ultrasound estimation of myometrial invasion of endometrial cancer by intrauterine radiologic scanning. J Clin Ultrasound. 1985; 13:397–404.
15. Park WN. Pathology and classification of trophoblastic tumors. In: Coppleson M, ed. Gynecologic

Oncology. New York: Churchill Livingstone; 1981; 2.

16. Perez C, Knapp RC, DiSaia PJ, et al. Gynecologic Tumors. In: De Vita VT, Hellman S, Rosenberg SA, eds. Cancer: Principles and Practice of Oncology. Philadelphia: JB Lippincott; 1982.

17. Plentyl A, Friedman E. Lymphatic System of the Female Genitalia. Philadelphia: WB Saunders; 1971.

18. Requard K, Wicks JD, Mettler FA. Ultrasonography in the staging of endometrial adenocarcinoma. Radiology. 1981; 140:781–785.

19. Shimamato K, Sakuma S, Ishigaki T, et al. Intramural blood flow: Evaluation with color Doppler echography. Radiology. 1987; 165:683–685.

20. Taylor KJW, Schwartz PE, Kohorn EI. Gestational trophoblastic neoplasia: Diagnosis with Doppler ultrasound. Radiology. 1987; 165:445–448.

21. Thigpen JT. Approaches to the evaluation and management of endometrial carcinoma. In: Forastiere AA, ed. Gynecologic Cancer. New York: Churchill Livingstone; 1984:219.

22. Waggenspack GA, Amparo EG, Hannigan EV, et al. MRI of cervical carcinoma. Semin Ultrasound CT MR. 1988; 9:158–166.

CHAPTER 8

Benign Masses of the Ovaries, Fallopian Tubes, and Broad Ligaments

DIANA KAWAI, REGINA RODRICK, MICHELLE LANIGAN

Today, ultrasound is the modality of choice for evaluating the female pelvis, including the uterus and adnexa. Diagnostic ultrasound permits multiplanar scanning of the pelvis without the harmful effects of ionizing radiation and plays a major role in the characterization of pelvic adnexal masses. Although ultrasound is of limited use for making definitive clinical diagnoses, a reliable diagnosis can usually be made through correlation with clinical information. In this chapter we focus on benign diseases of the adnexa, which includes the ovaries, fallopian tubes, and broad ligaments. The ovaries can be involved in a variety of benign entities, including ovarian cysts (physiologic, functional, miscellaneous), inflammatory processes (tuboovarian abscesses), and benign neoplasms (germ cell tumor, epithelial tumor, stromal tumor). Neoplasms are new tissue growths or tumors.[49] They may be cystic, mixed, or solid; benign or malignant. Malignant and inflammatory processes of the ovaries, fallopian tubes, and broad ligaments are discussed in other chapters, as are endometriomas, which may also present as adnexal masses.

Anatomy

The ovaries are usually located along the posterolateral aspect of the pelvic sidewalls, behind the broad ligaments, and lateral to the uterus. Other common locations include the posterior cul-de-sac, superior to the uterus, and adherent to the uterus. While performing the ultrasound scan care must be taken not to mistake the psoas muscle, obturator internus muscle, or bowel loops for ovaries. Identification of the ovaries may be facilitated by visualizing the ovarian follicles. The internal iliac artery and vein, key landmarks, should be visualized posterior to each ovary.[20,43] Other sonographic landmarks for the ovary are the ovarian artery and vein, which may be visualized as pulsatile, linear, anechoic structures measuring 3 to 10 mm in diameter and extending superiorly from the ovary.[20]

The ovaries are generally ellipsoid; therefore, the formula for volume calculation of a prolate ellipse (length × width × height/2) may be used to estimate ovarian volume.[22] Prepubertal ovarian volume gradually increases from less than 1 cm^3 at age 10 years. Normal ovarian volume in menstruating women averages around 6.5 cm^3, although it may be slightly less during the teenage and early adult years, and may increase to as much as 14 cm^3 as the patient matures.[39] The most common measurements given in the literature are 1 to 2 cm × 2 cm × 3 cm.[11] Ovarian size and shape may change with cyclic physiologic changes.

Various investigations into the average size of postmenopausal ovaries have been reported. The average size has ranged from 1.5 to 3.7 cm^3.[15,25,38] Atrophy of the ovaries generally occurs within 3 to 5 years after menopause.[38] Further evaluation has been recommended when any ovary in a postmenopausal woman measures twice the volume of the contralateral ovary or more than 7.1 cm^3.[15]

General Sonographic Technique

In the evaluation of an adnexal mass or masses, the clinician and sonographer must pay careful attention to patient history. An adequate history should include the patient's age, menstrual history, surgical history, complaints and symptoms (e.g., pain, fever, bleeding), use of contraceptive devices, pregnancy state, and history of previous pregnancies. Knowledge of significant findings on physical examination are also extremely important in the formation of a diagnosis.

Sonographic examination of the female pelvis usually begins with a real-time unit, using the transabdominal approach to obtain an overall view of the pelvic structures. Particular attention should be paid to the areas in which the referring physician reports palpating a mass and to areas where the patient feels pain. Real-time US enables the sonographer to avoid misinterpreting fluid-filled bowel as an adnexal mass, when peristalsis can be demonstrated. Mechanical and phased-array transducers allow the greatest degree of manipulation,[14] and are, therefore, ideally suited to angling the ultrasound beam around pelvic bones and through the urinary bladder to obtain as much sonographic information as possible.

When evaluating the adnexa, complete routine pelvic sonography is performed. The uterus and adnexa are thoroughly examined and the findings are documented. Any masses noted in the pelvis should be evaluated thoroughly. Documentation should include the location, size, and sonographic appearance of the mass. Whenever possible, anatomic landmarks such as the urinary bladder, uterus, and pelvic vessels should be included in images of a mass to verify the location of the mass. Labelling all images on a "hard copy" should also be done. Documentation should also be made of the origin of the mass by demonstrating whether or not the mass is continuous or contiguous with the ovary or uterus. The mass should be measured in all dimensions: anteroposterior, inferosuperior, and transverse. Characteristics such as mass contour, mass echo texture, degree of sound transmission, the presence of fluid-fluid or fluid-solid levels, septa, or nodular masses should be documented sonographically.

Adnexal structures are often difficult to visualize, so it may be helpful to reposition the patient after examining her in the supine position. Patient position may be changed to right side up or left side up, or the pelvis may be tilted anteriorly and supported by a pillow placed beneath the lower pelvis. Changing patient position redistributes fluid in the urinary bladder, thereby changing the position of the sonographic window relative to the structures the sonographer is attempting to image. The ultrasound beam may then be angled obliquely from one side of the pelvis to the other through the newly positioned urinary bladder. This allows manipulation of the beam so that it is perpendicular to the structure being imaged, to take advantage of the best possible axial resolution of the instrument.

Often, a loop of fluid-filled sigmoid or rectum can mimic a cystic or complex adnexal mass. In such cases, especially when peristalsis cannot be demonstrated, it is necessary to reevaluate the "mass" during or after a cleansing enema. A warm tap water or saline enema may also be used to identify the rectum, sigmoid colon, and cecum and to delineate the posterior cul-de-sac.[44]

Transvaginal ultrasound uses higher-frequency transducers and therefore provides better resolution of pelvic structures. The transvaginal approach is particularly useful when a retroverted uterus, bowel gas, patient obesity, inability to fill the urinary bladder, or pelvic adhesions limit the quality of the transabdominal ultrasound exam.[34] Due to limitations in the field of view, transvaginal ultrasound should be used as an adjunct to the routine transabdominal ultrasound examination.[30,34] The use of transvaginal color Doppler to distinguish malignant from benign ovarian neoplasms is currently under investigation. Increased vascularity appears to suggest malignancy.[29]

Articulated-arm (static) scanners may be used when a regional survey of the abdomen or pelvis is desired, for example, when evaluating the extent and relationship of adjacent structures to a large pelvic mass. Static scans enable the sonographer to document pelvic masses that are too large to fit onto a sector scan or onto two "aligned" images obtained with a linear-array transducer and displayed side by side.

Complementary Imaging Modalities

Although the examinations are more expensive, computed tomography (CT) and magnetic resonance imaging (MRI) may provide information ultrasound cannot. CT is often used to demonstrate the extent of known pelvic disease, such as pelvic inflammatory disease, endometriosis, or malignancy.[10,13,35] MRI is reportedly helpful in delineating the origins of pelvic masses by demonstrating connection to the ovary or uterus.[10] Tissue characterization by MRI has also been shown to be more specific than by ultrasound. Hemorrhagic fluid may be differentiated more reliably from protein-free fluid, fat, and solid lesions by MRI than by ultrasound. MRI is particularly useful in evaluating adnexal masses in pregnant women, because it does not use ionizing radiation.[50] Both CT and MRI are useful for evaluating pelvic disease in patients whose ultrasound examination results are suboptimal because of obesity or bowel gas.[10,35]

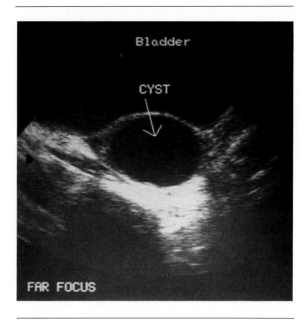

FIGURE 8-1. This cyst demonstrates the criteria for a simple cyst of the ovary: smooth walls, good acoustic transmission with posterior acoustic enhancement and no internal echoes.

Benign Cysts

Most cystic pelvic masses are ovarian in origin.[11] The sonographic criteria for simple cysts are (1) smooth, well-defined borders, (2) absence of internal echoes, and (3) increased posterior acoustic enhancement (Fig. 8-1). Thick, irregular walls or thick septations (>3 mm) may be associated with inflammation, endometriosis, or malignancy.[27,33] In sonographically complex adnexal masses, the risk of malignancy increases proportionally with the presence of echogenic components.[38] Adnexal cysts containing extremely echogenic foci are usually benign cystic teratomas; adnexal masses that are almost completely homogenously echogenic tend to be solid masses,[38,40] cysts with hemorrhage, or endometriomas.[11] Matted bowel loops and ascites have long been recognized as signs of malignancy.[27] A list of benign, noninflammatory cysts is presented in Table 8-1.

Ovarian cysts may be visualized sonographically in women at all reproductive stages, including pregnancy. Cysts measuring less than 3 cm in greatest diameter generally regress spontaneously and represent follicles. Sonographic follow-up is recommended for cysts between 3 and 5 cm; the vast majority regress spontaneously, but some continue to enlarge. Careful sonographic evaluation to detect septa or solid components is recommended for any ovarian cyst measuring more than 5 cm in its greatest dimension.[47] Up to 60% of cysts with thin septa and no solid components have been reported to regress spontaneously, usually within 3 months.[41] Even cysts that appear simple by sonographic criteria rarely resolve if they measure more than 10 cm in greatest diameter. Cysts of this size have a greater potential to become malignant or invasive and. so, are usually removed.[41] Cysts detected during pregnancy that measure more than 5 cm in diameter traditionally have been removed during the second trimester, as they may complicate the pregnancy or delivery and may represent a malignancy. However, J. G. Thornton and coworkers have suggested that, unless complications have occurred or are likely at delivery, simple cysts

TABLE 8-1. Benign cystic masses of the adnexa

Physiologic or Functional
    Ovarian follicles (physiologic cysts)
    Follicular cysts
    Corpus luteum cysts
    Theca lutein cysts
    Hyperstimulation syndrome

Miscellaneous
    Parovarian cysts
    Peritoneal inclusion cysts
    Hemorrhagic cysts
    Hydrosalpinx
    Polycystic ovary syndrome
    Inflammatory processes

measuring between 5 and 10 cm in diameter should be treated conservatively until the postnatal period, as they found the majority of these cysts to be benign.[47]

Traditionally ovarian cysts of any size found in postmenopausal women have been excised. Hall and colleagues reported that only one of 13 simple cysts excised from postmenopausal women in their facility was found to be malignant on histopathologic evaluation. Although the high incidence of ovarian cancer in postmenopausal women necessitates further investigation of any adnexal cyst, they suggested that their findings may reduce the anxiety experienced by postmenopausal women in whom adnexal cysts are discovered.[24] More recently, Goldstein and associates reported that postmenopausal, unilocular, ovarian cysts measuring less than 5 cm in largest dimension are usually benign (in the absence of ascites). They suggest that these cysts may safely be monitored with serial sonograms, particularly since transvaginal ultrasound is now available and provides superior resolution.[14]

FUNCTIONAL CYSTS

Functional or physiologic cysts of the ovary include ovarian follicles, follicular cysts, corpus luteum cysts, and theca lutein cysts. Ovarian follicles are visualized as anechoic structures in the relatively echogenic ovary. Follicles as small as 0.5 cm may be appreciated sonographically. Approximately 10 days prior to ovulation, the ovaries may contain several follicles. Not all of the follicles mature to the point of ovulation. A single follicle usu-

ally becomes dominant, measuring 2.0 to 2.5 cm in greatest dimension. One to three days before ovulation, the dominant follicle may appear sonographically as a "cloudy cone," with its wide end leading out to the periphery of the ovary.[31] During the midportion of the menstrual cycle, a release of luteinizing hormone leads to ovulation. During the second half of the menstrual cycle, the ovulatory follicle enlarges to become the corpus luteum.[22,23] If conception occurs, the corpus luteum produces progesterone until approximately the 11th or 12th week of pregnancy, when the placenta takes over production of progesterone. If conception does not occur, the corpus luteum generally regresses within 2 weeks.

FOLLICULAR CYSTS

Follicular cysts can occur through overdistention of a follicle that has failed to rupture.[11] They may be multiple but are usually unilateral. Ranging in diameter from 1 to 10 cm,[37] follicular cysts most commonly occur in female infants and women of childbearing age.[2] The large majority of patients with physiologic cysts experience no symptoms, as these cysts usually regress spontaneously. Sonographically, follicular cysts meet the criteria for a simple cyst, as described above. In general, any simple ovarian cyst measuring less than 5 cm in greatest dimension in an ovulating female should be reevaluated by ultrasound during the next menstrual cycle. A change in the size or appearance of the cyst or complete resolution generally will be seen. In some cases, patients with follicular cysts present with mild to severe pelvic pain.[28] The cyst may become symptomatic with the occurrence of hemorrhage, torsion, or rupture into the peritoneal cavity.[37] Sonographically, late hemorrhage is seen as an area of variable echo pattern (Fig. 8-2), whereas fresh hemorrhage appears echo-free. In the case of a ruptured cyst, changes in the appearance of the cyst may be associated with free fluid in the cul-de-sac.

CORPUS LUTEUM CYSTS

Corpus luteum cysts appear during the midluteal phase of the menstrual cycle. As the dominant follicle ruptures, the corpus luteum of menstruation may develop. The corpus luteum measures 1.5 to 2.5 cm and may appear echo-filled or possess irreg-

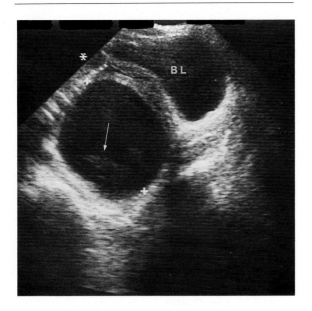

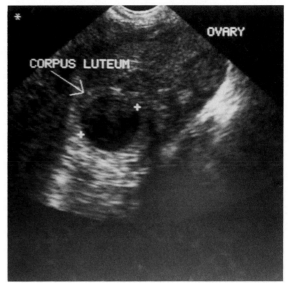

FIGURE 8-2. Hemorrhagic cyst located posterior to the urinary bladder (BL) containing debris in the dependent portion of the cyst (arrow).

FIGURE 8-3. Corpus luteum cyst of menstruation. Internal echoes in the anterior portion of the cyst represent hemorrhage. Remainder of ovary appears normal.

ular or thick borders around a central anechoic area.[31] Failure of absorption or excessive bleeding results in a functional corpus luteum cyst. Patients with corpus luteum cysts present with mild to severe pelvic pain.[40] Corpus luteum cysts generally are unilocular and unilateral and measure 5 to 11 cm in diameter. The sonographic appearance of the corpus luteum cyst is of a thin-walled cyst displaying good sonic through-transmission. The cyst may have irregular borders or internal echoes.[12] Unless torsion occurs, no treatment is required.[32] Involution usually occurs within 14 days.[2,18] Low-level echoes or a fluid-debris level may be seen if hemorrhage has occurred (Fig. 8-3). Rupture will result in fluid in the cul-de-sac and elsewhere in the abdomen. Hemorrhage and rupture frequently cause increased symptoms.

Should fertilization take place, a corpus luteum cyst of pregnancy may result.[21] In Figure 8-4, a corpus luteum cyst of pregnancy and a gravid uterus are demonstrated on a single sonographic image. During pregnancy, corpus luteum cysts may reach a maximum size of 3 cm at 8 to 10 weeks' gestation.

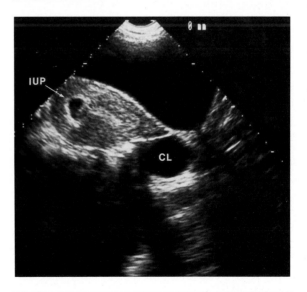

FIGURE 8-4. Corpus luteum cyst (CL) of pregnancy visualized posterior and inferior to a uterus containing an intrauterine pregnancy (IUP).

They generally resolve by 16 weeks' gestation.[2] At any point during this time, hemorrhage or rupture can occur, causing pelvic pain and a threat to both mother and fetus.[21]

Theca Lutein Cysts

Theca lutein cysts are the largest of the functional cysts and may range in size from 3 to 20 cm. They develop in response to excessive levels of the beta subunit of the hormone human chorionic gonadotropin (β-HCG). In 14 to 30% of cases, theca lutein cysts are associated with gestational trophoblastic diseases such as hydatidiform mole, chorioadenoma destruens, and choriocarcinoma. Montz and colleagues have observed an increased incidence of postmolar trophoblastic disease in hydatidiform mole patients who also had theca lutein cysts, particularly if the cysts became complicated or were bilateral.[36] Theca lutein cysts may also be seen with ovarian hyperstimulation syndrome, a complication of infertility drug therapy.[22,28] In rare instances, theca lutein cysts are seen with a normal singleton or multiple gestations.[1,22,28,36]

Sonographically, theca lutein cysts are multilocular, thin-walled, large, bilateral cystic masses (Fig. 8-5).[21] Bilateral development is thought to be a response to hormonal stimulation. Because of their association with gestational trophoblastic disease, it is important to evaluate the uterus carefully when theca lutein cysts are seen. A good patient history also is helpful in evaluating the cause of theca lutein cysts.[40]

Theca lutein cysts are generally treated conservatively, as they involute when the source of gonadotropin is removed, although they may persist for several months following trophoblastic evacuation. In some patients, the cysts persist long after the β-HCG levels are no longer detectable.[36] On occasion, theca lutein cysts, like other functional cysts, may undergo hemorrhage, torsion, or rupture, causing the patient pain. Surgery may be necessary if they become very large or in the event of intraperitoneal rupture or hemorrhage.

Parovarian Cysts

Parovarian cysts develop from the vestigial wolffian duct structures or arise from the tubal epithelium. The parovarium is located in the mesosalpinx, the

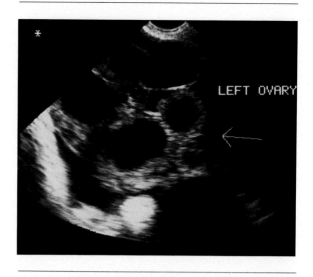

FIGURE 8-5. Hyperstimulated ovary contains multiple theca lutein cysts of varying sizes.

portion of broad ligament between the fallopian tube and the hilum of the ovary. These cysts account for about 10% of all adnexal masses and occur over a wide range of ages.[3] They are seen most commonly in the third and fourth decades and range in size from 1.5 to 19 cm.[1] Parovarian cysts are very difficult to distinguish from other ovarian lesions by physical examination. The large majority of symptomatic patients present with menstrual irregularities, increased lower abdominal girth, and pain if the cyst is large. Some small cysts remain asymptomatic and are found incidentally at surgery.

Parovarian cysts appear thin-walled, unilocular, and free of internal echoes on ultrasound. Since they do not respond to cyclic changes, their size does not change in relation to the menstrual cycle. Sonographically, parovarian cysts are indistinguishable from other cystic ovarian masses.[1,3] On occasion, a parovarian cyst may be recognized when a cyst is noted to be separate from an intact ovary with the fallopian tube draped or stretched over the cyst. As with other cystic masses, hemorrhage, torsion, and rupture alter the sonographic appearance.

PERITONEAL INCLUSION CYSTS

Cystic masses resulting from accumulations of serous fluid between adhesions or layers of peritoneum may be seen sonographically in patients following pelvic surgery. These cysts are referred to as peritoneal inclusion cysts.[11]

HEMORRHAGIC CYSTS

Any adnexal cyst or mass may twist, causing pain of sudden onset. The acute pain is caused by the vascular occlusion that results from the twisting of the base of the cyst or mass. When a pelvic ultrasound examination is requested for a nonpregnant patient with acute onset of pelvic pain (regardless of whether an adnexal mass is appreciated on physical exam), hemorrhage and torsion should be entertained as the primary diagnosis.

Hemorrhagic cysts generally display good through-transmission with variable sonographic features.[6,42] Fresh blood appears anechoic, progresses subacutely to a mixed echogenicity, and finally becomes anechoic again.[6] Any pattern or combination of these patterns may be seen. Debris may be seen in the posterior portion of a hemorrhagic cyst (Fig. 8-2). In some cases, septa may be present. Frequently, free fluid is seen in the cul-de-sac. The onset of pain and sonographic features are nonspecific, however, and can be encountered with other adnexal masses. A follow-up ultrasound examination may prove helpful in diagnosis in cases when clot lysis has taken place.

The ovary itself may also twist. Although torsion may occur with normal ovaries, most reported cases have involved children with ovarian masses or in women younger than 30 years of age. The fallopian tube is often involved as well. An increased incidence has been noted in pregnant patients. The clinical presentation is recurrent or acute sudden onset of localized pain and tenderness. If the torsion is incomplete and intermittent, the ovary may enlarge with edema. Areas of decreased and increased echogenicity may be appreciated in the ovary. These areas represent hemorrhage or infarct.[48] The only specific sonographic sign of torsion is the demonstration of multiple similar-sized cystic structures measuring as much as 25 mm in diameter in the cortical portion of a unilaterally enlarged ovary.[16,17] Multifollicular enlargement is

thought to result from fluid transudation into follicles due to the ovarian congestion caused by circulatory impairment.[17] Doppler evaluation may be useful in determining whether the ovary is receiving blood,[16] since torsion initially involves the ovarian vein but may progress to involve the ovarian artery as well.[48] Early diagnosis is extremely important, as surgical intervention may salvage the ovary.

HYDROSALPINX

Hydrosalpinx is a fluid collection in a scarred or blocked fallopian tube. Usually secondary to pyosalpinx, it evolves when the purulent material is replaced by serous fluid.[7] Both hydrosalpinx and pyosalpinx may result from pelvic inflammatory disease, which is discussed in Chapter 9. Patients with hydrosalpinx generally have symptoms related to distension of the fallopian tube.

Sonographically, hydrosalpinx appears as a tubular, cystic mass with smooth, well-defined walls (Fig. 8-6). Hydrosalpinx can be unilateral or bilateral and the tube may become quite large. This fluid collection may sonographically mimic an adnexal cyst or surrounding bowel. The distinguishing sonographic characteristic of a hydrosalpinx is that the end of the fusiform cystic structure tapers

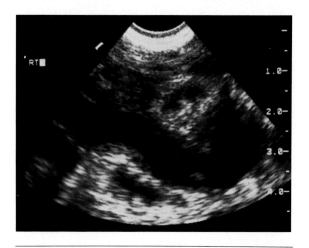

FIGURE 8-6. Anechoic tubular structure displays good through transmission, representing a hydrosalpinx.

as the tube enters the uterine wall.[11] Pyosalpinx may appear sonographically similar to hydrosalpinx, but there are low-level internal echoes representing pus. If the ovary can be visualized as one wall of the abscess, the diagnosis of tuboovarian abscess may be entertained.[11] Fluid-filled bowel, bladder diverticulum, urachal cyst, and mesenteric cyst are some of the nongynecologic entities that can also appear as cystic pelvic masses.

POLYCYSTIC OVARY DISEASE

Polycystic ovary disease (Stein-Leventhal syndrome) is an endocrine disorder associated with obesity, oligomenorrhea, hirsutism, and infertility. Infertility is thought to result from the unusually thick capsule surrounding the ovaries in these patients. The clinical presentation varies greatly with the degree and duration of the hormone imbalance. Since certain adrenal tumors can also cause oligomenorrhea and infertility, adrenal tumor should be considered in the clinical differential diagnosis of these patients.

The sonographic appearance of the ovaries in patients with polycystic ovary disease varies widely. In classic cases, the ovaries are enlarged bilaterally and contain multiple tiny peripheral cysts (Fig. 8-7).[26] The cysts may range in diameter from 2 to 6 mm.[46] Because they can be quite small, often only the echogenic linear walls may be visualized. Up to 25% of pelvic sonograms performed on patients with the clinical findings of polycystic ovary syndrome reveal sonographically normal ovaries.[22,46] High-resolution real-time scanners and the transvaginal approach have proven to be beneficial in the diagnosis of this disease.

Women with true polycystic ovary disease may have no clinical manifestations, however, the cysts are always bilateral. The sonographic appearance of polycystic ovaries may also be seen in women being treated with follicle stimulating hormones or in newborn girls whose ovaries are responding to maternal hormones.[22]

Inflammatory Processes

Inflammatory processes in the pelvis include pelvic inflammatory disease (pyosalpinx and tuboovarian abscess) and nongynecologic abscesses. Pelvic in-

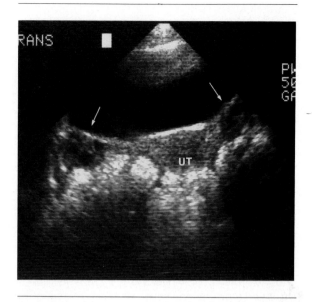

FIGURE 8-7. Polycystic ovaries (*arrows*) are demonstrated bilaterally on this transverse scan through the uterus (UT). Note the peripheral placement of the cysts.

flammatory disease is associated with the use of intrauterine contraceptive devices and with gynecologic infections. A complete discussion of pelvic inflammatory disease is presented in Chapter 9. Pelvic abscesses are usually symptomatic: Patients present with fever, pain, and elevated white blood cell counts.

A variety of sonographic patterns can be displayed by pelvic abscesses. Such collections usually demonstrate good through-transmission and may have irregular borders, internal septae, debris levels, and air. Gas within an abscess produces bright echoes and may shadow. The differential diagnosis should include hematoma, endometrioma, ectopic pregnancy, necrotic gynecologic tumor, and abscess of nongynecologic origin (e.g., diverticular abscess, periappendiceal abscess, Crohn's disease (Fig. 8-8), psoas abscess, postsurgical abscess). Because many of these entities have similar sonographic appearances, a complete patient history is critical for distinguishing which disease process most likely has been demonstrated.

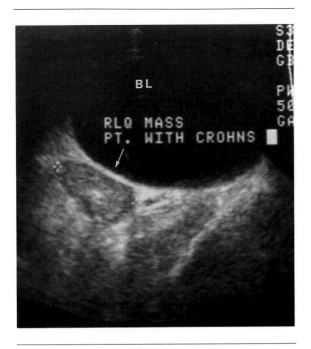

FIGURE 8-8. Crohn's abscess *(arrow)* located posterior to the urinary bladder (BL). The mass appears sonographically solid, but displays good acoustic transmission.

Benign Neoplasms

Eighty percent of all ovarian tumors are benign. Benign ovarian neoplasms may be categorized as germ cell tumors, epithelial tumors, or stromal tumors, depending on the ovarian tissue elements and derivation of these tumors. The most common benign adnexal neoplasms are benign cystic teratomas (germ cell tumor) and cystadenomas (epithelial tumors). Stromal tumors include fibroma and thecoma.[28] Benign neoplasms are summarized in Table 8-2.

Benign Cystic Teratoma

Benign cystic teratomas are the most common of the germ cell tumors. They are also the most frequently seen ovarian tumor in women under age 20. Although teratomas may occur in any age group, they are most often seen during the second and third decades. The terms "dermoid tumor" and "teratoma" are often used interchangeably, al-

though teratomas contain tissue of all three germ layers (ectoderm, mesoderm, endoderm) whereas dermoids are composed of ectodermal tissue only.[22] Pathology specimens of teratomas include teeth, hair, and glandular tissues (sweat, apocrine, sebaceous). Neural and thyroid tissue have also been seen on histopathologic examination. The malignant potential of a teratoma is based on its tissue maturity, but malignant change rarely occurs (<1%) in benign cystic teratomas.

Although patients with teratomas usually have no symptoms, they may present with pain or a palpable mass. Teratomas may twist, but they rarely rupture, due to their thick capsules. If the tumor does rupture, the patient may present as a surgical emergency with signs of peritonitis.

Teratomas are often first detected as incidental findings during sonographic examination. Most teratomas are located superior to the fundus of the uterus, because they are often connected to the ovary by a stalk, or pedicle.[11] They are bilateral in approximately 8 to 15% of patients. There is a wide spectrum of sonographic appearances of teratoma, including predominantly cystic mass, complex mass with calcifications, fat-fluid level within a complex mass, and diffusely echogenic mass without shadowing. Most commonly, teratomas appear sonographically as complex masses that are predominantly solid, containing echogenic foci that represent calcium or fat with or without acoustic shadowing.[11] This type of teratoma is the most difficult to detect, as the sonographic appearance mimics that of bowel gas. Occasionally, the "tip of the iceberg" sign is demonstrated; this refers to a very echogenic anterior component with poor through transmission, which prevents visualization of the more posterior portion of the mass (Fig. 8-9A).[19] When a fat-fluid level is identified, the fluid component is seen in the more dependent position while the echodense fat floats on top of the fluid (Fig. 8-9B). The sonographic appearance of a teratoma varies according to its elemental components—skin, hair, teeth, bone, fat. In Figure 8-9C, balls of hair may be seen floating on fluid. With the presence of significant bone and teeth components, echogenic foci with distal shadowing should be demonstrated on ultrasound examination. It is important to consider the possibility of a teratoma if

TABLE 8-2. Benign ovarian neoplasms

NEOPLASM	AGE GROUP	LATERALITY	SONOGRAPHIC CHARACTERISTICS
Germ Cell Tumors			
Benign cystic teratoma	Any age, usually younger than 20 years	15% bilateral	Varied: predominantly cystic, complex with calcifications, fat-fluid level, diffusely echogenic, predominantly solid with echogenic foci, with or without shadowing
Epithelial Tumors			
Serous cystadenoma	40s and 50s	25% bilateral	Usually unilocular; may have thin septations; may have papillary projections
Mucinous cystadenoma	40s and 50s	5% bilateral	Usually multilocular; may reach 30 cm diameter, may contain debris
Brenner tumor	Any age, usually around 50 years	6.5% bilateral	Solid; echogenic; size ranges from microscopic to 8 cm diameter
Stromal Tumors			
Fibroma	40s and 50s	Unilateral	Hypoechoic, attenuates acoustic beam, measures 5 to 16 cm; multiple in 10% of cases
Thecoma	Postmenopausal	Unilateral	Hypoechoic; attenuates sound; measures up to 30 cm diameter
Sertoli-Leydig cell tumor	Usually younger than 30 years	Unilateral	Echogenic mass

a pelvic mass is palpated but cannot be demonstrated sonographically. Radiography of the pelvis may prove helpful in demonstrating the presence of fat, bone, or teeth.

Technique. Decubitus sonographic scanning may aid in demonstrating fat-fluid or fluid-debris levels, as these levels should shift as different parts of the mass become dependent. Carefully shaking the patient may even produce wave forms in the fat-fluid interface that are visible by ultrasound.[38] Water enemas may help differentiate a teratoma from bowel. In such procedures, the rectum is distended with 100 to 200 ml of lukewarm tap water introduced slowly. The microbubbles in the tap water provide sonographic "contrast," which helps to distinguish rectum from pelvic masses. The urinary bladder must be moderately distended for optimal visualization of pelvic structures with the water enema technique.[11]

Other Imaging Modalities. A pelvic radiograph may show the fat, teeth, or bony components of teratomas. CT and MRI also display some characteristic findings of benign cystic teratoma. Fat has a characteristic appearance on CT, and CT can demonstrate fat-fluid or fluid-debris levels in these tumors. Benign cystic teratomas with high fat content have been demonstrated with MRI: The fat component in the tumors gives very high signal intensity on T1-weighted images.[22]

Treatment. Surgical removal of benign cystic teratomas is usually indicated. Since the patients are generally young, it is important that ovarian function be preserved. It is often possible to resect the teratoma without removing the entire ovary.[44]

EPITHELIAL TUMORS

Epithelial tumors arise from the ovarian epithelium. The benign epithelial tumors include serous

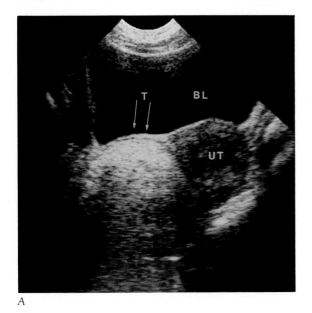

A

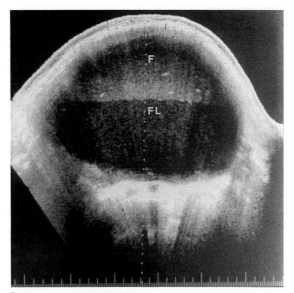

B

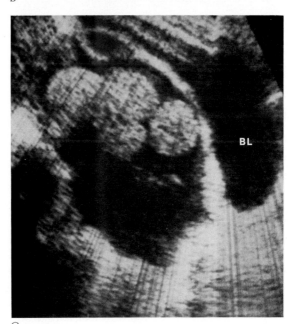

C

Figure 8-9. (A) Teratoma (T) located posterior to the urinary bladder (BL) and to the right of the uterus (UT) on transverse scan. The teratoma appears brightly echogenic anteriorly and simulates bowel gas. (B) Teratoma with a fat-fluid level is demonstrated on a static scan. The fatty component (F) is floating on the dependently located fluid (FL). (C) Teratoma located posterior to the urinary bladder on longitudinal scan. Echogenic "balls" of hair appear to float on fluid located in the dependent portion of the teratoma.

cystadenoma and mucinous cystadenoma (their malignant counterparts are serous cystadenocarcinoma and mucinous cystadenocarcinoma, respectively.) Less common benign epithelial tumors include Brenner tumors and mixed epithelial tumors.

Cystadenomas. As the names suggest, serous cystadenomas contain thin, serous fluid, and mucinous cystadenomas contain thicker mucin. In general, cystadenomas may grow very large and are seen in females during the fifth and sixth decades of life.

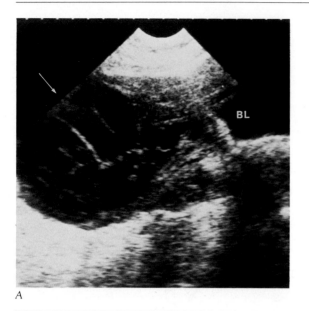

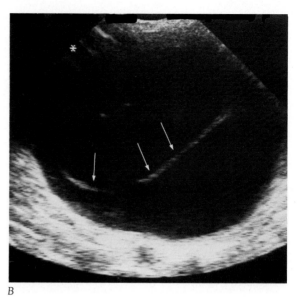

A

B

FIGURE 8-10. (A) Cystadenoma (*arrow*) is demonstrated superior to the urinary bladder (BL). Multiple septations may be appreciated within the cyst. (B) Arrows point to a single thin septum in the cyst.

As these masses become larger, septations and papillae tend to develop internally (Fig. 8-10A).[11] It is very difficult to differentiate sonographically between benign and malignant forms of cystadenoma, so it is important to look for secondary signs of malignancy, such as ascites or fixation of the mass. It is sometimes possible to differentiate mucinous from serous cystadenomas based on the echogenicity of fluid demonstrated. Serous cystadenomas are more common than mucinous cystadenomas. They are usually unilocular and may be bilateral in 25% of cases. Serous cystadenomas may contain very thin septations (Fig. 8-10B), and on occasion, papillary projections.[40] Mucinous cystadenomas are bilateral less than 5% of the time and can grow extremely large (15 to 30 cm) with multiple prominent septations and debris.[1,22] Histopathologic analysis is required for a definitive diagnosis.

Brenner Tumors. Brenner tumors are solid ovarian tumors arising from the ovarian surface epithelium.[5] They account for 1.7% of all ovarian neoplasms.[8] Brenner tumors can be seen in any age group but generally are found in women in the fifth and sixth decades who present with abnormal uterine bleeding. The tumors are bilateral in 6.5% of cases and range in size from microscopic to about 8 cm in diameter.[8] The usual sonographic presentation is an echogenic mass that may contain small cystic spaces (Fig. 8-11).[2,51] Brenner tumors often are diagnosed histopathologically as incidental findings in specimens of associated pelvic disease. Malignant changes rarely occur in Brenner tumors. Malignant forms of this tumor are generally large and cystic.[8]

Stromal Tumors

Benign stromal tumors include fibromas, thecomas, and Sertoli-Leydig cell tumors (also referred to as androblastomas and arrhenoblastomas).[40] Fibromas, thecomas, and Sertoli-Leydig cell tumors are all sonographically hypoechoic adnexal masses and cannot be distinguished from one another or from other solid benign and malignant ovarian disease.[4,40] The differential diagnosis of uterine fibroids may be ruled out by establishing the ovarian origin of the mass.[40,52]

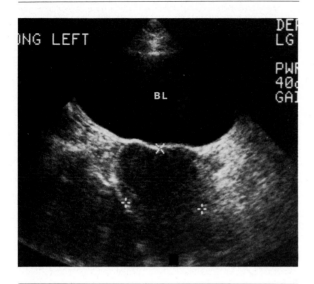

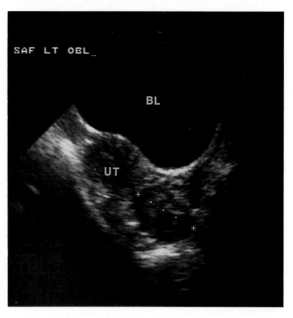

FIGURE 8-11. Brenner tumor is located posterior to the urinary bladder (BL) on longitudinal scan. Borders of the solid tumor are marked by the mechanical measuring device. The posterior border is not well-delineated. An acoustic shadow may be appreciated posterior to the mass.

FIGURE 8-12. Thecoma located posterior to the cervix on a longitudinal scan. Diameter of solid tumor measured by mechanical measuring device. (BL, urinary bladder; UT, uterus.)

Fibromas constitute about 5% of ovarian tumors and generally are found in women in the fifth or sixth decades.[45] Ranging in size from 5 to 16 cm, they are multiple in 10% of cases.[40] Fibromas are calcified in less than 10% of cases.[53] Bilateral, calcified, multinodular fibromas are atypical and generally are associated with basal cell nevus syndrome, a hereditary disorder. Very small fibromas are relatively common and often are associated with other ovarian neoplasms.[53] Sonographically, fibromas appear homogeneously hypoechoic and attenuate the sound beam, producing an acoustic shadow posterior to the mass. Ascites and right-sided pleural effusion may accompany fibromas in 1 to 3% of cases. This triad is called Meig's syndrome.[40] Fibromas larger than 10 cm in diameter may be associated with ascites in the absence of a pleural effusion in 10 to 15% of cases.[53]

Thecomas are estrogen-producing, solid ovarian masses that account for 1 to 2% of ovarian tumors. They are usually unilateral[53] and may measure up to 30 cm in diameter. The chief patient complaint is abnormal uterine bleeding, which results from estrogen production.[9] Thecomas occur most frequently in postmenopausal women and in young girls. The characteristic sonographic appearance of a thecoma is that of a pelvic mass that casts an acoustic shadow corresponding to the entire mass. Figure 8-12 is a sonographic image of a small thecoma confirmed by histopathologic examination. Although they are not considered to be malignant, they may become invasive and may place the patient at increased risk of endometrial cancer.[40,52]

Sertoli-Leydig cell tumors are unilateral neoplasms. They account for less than 0.5% of all ovarian neoplasms. Patients often present with pain or abdominal swelling, and one-third suffer masculinization effects. Seventy-five percent of cases occur in women less than 30 years of age.[53] Sertoli-Leydig cell tumors appear sonographically as echogenic masses and may not be distinguished from other solid ovarian tumors. Up to 20% are malignant.[40]

TABLE 8-3. Differential diagnoses for benign adnexal masses

Cystic Adnexal Masses
  Follicular cyst
  Corpus luteum cyst
  Parovarian cyst
  Peritoneal inclusion cyst
  Hemorrhagic cyst
  Hydrosalpinx
  Endometrioma
  Benign cystic teratoma

*Predominantly Cystic Adnexal Mass with
Septations and/or Debris*
  Theca lutein cyst
  Hemorrhagic cyst
  Cystadenoma
  Tuboovarian abscess
  Ectopic pregnancy
  Cystic adnexal masses

Solid Adnexal Mass
  Endometrioma
  Hemorrhagic cyst
  Brenner tumor
  Thecoma
  Fibroma

Differential Diagnoses

The sonographic presentation of ectopic pregnancy and endometriosis ranges from predominantly cystic to complex pelvic masses. In the proper clinical setting, it is imperative that ectopic pregnancy and endometriosis be included in the differential diagnosis of the pelvic mass. These entities are discussed in detail in Chapters 9 and 21.

The differential diagnoses for benign cystic and solid ovarian masses are presented in Table 8-3. Fluid-filled bowel or abnormal bowel may mimic cystic, complex, or solid adnexal masses. Sonography cannot differentiate between benign and malignant masses.[27,38] Solid adnexal tumors tend to be more malignant, as do cysts with multiple septations or solid mural nodules.[24,32] Associated ascites, peritoneal implants, or visceral metastases also favor malignancy. Since functional cysts are virtually nonexistent in postmenopausal women, any adnexal mass is worrisome and should be evaluated.

Ultrasound continues as the primary imaging modality in the evaluation of a pelvic mass. A sonographic examination by a skilled sonologist or sonographer in conjunction with the appropriate clinical findings should generate a working diagnosis or differential for any pelvic mass.

References

1. Alpern MB, Sandler MA, Madrazo BL. Sonographic features of parovarian cysts and their complications, AJR. 1984; 143:157–160.
2. Athey PA. Adnexa: Nonneoplastic cysts. In: Athey PA, Hadlock FP. Ultrasound in Obstetrics and Gynecology. 2nd ed. St. Louis: CV Mosby; 1985; 206–221.
3. Athey PA, Cooper NB. Sonographic features of parovarian cysts. AJR. 1985; 144:83–86.
4. Athey PA, Malone RS. Sonography of ovarian fibromas/thecomas. J Ultrasound Med. 1987; 6:431–436.
5. Athey PA, Siegel MF. Sonographic features of Brenner tumor of the ovary. J Ultrasound Med. 1987; 6:367–372.
6. Baltarovich OH, Kurtz AB, Pasto ME, et al. The spectrum of sonographic findings in hemorrhagic ovarian cysts. AJR. 1987; 148:901–905.
7. Berland LL, et al. Ultrasound evaluation of pelvic infections. Radiol Clin North Am. 1982; 20:367.
8. Czernobilsky B. Common epithelial tumors of the ovary. In: Kurman RJ, ed. Blaustein's Pathology of the Female Genital Tract. 3rd ed. New York: Springer-Verlag; 1987; 560–606.
9. Diakoumakis E, Vieux U, Seife B. Sonographic demonstration of thecoma: Report of two cases. Am J Obstet Gynecol. 1984; 150:787–788.
10. Dooms GC, Hricak H, Tscholakoff D. Adnexal structures: MR imaging. Radiology. 1988; 158:639–646.
11. Fleischer AC. Gynecologic sonography. In: Fleischer AC, James AE, eds. Diagnostic Sonography. Principles and Clinical Applications. Philadelphia: WB Saunders; 1989; 221–340.
12. Fleischer AC, Daniell JF, Rodier J, et al. Sonographic monitoring of ovarian follicular development. J Clin Ultrasound. 1981; 9:275–280.
13. Fleischer AC, Walsh JW, Jones HW, et al. Sonographic evaluation of pelvic masses: Method of examination and role of sonography relative to other imaging modalities. Radiol Clin North Am. 1982; 20:397–412.
14. Goldstein SR, Subramanyam B, Synder JR, et al. The postmenopausal cystic adnexal mass: The potential role of ultrasound in conservative management. Obstet Gynecol. 1989; 73:8–10.
15. Goswamy RK, Campbell S, Whitehead MI. Screening for ovarian cancer. Clin Obstet Gynecol. 1983; 10:621.

16. Graif M, Itzchak Y. Sonographic evaluation of ovarian torsion in childhood and adolescence. AJR. 1988; 150:647–649.

17. Graif M, Shalev J, Strauss S, et al. Torsion of the ovary: Sonographic features. AJR. 1984; 143:1331–1334.

18. Green TH. Gynecology: Essentials of Clinical Practice. Boston: Little, Brown & Co; 1965.

19. Gutman PH Jr. In search of the elusive benign cystic ovarian teratoma: Application of the ultrasound "tip of the iceberg" sign. J Clin Ultrasound. 1977; 5:403.

20. Hackeloer BJ, Nitschke-Dabelstein S. Ovarian imaging by ultrasound: An attempt to define a reference plane. J Clin Ultrasound. 1980; 8:497–500.

21. Hall DA. Sonographic appearance of the normal ovary, of polycystic ovary disease and of functional ovarian cysts. Semin Ultrasound. 1983; 4:149.

22. Hall DA, Hann LE. Gynecologic radiology: Benign disorders. In: Taveras JM, Ferrucci JT. Radiology. Diagnosis—Imaging—Intervention. Philadelphia: JB Lippincott; 1988; 4:1–9.

23. Hall DA, Hann LE, Ferrucci JT Jr, et al. Sonographic morphology of the normal menstrual cycle. Radiology. 1979; 133:185.

24. Hall DA, McCarthy KA. The significance of the postmenopausal simple adnexal cyst. J Ultrasound Med. 1986; 5:503–505.

25. Hall DA, McCarthy KA, Kopans DB. Sonographic visualization of the normal postmenopausal ovary. J Ultrasound Med. 1986; 5(1):9–11.

26. Hann LE, Hall DA, McArdle CR, et al. Polycystic ovarian disease: Sonographic spectrum. Radiology. 1984; 150:531–534.

27. Herrmann UJ, Locher GW, Goldhirsch A. Sonographic patterns of ovarian tumors: Prediction of malignancy. Obstet Gynecol. 1987; 69:777–781.

28. Jones HW, Jones GS. Novak's Textbook of Gynecology. Baltimore: Williams & Wilkins; 1981.

29. Kurjak A. Transvaginal color Doppler. Presented at Leading Edge in Ultrasound Conference. Atlantic City, NJ, April 1989.

30. Lande IM, Hill MC, Cosco FE, et al. Adnexal and cul-de-sac abnormalities: Transvaginal sonography. Radiology. 1988; 166:325–332.

31. Lenz S. Ultrasonic study of follicular maturation, ovulation and development of corpus luteum during normal menstrual cycles. Acta Obstet Gynecol Scand. 1985; 64:15–19.

32. Leopold GR. Pelvic ultrasonography. In: Sarti DA, ed. Diagnostic Ultrasound. Text and Cases. Chicago: Year Book Medical Publishers. 1987; 692–695.

33. Meire HB, Farrant P, Guha T. Distinction of benign from malignant ovarian cysts by ultrasound. Br J Obstet Gynecol. 1978; 85:893–899.

34. Mendelson EB, Bohm-Velez M, Joseph N, et al. Gynecologic imaging: Comparison of transabdominal and transvaginal sonography. Radiology. 1988; 166:321–324.

35. Mitchell DG, Mintz MC, Spritzer CE, et al. Adnexal masses: MR imaging observations at 1.5 T, with US and CT correlation. Radiology. 1987; 162:319–324.

36. Montz FJ, Schlaerth B, Morrow CP. The natural history of theca lutein cysts. Obstet Gynecol. 1988; 72:247–251.

37. Morley P, Barnett E. The ovarian mass. In: Sanders RC, James AE, eds. The Principles and Practice of Ultrasonography in Obstetrics and Gynecology. 2nd ed. Norwalk, CT: Appleton-Century-Crofts; 1980; 357.

38. Moyle JW, Rochester D, Sider L, et al. Sonography of ovarian tumors: Predictability of tumor type. AJR. 1983; 14:985–991.

39. Munn CS, Kiser LC, Wetzner SM, et al. Ovary volume in young and premenopausal adults: US determination. Radiology. 1986; 159:731–732.

40. Neiman HL, Mendelson EB. Ultrasound evaluation of the ovary. In: Callen PW, ed. Ultrasonography in Obstetrics and Gynecology. 2nd ed. Philadelphia: WB Saunders; 1988:423–447.

41. Pinotti JA, Marussi EF, Zeferino LC. Evolution of cystic and adnexal tumors identified by echography. Int J Gynecol Obstet. 1988; 26:109–114.

42. Reynolds T, Hill MC, Glassman LM. Sonography of hemorrhagic ovarian cysts. J Clin Ultrasound. 1986; 14:449–453.

43. Rodriguez MH, Platt LD, Medearis AL, et al. The use of transvaginal sonography for evaluation of postmenopausal ovarian size and morphology. Am J Obstet Gynecol. 1988; 159:810–814.

44. Rubin C, Kurtz AB, Goldberg BB. Water enema: A new ultrasound technique in defining pelvic anatomy. J Clin Ultrasound. 1978; 6:28–33.

45. Stephenson WM, Laing FC. Sonography of ovarian fibromas. AJR. 1985; 144:1239–1240.

46. Swanson M, Sauerbrei EE, Cooperberg PL. Medical implications of ultrasonically detected polycystic ovaries. JCU. 1981; 9:219–222.

47. Thornton JG, Wells M. Ovarian cysts in pregnancy: Does ultrasound make traditional management inappropriate? Obstet Gynecol. 1987; 69:717–721.

48. Warner MA, Fleischer AC, Edell SL, et al. Uterine adnexal torsion: Sonographic findings. Radiology. 1985; 154:773–775.

49. Webster's New Collegiate Dictionary. Springfield, MA: G & C Merriam; 1976.

50. Weinreb JC, Brown CE, Lowe TW, et al. Pelvic masses in pregnant patients: MR and US imaging. Radiology. 1986; 159:717–724.

51. Williams CO. Radiologic Seminary CL XXXIV: Brenner tumor of the ovary—Ultrasound findings. J Miss State Med Assoc. 1978; 19:168.

52. Yaghoobian J, Pinck RL. Ultrasound findings in thecoma of the ovary. J Clin Ultrasound. 1983; 11:91–93.

53. Young RH, Scully RE. Sex cord-stromal, steroid cell, and other ovarian tumors with endocrine, paraendocrine and paraneoplastic manifestations. In: Kurman RJ, ed. Blaustein's Pathology of the Female Genital Tract. 3rd ed. New York: Springer-Verlag; 1987:607–658.

CHAPTER **9**

Pelvic Inflammatory Disease and Endometriosis

REBECCA HALL, KATHLEEN S. HOWE

Endometriosis and pelvic inflammatory disease (PID) are diffuse disease processes of the female pelvis that cause inflammatory changes. Progressive diseases, they display a varied pattern of tissue involvement and clinical presentation. Clinical presentation in the early stages of both diseases is frequently nonspecific and may mimic functional bowel disease. The picture is further complicated because these very different entities may have similar sonographic findings. For these reasons, sonography of PID and endometriosis can be discussed together, although their causes, clinical presentations, and progression are distinctive. Close correlation of patient history, clinical findings, and sonographic findings should enable the clinician to distinguish between PID and endometriosis. In this chapter we consider endometriosis and PID separately in terms of etiology, clinical findings, and sonographic findings. Table 9-1 summarizes the differences and similarities of the two.

Pelvic Inflammatory Disease

PID is a nonspecific term that refers to inflammation caused by infection in the upper genital tract. Locations affected by PID include the endometrium (endometritis), the uterine wall (myometritis), the uterine serosa and broad ligaments (parametritis), and the ovary (oophoritis). The most common location of infection is the oviducts, or fallopian tubes (salpingitis).

Salpingitis is a disease with major economic and health consequences. Approximately 1 million cases of salpingitis are diagnosed each year in the United States, at an estimated cost of care in excess of $3 billion. It is expected that the incidence of PID will increase directly with the current rise in the number of sexually active persons.[15] Twenty percent of patients who have had salpingitis become infertile and those who do conceive have a six to ten times greater risk of ectopic pregnancy. In addition, tuboovarian abscess (TOA) is a common sequela of salpingitis. As many as 34% of patients hospitalized with salpingitis progress to TOA.[10,27]

ETIOLOGY

The cause of PID is almost invariably (99%) multifactorial, by bacterial invasion ascending from the mixed flora of the vagina and cervix. The most common bacteria that cause PID are (in descending order) *Chlamydia trachomatis* and *Neisseria gonorrhoeae* (gonococcus). Endogenous anaerobic bacteria (*Bacteroides*, *Peptostreptococcus*, and *Peptococcus* species) and aerobic bacteria (*Streptococcus*, *Escherichia coli*, and *Staphylococcus* organisms) have also been implicated.

In the past, *N. gonorrhoeae* was considered "the major pathogen" in salpingitis. However, Landers and colleagues state that gonococci may initially penetrate the endocervical barrier, thus affording other organisms access to the upper genital tract.

143

TABLE 9-1. Characteristics of PID and endometriosis compared

	PID	ENDOMETRIOSIS

Etiology	Variable:
	Bacterial infection
	Neisseria gonorrhoeae
	
	Chlamydia species
	Anaerobic bacteria
	   Bacteroides
	   Peptostreptococcus
	   Peptococcus
	Aerobic bacteria
	   Streptococcus
	   Escherichia coli
	   Staphylococcus
		Presence of endometrial tissue in
		   abnormal locations outside uterus.
		Most commonly held mechanism is
		   retrograde menstruation.
		Can be diffuse or focal (endometrium).

Clinical
Findings
	Stage 1, early PID or endometriosis 50 to 80%
	   asymptomatic
	Gonococcus culture may still be positive.
	History of venereal disease, IUD, or pelvic
	   surgery
	Pelvic tenderness
	Vaginal discharge
	Urethral burning
	Stage 2, salpingitis (with or without formation
	   of pyosalpinx and resolution to
	   hydrosalpinx)
	Fever
	Chills
	Acute abdominal complaints
	Abnormal vaginal bleeding
	Stage 3, TOA or pelvic peritonitis with or
	   without pelvic abscess
	Fever with shaking chills
	Acute abdominal pain
	Significantly increased WBC
	Fitzhugh-Curtis syndrome
		May be asymptomatic. Symptom
		   characteristics:
		Involuntary infertility
		Cyclic dysmenorrhea
		Pelvic pain
		Dyspareunia
		Radiating back, leg, or groin pain

The initial gonorrheal infection may then be replaced by competing anaerobic or aerobic infective processes.[5,15] The predominant organisms isolated from TOA aspirates were found to be *E. coli, B. fragilis* and other *Bacteroides* species, aerobic streptococci, peptococci, and peptostreptococci. PID does occur in some patients without gonorrhea, chlamydia, or an intrauterine contraceptive device (IUD). It has been suggested that such patients have vaginitis with high concentrations of anaerobic bacteria, which may cause alterations in the physiologic or immunologic defense system. This in turn promotes invasion of the upper genital tract by normal vaginal and cervical flora.[15]

Although the vast majority (85%) of patients with PID become infected through sexual transmission, there are other routes of infection. The pathogen in PID may be introduced into the upper genital tract through curettage, hysterosalpingography, endometrial biopsy, or an IUD. Women who use an IUD have a greater risk of contracting PID than women who use oral or barrier forms of contraception. It has been postulated that the IUD string protruding from the uterus through the cer-

TABLE 9-1. (*continued*)

	PID	ENDOMETRIOSIS
Sonographic Characteristics	Stage 1, early PID Nonspecific findings: 　Thickened, hyperechoic endometrium surrounded by hypoechoic fluid 　May see fluid within endometrial cavity 　May see highly reflective interface within endometrial cavity representing gas with "dirty" acoustic shadow 　May see cul-de-sac fluid (anechoic or complex) Stage 2, Salpingitis 　Serpiginous swollen tubes appear as tubular or beaded adnexal masses 　Pointed beak (tapered end) of swelling, the proximal end of the tube 　Distended end the distal fimbriated end of the tube 　Pyosalpinx appears hypoechoic or complex, eventually becoming anechoic as resorption occurs and as hydrosalpinx develops 　Hydrosalpinx appears as sausage-shaped or ovoid adnexal structure with distinct borders and enhanced through-transmission; tail points toward uterus 　Ampullary segment is expanded portion of cyst	Variable appearance: May see nonspecific contour changes of pelvic structures or indistinct normal tissue planes Diffuse endometriosis can appear as solid homogeneous adnexal mass or complex Focal endometriosis appears as a cystic or complex, primarily cystic, spherical structure with discrete, thick, irregular walls; commonly exhibits uniform dispersion of low-level internal echoes; enhanced through-transmission
Differential Diagnoses by Ultrasound	Endometriosis Hemorrhagic ovarian cyst Ectopic pregnancy Neoplasm	PID Ectopic pregnancy Hemorrhagic ovarian cyst Neoplasm

vix into the vagina provides a route of infection. Less than 1% of all cases of PID result from hematogenous or lymphatic spread or from transperitoneal spread as a result of perforated appendix or intraabdominal abscess.[8]

PROGRESSION

PID is a progressive disease whose stages are determined by the upward migration of surface-invading bacteria from cervix to endometrium to salpinges to pelvic peritoneum. The initial spread of infection past the cervical barrier results in endo-

metritis, or early PID. In early PID, although the endometrial surface is infected with the pathogen, the uterus itself is generally immune to the inflammatory impact of the infection.[21] Rather, the endometrial cavity serves as a conduit for the organisms to reach the fallopian tubes. Varying degrees of salpingitis resulting from the spread of infection characterize the later stages of PID.

The second stage of pelvic inflammatory disease is characterized by acute or subacute salpingitis in which the tube becomes swollen or edematous. With acute gonorrheal salpingitis, a purulent exudate develops within the lumen of the tube, causing it to distend. With pyogenic salpingitis, the tube walls become grossly edematous and thickened, causing a much greater enlargement of the tube than with gonorrheal salpingitis.[21] If the lumen of the tube becomes blocked at the fimbriated orifice, purulent material builds up within the lumen, producing pyosalpinx (pus-filled tube). The development of pyosalpinx is usually associated with a chronic tubal infection or reinfection of a previously scarred tube.[21] Hydrosalpinx is a sequela of pyosalpinx: With the resolution of the acute infection, the purulent exudate is resorbed and a clear, watery fluid remains.[21] The walls of the tube remain distended and stretched, resulting in a thin-walled structure.

Extension of the inflammation from the salpinges may involve the broad ligaments (parametritis) and the ovaries (oophoritis). If the purulent material formed in the tube oozes from the fimbriated opening and over the adherent ovary, an abscess involving both the tube and the ovary may form a TOA. If pus escapes from the tube into the peritoneal cavity, a pelvic peritonitis develops, which may give rise to pelvic abscess.[21] Abscess formation may cause adhesions to form between uterus, bladder, adnexa, and bowel.[11,15]

The stages of extension of disease may be summarized as follows: (1) early PID or endometritis, (2) salpingitis with or without formation of pyosalpinx and resolution to hydrosalpinx, and (3) severe PID with TOA, or pelvic peritonitis with or without pelvic abscess. The course of the disease seems to be related to the type and virulence of the infecting organism, individual response to the infection, and a history of previous infection.[21]

CLINICAL FINDINGS
The patient with pelvic infection is often a young, sexually active woman with a wide range of nonspecific complaints. The clinical presentation ranges from minor complaints to acute life-threatening illness.[8,9] The most frequent symptoms are lower abdominal pain and pelvic tenderness, usually diffuse and bilateral, and constant dull pain, usually described as accentuated by movement or sexual activity. Onset of symptoms may be rapid (associated more often with *N. gonorrhoeae*) or insidious (associated more often with *C. trachomatis*).[8] Physical examination may reveal cervical or ad-

nexal tenderness, abdominal rebound and tenderness, and adnexal masses.[8,9] Seventy-five percent of patients with PID have associated endocervical infection with coexisting purulent vaginal discharge on physical examination.[8,9] Forty percent have abnormal vaginal bleeding and only 30% have fever. This spectrum of clinical findings contributes to the high rate of misdiagnoses when diagnosis is based on clinical criteria alone.

Laboratory findings play only a minor role in the diagnosis of PID. While 50% of PID patients have leukocytosis and may have an elevated erythrocyte sedimentation rate, this finding is nonspecific. It is significant to note that many patients, even with advanced abscess, may have no fever or elevated white blood cell count.[8,15] A small percentage (3 to 4%) have acute appendicitis with corresponding laboratory findings coexistent with PID.

Some patients may present with pelvic and right-sided upper quadrant pain. Fitzhugh-Curtis syndrome is a constellation of clinical findings that includes right-sided pleuritic pain and right-sided upper quadrant pain and tenderness on palpation. Fitzhugh-Curtis syndrome is experienced by 5 to 10% of patients with PID and is due to perihepatic inflammation from peritonitis, as the infected fluid tracks into the subhepatic space from the lower pelvic peritoneal compartments.

Although laboratory findings generally are of little help in establishing the diagnosis of PID, the detection of human chorionic gonadotropin (HCG) has major implications.[8,15] A small number (3 to 4%) of patients who present with symptoms of pelvic infection test positive for HCG, indicating pregnancy. Because there is a strong association of PID and ectopic pregnancy, particularly in patients who have a history of PID and TOA,[2] patients suspected of having PID who test positive for HCG should have an ultrasound examination to determine the location of the gestation and the extent of possible pelvic infection.

The gold standard for accurate diagnosis of PID has been direct visualization of pelvic structures by laparoscopic examination. In Sweden, for example, laparoscopy is performed on all patients with pelvic infections. In the United States, the most common method of diagnosis is the clinical history in conjunction with sonographic findings. Usually, only equivocal cases and patients who do not respond to antibiotic treatment are examined by laparoscopy.[8,16]

TREATMENT

Empiric antimicrobial therapy options initially include penicillin and tetracycline, and then combinations of cephalosporin, aminoglycoside, clindamycin, chloramphenicol, and cefotoxamine. For patients who do not respond, surgical therapy to drain the abscess or remove affected tubes or ovaries may be required. Percutaneous drainage of TOAs under ultrasound guidance has been reported, which has obviated the necessity for surgical intervention.[4]

ULTRASOUND IN THE MANAGEMENT OF PELVIC INFLAMMATORY DISEASE

As the ascending infection travels from cervix to endometrium to salpinges to pelvic peritoneum, ultrasound contributes increasingly to the diagnosis of PID. The early manifestations of the disease present nonspecific ultrasound findings; however, the progression to TOA and pelvic abscess is detected by ultrasound imaging with a high degree of specificity and sensitivity. Once the diagnosis has been made and treatment has been instituted, serial ultrasound examinations may be performed to monitor treatment response. Ultrasound examination confirms the presence and location of masses that may require surgical intervention.

The vast majority of PID patients are young women with many years of reproductive life ahead. The scarring of the fallopian tubes, which may be a result of pelvic infection, puts them at increased risk for ectopic pregnancy and sterility. Ultrasound examination is useful for determining the location of early gestation in patients with a history of PID (see Chapter 21).

ULTRASOUND FINDINGS IN PELVIC INFLAMMATORY DISEASE

The sonographic presentation of PID varies with the extent of the infection. Findings are dynamic, changing rapidly over a short time.[25] This discussion will consider the sonographic appearance of the various stages of infection and their sequelae.

Early Pelvic Inflammatory Disease. Early sonographic findings are too nonspecific to provide a firm diagnosis of PID; however, a constellation of sono-

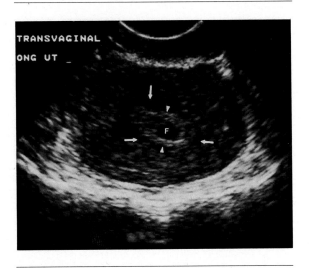

FIGURE 9-1. Transvaginal sonogram demonstrates changes in the endometrium as a result of endometritis. Note echogenic endometrium (*arrowheads*) enveloping a definite fluid collection (F). This prominent endometrium is surrounded by hypoechoic ring (*arrows*).

graphic findings may be present. Because the infection affects the endometrium, early findings include changes associated with endometritis or myometritis (Fig. 9-1). The endometrium may appear prominent and hyperechoic and may be surrounded by a hypoechoic ring or may contain a definite fluid collection. A subtle hypoechogenicity of the uterus may signal early uterine infection.[15,24,25] Postpartum endometritis as a result of retained products of conception, IUD perforation, or ascending microorganisms from the vagina such as *E. coli* and *Clostridium perfringens* (*welchii*) can result in a gas containing abscess in the endometrial cavity. Typical "dirty acoustic shadow" appearance behind high-level reflectors within the endometrial cavity may appear on ultrasound.[11,24,25] Other early findings are indistinct borders of the pelvic structures[1,24] and posterior cul-de-sac fluid. The amount of fluid, whether transudate or exudate, must be greater than that found midcycle in normal subjects, more than 4 to 6 ml.[24] The fluid may appear complex if it contains blood or pus. A distended bladder can displace cul-de-sac fluid, result-

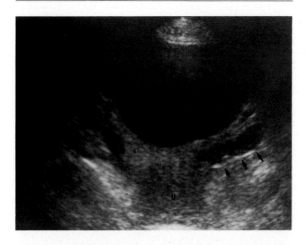

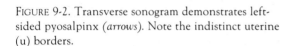

FIGURE 9-2. Transverse sonogram demonstrates left-sided pyosalpinx (*arrows*). Note the indistinct uterine (u) borders.

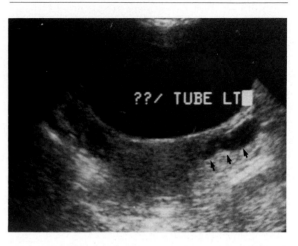

FIGURE 9-3. Transverse sonograms of salpingitis. Note the serpiginous configuration of the edematous tube (*arrows*).

ing in underestimation of pelvic fluid volume. The presence of cul-de-sac fluid cannot be correlated directly with the severity of disease.[2]

Pyosalpinx. As the infection ascends the genital tract, acute salpingitis results. Tubal infection has a destructive effect on the tubal mucosa that can result in the formation of purulent exudate. Pyosalpinx (pus-filled fallopian tubes) may develop and distend the oviducts. These will appear as tubular adnexal masses or as a string of beadlike adnexal masses (Fig. 9-2). This appearance is due to the blockage of the tubal lumen at the fimbriated end or at various points along the tube and resultant retention of the purulent exudate.[20] These masses are primarily cystic structures, but their sonographic appearance ranges from anechoic simple cysts to complex, primarily cystic structures with relatively smooth borders due to edema from the inflammatory process (Fig. 9-3). The stage of pus formation and the presence of debris and fluid determine the sonographic characteristics along that spectrum. Usually the walls of the pyosalpinx are relatively smooth, but they may appear shaggy.[2,24,27] Pyosalpinx is usually a unilateral process, but it may be bilateral.[11,24]

Severe Pelvic Inflammatory Disease with Tuboovarian Abscess. Severe PID results from the escape of purulent exudate into the peritoneal cavity and in the formation of TOAs. TOA is usually a bilateral process of varying size and echogenicity. Bilateral TOAs may completely fill the pelvis, obscuring the uterine borders. TOA should be suspected when cystic adnexal masses with indistinct, thick walls, internal septations, or complex internal echoes appear (Figs. 9-4, 9-5). The sonographic characteristics of these masses vary according to the stage of abscess formation. Severe PID may appear as an indistinct complex mass (Fig. 9-6), while a resorbing mass will result in a more cystic appearance. As treatment causes healing, pelvic structures begin to regain their normal appearances.

Peritonitis. As diffuse infectious involvement of the pelvis occurs, the borders of all the pelvic structures, including ovaries and tubes, become indistinct owing to parametrial inflammation (Fig. 9-7). This is due to the development of multiple abscesses forming septa. Some of the bacteria implicated in PID cause gas-forming abscesses, which further obscure tissue planes,[24] including the posterior cul-de-sac. In addition, the gas-forming or-

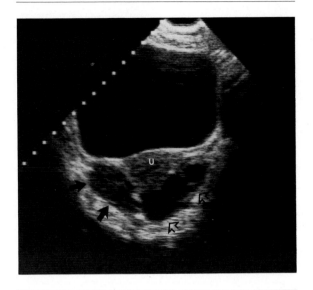

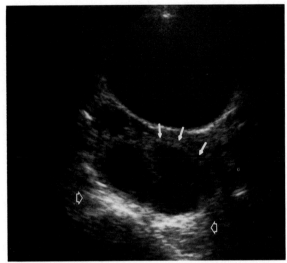

FIGURE 9-4. Transverse sonogram of bilateral TOA. Right TOA (*arrows*) with complex internal echoes. Left TOA (*open arrows*) is primarily cystic with thick walls and internal septations.

FIGURE 9-5. Oblique sonograms of left adnexal TOA. Note the indistinct thick walls (*closed arrows*) and enhanced through-transmission (*open arrows*) of this complex, primarily cystic mass.

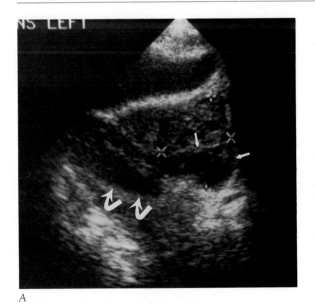

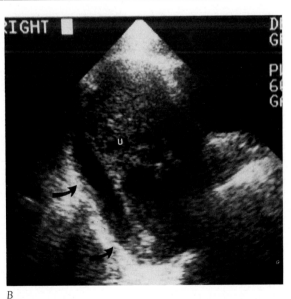

A

B

FIGURE 9-6. (A) Severe PID with posterior fluid collection (*curved arrows*). Transverse scan demonstrates indistinct complex mass in left adnexa (*straight arrows*). (B) Midline sagittal section, after partial voiding. Heterogeneous appearance of uterus (U) indicates myometritis.

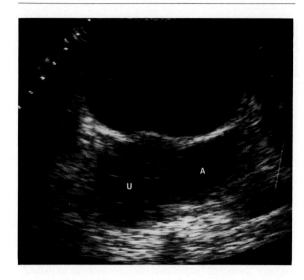

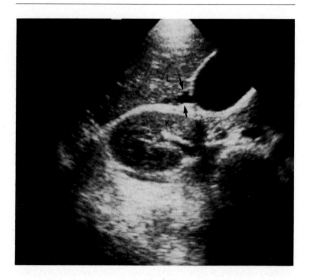

FIGURE 9-7. Severe PID in transverse section in which the uterus (U) can barely be distinguished from enlarged left adnexa (A).

FIGURE 9-8. Transverse sonogram of right upper quadrant demonstrates perihepatic fluid collection in Morison's pouch (*arrows*) between kidney (K) and liver (L). Associated with Fitzhugh-Curtis syndrome.

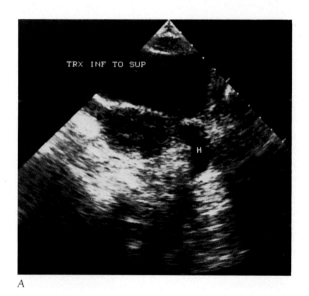

A

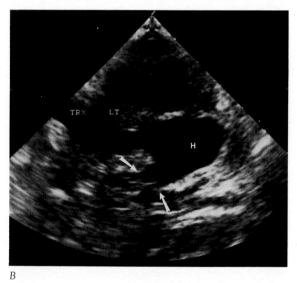

B

FIGURE 9-9. Left hydrosalpinx (H) demonstrated in (A) transabdominal sonogram and (B) transvaginal sonogram. Note the dilatation of fimbriated end of tube on (B) (*arrows*). Transvaginal sonography provides clearer delineation of small pelvic structures.

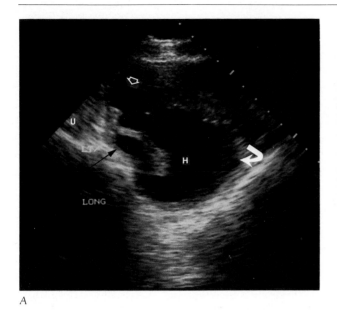
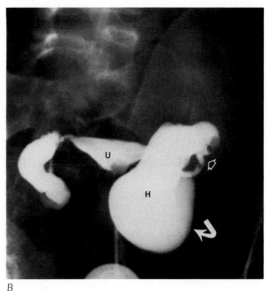

A   B

FIGURE 9-10. Left hydrosalpinx by sonography (A) and hysterosalpingography (B). Uterus (U), hydrosalpinx (H). The proximal end of the fallopian tube is obscured because of the folding over of the ampullary portion (*curved arrow*) on this view. The fimbriated end of the tube is represented by the *open arrow*.

ganisms may create a complex, reflective, echogenic appearance.[9] With abscess formation and the development of peritonitis, loculated fluid collections appear in the pelvis. These loculations may displace adjacent organs or compartments. Some of the infected fluid may not be loculated but may flow freely in the pelvis, paracolic gutters, and mesenteric reflections, shifting with changes in the patient's position. If it flows to the perihepatic space, the patient might experience Fitzhugh-Curtis syndrome (Fig. 9-8). Once fluid is discovered, the sonographer should note changes in appearance of the free-fluid by moving the patient from supine to right posterior oblique (RPO) and left posterior oblique (LPO) positions. It should be noted that pelvic peritonitis may lead to ileus, which will further complicate the sonographic findings by distending the bowel.

Chronic Pelvic Inflammatory Disease. Chronic PID refers to both the residue of acute infection and the subacute recurrence of previous PID. Hydrosalpinx, sterile fluid in a scarred fallopian tube, can occur as a result of long-standing PID. It appears as a sausage-shaped or ovoid, anechoic adnexal structure with enhanced acoustic transmission (Fig. 9-9). It has distinct borders and thin walls, owing to long-standing enlargement. In hydrosalpinx there is typically a tail-shaped structure pointing toward the uterus as the ampullary portion of the tube expands more than the proximal portion (Fig. 9-10).[24] Hydrosalpinx may be difficult to differentiate from an ovarian cyst or small cystadenoma.[25] Like ovarian cysts, hydrosalpinges occasionally undergo torsion.[21]

When adhesions have developed as the result of long-standing severe PID, the borders of pelvic structures may become obliterated or ill-defined because of fixation of organs by widespread fibrosis.[24] As in all pelvic examinations, it is important to distinguish bowel from possible PID, as bowel may mimic pelvic masses. If peristalsis is not evident, bowel may be differentiated from a "mass" by using the water enema technique.

Following treatment, serial ultrasonographic examinations will demonstrate resolution of pelvic infection by documenting changes in size and appearance of pelvic structures. This may be as simple as documenting the reduction in the size of masses or the amount of free fluid or as complex as judging the changes in the appearance of pelvic structures as they return to normal.[26] If the disease does not respond to conservative therapy, the ultrasound examination provides valuable information on the size and location of abscesses for surgical drainage.[24] With appropriate treatment, sonographic evidence of resolution should be seen within 6 to 8 weeks after antibiotic therapy begins.[2]

OTHER IMAGING MODALITIES

Although ultrasound is the standard diagnostic imaging procedure in the evaluation of PID, other noninvasive imaging techniques utilized to differentiate TOA from other masses include computed tomography (CT), magnetic resonance imaging (MRI), and radionuclide scanning.[15,19] Mitchell and coworkers recommend MRI as a useful supplement to ultrasound or CT if clearer documentation of the presence or absence of blood, fluid, fat, or protein components in the adnexal masses will increase the physician's confidence in diagnosis.[5,20] It is the opinion of some investigators that gallium-67 imaging in conjunction with sonographic examination or CT can lead to early diagnosis and treatment of occult infections.[19] Because sonography is inexpensive, readily available, does not expose the patient to ionizing radiation, and lends itself to serial scanning to follow treatment efficacy, it is recommended as the primary diagnostic modality.[15]

Endometriosis

Endometriosis is defined as heterotopic growth of the glands and stroma of the uterine lining (endometrium) which continue to respond to the hormonal influence of the ovulatory cycle.[7,8] Although the disease is generally regarded as a benign process, its chronic progression can produce a wide range of clinical consequences, such as excruciating cyclic pain and infertility.

ETIOLOGY

The etiology of endometriosis is uncertain, but several theories have been advanced. The dissemination of endometrial tissue throughout the pelvis via retrograde menstruation is the most popular theory. Other theories postulate vascular or lymphatic spread, metaplasia caused by the stimulation of menstrual debris by estrogen and progesterone, genetic predisposition, immunologic defects and contributing environmental factors.[8,29]

Endometriosis is directly related to the cyclic hormonal stimulation of the reproductive years. Natural menopause gradually brings relief of symptoms. Patients who have had transabdominal hysterectomy with bilateral oophorectomy experience prompt and complete regression of ectopically located endometrial tissue and relief of symptoms, although scar tissue may persist. It is assumed that intrapelvic bleeding and the development of adhesions cease when hormonal stimulation of ectopic endometrium ceases.[8,14]

Endometriosis can be diffuse or focal; 66% of implants are located in the pelvis. Focal implants involving the ovaries are called endometriomas. The term "chocolate cyst" is used to describe the characteristic appearance of an endometrioma filled with old blood from repeated episodes of hormonally stimulated endometrial sloughing within the implant. These are generally small, measuring 2 to 5 cm.[24] The most common site for endometrial implantation is the ovaries, usually bilaterally. Other locations include the anterior and posterior cul-de-sac, the broad ligaments, pelvic lymph nodes, the cervix, vagina, vulva, and fallopian tubes (Fig. 9-11).[8,23,29] Rarely, implantation occurs in areas of previous surgery, the umbilicus, bladder, kidney, arms, legs, and urinary tract. Pleural endometriosis which has spread from the pelvis through diaphragmatic defects has been documented.[8,13]

The color, shape, size, degree of inflammation, and associated fibrosis of the endometrial implants vary. The differences are associated with cyclic hormonal changes and how long the implant has been active. New lesions are small (<1 cm diameter), blood-filled, and raised above the surface of surrounding tissue. Lesions within the ovaries may range from these small, 1-mm, "new" implants to larger chocolate cysts, which may be 8 to 14 cm in diameter.[8,23,24]

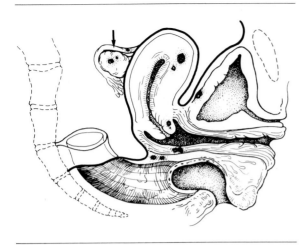

FIGURE 9-11. Schematic diagram of female pelvis shows sites for focal implants of ectopic endometrial tissue. The most common site of implantation is the ovary (*arrow*).

CLINICAL FINDINGS

It is estimated that 30 to 40% of infertility patients have endometriosis. The symptoms are common to several conditions, including chronic PID, ovarian malignancy, degeneration of uterine myoma, adenomyosis, primary dysmenorrhea, and functional bowel disease, so diagnosis is difficult.[8,17] It is further complicated by the fact that 5 to 10% of female laparotomy patients of childbearing age have been found incidentally to have endometriosis and that as many as 30% of all women may have no symptoms but evidence of endometriosis.

The typical endometriosis patient is nulliparous and in her 30s. The variety of symptoms is wide: asymptomatic involuntary infertility, dysmenorrhea, incapacitating pelvic pain, and dyspareunia, among others.[7,8,17,24,28] Endometriosis is rare in women under 20 years.[17]

One of the most common presenting symptoms is pelvic pain, but there is no direct relationship between the degree of pain and extent of the disease. A minimal amount of tissue implantation may result in excruciating pain if it causes peritoneal stretching, while extensive endometrial implants in less sensitive locations may create no symptoms. In fact, pain may be inversely related to the extent of disease. Patients with pelvic pain present with secondary dysmenorrhea (due to successive periods of swelling and extravasation of blood and menstrual debris into the surrounding tissue) and dyspareunia (either due to direct pressure of implants on the uterosacral ligaments or in the cul-de-sac or as a result of the immobilization of adherent structures).[7,8,23]

Pelvic pain usually begins 24 to 48 hours before menstruation and lasts several days; or it may be chronic, worsening during menses.[8,25] Descriptions of the pain range from a dull ache to severe unilateral or bilateral pain, which may radiate to the lower back, legs, or groin. Patients also report "pelvic heaviness," described as a feeling of swelling or congestion in the pelvic region. Fifteen to twenty percent of patients with endometriosis also have menorrhagia or abnormal premenstrual spotting.[8,23]

Endometriosis is a chronic and progressive disease of the childbearing years. The prognosis for pain and fertility is variable; some infertile patients remain otherwise asymptomatic throughout the course of the disease.

TREATMENT

Treatment of endometriosis may take two basic forms: The implant site may be excised or the hormonal stimulation that causes the cyclic growth and swelling may be ablated. Treatments for endometriosis include the following:

1. The synthetic steroid Danazol inhibits ovulation, causes amenorrhea, and produces atrophic changes in both the endometrium and the ectopic endometrial implants.
2. Continuous therapy with oral contraceptives and/or progesterone promotes a pseudopregnant state (anovulatory-acyclic hormonal environment), causing ectopic endometrial tissue to be resorbed.
3. Surgical intervention is necessary to excise large endometriomas or relieve ureteral obstruction, compromised bowel function, or adnexal masses.
4. Complete hysterectomy with oophorectomy is an option for patients who have completed childbearing.[7,8,23,24]

Laser surgery appears to hold promise for the future treatment of all types of endometriosis. Treat-

Table 9-2. Ultrasound examination for endometriosis or PID

Examination	
Uterus	*Size* is measured and documented on midline sagittal and AP miduterus and transverse. *Echogenicity* is noted; echo patterns are compared to normal homogeneous appearance, especially when performing serial exams. *Architecture* and border definition are noted.
Endometrium	Changes of normal echogenic patterns throughout the ovulatory cycle must be understood by the sonographer (see Normal Menstrual Cycle, Chapter 3). For example, a 6-mm echogenic endometrium surrounding a small amount of sonolucent endometrial cavity fluid is the normal premenses appearance of the late secretory phase but is abnormal for the first-week proliferative phase.
Adnexa	Delineation and measurement of ovaries in two planes must be consistently documented.

If Abnormalities Are Found:

If "masses" are seen, the following parameters are characterized in two planes:

Size is marked by caliper measurements.

Shape of "mass(es)." Spherical, ovoid, sausage-shaped? Where is it in relation to the ovaries? Could it be tubal? If you suspect it is tubal, is it dilated? Can you follow tube to the fimbriated end?

Internal definition. Is it sonolucent, hypoechoic, complex? Are there septa?

Adjacent structures. Is there indentation or displacement of normal adjacent structures, such as uterus or bladder?

Wall thickness. If the wall is thick, document with measurements. Is there fluid surrounding the border?

Posterior cul-de-sac. Is there free fluid? Is it sonolucent or is there debris in it? If fluid is present, is there also free fluid in Morison's pouch in the right-side upper quandrant? If so, document it.

Patient position. How does the appearance of such "mass(es)" change when the patient is moved to oblique positions, or following partial voiding and complete voiding? If the patient can tolerate transvaginal scanning, how do the "masses" appear in comparison? Do the findings confirm or clarify the transabdominal finding?

Pre- and postprocessing. Proper use of pre- and postprocessing capabilities should help. For example, changing the postprocessing curve on a poorly defined mass may accentuate the borders more effectively.

Remember: The key to a successful serial scanning technique is consistent documentation of all of the above.

---

ment may be monitored by second-look laparoscopy.

Role of Ultrasound. The goal of ultrasound in the management of endometriosis is to add as much detail as possible to the clinical picture, such as location and extent of disease. Ultrasound findings are most useful in the clinical management of advanced stages of the disease.

As in all scanning protocols for pelvic sonography, the examination should include visualization of the uterus and all its borders, the bilateral muscle groups that surround the uterus (iliopsoas, piriformis, obturator internus, and levator ani), the ovaries, pelvic vasculature, bladder, and ureters, all in at least two planes. The careful delineation of structures is particularly important when attempting to diagnose diffuse processes such as endometriosis or PID, which may produce subtle sonographic changes. Additionally, the blurring of

tissue planes associated with progressive PID or endometriosis necessitates more careful scanning in order to distinguish the mass from neighboring structures (Table 9-2).[24]

It must be noted that a negative ultrasound examination in the presence of clinical findings suggestive of endometriosis does not exclude an active, developing process.[3] Some authors assert that ultrasound plays only a minor role in the diagnosis of endometriosis because it is neither sensitive nor specific.[29]

Ultrasound Findings

The sonographic findings in endometriosis are variable.[8,24] Endometrial implants may exhibit sonographic patterns ranging from cystic to solid to complex. Generally, there must be a large volume of abnormal endometrial tissue if it is to be detected on ultrasound examination (Fig. 9-12). This volume of tissue may exist in large focal deposits or

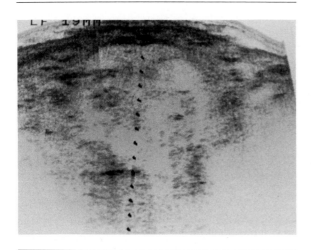

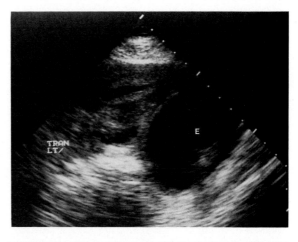

FIGURE 9-12. Diffuse endometriosis completely obliterates pelvic tissue planes.

FIGURE 9-13. Endometrioma (E) with characteristic complex, primarily cystic, appearance.

in widespread, diffuse sites of implantation. Solid echo patterns representing organized blood or fibrin deposits may appear as uniform homogeneous masses, but differentiation from other adnexal disease processes such as PID, neoplasms, hemorrhagic corpus luteum cysts, or ectopic pregnancy is difficult because normal tissue planes become indistinct as the disease progresses.[11,17,24]

The ultrasound diagnosis of focal endometriosis is made by visualization of complex, primarily cystic, structures representing chocolate cysts or endometriomas (Fig. 9-13). These are discrete, thick-walled, spherical pelvic masses (Fig. 9-14). Most commonly they exhibit uniform dispersion of low-level internal echoes (Fig. 9-15). In a minority of patients, they may be totally sonolucent or septated with enhanced through transmission (Fig. 9-16).[11,17,25] The walls of endometrial cysts are irregular, unlike the smooth walls of simple ovarian cysts. They may create bladder displacement by mass effect.[7,17,23,24]

Endometrial chocolate cysts are easily visualized by transvaginal sonography as uniformly echogenic masses when still recognizable as part of the ovary (Fig. 9-17). When the endometriomas are larger they may be difficult to visualize because of the limited field of view associated with transvaginal sonography. Their echo pattern may resemble that of sebaceous dermoid cysts and hemor-

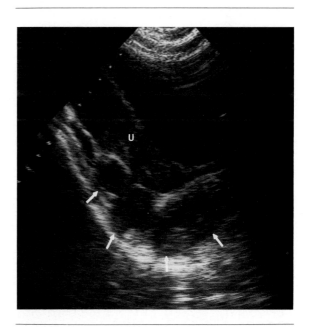

FIGURE 9-14. Longitudinal sonogram demonstrates multiple endometriomas (*arrows*) posterior to uterus (U). Note the irregular thick walls of these spherical masses and the different levels of echogenicity due to the various stages of aging.

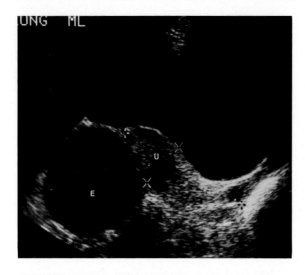

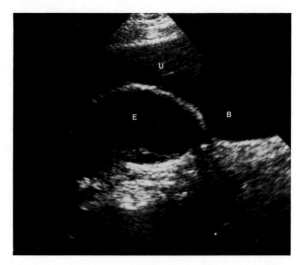

FIGURE 9-15. Longitudinal sonogram shows the classic low-level echoes within this endometrioma (E) located superior to the uterus (U).

FIGURE 9-16. Oblique sonogram demonstrates the less common sonographic appearance of endometriomas (E) adjacent to bladder (B) and uterus (U). Note the septae and enhanced through-transmission.

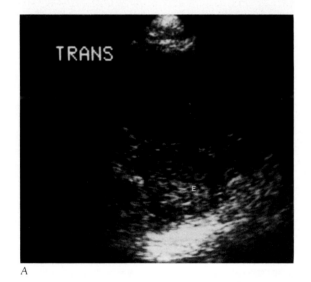

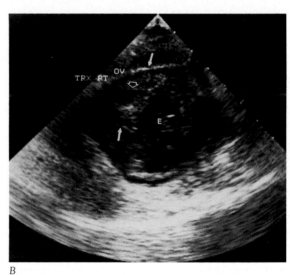

A

B

FIGURE 9-17. Comparison of transabdominal sonogram (A) and transvaginal sonogram (B) of the same endometrioma (E). Note the improved distinction of the endometrioma from the ovary (*closed arrows*) on the transvaginal sonogram. A small follicle is noted in the ovary (*open arrows*).

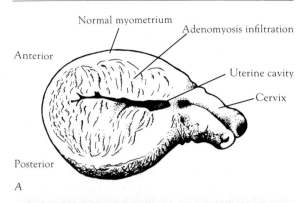

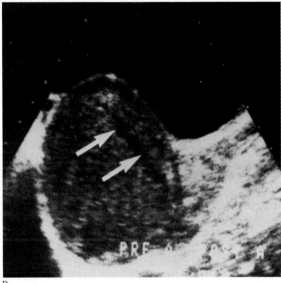

FIGURE 9-18. (A) Diagram of longitudinal section of uterus shows gross appearance of diffuse adenomyosis. (B) Longitudinal sonogram shows adenomyosis of uterus. Note thickened posterior wall and eccentric displacement of uterine cavity (*arrows*). (From Bohlman M, et al. Sonographic findings in adenomyosis of the uterus. AJR. 1987;148:765–766.

rhagic corpus luteum cysts.[14,28]

As with all pelvic scans, it is especially important to distinguish bowel from areas of possible pathology when examining a patient whose clinical presentation suggests endometriosis. If peristalsis is not evident in a suspicious area, bowel should be differentiated from mass by use of a water enema. Bowel involvement may also produce changes on barium studies.[6,7]

Diagnosis and treatment of endometriosis is based primarily on clinical findings. Other common diseases that involve the pelvic organs, however, must be included in the differential diagnosis because of overlapping patterns of clinical presentation. These include PID, ectopic pregnancy, abscess, neoplasm, hemorrhagic corpus luteum cyst, leiomyoma, ovarian cyst, and cystadenoma.[7,25] Ultrasonographic findings may add valuable information such as the extent and progress of the disease and it may contribute to narrowing the differential diagnosis.

Adenomyosis

DEFINITION

Adenomyosis is often described as "internal endometriosis," where growth of endometrial glands and stroma occurs within the uterine myoma at a depth of at least 2.5 mm from the basalis layer of the endometrium (Fig. 9-18).[8,25,29] The aberrant growth of endometrial tissue within the uterine wall differs from endometriosis in that it does not undergo the cyclic changes resulting from ovarian hormone production. The cul-de-sac and ovaries are not involved. The most common clinical manifestations of adenomyosis are pelvic pain, hypermenorrhea, and intermenstrual spotting.[22]

CLINICAL FINDINGS

Patients with adenomyosis are older than those with endometriosis, are parous, and have a history of hypermenorrhea and dysmenorrhea. Pain associated with adenomyosis is noticed immediately before or during menstruation. On physical examination, the uterus is found to be enlarged, often two or three times normal size. The clinical presentation and physical findings may mimic those of leiomyoma.[22] Hysterosalpingography may show an enlarged uterus, or results may be normal.[5]

TREATMENT

Adenomyosis is treated surgically by total hysterectomy with or without removal of the ovaries. Hormone treatments utilized for endometriosis have been uniformly unsuccessful.[14]

ULTRASOUND FINDINGS

The primary ultrasound finding in adenomyosis is a symmetrically enlarged fundus and body of the uterus due to endometrial hyperplasia and hypertrophy of the uterine muscle.[1,2,3,25] The sonographic texture of the uterus is uniform; echogenicity is normal or slightly decreased. The endometrial cavity may be displaced by thickened posterior myometrium.[3] This thickened area may have a "Swiss cheese" appearance owing to areas of focal hemorrhage and clot within the uterine muscle.[3,7,24]

These findings are also consistent with uterine myomas and endometrial carcinoma. Care must be taken to further evaluate the disease process by utilizing signal-processing capabilities to better distinguish myometrium from endometrium. Transvaginal sonography may prove to be helpful as it is used more commonly to differentiate uterine pathology.

MRI may offer some assistance in the difficult task of distinguishing adenomyosis from leiomyoma. MRI researchers believe that the difference in signal intensities between the two entities as well as the comparison of border definition and effect on surrounding structures may hold a key to this diagnostic problem. The differentiation is important for patients who wish to preserve their reproductive capacity. Presurgical diagnosis of leiomyoma may permit myomectomy instead of hysterectomy. Diagnosis must be confirmed histologically.[18]

References

1. Berland L, Lawson T, Roley W, et al. Ultrasound evaluation of pelvic infections. Radiol Clin North Am. Philadelphia: WB Saunders; 1982.
2. Bernstine R, Kennedy W, Waldron J. Acute pelvic inflammatory disease: Clinical follow-up. Int J Fertil. 1987; 32:229–332.
3. Bohlman M, Ensor R, Sanders R. Sonographic findings in adenomyosis of the uterus. AJR. 1987; 148:765–766.
4. Casola G, et al. Percutaneous drainage of tubo-ovarian abscesses. Presented at the 74th Scientific Assembly and Annual Meeting of the Radiologic Society of North America, Chicago, Nov. 27–Dec. 2, 1988.
5. Chinn D, Callen P. Ultrasound of the acutely ill obstetrics and gynecology patient. Radiol Clin North Am. Philadelphia: WB Saunders; 1983.
6. Dallenbach-Hellweg G. Histopathology of the Endometrium. New York: Springer-Verlag; 1987.
7. Deutsch A, Gosink B. Nonneoplastic gynecologic disorders. Semin Roentgenol. 1982; 17:269–283.
8. Droegemueller W, Herbst A, Michell D, et al. Comprehensive Gynecology. St. Louis: CV Mosby, 1987.
9. Galask R, Larsen B. Infectious Diseases in the Female Patient. New York: Springer-Verlag; 1986.
10. Hager W. Follow-up of patients with tuboovarian abscess(es) in association with salpingitis. Obstet Gynecol. 1983; 61:680.
11. Hall R. The Ultrasound Handbook. Philadelphia: JB Lippincott; 1988.
12. Hemsell D, Santos-Ramos R, Cunningham G, et al. Cefotaxime treatment for women with community-acquired pelvic abscesses. Am J Obstet Gynecol. 1985; 151:771–777.
13. Kang H, Choi B, Park J, et al. Endometriosis: CT and sonographic findings. AJR. 1987; 148:523–524.
14. Kistner R. Gynecology Principles and Practice. 4th ed. Chicago: Year Book Medical Publishers; 1986.
15. Landers D, Sweet R. Current trends in the diagnosis and treatment of tuboovarian abscess. Am J Obstet Gynecol. 1985; 151:1098–1110.
16. Ledger W. Infection in the Female. 2nd ed. Philadelphia: Lea & Febiger; 1986.
17. Manor WF, Zwiebel WJ, Hanning RV Jr, et al. Ectopic pregnancy and other causes of acute pelvic pain. Semin Ultrasound, CT MR. 1985; 6:181–184.
18. Mark A, Hricak H, Heinrichs L, et al. Adenomyosis and leiomyoma: Differential diagnosis with MR imaging. Radiology. 1987; 163:527–529.
19. Mettler FA, Guiberteau M. Essentials of Nuclear Medicine Imaging. 2nd ed. Orlando, FL: Grune and Stratton; 1986.
20. Mitchell D, Mintz M, Spritzer C, et al. Adnexal masses: MR imaging observations at 1.5T, with US and CT correlations. Radiology. 1987; 162:319–324.
21. Novak E. Novak's Textbook of Gynecology. 9th ed. Baltimore: Waverly Press; 1975.
22. Nyberg D, Laing F, Jeffrey B. Sonographic detection of subtle pelvic fluid collections. AJRF. 1984; 143:261–263.
23. Rosenwaks Z, Benjamin F, Stone M. Gynecology: Principles and Practice. New York: Macmillan; 1987.
24. Sanders R, James E. The Principles and Practice of Ultrasonography in Obstetrics and Gynecology. 3rd ed. Norwalk, CT: Appleton-Century-Crofts; 1985.
25. Sarti D. Diagnostic Ultrasound: Text and Cases. 2nd ed. Chicago: Year Book Medical Publishers; 1987.
26. Spirtos N, Bernstine R, Crawford W, et al. Sonography in acute pelvic inflammatory disease. J Reprod Med. 1982; 27:312–320.
27. Swayne L, Love M, Karasick S. Pelvic inflammatory disease: Sonographic-pathologic correlation. Radiology. 1984; 151:751–755.
28. Timor-Tritsch I, Rottem S. Transvaginal Sonography. New York: Elsevier; 1988.
29. Wilson E. Endometriosis. New York: Alan R. Liss; 1987.

CHAPTER 10

Ovarian Malignancies

RUTH ROSENBLATT

The role of ultrasound (US) imaging with regard to ovarian malignancy is threefold. First, it permits the accurate evaluation of the patient with a suspected pelvic mass. Second, in a patient with the diagnosis of ovarian carcinoma, the US examination helps determine the presence of recurrent or persistent disease after surgery and chemotherapy. Finally, US is currently being explored as a potentially useful screening tool for ovarian malignancy.

Incidence and Prognosis

Ovarian malignancy is a disease of low prevalence, accounting for only 4% of all cancers in women.[1] Yet, it causes more deaths than any other cancer of the female reproductive system (trailing behind cancer of the breast, lung, and colon) and is the fourth leading cause of cancer deaths among women. The relatively high mortality of ovarian malignancy is a reflection of its low cure rate. The American Cancer Society estimates that approximately 17,000 to 19,000 new cases are diagnosed each year in the United States and that one out of every 70 newborn girls will develop ovarian cancer during her lifetime.[1] While mortality rates for other gynecologic malignancies are declining, there is evidence to suggest that both the incidence and mortality of ovarian cancer are increasing.[2,10,12,15] There are global variations in the incidence of ovarian cancer. For instance, it is much more com-

mon in the Scandinavian countries and the United States than in India and Japan, where it is rare.[17]

The poor prognosis of ovarian malignancy is in great measure related to the fact that the disease is often diagnosed at a late stage. In such cases the overall 5-year survival rate is about 22%. Ovarian malignancy is, unfortunately, found late because early in its course the disease is usually silent. When symptoms appear, they are often vague. On the other hand, if the disease happens to be detected and treated in its early phase the 5-year survival rate may reach 85 to 90%.[1] Factors that determine the prognosis are: (1) stage, the extent of the disease when it is first diagnosed; (2) tumor grade, the histopathologic classification or the degree of cellular differentiation; and (3) the extent of residual disease following initial surgical excision.

Early detection of ovarian malignancy offers the most effective means of reducing the current high mortality rate. Research in a number of medical disciplines, including epidemiology, gynecologic oncology, and radiologic imaging, has been directed toward this goal. Extensive epidemiologic studies have helped to define the population at risk.[28] It is possible that such data will be useful in making screening economically more feasible because of the low prevalence of the disease. Biochemical research in the field of oncology has involved immunologic studies in an effort to detect the presence of even a small population of malignant cells by means of tumor markers.[28] Finally, the ongoing improvement in imaging techniques enables the visualization of even minimal ovarian enlargement.

Epidemiology and Risk Factors

A number of recent studies in the epidemiology of ovarian cancer have shed some light on risk factors for this disease. Age is the major risk factor for the most common ovarian malignancies. The peak incidence is between 55 and 59 years.

A direct relationship has been observed between the number of years of ovulatory activity and the risk of developing epithelial ovarian cancer, the most common type. A woman whose ovulatory activity extends for more than 40 years is considered at high risk.[28] Conversely, there appears to be a protective influence against developing ovarian cancer when ovulatory activity is reduced. For example, pregnancy, lactation, oral contraceptives, and a shorter reproductive span due to late menarche or early menopause are all factors that decrease the number of years of ovulatory activity. An animal model for ovulatory activity and ovarian cancer has been provided by studies of domestic fowl. It appears that a significantly greater incidence of ovarian cancer occurs among chickens reared for egg-laying capacity than among broiler chickens, and further, the cancer affects the left ovary only, which is, in fact, the one producing the ova.[17] An interesting theory regarding the relationship of ovulation and the development of ovarian cancer has been postulated. Ovulation involves minor but repeated trauma to the surface epithelium of the ovary with exposure to estrogen-rich follicular fluid and the formation of inclusion cysts as a reparative process in follicular rupture. This incessant ovulation may predispose to carcinogenesis.[7]

As with breast cancer, a strong family history of ovarian cancer (maternal or sibling) places a woman at high risk, making this genetic risk factor a criterion for screening studies.[12] A strong family history of breast cancer may also increase the risk of developing an ovarian malignancy.[15]

Certain environmental factors have been linked to ovarian cancer risk. A three- to fivefold higher incidence of ovarian cancer and mortality has been observed in industrialized countries than in developing nations.[28] A notable exception is Japan, an industrialized country with a low incidence of ovarian cancer. Countries with the highest incidence of ovarian cancer are Sweden, Norway, and the United States. Global variations have led epidemiologists to postulate that carcinogens in the air, water, or diet of industrialized communities play a role in the higher incidence of this disease.[15]

Talcum powder used for perineal hygiene has also been implicated as a possible causal factor. It has been postulated that insoluble, finely divided powder particles may migrate to the peritoneal cavity via vagina, uterus, and tubes and act as irritants, promoting cancer growth.[15]

Pathology

HISTOLOGIC CLASSIFICATION

The pathology and pathophysiology of ovarian malignancy are extremely complex. The ovary has both endocrine and reproductive functions and is composed of at least four different cell populations, each of which may undergo malignant transformation. A classification of ovarian tumors has been proposed by the World Health Organization.[14] There are nine broad categories of tumors based on the cell of origin. Each of these categories of neoplasms is further divided into histologically distinguishable lesions which may be benign, borderline malignant, or frankly malignant. Varying degrees of histologic differentiation can be found in different sections of one lesion. While the most differentiated area of the lesion determines the cell type, the least differentiated portion determines its malignant potential. The degree of cellular differentiation is used for tumor grading and represents an important criterion in assessing the severity of the disease, and therefore the prognosis. Poorly differentiated cancers have a higher likelihood of aggressive growth, and occult metastases may be present even when the primary lesion is small.

Tumors originating from the *epithelium* covering the ovaries account for 90 to 95% of ovarian malignancies, the serous and mucinous cystadenocarcinomas. A much less common group of lesions are the gonadal stromal, or *sex cord,* neoplasms, some of which may be endocrinologically active and therefore be diagnosed when smaller in size. The least common group are the *germ cell* lesions. Me-

TABLE 10-1. Most common malignant ovarian neoplasms: Correlation of clinical and sonographic findings*

Pathology (Frequency)	Clinical Features	Sonographic Findings
Epithelial (90–95%)		
Cystadenocarcinoma, serous (more common) or mucinous	Peri- and postmenopausal; abdominal pain; distension; GI symptoms	Large (10- to 30-cm), complex cysts with clear or echogenic fluid; thick septa and papillations; 25–60% are bilateral
Undifferentiated adenocarcinoma		Fixation; ascites common; echogenic ascites suggests pseudomyxoma peritonei
Endometrioid	May be associated with benign endometriosis and endometrial cancer	Mixed cystic and solid pattern; 30% are bilateral; may be seen associated with endometrial echo abnormality
Sex Cord Neoplasms (2%)		
Granulosa-theca cell tumor	Wide age range; associated with hyperestrinism; vaginal bleeding due to endometrial hyperplasia or carcinoma	Predominantly solid; unilateral; homogenous; may see endometrial thickening
Androblastoma (Sertoli-Leydig cell tumor)	Common in adolescence; may have masculinizing effect	Usually solid and unilateral
Germ-Cell Neoplasms (1%)		
Dysgerminoma	Often seen in adolescence; radiosensitive; may be cause of primary amenorrhea	Usually solid; variable in size; 10-20% are bilateral
Choriocarcinoma	May cause precocious puberty; associated with high levels of HCG; aggressive growth	Variable consistency
Teratocarcinoma	Rare tumor; often seen in young adulthood	Variable appearance with cystic and highly echogenic areas with acoustic shadow
Endodermal sinus tumor	May be seen in association with teratoma; highly malignant; young adulthood	Predominantly solid, with areas of necrosis
Metastases to Ovary (4–8%)		
Krukenberg tumor (primary in gastrointestinal tract) or from other sites: breast, lung, pancreas, lymphoma	Peri- and postmenopausal; may be first manifestation of extraovarian malignant disease; search for GI primary	Large masses; usually complex texture and bilateral; more common on right if unilateral; often indistinguishable from ovarian primary malignancy

*For a complete World Health Organization classification of ovarian tumors the reader is referred to Jones H, Jones G, eds. Novak's Textbook of Gynecology. 11th ed. Baltimore: Williams & Wilkins; 1988:507.

tastases to the ovary account for about 4 to 8% of ovarian malignancies. Although the sonographic specificity for a particular histologic type of ovarian malignancy is poor, correlation of the clinical features and the sonographic appearance may lead to a more accurate diagnosis. Table 10-1 summarizes the pathologic, clinical, and sonographic features of the most common ovarian malignancies.

PATHOPHYSIOLOGY

A characteristic feature of most epithelial cancers is the tendency to form cystic masses with multiple septa. The masses are often enormous, reaching 30 to 40 cm in diameter and weighing 10 to 15 kg and, of course, extending into the abdomen. The cysts contain serous or mucinous fluid; nodular or papillary growths project into the fluid and may also be present on the external surface of the cyst (Fig. 10-1). The tissue is friable, and thin-walled blood vessels of the lesion predispose to intracystic bleeding. Areas of the lesion devoid of adequate blood supply may undergo necrosis. Bleeding and necrosis add to the fluid content of the lesion (Fig. 10-2). Dystrophic calcification often occurs within areas of cellular degeneration. These microcrystals, or psammoma bodies, may be seen radiographically. The epithelial tumors which do not secrete fluid are generally smaller but may still have within them irregular fluid collections secondary to hemorrhage and necrosis.

Ascites is often associated with ovarian malignancy. At postmortem it is found in 60 to 70% of cases. Typically the fluid has a high protein content. Protein-rich fluid exudes from the tumor-bearing surfaces of the peritoneum, since tumor vessels are more permeable to protein.[8] Fluid accumulates first in the dependent portion of the peritoneal cavity, such as the cul-de-sac in the pelvis. Subsequently the fluid ascends into both paracolic gutters but predominantly on the right because this space is broader and forms a better communication between the right upper quadrant and the pelvis (Fig. 10-3A).

When spontaneous leakage or rupture of a mucinous cystadenocarcinoma occurs, the peritoneal cavity is contaminated with the sticky gelatinous fluid, leading to massive abdominal distension, a condition known as pseudomyxoma peritonei (Fig. 10-4). Rupture of mucinous neoplasm of the appendix (most often malignant) is also a cause of this condition.

Spread and Staging of Ovarian Malignancy

The major patterns of spread of ovarian malignancy are direct extension to involve contiguous organs in the pelvis, peritoneal seeding, and lymphatic spread. Ovarian cancer is the most common

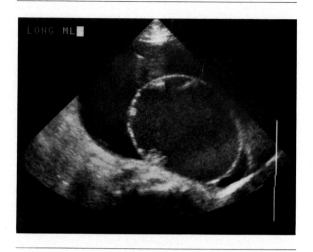

FIGURE 10-1. Papillary serous cystadenoma of low-grade malignancy, stage Ia, in an 80-year-old woman with abdominal discomfort. Midline sagittal scan demonstrated a cyst within a cyst. Note the papillations on the inner cyst wall and the echogenic fluid, which contained fine particulate debris and residua of previous bleeding. The entire lesion was 21 × 17 × 11 cm, unilateral, and confined to the ovary.

tumor responsible for peritoneal malignancy in women. Intraperitoneal dissemination occurs when tumor cells are shed from the lesion and establish growth on peritoneal surfaces within the abdomen, particularly the diaphragmatic leaflets, liver capsule, bowel serosa, and omentum. This occurs relatively early in the disease and is often, but not always, associated with ascites. There are several pathways for the lymphatic spread of tumor cells: peritoneal lymphatics draining toward the diaphragm and pelvic lymphatics draining to the retroperitoneum. The pattern of spread of ovarian tumor is not predictable. Since the diaphragmatic lymphatics are the major pathways of peritoneal fluid drainage, blockage of this pathway by tumor may also produce ascites. The diaphragmatic lymphatics that drain to the retrosternal and mediastinal nodes constitute a major avenue of spread of the disease to the chest.

In advanced cases of ovarian malignancy, antegrade spread or distal migration of tumor cells to the uterus may be manifested by positive vaginal

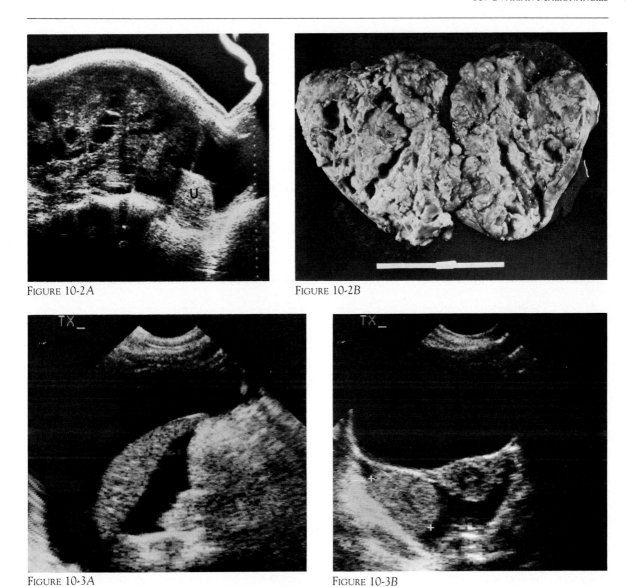

FIGURE 10-2A

FIGURE 10-2B

FIGURE 10-3A

FIGURE 10-3B

FIGURE 10-2. Endometrioid carcinoma, stage III, in a 59-year-old woman with increased abdominal girth, weight loss, and mild abdominal discomfort. (A) Sagittal view of pelvis and abdomen with minimal bladder distension. The large mass, predominantly solid, contains numerous cystic spaces (U, uterus). (B) Cut surface of an 11 × 10-cm tumor, predominantly solid, with areas of necrosis. At surgery, metastatic nodules were found on the mesentery and omentum.

FIGURE 10-3. Granulosa-theca cell tumor in an 18-year-old woman with abdominal distension. (A) Transverse view of the right upper quadrant demonstrating a large amount of ascites, predominantly on the right and surrounding the liver. (B) Transverse view of the pelvis showing a right adnexal solid mass, 8 × 7 × 6 cm, homogeneous in texture.

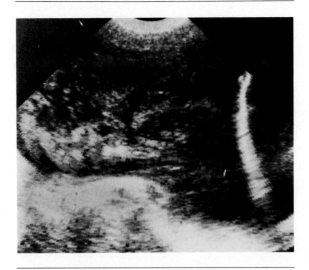

FIGURE 10-4. Pseudomyxoma peritonei in a 62-year-old woman with increasing abdominal girth. Midline sagittal scan above the bladder. Echogenic fluid was noted floating between loops of bowel.

TABLE 10-2. FIGO staging system for ovarian cancer

Stage I. Growth limited to the ovaries
    Ia. Only one ovary involved, no ascites
    Ib. Growth limited to both ovaries, no ascites
    Ic. Growth limited to ovaries but ascites or positive cytology present
Stage II. Growth beyond ovaries but limited to the pelvis
    IIa. Extension to uterus/tubes
    IIb. Extension to other pelvic structures, including uterus
    IIc. Extension within pelvis and ascites
Stage III. Growth beyond the pelvis. Retroperitoneal nodal and/or intraperitoneal omental spread, excluding deep liver metastases
Stage IV. Distant metastases or pleural involvement. Liver parenchymal metastases.

Adapted from Jones H, Jones G, eds. Novak's Textbook of Gynecology. 11th ed. Baltimore: Williams & Wilkins; 1988:797.

cytology. Not infrequently, distant metastases occur in the liver. Sonographically, these lesions may have a complex cystic appearance, reflecting the presence of fluid and mucin within them.

The extent of tumor spread or stage of disease at time of diagnosis is an important parameter in the patient's clinical course. A staging scheme proposed by the International Federation of Gynecologists and Obstetricians (FIGO) is a widely accepted classification (Table 10-2). The stage of disease is determined at the time of laparotomy. Imaging techniques such as computed tomography (CT) and US add further information to increase accuracy of staging.[19,26]

Clinical Considerations

Symptoms

Ovarian carcinoma is mainly a disease of peri- and postmenopausal women: Mean age at diagnosis is 52 years. The insidious, sometimes vague, symptoms of ovarian cancer often contribute to delay in diagnosis. When symptoms do appear they are related to pressure from an enlarging pelvic mass or from accumulation of ascites. Less frequently, man-ifestation of hormone activity (feminizing or masculinizing symptoms) provide a clue to the presence of a lesion. Rarely, the diagnosis is made only when the tumor undergoes torsion and the patient presents with an acute abdomen, requiring surgical intervention.

An analysis of ten clinical studies from the literature, comprising over 2000 patients, disclosed that 50% of ovarian cancer patients presented with pain.[22] An almost equally common complaint was abdominal distension (49%). Gastrointestinal symptoms such as indigestion or bloating were present in 21% of cases. Such complaints are often treated symptomatically, diverting attention from the pelvis and delaying diagnosis. It has been emphasized that undiagnosed, persistent gastrointestinal symptoms in women over 40 should prompt a search for an ovarian lesion. The pressure from mass and ascites accounts for urinary symptoms of urgency and frequency seen in 17% of patients. The mass may produce backache, pelvic pressure, or simply a vague feeling of pelvic unrest. Despite increase in abdominal girth, 17% of patients may complain of weight loss.

A significant number of patients with ovarian malignancy present with or develop vaginal bleeding (17%). Bleeding may be secondary to estrogen secretion by the lesion (see below), concurrent endometrial and ovarian carcinoma, or, rarely, direct spread of the lesion to the endometrium (Fig. 10-

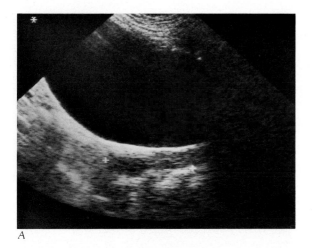

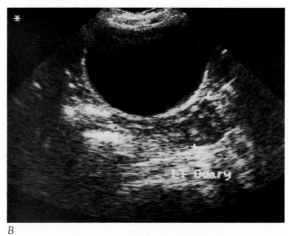

A   *B*

FIGURE 10-5. Serous papillary carcinoma in a 79-year-old woman. Results of abdominal Pap smear and findings at dilation and curettage were compatible with adenocarcinoma. No mass was palpated on pelvic examination. (A) Sagittal view of the uterus demonstrates a normal-sized uterus for patient's age. Despite this, findings at dilation and curettage were positive for papillary carcinoma. (B) Transverse view of pelvis shows a 4.4-cm solid left adnexal mass with good sound transmission. This proved to be an ovarian serous papillary carcinoma.

5). Not infrequently, the cause of bleeding is undetermined.

Symptoms of abnormal endocrine activity are sometimes a clue to the presence of an ovarian malignancy that is hormonally active or stimulates the normal ovarian tissue to increased hormone production. Feminizing effects due to overproduction of estrogen by a granulosa cell tumor are often associated with vaginal bleeding in the postmenopausal patient. In young girls the rare primary ovarian choriocarcinoma may be a cause of precocious puberty. Conversely, a rare cause of primary amenorrhea in adolescents is dysgerminoma, which is the counterpart of, and histopathologically resembles, the seminoma of the testis. A lesion that often produces defeminizing or masculinizing effects is the androblastoma or Sertoli-Leydig cell tumor. This lesion is more commonly seen in adolescents or young women and is often solid (Fig. 10-6). Other endocrinelike effects, such as Cushing's syndrome, hypoglycemia, hypercalcemia, and hyperthyroidism, may be seen in association with ovarian malignancy. One consequence of hor-

monal activity by the ovarian lesion is the possibility of earlier diagnosis. Inappropriate hormonal activity is not diagnostic of ovarian malignancy, however. A variety of benign ovarian neoplasms as well as ovarian or adrenal hyperplasia may also manifest such abnormalities.

Any mass may undergo sudden compromise of its blood supply due to torsion or incarceration. Such an event is likely to produce acute abdominal symptoms that may mimic inflammatory disease. In the pediatric age group, ovarian malignancy is likely to present as a pelvic or abdominal mass, with or without torsion. Torsion is also more likely to occur in the second or third trimester of pregnancy.[28]

TREATMENT

Treatment options include surgery, radiotherapy, and chemotherapy. Surgery plays a crucial role in the diagnosis and treatment of ovarian cancer. Surgical planning and management is decisive in the prognosis of ovarian malignancy, and maximum information regarding staging prior to initial on-

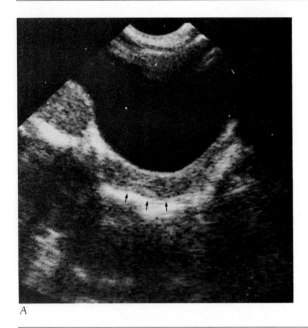
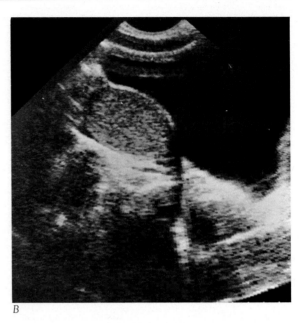

A

B

FIGURE 10-6. Androblastoma (Sertoli-Leydig cell tumor). A 17-year-old girl with clinical signs of virilization and primary amenorrhea. (A) Sagittal view of the small uterus (*arrows*), which is infantile in shape. (B) Sagittal view of the right adnexa showing a unilateral solid lesion measuring 7 × 3 cm. Note good sound transmission through the mass.

cologic surgery is important. Surgical excision provides the specimen for histologic confirmation. An attempt is made to remove the bulk of the tumor, in order to minimize residual disease and enhance the effectiveness of radiation and chemotherapy. Initial inspection at surgery also provides information for staging the disease. Surgical treatment usually includes bilateral salpingo-oophorectomy, total hysterectomy, and omentectomy. In young women with stage I disease, only the involved ovary may be removed. Following surgery a cyclic course of chemotherapy, and in some cases radiation therapy, may be given, especially for stage II through stage IV disease. A repeat laparotomy (second-look operation) is sometimes performed after a course of chemotherapy, to determine the presence or absence of residual disease and to plan possible further treatment accordingly.

LABORATORY TESTS

Much work has been done on laboratory detection of malignancies, including ovarian carcinoma.[28] The work is based on the principle of finding telltale substances in the serum or plasma of patients who harbor a malignancy. Such substances, which may be proteins, hormones, or enzymes, are produced by cancer cells, or by the sensitized nonmalignant tissue of the patient's immune system in response to the presence of cancer cells. These substances (antigens) have been termed "tumor markers."

While significant elevations in certain tumor markers have been described in ovarian carcinoma patients, none has been sensitive enough to be practical as a screening test; however, in a patient with a known pelvic mass, certain laboratory tests may be helpful in the diagnosis. For example, a serum radioimmunoassay has been developed for an antibody called CA 125. Serum elevations of this monoclonal antibody may be found in most nonmucinous ovarian epithelial cancers.[4]

Cytologic examination of ascitic fluid is often helpful in the diagnosis of ovarian malignancy. When ascites is only minimal, ultrasound may be used to guide fluid aspiration.

Imaging Diagnosis

CONVENTIONAL RADIOLOGY

Important information is often gained from a plain radiograph of the abdomen and a barium enema study.

The principal value of the *radiograph* of the abdomen, the simplest and least expensive radiographic examination, is that it detects calcifications and abnormal soft tissue masses in patients with abdominal distension. The most common ovarian lesion, serous cystadenoma, and its malignant counterpart, cystoadenocarcinoma, may contain fine granular calcifications termed psammoma bodies, which may coalesce to form cloudlike aggregates. The calcifications occur in approximately 12% of ovarian cystadenomas and cystadenocarcinomas and may be found in the primary lesion or its metastatic deposits. Coarse, sometimes curvilinear calcifications are seen more often with mucinous cystadenocarcinoma and in pseudomyxoma peritonei. A wide range of plain film densities, sometimes quite specific, may be present in cystic teratomas, including their far less common malignant counterpart, the teratocarcinoma. Malignant teratomas, which are typically seen in adolescents or very elderly patients, may contain areas of coarse calcification.

The *barium enema* has a significant role in patients with suspected ovarian malignancy. It may demonstrate extrinsic displacement or encasement of the colon or abnormalities of contour that raise the suspicion of serosal involvement. In addition, the barium enema may demonstrate a primary colonic malignancy, which may be coincidental to the ovarian primary or the source from which metastases to the ovary have spread.

COMPUTED TOMOGRAPHY

Specific strengths of the CT examination include

the demonstration of pelvic side wall masses, nodal enlargement in the retroperitoneum, liver metastases, and calcifications.[20]

When intravenous contrast and oral contrast are given, the CT examination provides accurate anatomic information about the urinary tract, the opacified portions of the gastrointestinal tract, and the presence of ascites, in addition to demonstrating the mass. Deep and subcapsular liver metastases that may be difficult or impossible to detect at surgery are readily visualized. Therefore, CT together with the ultrasound examination are complementary to laparotomy as means of staging the disease.

Following surgery, CT is used to assess residual disease; following chemotherapy, CT is frequently used to assess response to treatment. In evaluating recurrent disease, the CT scan may show extensive unresectable tumor, thereby obviating unnecessary surgery.[27] The main limitation of CT is the difficulty in detecting small foci of disease, that is, peritoneal implants and lymph nodes smaller than 2 cm.

MAGNETIC RESONANCE IMAGING

Initial reports of magnetic resonance imaging (MRI) of adnexal masses suggest that this modality offers some refinements in tissue characterization over CT and ultrasound.[21] Fat and blood have high signal intensity, but tissue specificity is not sufficient to distinguish ovarian malignancy from benign or inflammatory lesions. In one study that compared staging of ovarian cancer with MRI and CT, the authors suggested that MRI offers no particular advantage over CT.[5] In fact, the MRI study failed to demonstrate calcified peritoneal implants that were noted on CT. On the other hand, like US, MRI has the capability of multiplanar imaging, and this feature, together with the good spatial resolution of pelvic anatomy, makes MRI a good tool for determining the origin of a pelvic mass. MRI may therefore be used when US or CT findings are suboptimal or indeterminate.[9]

ULTRASOUND

Screening for Ovarian Malignancy. Normally, significant regression in ovarian size as well as changes in texture and surface characteristics occur in the perimenopausal period. Ovarian dimensions change from approximately 3.5 × 2 × 1.5 cm to 2

$\times$ 1 $\times$ 0.5 cm, making the ovary impalpable in most cases. Diminished blood supply and absence of folliculogenesis produce a wrinkled surface and a change in texture. Absence of this normal regression 3 to 5 years after menopause is considered pathologic and has been termed the postmenopausal palpable ovary (PPO) syndrome, which needs prompt investigation.[3] Early detection of an adnexal mass in peri- and postmenopausal patients is currently considered the most promising means of favorably influencing the prognosis of ovarian cancer. The yield of detecting asymptomatic ovarian carcinoma in women by means of physical examination is only 1 per 10,000 examinations.[3] Some limitations to a reliable physical examination include obesity, vaginal atrophy, and muscle tension. These limitations are often overcome with pelvic US, so the yield of ovarian carcinoma in a high-risk population using US may be much greater.

Ultrasound screening of postmenopausal women for ovarian carcinoma is currently being explored. In a recent ovarian carcinoma screening study of 115 women (of whom 35 were in the postmenopausal age group), the ultrasound examination was found to be a more sensitive tool than the physical examination in measuring ovarian volume and size.[12] In this limited series of women with a family history of ovarian carcinoma, one case of bilateral serous cystadenoma was found in a patient whose daughter had ovarian cancer. One case of ovarian carcinoma was found in each of several larger screening studies of 1084 and 804 women.[2,10] In order to increase the specificity of the screening test for ovarian carcinoma, some authors have suggested using a multimodality approach that combines the serum antibody test CA 125 with pelvic ultrasound and the physical examination.[16]

When screening patients for ovarian malignancy, size as well as consistency are important features to note. To date, ultrasound studies of ovarian volume in postmenopausal women have suggested a range of 2.5 to 3.7 cm^3 as the upper limit of normal.[10,13] Significant size inequality is another criterion for ovarian enlargement. It has been suggested that one ovary should not be more than twice the size of the contralateral one,[6] but in postmenopausal women less dramatic size discrepancies should raise a suspicion. A predominantly solid or complex consistency is more suspicious than a purely cystic mass (Fig. 10-3). Benign inclusion cysts are not rare in postmenopausal women. It is likely that the use of transvaginal ultrasound will allow distinctions in tissue texture to be made with greater confidence and will provide further refinements in the assessment of ovarian size. To date, the best approach combines information from transabdominal and endovaginal studies.[11]

A significant limitation in ultrasound study of postmenopausal patients is the difficulty in identifying normal postmenopausal ovaries, which are devoid of follicles, a characteristic feature that aids ovarian identification in premenopausal women. Greater experience, careful scanning technique, and transvaginal scanning will overcome some of the difficulty. In addition, when ovarian enlargement is due to a neoplasm it is likely that a portion of the mass will be composed of cystic elements containing septa, thereby aiding in its recognition.

Sonographic Diagnosis

US is often the initial imaging study for patients with ovarian malignancy. The object of the US examination is to characterize the mass, define its contours, and measure it. The ovarian origin of the mass can usually be suspected, particularly if a normal uterus is identified. The gross anatomy of the most common form of ovarian malignancy, cystadenocarcinoma, lends itself well to ultrasound depiction because of the propensity of the lesion to form cystic masses with internal septa and soft tissue protrusions (Fig. 10-1). Diffuse low-amplitude signals within the cystic mass or a portion thereof suggest the presence of mucin, as is seen in mucinous cystadenoma and cystadenocarcinoma. It should be noted, however, that this finding is not specific for mucin, as it may be seen with fresh blood or purulent material. High-amplitude reflections associated with acoustic shadowing are often a clue to the presence of calcifications within the mass.

The US examination does not have the specificity to distinguish between benign and malignant disease, but a number of sonographic features, if present, favor the diagnosis of ovarian malignancy. As the proportion of solid component of the lesion increases, so does the likelihood of its being malig-

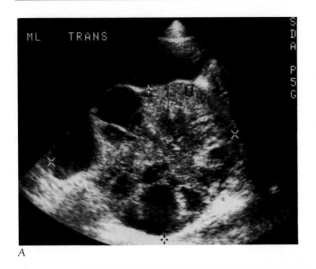

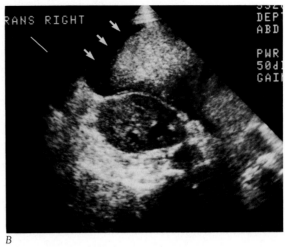

FIGURE 10-7. Metastatic disease to both ovaries in a 42-year-old woman who presented with weight loss and hepatomegaly. (A) Complex, multicystic mass distending the cul-de-sac, adherent to posterior surface of the uterus (U), which is compressed. (B) Transverse scan of the right upper quadrant demonstrates ascites and nodularity on the liver capsule representing serosal metastases (arrows).

nant. Solid portions of the lesion consist of irregular septations, 2 mm or more thick, and papillations.[23] Not infrequently an ovarian malignancy has a predominantly or completely solid texture (Figs. 10-3, 10-6). Good to excellent sound transmission may be observed in such cases. This is undoubtedly due to the friable necrotic tissue and high fluid content in the lesion. Nodularity and poor definition of the outer margin of the mass favor malignancy. Immobility or noncompressibility implies fixation of a mass and suggests malignancy. In addition, bilateral disease also favors malignancy. This finding is often difficult to ascertain. If the lesions are large, they may coalesce in the cul-de-sac to form one large mass (Fig. 10-7). Although ascites can be a feature of a benign ovarian lesion, notably the ovarian fibroma, presence of ascites together with a cystic pelvic mass raises the suspicion of malignancy. In some cases ascites is the only clue to the presence of ovarian malignancy and the ovarian lesion may not be visualized. In such cases use of a transvaginal probe may be of diagnostic value (Fig. 10-8). The ultrasound appearance of the ascitic fluid in pseudomyxoma peritonei is usually echogenic as a result of the thick globular consistency of the fluid (Fig. 10-4).

A limitation of ultrasound is the difficulty in detecting small-volume disease involving retroperitoneal nodes, peritoneal surfaces, and omentum.[18] Lesions situated high in the pelvis are partially or entirely outside the field of view of the transvaginal probe. Despite these limitations, ultrasound provides reasonably accurate information for initial staging and evaluation for recurrent disease, with a reported accuracy of 90%.[19,26]

Sonographic Monitoring

Ultrasound is often used to monitor for persistent or recurrent disease following surgery and during treatment (Fig. 10-9). A scan shortly after surgery may serve as a baseline study. In scanning the patient following total hysterectomy it is important to adjust the gain settings so that the increased sound transmission through the urinary bladder does not obscure a small pelvic mass. Transvaginal scanning may clarify any question in the presence of a mass in the true pelvis. Survey of the liver and

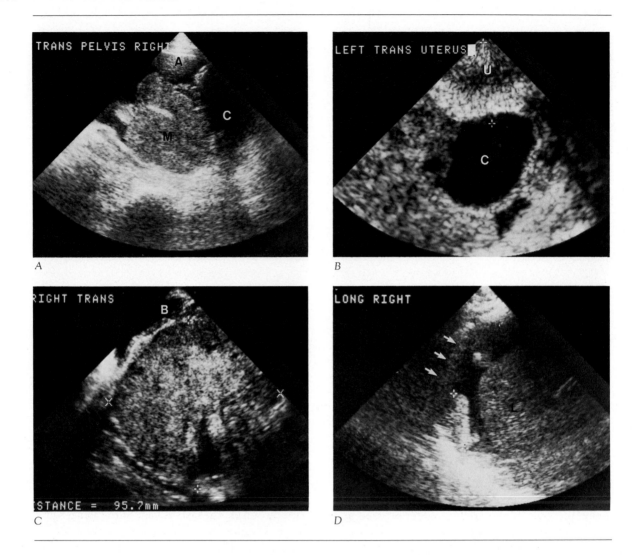

FIGURE 10-8. Undifferentiated adenocarcinoma, stage IV, in a 68-year-old woman with progressive abdominal distension. (A) Transverse view of the pelvis shows a lobulated mass on the right (M) with a cystic component on the left (C). Ascites (A) is seen anteriorly. The patient could not maintain a filled bladder. (B) Transvaginal view in the transverse plane shows a partial view of the uterus (between calipers). The cystic component of the mass (C) is seen posterior to the uterus (U). In this case the transvaginal scan was able to resolve the uterus and adnexal mass as separate structures. (C) Transvaginal transverse view of the right adnexa shows a 9- to 10-cm, predominantly solid mass representing the right ovarian carcinoma (B, portion of the bladder). (D) Longitudinal view of the right subphrenic area (arrows on portions of diaphragm) shows a metastatic nodule on the inferior surface of the right hemidiaphragm (between calipers).

retroperitoneal areas should be part of the postoperative examination as well. If pelvic masses, peritoneal nodules, or loculated areas of ascites are observed, ultrasound may be used to guide needle aspiration.

Ultrasound Scanning Protocol

The examination consists of a systematic survey of the pelvis in the sagittal and transverse planes with identification of the bladder, uterus, and adnexal and cul-de-sac areas (Table 10-3). In studying a pelvic mass, depth gain curve, focal zone, and depth of view need to be adjusted in order to optimize the image and to demonstrate degree of sound transmission through the mass.

Often it is not possible to perform the ideal pelvic sonographic examination in the presence of a large pelvic mass because it is difficult for the patient to maintain a full bladder. It is important, however, to have enough fluid in the bladder so that it can be identified, used as a landmark, and not mistaken for the cystic mass (Fig. 10-9). In some cases instillation into the bladder of 300 to 500 ml of normal saline via a Foley catheter may be required. Transvaginal US is an important adjunct to the examination, especially when an adequate transabdominal scan is not possible. Usually transvaginal US improves delineation of the adnexal mass and better defines the uterus (see Fig. 10-8B). It is important to identify uterine texture and contour. Abnormalities in the endometrial canal reflection suggest hyperplasia or associated endometrial carcinoma (Table 10-1).

When ovarian malignancy is suspected based on the sonographic appearance of the mass, a complete pelvic *and* abdominal study should be done in order to provide information for staging (Table 10-2). Search for ascites is directed to the cul-de-sac, paracolic gutters, especially on the right, and around the liver edge (Fig. 10-10). The inferior surfaces of the diaphragmatic leaflets may be visualized in the presence of moderate ascites. This enables the sonographer to demonstrate nodules on the liver capsule or on the diaphragmatic surface, which suggest stage-IV disease (Fig. 10-8D). Attention should be directed to the peritoneal surfaces to detect tumor implants (Figs. 10-7B and 10-8D). Observation of peristalsis is of course an important

TABLE 10-3. Summary of ultrasound protocol for ovarian malignancy

PURPOSE	SONOGRAPHY CHECKLIST
Screening	Note any ovarian enlargement. In peri- and postmenopausal women, ovarian linear dimension should not exceed 3 cm in length and 1.5 cm in thickness. Note significant asymmetry in ovarian size.
Diagnosis	Observe texture, contour, size, and sound transmission of mass. Determine whether it is unilateral or bilateral. Note uterine contours and endometrial reflection. Check for ascites. Identify liver, retroperitoneal, or omental masses. Check kidneys for hydronephrosis.
Monitor	Compare to baseline study to exclude new masses. Check for ascites, retroperitoneal nodes, and liver masses. Survey pelvis, abdomen, and retroperitoneum prior to second-look operation.

aspect of real-time scanning and may avoid confusion between tumor nodules and loops of bowel. The sonographer also has the opportunity of a "hands on" maneuver of exerting gentle pressure on the cystic mass (if it is superficially located) in order to assess it for compressibility, which is a feature of bowel and is usually not present in cystic malignant lesions. Evaluation of liver parenchyma is an integral part of the ultrasound study in the search for metastases. The costophrenic angles are also evaluated for the presence of pleural effusion. Both kidneys should be studied to assess the presence or absence of hydronephrosis. In the presence of massive ascites, it may be difficult to image the para-aortic area to demonstrate retroperitoneal adenopathy; in such cases, oblique and coronal scanning should be attempted.

Differential Diagnosis

The differential diagnosis of ovarian malignances includes a variety of benign ovarian neoplasms. No imaging modality has yet been able to provide the tissue specificity necessary to distinguish between benign and malignant lesions. Most ovarian neo-

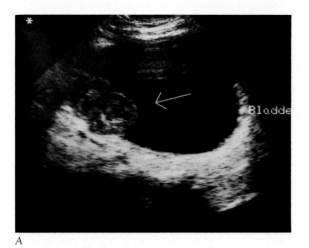

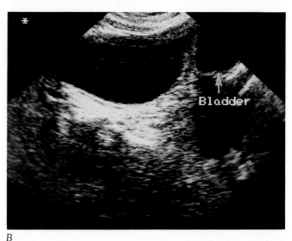

A   B

FIGURE 10-9. Recurrent cystadenocarcinoma in a 69-year-old woman, who underwent total abdominal hysterectomy and bilateral salpingo-oophorectomy for adenocarcinoma of the ovary. (A) Sagittal view of the pelvis with a nondistended bladder shows a cystic mass, which was initially mistaken for the urinary bladder. Note reverberation artifact anteriorly and nodularity (*arrow*) in the superior aspect of the cyst. (B) Repeat scan with minimal bladder distension confirmed the supravesical location of the cystic mass, which proved to be a recurrent cancer.

plasms are benign, and their gross pathology is often indistinguishable from that of their malignant counterparts. In the menstruating woman, nonneoplastic cystic lesions of the ovaries such as large follicular cysts, corpus luteum, and theca luteum cysts are also considered in the differential diagnosis. These lesions have a mixed echogenic pattern, particularly when intracystic hemorrhage occurs. Nonneoplastic cystic masses of the ovary in the postmenopausal age group that may resemble neoplasms are inclusion or parovarian cysts.

Pedunculated leiomyomas may mimic an ovarian neoplasm, particularly when degeneration due to vascular compromise results in the formation of cystic spaces.[24]

Neoplasms of the fallopian tube are exceedingly rare and often malignant. These lesions are usually mistaken for ovarian malignancies.

Tumorlike conditions that are morphologically similar to ovarian neoplasms include endometriosis and pelvic inflammatory disease. Ectopic pregnancy should always be considered in menstruating women. Gastrointestinal diseases such as diver-

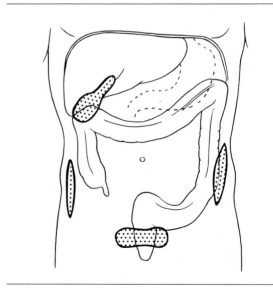

FIGURE 10-10. Diagrammatic view of the peritoneal cavity. Dotted areas represent the most common sites of ascites fluid collection.

ticulitis and colitis often produce inflammatory masses and fluid collections in the pelvis and should be considered, particularly in postmenopausal patients.

Distended, fluid- and stool-filled loops of bowel in the pelvis may appear tumorlike. While the observation of peristalsis identifies the bowel, absence of peristalsis need not exclude it. For example, ischemic disease of the bowel may be associated with adynamic ileus, and a small amount of ascites may also be observed.

The sonographer faces a number of diagnostic challenges in the presence of a pelvic mass. The first is to determine the origin of the mass: Is it ovarian, uterine, or nongynecologic? The second is to identify characteristics that are consistent with a benign or malignant neoplasm. Awareness of the differential diagnosis is important because of the morphologic similarity of many pelvic disorders.

References

1. American Cancer Society. Cancer Statistics 1988. Cancer J Clin. 1988; 38:1:5–22.
2. Andolf E, Svalenius E, Astedt B. Ultrasonography for early detection of ovarian carcinoma. Br J Obstet Gynecol. 1986; 19:1286–1289.
3. Barber HRK, Graber EA. The PMPO syndrome (postmenopausal palpable ovary syndrome). Obstet Gynecol. 1971; 38:921–923.
4. Bast RC Jr, Klug TL, St. John E, et al. A radioimmunoassay using a monoclonal antibody to monitor the course of epithelial ovarian cancer. N Engl J Med. 1983; 309:883–887.
5. Bies JR, Ellis JH, Kopecky KK, et al. Assessment of primary gynecologic malignancies: Comparison of 0.15T resistine MRI with CT. AJR. 1984; 143:1249–1257.
6. Campbell S, Goswamy R, Goessens L. Real-time ultrasonography for determination of ovarian morphology and volume. Lancet. 1982; 1:425–426.
7. Casagrande JT, Pike MC, Ross RK, et al. "Incessant ovulation" and ovarian cancer. Lancet. 1979; 2:170–173.
8. Coates G, Bush RS, Aspin N. A study of ascites using lymphoscintigraphy with ^{99m}Tc sufur colloid. Radiology. 1973; 107:577–583.
9. Dooms GC, Hricack H, Tschalakoff D. Adnexal structures: MR imaging. Radiology. 1986; 158:639–646.
10. Goswamy RK, Campbell S, Whitehead ML. Screening of ovarian cancer. Clin Gynecol Obstet. 1983; 10:621–643.
11. Granberg S, Wikland M. Comparison between endovaginal and transabdominal transducers for measuring ovarian volume. J Ultrasound Med. 1987; 6:649–653.
12. Granberg S, Wikland M. A comparison between US and gynecologic examination for detection of enlarged ovaries in a group of women at risk for ovarian cancer. J Ultrasound Med. 1988; 7:59–64.
13. Hall DA, McCarthy KA, Kopans DB. Sonographic visualization of the normal postmenopausal ovary. J Ultrasound Med. 1986; 5:9–11.
14. Hart WR. Pathology of malignant and borderline epithelial tumors of the ovary. In: Coppleson M, ed. Gynecologic Oncology—Fundamental Principles and Clinical Practice. New York: Churchill Livingstone; 1981; 2:633–654.
15. Heintz APM, Hacker NF, Lagasse LD. Epidemiology and etiology of ovarian cancer: A review. Obstet Gynecol. 1985; 66:127–135.
16. Jacobs I, Bridges J, Reynolds C, et al. Multimodal approach to screening for ovarian cancer. Lancet. 1988; 1:268–271.
17. Jones HW, Jones GS. Novak's Textbook of Gynecology. 11th ed. Baltimore: Williams & Wilkins; 1988; 507–558.
18. Khan O, Cosgrove DO, Fried AM, et al. Ovarian carcinoma follow-up: US versus laparotomy. Radiology. 1986; 159:111–113.
19. Khan O, Wiltshaw E, McGready VR, et al. Role of US in the management of ovarian CA. J Soc Med. 1983; 76:821–827.
20. Mitchell DG, Hill MC, Hill S, et al. Serous carcinoma of the ovary: CT identification of metastatic calcified implants. Radiology. 1986; 158:649–652.
21. Mitchell DG, Mintz MC, Spritzer CE, et al. Adnexal masses: MR imaging observations at 1.5T with US and CT correlation. Radiology. 1987; 162:319–324.
22. Morrow CP. Malignant and borderline epithelial tumors of ovary: Clinical features staging diagnosis. Intraoperative assessment and review of management. In: Coppleson M, ed. Gynecologic Oncology—Fundamental Principles and Clinical Practice. New York: Churchill Livingstone; 1981; 2:655–679.
23. Moyle JW, Rochester D, Sider L, et al. Sonography of ovarian tumors: Predictability of tumor type. AJR. 1983; 241:985–991.
24. Nocera RM, Fagan CJ, Hernandez JC. Cystic parametrial fibroid mimicking ovarian cystadenoma. J Ultrasound Med. 1984; 3:183–187.
25. Requard CK, Mettler FA Jr, Wicks JD. Preoperative sonography of malignant ovarian neoplasms. AJR. 1981; 137:79–82.

26. Sanders RC, McNeil BJ, Finberg HJ, et al. A prospective study of CT and US in the detection and staging of pelvic masses. Radiology. 1983; 146:439–442.

27. Silverman PM, Osborne M, Dunnick NR, et al. CT prior to second-look operation in ovarian cancer. AJR. 1988; 150:829–832.

28. Smith LH. Ol RH. Detection of malignant ovarian neoplasms: A review of the literature. Obstet Gynecol Survey. 1984; 39:313–360.

CHAPTER 11

Role of Sonography in Infertility Management and in Contraception

KATHARINE STEURER, ROGER C. SANDERS

Infertility has been defined as failure to conceive for at least 1 year. More than one out of eight couples in the United States of America are classified as infertile. It is estimated that there are 2.8 million couples in the United States of America who want to have children but are unable to conceive. Factors such as age, life-style, and biologic problems can dramatically lower chances of conception.[12] The process of conception is such an intricate one that even the most fertile couple has only one chance in four of conceiving each month.[31] For fertilization, implantation, and maintenance of pregnancy to take place, a series of complex and interrelated events must occur. The male must produce an adequate number of sperm and deposit them in the upper vagina at the approximate time of female ovulation. The female's ovulatory mechanisms must be normal. Sufficient estrogen is needed in the periovulatory phase to stimulate the production of cervical mucus of the quality and quantity that will permit the passage of sperm into the uterus. The fallopian tubes must be patent and mobile, to allow fertilization to take place and to enable the ovum to travel to the uterus. The uterus must be capable of supporting implantation and fetal growth throughout pregnancy.[12]

There are many reasons why a couple may have difficulty conceiving. Medical problems responsible for infertility may be present in both male and female. Each partner may have a minor medical problem; when combined they may impair fertility. In some couples the reasons for infertility cannot be explained.[31]

The role of ultrasound in this complex process of fertilization is diverse. First, ultrasound is used for diagnosing disease or structural barriers in either partner that may be hindering fertilization. Second, ultrasound may be used in conjunction with therapy for patients in whom ovulation must be hormonally induced. Ultrasound is used to confirm and follow the pregnancy through implantation and its early growth. Third, ultrasound is used when ova are obtained for in vitro fertilization and to guide optimal positioning of the fertilized ovum.[5,6]

Male Infertility Factors

The male factor may be responsible or partly responsible for failure to conceive. In order to conceive, the quality and quantity of sperm must be adequate. Male impotence with lowered sperm count may stem from specific childhood problems such as undescended testicles or torsion or from the sequelae of mumps in the testicles and atrophic gonads which may decrease fertility. Other causes, including previous injury or surgery, infections of the reproductive tract, and venereal disease, may be associated with urethral strictures, or vasoepididymal obstruction. Ultrasound is not used in the

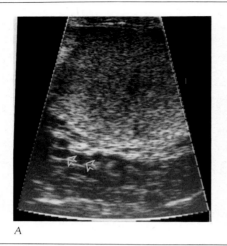
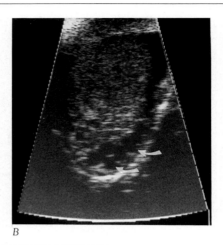

A

B

FIGURE 11-1. (A) Prominent vessels can be seen posterior to the testicle (open arrow). (B) When the patient performed Valsalva's maneuver, this varicocele dilated (curved arrows).

investigation of most causes of male infertility; however, varicoceles, which are common, may cause infertility. Small varicoceles can be detected by ultrasound when they cannot be found clinically (Fig. 11-1). Varicocelectomies have improved the fertility rate.[12]

Female Factors

The factors that contribute to the problem of female infertility are age, infection or surgery, disease, congenital anomalies, and hormone imbalance. These problems can be divided into mechanical and biologic categories.

Mechanical problems produced by infection or surgery are summarized in Tables 11-1 and 11-2. The sonographic appearances are considered in other chapters.

Biologic problems such as extremes of age and hormone imbalance are other factors in infertility. A woman who postpones childbearing until later in life increases her risk of infertility. Fertility naturally declines 10 years prior to menopause, owing to hormonal changes. Using contraception for a long time before childbearing decreases fertility. There is also an increased incidence of endometriosis in older premenopausal women.[16]

HORMONAL CAUSES OF INFERTILITY

Infertility from hormone imbalance is due to a defect of the pituitary-hypothalamic-ovarian axis. This dysfunction may be caused by disease or tumors of the hypothalamus, pituitary, or ovary. Obesity, anorexia, and stress also contribute to hormone imbalance. If the pituitary, hypothalamus, or ovaries are not functioning or are functioning improperly, irregular ovulation, anovulation, or amenorrhea may result.[12]

Ovulation Induction

Before a patient begins ovulation induction therapy, the cause of the infertility must be discovered. Pathology that may be reversible, such as endometriosis or uterine synechiae, or other factors such as tubal obstruction and sperm inadequacy should be ruled out or corrected (see Tables 11-1 and 11-2), and evidence of absent ovulation should be established by hormone assay and basal body temperature documentation.

Ovulation induction with hormone therapy is used to treat ovulatory disorders caused by a dysfunction of the pituitary-hypothalamic-ovarian axis. The aim of ovulation induction therapy is to stimulate early growth of many follicles so that one

TABLE 11-1. Mechanical causes of female infertility

Uterus
    Synechiae (Ascherman's syndrome)
    Fibroids
    Congenital anomalies
Tubes
    Endometrial implants
    Blocked tubes due to PID
    Congenital anomalies and adhesions
Ovaries
    Polycystic ovary
    Adhesions

or more may reach ovulation. Increased growth of the dominant follicles that will ovulate begins on days 3 to 5 of the cycle. Drugs such as Clomid or Perganol (HMG), which are used to stimulate follicular growth, can cause other follicles to become "dominant," if they are taken at this early stage. Human chorionic gonadotropin (HCG) is administered to induce ovulation. It stimulates the midcycle lutenizing hormone (LH) ovulatory surge that initiates ovulation.[35]

Ovulation induction therapy is also used for patients who will undergo artificial insemination or in vitro fertilization procedures. Ovulation induction therapy aids in optimal timing of artificial insemination. In vitro fertilization employs ovulation induction therapy to produce a number of mature oocytes simultaneously, so that oocytes can be retrieved.[5]

MONITORING OVULATION INDUCTION
The parameters used to monitor and predict follicle growth and ovulation are basal body temperature (BBT), cervical mucus, estrogen levels, and the sonographic appearance of ovarian follicles. The BBT is taken daily and charted; a temperature increase is seen at the time of ovulation. There is a significant rise in BBT following ovulation, owing to the high level of progesterone secreted from the corpus luteum. Quality and quantity of cervical mucus are measured to assess its viscosity. Before ovulation it develops a stringy texture suitable for sperm transport. Estrogen levels are measured daily by serum estradiol (E_2) levels in the blood. Measurements of LH and progesterone may also be taken before ovulation. The standard laboratory and clinical parameters, including BBT charting, cervical mucus assessment, and estrogen-hormone assays, provide useful indirect information about follicular growth and ovulation.[12]

TABLE 11-2. Features of obstructive lesions that cause infertility

LESIONS	PATHOLOGY	ETIOLOGY	RESULTS
Adhesions			
PID	Scar tissue forms around tubes and ovaries	Sexually transmitted diseases IUD wear Incomplete spontaneous abortion	Tubes and ovaries covered by scar tissue; ectopic pregnancy may result
Endometriosis	Endometrial implants, loculations of old blood in pelvis	Ectopic growth of endometrial tissue stimulated by ovarian hormones	20–60% infertility; tubes blocked by adhesions
Surgery	Scar tissue around tubes and ovaries; intrauterine synechiae (endometrial adhesions)	Any pelvic surgery; D and C with or without previous elective abortion	Sperm passage impeded by synechiae
Uterine Cavity Distortion			
Myoma	Submucosal fibroids	Older patient	Mass impinges on uterine cavity
Congenital anomaly	Bicornuate, unicornuate, or double uterus	Congenital	Early abortion due to abnormal shape
DES exposure	T-shaped uterus, hypoplastic cavity, short cervix	Woman was exposed to DES in utero	Lowered conception, spontaneous abortion frequent

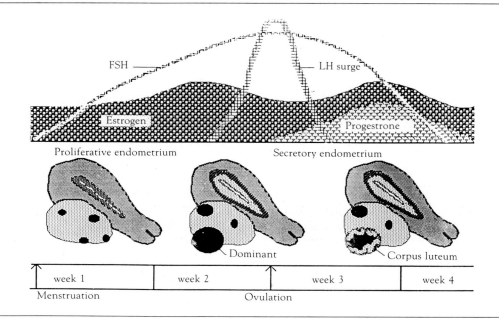

FIGURE 11-2. Throughout the 28-day cycle, ultrasound appearances are related to hormonal changes.

ROLE OF ULTRASOUND IN OVULATION INDUCTION

Diagnostic ultrasound provides direct information about the physiology of the ovarian cycle in a convenient, noninvasive manner by demonstrating follicular growth (Fig. 11-2). If ultrasound is utilized in combination with laboratory and clinical values, detailed and precise information may be gained that improves the accuracy, safety, and efficacy of ovulation induction.[6]

A baseline sonogram is made at the beginning of a patient's cycle to evaluate the status of the ovaries, exclude residual cysts from earlier cycles, and rule out pathologic conditions that might hinder fertility. The entire pelvis is examined transabdominally, utilizing the full bladder technique. Then a transvaginal scan is performed with the bladder empty to examine the tubes and ovaries more closely. If the results of the baseline sonogram are normal, the patient begins hormone therapy with Clomid or Perganol (Table 11-3). Serial transvaginal ultrasound examinations are initiated when the estrogen level rises. The increase relates to induced follicular growth, which occurs about days 5 to 7 of the cycle. The patient is then scanned daily.

Follicular development is correlated with daily increase in the serum estradiol level.[1]

On day 5, 6, or 7 of the induced cycle, when the second transvaginal examination is performed, the follicles appear as small cystic structures within the ovary (Fig. 11-3). At this time, the follicles may be numerous and measure 8 to 10 mm in diameter. The three largest follicles in each ovary are measured. Measurements are taken from inside wall to inside wall of the follicle in sagittal and coronal planes. For serial measurements, comparison volume calculation is worthwhile (Fig. 11-4); if a single diameter is used, it may be accidentally altered if the follicle is flattened or elongated by transducer

TABLE 11-3. Ovulation induction protocol

Day 1	First day of menstrual cycle.
	Baseline transabdominal and
	transvaginal ultrasound studies.
	Begin Clomid or Perganol.
Day 2	Daily hormonal assays commence.
Day 5	Daily transvaginal ultrasound until
	ovulation to monitor follicular growth.

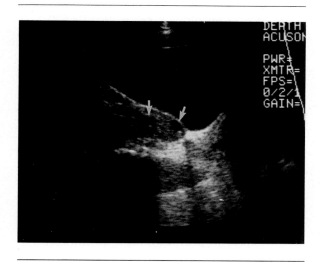

FIGURE 11-3. Longitudinal transabdominal scan of ovary with small follicles early in cycle (*arrows*).

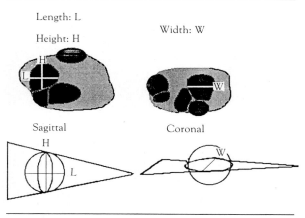

FIGURE 11-4. One follicle at a time is measured in the sagittal and coronal plane using the transvaginal transducer.

pressure. The number, size, and rapidity of follicle growth vary with each patient, depending on her response to the hormone therapy. By the 8th to 12th day of the cycle, a dominant follicle or multiple dominant follicles reach 14 to 18 mm in diameter, outdistancing the growth of other follicles in both ovaries (Fig. 11-5). The dominant follicle or follicles grow rapidly, 2 to 3 mm per day, 3 to 4 days before ovulation. The optimal follicle size for HCG administration is 18 mm. Patients ovulate 24 to 36 hours after HCG is given. The dominant follicle or follicles reach 20 to 24 mm by the time of ovulation.[1]

A sonographically detectable sign of impending ovulation that occasionally is seen is the cumulus oophorus, a dense layer of granulosa cells that surrounds the oocyte within the follicle. The cumulus is occasionally seen as a small echogenic cone projecting into the follicle (Fig. 11-6). The presence of the cumulus oophorus indicates that ovulation will occur within 36 hours.[25]

With the associated elevation of the estrogen level, the endometrium thickens, appearing more echogenic as ovulation approaches. The endometrium is moderately thick and echogenic after ovulation, in the secretory phase (Fig. 11-7B). The endometrium should be measured from anterior to

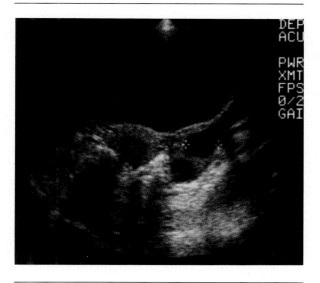

FIGURE 11-5. A transabdominal scan demonstrates the dominant follicle in the left ovary (asterisks).

posterior wall (Fig. 11-7). In the preovulatory or proliferative phase, it measures 2 to 4 mm, and in the postovulatory or secretory phase, 5 to 6 mm.[11] Sometimes a small hypoechoic layer is seen surrounding the echogenic layer. This is thought to

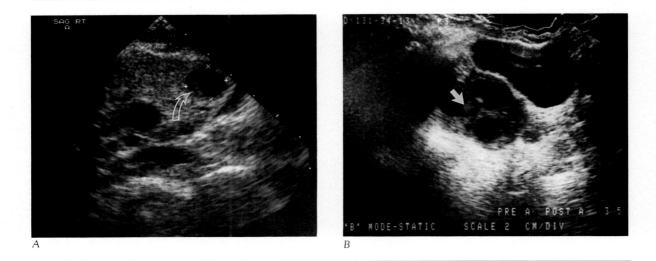

FIGURE 11-6. (A) An endovaginal scan of an ovary with a follicle containing an echogenic cumulus oophorus (*curved arrow*) projecting into the follicle. (B) A transabdominal scan of an ovary with a follicle containing a cumulus oophorus (*arrow*).

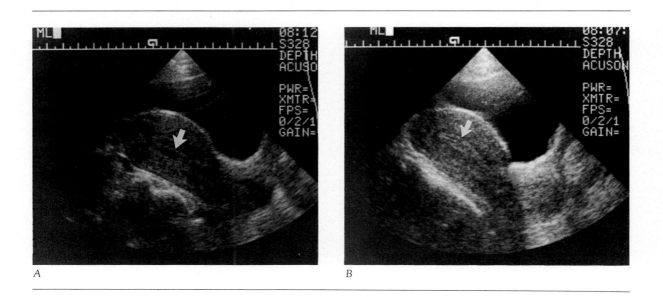

FIGURE 11-7. Transabdominal sagittal midline scans of the uterus. (A) A thin endometrial cavity (*arrow*) is surrounded by echolucent halo of endometrium during the proliferative phase of the cycle. (B) The endometrial echo is more prominent in the secretory phase of the cycle (*arrow*).

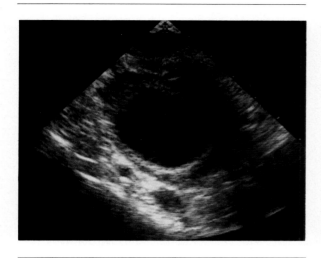

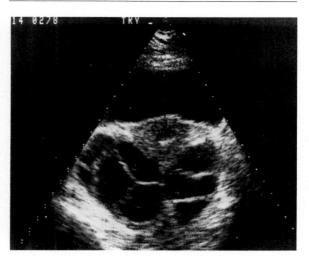

FIGURE 11-8. Corpus luteum cyst shows a few internal echoes and a slightly irregular border.

FIGURE 11-9. Transverse, transabdominal scans of mild ovarian hyperstimulation syndrome. The ovaries are enlarged and contain numerous large cysts.

represent a network of capillaries and veins and has been termed the "ring" sign.[17] Patients undergoing Clomid treatment, despite a high estrogen level, have relatively little thickening of the endometrium. It has been suggested that this is due to an antiestrogen effect of high doses of Clomid on the endometrium. The effect of Clomid and Perganol on the endometrium remains speculative.[32]

After ovulation occurs the sonographic signs are of a sudden decrease in follicle size, disappearance of the large echo-free follicle or follicles, and the appearance of internal echoes or blurred margins to the follicle. With collapse, follicles may develop a crenated contour. A fluid collection may develop in the region of the ovary or in the cul-de-sac. Small amounts of fluid may be seen in the cul-de-sac before ovulation, but there is an abrupt increase in fluid once the follicle leaves the ovary.

A corpus luteum cyst may be seen following ovulation, appearing as a small irregular cyst with low-level internal echoes (Fig. 11-8). In a few patients, a well-defined cyst as large as 40 mm has been seen. Corpus luteum cysts should resolve early in the next cycle.[25]

COMPLICATIONS

Multiple Pregnancy. Ovulation induction is associated with an increased risk of multiple pregnancy.

The decision to withhold HCG or not to proceed with artificial insemination may be made when there is sonographic evidence of multiple mature follicles; however, not all multiple ovulations lead to multiple pregnancy and the number of successful pregnancies cannot be predicted by ultrasound or serum estradiol assay (or homone assay).[7]

Hyperstimulation. Ovarian hyperstimulation syndrome (OHSS) is a serious potential complication of ovulation induction (Fig. 11-9). In OHSS, multiple follicles are induced, and multiple theca lutein cysts develop. The ovaries become extremely large, owing to the presence of numerous large follicles, and edema of the stroma is produced by the increased levels of HCG. The estrogen level is very high.

OHSS may be mild, moderate, or severe, and can be detected by a combination of ultrasound and clinical and laboratory parameters. Mild hyperstimulation is characterized by lower abdominal pain or discomfort with ovarian enlargement with multiple cysts representing follicles no greater than 5 cm in diameter (Fig. 11-9). In severe hyperstimulation, the ovaries are grossly enlarged to more than 10 cm in diameter. There is an increased risk of ovarian rupture or torsion. The ovaries contain large, thin-walled cysts that replace most of the parenchyma. Ascites or pleural effusions are additional changes associated with severe hyperstimulation. If the patient does not become pregnant, the syndrome resolves within 3 to 7 days following the next menstrual cycle. If pregnancy occurs, symptoms may persist for about 6 to 8 weeks.[1]

In Vitro Fertilization with Embryo Transfer (IVF-ET)

If the fallopian tubes are blocked pregnancy can be achieved by removing the ova from the ovary, fertilizing them in a test tube, and placing the fertilized eggs in the uterus. The sperm obtained from the husband or donor is added to a culture dish containing the ova to allow fertilization to take place. After fertilization has occurred the embryo or embryos are transferred to the uterus for implantation and the pregnancy is allowed to progress naturally. The success rate is between 10 and 25%. Hormonal stimulation promotes the development of many mature follicles so that several oocytes can be retrieved.[5] Ovarian response to hormone therapy is monitored daily by ultrasound and prior to ovum retrieval by estrogen level assays. The number and size of the mature follicles are assessed with ultrasound so that administration of HCG can be timed properly.

When at least two—and preferably three or more—follicles reach 1.8 mm in diameter, HCG is administered. Ovulation occurs 36 to 38 hours after HCG is given. The patient is scheduled for oocyte retrieval 34 to 35 hours after HCG administration; when the follicles have matured the oocytes are aspirated from the follicles. Ultrasound is performed immediately before oocyte retrieval, to ensure that premature ovulation has not occurred. The cycle may be cancelled if this is the case, unless only the largest follicle has collapsed while the others have remained intact.[6]

There are two approaches to ovum retrieval. Laparoscopy has been the standard method of ova retrieval in most IVF programs; however, ultrasonically guided retrieval of ova—by the transabdominal-transvesical, transurethral, or transvaginal method—is rapidly gaining acceptance.[7]

The transvesical ultrasound-guided follicle aspi-

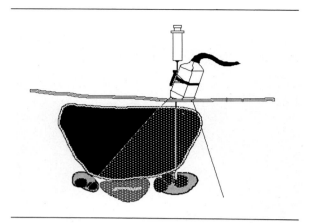

FIGURE 11-10. The transvesical ultrasound-guided follicle aspiration procedure with sector scanner and biopsy guide. The needle is inserted into the abdominal wall through the bladder and enters the follicle. The ultrasound image is monitored so the needle course can be optimized.

ration procedure is performed in the operating room using a real-time 3.5- or 5-MHz linear array or sector scanner with a biopsy guide attachment (Fig. 11-10). The bladder is filled with 200 to 400 ml of sterile saline. In addition to the guidance system to attach to the transducer, a 20- or 25-cm-long 17- or 18-gauge needle is required. The ultrasound transducer is placed in a sterile plastic bag to which a sterilized needle is attached. The sonographer scans the patient transabdominally and locates the ovary containing the mature follicles (Fig. 11-10). The follicle to be punctured first is located, and the needle course is aligned with the puncture line on the monitor. The aspiration needle is connected to a flask and vacuum pump apparatus for suction. The sonographer holds the transducer steadily in alignment with the follicle, so the course of the aspiration needle can be followed along the puncture line on the monitor. After the needle is inserted into the follicle, suction is applied and the follicle is seen on the TV monitor to collapse. In some patients the ovaries may be inaccessible and fixed behind the uterus in the cul-de-sac. Obesity may pose technical difficulties, and such patients may be better approached vaginally.[24,27]

Inserting the needle through the vagina or ure-

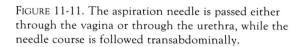

FIGURE 11-11. The aspiration needle is passed either through the vagina or through the urethra, while the needle course is followed transabdominally.

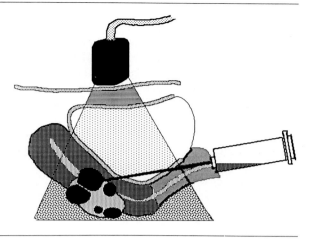

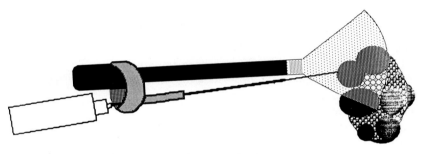

FIGURE 11-12. The transvaginal sector scanner with needle guide. The needle follows the path determined by the needle guide. The puncture line is seen on the monitor. By moving the transducer one can angle the needle track through the follicle.

thra with ultrasound monitoring is an alternative (Fig. 11-11). The bladder is filled with 200 to 400 ml of sterile saline. The sonographer locates the ovaries with follicles and visualizes the vagina on the same image.

When the vaginal route is used, the vagina is cleansed and the vaginal fornix is injected with local anesthetic. The clinician inserts the aspiration needle through the posterior vaginal fornix as the sonographer follows and directs the needle tip transabdominally toward the follicular wall. When the wall of the follicle is seen to bulge under the pressure of the needle, the clinician firmly inserts the needle into the follicle and aspiration is performed. The transurethral approach is much the same, but the needle is passed through the urethra

and posterior wall of the bladder into the follicle.[27]

The use of a transvaginal sector scanner with a needle guide (Fig. 11-12) is becoming the most popular technique, as it can be used in obese patients and those with adhesions. Transvaginal probes have a needle guide attachment. The route of the needle is shown by a series of dots on the screen, so that the needle can be inserted into the follicle. As the clinician scans while inserting the needle, the sonographer operates the controls of the ultrasound equipment and assists. No bladder filling is required, so the ovaries fall into a position close to the fornix.[8]

Depending on factors such as position of the ovary, presence of a vaginal infection, or availability of ultrasound equipment, the ultrasound guidance method of choice for ovum retrieval is determined. A major advantage of ultrasound over laparoscopic ovum retrieval is that there is no need for general anesthesia, so the risk and the cost of the procedure are reduced. Additionally, repeated attempts may be made at IVF with ultrasound methods, which is not possible with laparoscopy. Ultrasound also eliminates the possibility of adverse side affects on the oocytes from the gas phase of carbon dioxide insufflation during laparoscopy.

Embryo transfer is performed 48 to 72 hours after the retrieved ova have been fertilized.[5] Ultrasound may be used to guide optimal placement of fertilized embryos in the uterine cavity.[27]

Initially IVF-ET was available only to women with inoperable tubal damage or no tubes. Now the technique is also employed for infertility problems such as severe endometriosis, cervical mucus abnormalities, oligospermia, or other male infertility factors. IVF-ET is also used with couples who have immunologic (i.e. antisperm antibodies), or prolonged or unexplained infertility. Patients with problems of oligospermia may accept IVF-ET as an alternative to artificial insemination (AID) because they want the child to be genetically their own.[7]

Gamete intrafallopian transfer (GIFT) is an alternative to IVF-ET if tubal patency of at least one fallopian tube is demonstrated. The indications for GIFT are endometriosis (provided that the fallopian tubes are free of disease), cervical stenosis, oligospermia, immunologic infertility, or unexplained infertility of two years' duration or more. In the GIFT procedure, both gametes, sperm and oocyte, are placed into the fallopian tubes through a laparoscope (Fig. 11-13). This is a more physiologic approach than IVF-ET, as the ampullary region of the fallopian tube is the normal site of fertilization. GIFT is similar to the IVF program, except for a few distinguishing features: The patient is on the ovulation induction regimen and is monitored with the usual parameters, including daily ultrasound examinations and blood estrogen levels. Oocytes are retrieved laparoscopically and a semen specimen is obtained. Spermatozoa are treated as in the IVF procedure. As soon as follicular aspiration and oocyte inspection is completed the sperm and oocytes are loaded into a catheter, which is inserted into the aspirating needle of the laparoscope. The

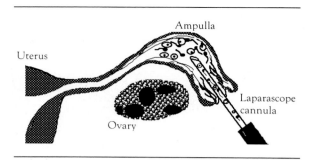

FIGURE 11-13. Gamete intrafallopian transfer (GIFT). Sperm and ovum are deposited in ampullary region of the fallopian tube.

catheter tip is placed 1.5 cm into the fimbriated end of the fallopian tube, and the contents are injected. Usually no more than two oocytes are placed in each fallopian tube. The pregnancy rate for GIFT is the same as or slightly higher than for IVF-ET.[6]

Elective Abortion

When a patient has made the decision to undergo elective abortion, ultrasound is often used in clinical management before, during, and after the operation.

DATING

Preoperative ultrasound is used to confirm an intrauterine pregnancy and to determine gestational age. Dates by pelvic examination may conflict with the patient's alleged dates by menstrual period and may be difficult to establish by examination if the patient is uncooperative, obese, or has a fibroid uterus. Pelvic examination is not as accurate as ultrasound at any stage of pregnancy, particularly at 14 to 24 weeks. An ultrasound study is unnecessary if the dates derived from pelvic examination and menstrual history correspond, but it is worthwhile if these do not agree or if the patient is close to the abortion time limit. Earlier in the pregnancy, at the 12- to 16-week stage, ultrasound is often done to establish whether dilation and curettage (D and C) can still be performed. In many institutions it is considered safer after 14 weeks to perform amnioinfusion rather than dilation and evacuation.[29]

UTERUS TOO LARGE BY EXAMINATION

Multiple pregnancy or fibroids may be responsible for an apparently large uterus in a woman who appears to be over the abortion limit by clinical examination. For example, the uterus of a patient carrying 18-week twins may look like the uterus usually does at 23 weeks.

FINDINGS THAT ALTER THE PERFORMANCE OF A DILATION AND CURETTAGE

Early-pregnancy abortion is usually performed by D and C. Ectopic pregnancy is a contraindication to D and C, as the pregnancy lies outside the uterus and laparotomy is required. Although hydatidiform mole is treated by D and C, a different approach, with scraping of the molar tissue from the uterine wall, is used when a mole is present, so it is desirable to know about the existence of a mole in an abortion candidate prior to the D and C. Fetal demise may obviate D and C because spontaneous abortion may occur.[26]

GUIDANCE OF CANNULA INSERTION

Uterine congenital anomalies, such as a double uterus with a pregnancy or a pregnancy in one horn of a bicornuate uterus, need to be identified because the D & C catheter may be inserted into the wrong uterus or the wrong side of a bicornuate uterus. Fibroids may make it impractical to perform a D & C if the fibroid is so large that the distance between the cervix and the gestational sac exceeds the length of the cannula.

Ultrasound may be called upon to assist in the operative procedure, to guide the insertion of the needle into the amniotic sac for amnioinfusion if the patient is obese or there are fibroids. If the abortion is performed prior to 14 weeks but fibroids make D and C difficult, ultrasound may be used to guide the suction cannula and to observe how far it can be placed into the uterus without perforating the fundus.[29]

POSTOPERATIVE

A postoperative ultrasound study may be requested to reveal a remaining gestational sac if the pathologic findings do not show evidence of a fetus. If pain and bleeding occur following a D and C, an ultrasound study may be ordered to exclude retained products of conception; pelvic ultrasound may reveal echogenic debris in the uterine cavity. In most instances it is not possible to distinguish between blood and retained fetal material; however, absence of material in the endometrial cavity may indicate that D and C need not be repeated.[15]

Intrauterine Contraceptive Devices

Numerous contraceptive techniques exist; most have no sonographic features. A diaphragm may be visible as an echo with a shadow just below the cervix; oral contraceptives although without obvious effect on the pelvic structures may have complications that are visible sonographically, such as splenomegaly with portal vein thrombosis or adenoma of the liver. Our discussion of contraceptive devices concentrates on intrauterine devices (IUDs; Fig. 11-14). The term IUD describes any contraceptive technique that uses foreign material placed in the uterine cavity to prevent pregnancy. IUDs are designed to prevent the development of a pregnancy without causing permanent loss of reproductive capability (as tubal ligation does). Many women still have IUDs in place that were inserted in the past, but most manufacturers have stopped producing the devices. The Dalkon shield was abandoned owing to its high incidence of midtrimester abortion and a pelvic inflammation rate four to five times higher than those of other IUDs. The Copper 7 and Copper T had no significant complications but were removed from the marketplace by manufacturers unable to afford product liability litigation in the wake of a tarnished IUD reputation. A new Copper T IUD, Paragard, was introduced in 1988.

IUDs are not risk-free. The following contraindications to their use have been established: pregnancy or suspected pregnancy, pelvic inflammatory disease, cervicitis, myoma, abnormal uterine bleeding, uterine cancer, and congenital uterine anomalies. IUD use is considered undesirable for teenagers and other nulliparous patients and in the immediate postpartum period, because the consistency of the uterus is softer and, so, prone to perforation. "The IUD is intended for women who are over 25, plan to stay in a monogamous relationship, and already have children. For these women,

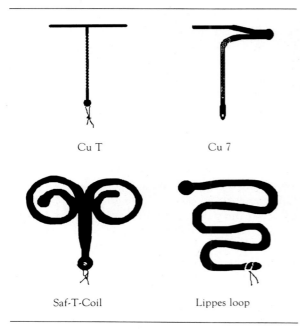

Cu T   Cu 7

Saf-T-Coil   Lippes loop

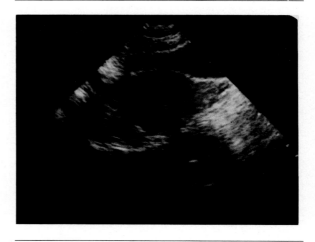

FIGURE 11-15. Transverse of Lippes loop IUD shows entrance and exit echoes.

FIGURE 11-14. Diagram of the most common IUDs. The Paragard and the Progestasert look like the Copper T.

the risks of pelvic infection and resultant sterility are extremely low."[3]

Some women are still carrying first-generation IUDs that should be replaced or removed when their time limit has expired.[3]

FUNCTION

IUDs do not prevent ovulation, sperm transport, or fertilization from taking place. The IUD acts directly on the uterus to prevent implantation. Copper-releasing IUDs cause the endometrial tissues to be premature and out of phase with ovulation. Progestin-releasing IUDs, such as the Progestasert, liberate 65 mg of progesterone daily into the uterine cavity. This has local antifertility effects such as increased viscosity of the cervical mucus, and it retards endometrial development. Since it is a relatively weak progestogen, ovulatory cycles are unchanged. The fertilized ova, too small to be seen with ultrasound, are then expelled from the uterus. Fibrosis and edema are found adjacent to the IUD. IUDs are also thought to cause a response similar to a foreign body reaction in other tissues. They cause macrophages to be mobilized, which attack

foreign protein such as spermatozoa, and possibly ova.[19]

Large IUDs that fill the intrauterine cavity are considered to have the greatest efficiency; however, they are associated with increased rates of pain and bleeding. The uterine cavity has a smaller antero-posterior than transverse dimension plane, and IUDs are designed to fit this configuration.[14]

When an IUD is removed, its contraceptive effects on the uterus are reversed and pregnancy may follow shortly. Fertility rates of women who involuntarily discontinue IUD use (i.e., pain, bleeding, infection) have not been evaluated.[16]

The IUD exhibits higher-amplitude echoes and is responsible for two echoes, an entrance and an exit reflection (Fig. 11-15). When the sound beam is perpendicular to the IUD, an acoustic shadow is demonstrated if the IUD falls within the narrow portion of the beam. To narrow the beam, a high-frequency or focused transducer is used. The gain is adjusted to a lower setting so noise does not obscure the image.

SONOGRAPHIC TECHNIQUE AND APPEARANCE

The IUD should be positioned correctly in the fundus of the uterine cavity, well above the internal os (Fig 11-16). The IUD string is attached to the proximal end and protrudes 1 inch from the cervix into

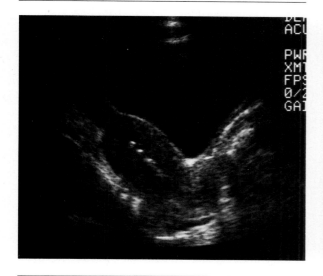

FIGURE 11-16. Echoes from the rings of a Lippes loop. Each ring has a double echo, an entrance and an exit echo.

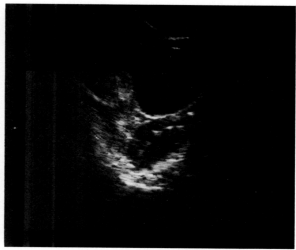

FIGURE 11-17. Longitudinal image of a retroverted uterus with a Lippes loop. The IUD is too large for the uterus and protrudes through the cervix.

the vagina. It should be palpable by or visible to the patient. The IUD should be positioned appropriately within the endometrial cavity of the uterine fundus and not at the cervix (Fig. 11-17). The IUD echoes should be in a central position in both transverse and long views of the uterus. The echo pattern should be easily obtained and reproducible. The IUD can be differentiated from normal endometrial echoes by the high-amplitude centrally located echoes, acoustic shadowing, and entrance and exit echoes.[4,10,14,21]

Each type of IUD has a characteristic echo pattern. In long axis the Lippes loop appears as two to five evenly spaced double echoes with moderate- to high-amplitude echoes, provided that the view is through the long axis of the IUD (Figs. 11-16, 11-17). On a transverse view, each rung of the IUD appears as an echogenic line (see Fig. 11-15). Entrance and exit reflections are demonstrated in both short and long axis.[4,10,21]

The Saf-T-Coil (Fig. 11-14) is a double coil with one central arm exhibiting a linear echo pattern in the long axis. In the transverse view, it has a pattern of interrupted echoes similar to the Lippes loop.

The Copper 7 and Copper **T** (Fig. 11-14) have similar ultrasound characteristics.[17] Both have a fine copper wire wound around their long arm; the short arm of each has a slightly different shape. In the long axis, a high-amplitude linear echo with a reverberation artifact from copper wound around the long limb may be seen, and there are moderate-amplitude echoes at the upper end from the short limb. In transverse view, the IUD appears as an echogenic dot. The Progestasert **T**-shaped IUD is visualized as an echogenic line with entrance and exit echoes seen in transverse and longitudinal axis with a similar shape to the Copper 7. The Paragard IUD also has an appearance similar to that of a Copper 7 (Fig. 11-18).[4,10,21]

Transvaginal scanning can be utilized for more specific visualization of the IUD position in the uterus. The position of the IUD in the endometrial cavity is well demonstrated, even in the secretory phase.

Patients with IUD problems present with pregnancy, a missing string, or lower abdominal pain and fever.

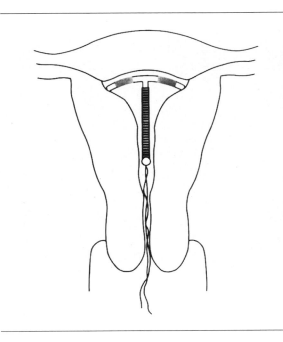

FIGURE 11-18. Diagram of Paragard IUD (taken from manufacturer's advertising material).

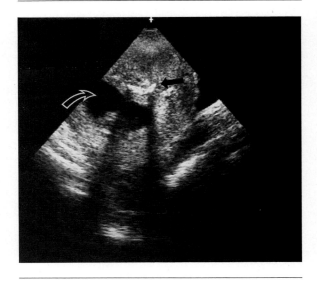

FIGURE 11-19. Pregnancy with IUD, which can be seen embedded in the placenta (*arrow*). Open arrow points to contents of gestational sac.

Pregnancy and IUD

IUDs are not 100% effective. Pregnancy may occur even when an IUD is in the correct location. It is alleged that pregnancy with an IUD in place may result in complications such as spontaneous abortion, sepsis, and septic abortion. Most institutions choose to remove the IUD if it is within the lower uterine segment and the marker thread is still visible. Pregnancy can cause the marker to migrate up into the uterus.[10,13,16] This procedure may increase the chance of spontaneous abortion, depending on the relationship of the IUD to the pregnancy. If the patient wishes to continue the pregnancy with the IUD, she must be monitored carefully for signs of sepsis or spontaneous abortion. The long-term effect on the fetus and the rate of congenital anomalies with a concomitant IUD have not been established.[16]

Intrauterine pregnancy may result from perforation of an IUD or unnoticed expulsion; however, intrauterine pregnancies do occur with IUDs in a suboptimal position or even in the proper location. The position of the IUD in relation to the gestation should be determined (Fig. 11-19). It is easier to detect an IUD in the first trimester of pregnancy than in the second or third trimester. An IUD may be visualized adjacent to a coexisting intrauterine pregnancy or low in the cervix. Usually the IUD is at a distance from the pregnancy.

In later pregnancy, the gestation occupies most of the uterine cavity. It may be impossible to determine whether the IUD is present in the cavity; fetal part echoes can be indistinguishable from those of an IUD.

Complications of IUD Use

Pelvic Inflammatory Disease. The use of an IUD is associated with an increased risk of PID. The use of any type of IUD with a string marker provides a potential route for infection into the uterine cavity. Most commonly, abscesses are seen as an echopenic collection between the uterus and ovary (Fig. 11-20).[4,10,16,21]

Lost IUD. If the string is not visible, there are several possibilities: The IUD may have been spontaneously expelled, the thread may have become detached or may have migrated up into the uterus, or

FIGURE 11-20. Copper 7 IUD within the uterus (*open arrow*). There is an abscess due to pelvic inflammatory disease in the right adnexa (*black arrow*).

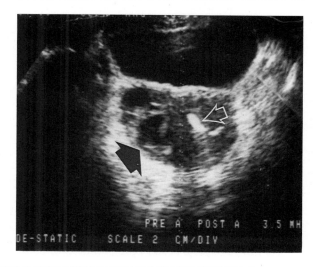

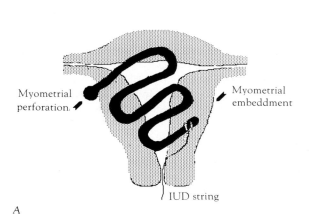

A

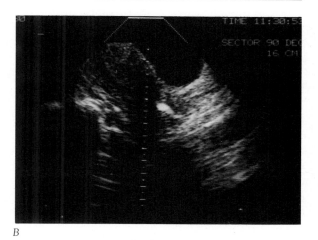

B

FIGURE 11-21. (A) Diagram of malpositioned Lippes loop shows perforation and embedment. (B) Sonogram shows Copper T embedded in the myometrium in the cervical region.

the IUD may have perforated the myometrium or cervix (Fig. 11-21). IUD perforation may be without symptoms. The presence of the string does not ensure that perforation has not taken place.[4,10,21]

Perforation. An IUD that has perforated the uterus and projects into the surrounding bowel is not sonographically visible. Perforation into the myometrium is seen in the wall rather than in the endometrial cavity (Fig. 11-21). Partial or total perforation of the uterus may occur during or after IUD insertion. Perforated IUDs must be removed because they may cause intestinal obstruction, peritonitis, abdominal adhesions, pregnancy, and serious infections that can lead to infertility or death. Surgical removal of an intraabdominal IUD may be a complicated and extensive procedure. Extrauterine perforated IUDs are rarely visible with ultrasound.[4,10,16]

If no IUD is seen on ultrasound examination

and there is no intrauterine pregnancy, a plain film radiograph is taken. Absence of the IUD confirms unnoticed expulsion. The presence of an IUD outside the uterus confirms that it is in the abdomen and has silently perforated the uterus. If the echo pattern from the sonogram is incomplete or eccentric, the device may be broken and CT is recommended to locate it. An intrauterine extracavitary location can often be diagnosed with ultrasound if the endometrial cavity and the IUD can be demonstrated separately.[4,10,21]

Ectopic Pregnancy. Ectopic pregnancy may be associated with IUDs. In the United States ectopic pregnancy occurs in about 1 in 200 pregnancies. This incidence is related to certain factors, such as a history of PID, prior ectopic pregnancy, and a history of induced abortion. The risk of ectopic pregnancy is thought to be 5 to 10 times greater for IUD users than for other women, and the risk of ectopic pregnancy may persist after an IUD is removed.[16]

ULTRASOUND PITFALLS

While ultrasound is the method of choice for identification and localization of IUDs, the technique has certain pitfalls. IUD morphology may be difficult to recognize in a retroverted uterus. Uterine fibromas and leiomyomas may displace the uterine cavity and cause an eccentric endometrial cavity echo. During the secretory phase, the endometrial cavity echoes are prominent and may mask an IUD unless a transvaginal transducer is used.

Conclusion

Diagnostic ultrasound is an essential component of the successful management of infertility problems. There is no other way to directly visualize follicle growth, and it is evident that sonographic guidance for removal of oocytes from the follicles will be the preferred method. Ultrasound is also a valuable aid in the management of elective abortion; however, the only method of contraception in which ultrasound has a large role is IUDs. Here it is helpful in showing that the IUD is in the optimal location and that none of the complications associated with IUDs are present.

References

1. Austin C. The role of ultrasound in infertility. In: Sciarra JJ, Walkins TJ, eds. Gynecology and Obstetrics: Reproductive Endocrinology, Infertility, Genetics. Philadelphia: Harper and Row; 1982; 5:1–13.

2. Bergquist T, Burkman R, Atienza M, King TM. The use of ultrasonography for elective abortion. In: Sanders RC, James AE, eds. The Principles and Practice of Ultrasonography in Obstetrics and Gynecology. 3rd ed. New York: Appleton-Century-Crofts; 1984:291–296.

3. Bor J. IUD, with caveat on consent, to be on sale in April. Baltimore Sun, March 16, 1988.

4. Cochrane WJ. The value of ultrasound in the management of intrauterine devices. In: Sanders RC, James AE, eds. The Principles and Practice of Ultrasonography in Obstetrics and Gynecology. 3rd ed. New York: Appleton-Century-Crofts; 1984:335–343.

5. Damewood MD, Wallach EE. Latest techniques improve IVF success rates. Contemporary Ob Gyn. 1986; 28:41–52.

6. Damewood MD, Wallach EE. *In vitro* fertilization update. Postgrad Obstet Gynecol. 1986; 6:1–6.

7. Diamond MP, DeCherney AH. Ovulation induction and oocyte recovery for in vitro fertilization. In: Sciarra JJ, Walkins TJ, eds. Gynecology and Obstetrics: Reproductive Endocrinology, Infertility, Genetics. Philadelphia: Harper and Row; 1982; 5:1–8.

8. Evers JLH, Larsen JF, Gnany GG, et al. Complications and problems in transvaginal sector scan-guided follicle aspiration. Fertil Steril. 1988; 49:278–282.

9. Fleisher AC, Wentz AC, Jones HW, et al. Ultrasound evaluation of the ovary. In: Callen PW, ed. Ultrasonography in Obstetrics and Gynecology. Philadelphia: WB Saunders; 1983:209–225.

10. Gross BH, Callen PW. Ultrasonography in the detection of intrauterine contraceptive devices. In: Callen PW, ed. Ultrasonography in Obstetrics and Gynecology. Philadelphia: WB Saunders; 1983:249–258.

11. Gross BH, Callen PW. Ultrasound of the uterus. In: Callen PW, ed. Ultrasonography in Obstetrics and Gynecology. Philadelphia: WB Saunders; 1983:227–247.

12. Hammond MG, Talbert LM, eds. Infertility. A Practical Guide for the Physician. Oradell, NJ: Medical Economics Books; 1985.

13. Harnsberger HR, Lee TG, Dwight HM, et al. Unusual intrauterine objects: Potential pitfalls in ultrasonographic identification. J Ultrasound Med. 1983; 2:169–172.

14. Hasson HM. The uterine cavity and intrauterine con-

traception. In: Sciarra JJ, Walkins TJ, ed. Gynecology and Obstetrics: Fertility Regulation, Psychosomatic Problems, Human Sexuality. Philadelphia: Harper and Row; 1982:6:1–11.

15. Hern WM. First trimester abortion: Complications and their management. In: Sciarra JJ, Walkins TJ, eds. Gynecology and Obstetrics: Fertility Regulation, Psychosomatic Problems, Human Sexuality. Philadelphia: Harper and Row; 1982; 6:1–9.

16. Keith LG, Berger GS, Edelman DA. Health risks of intrauterine contraception. In: Sciarra JJ, Walkins TJ, eds. Gynecology and Obstetrics: Fertility Regulation, Psychosomatic Problems, Human Sexualtiy. Philadelphia: Harper and Row; 1982; 6:1–7.

17. Kurtz AB, Rifkin MD. Normal anatomy of the female pelvis. In: Callen PW, ed. Ultrasonography in Obstetrics and Gynecology. Philadelphia: WB Saunders; 1983:193–208.

18. Lippes J. The use of intrauterine devices as pregnancy interceptives. In: Sciarra JJ, Walkins TJ, eds. Gynecology and Obstetrics: Fertility Regulation, Psychosomatic Problems, Human Sexuality. Philadelphia: Harper and Row: 1982; 6:1–5.

19. Maxwell R. Intrauterine contraceptive devices. In: Friedman EA, ed. Response to Contraception. Philadelphia: WB Saunders; 1973; 111–132.

20. Meldrum DR, Chetkowski R, Steingold KA, et al. Evolution of a highly successful in vitro fertilization-embryo transfer program. Fertil Steril. 1987; 48:86–93.

21. Najarian KE, Kurtz AB. New observations in the sonographic evaluation of intrauterine contraceptive devices. J Ultrasound Med. 1986; 5:205–210.

22. Novy MJ. Infections as a cause of infertility. In: Sciarra JJ, Walkins TJ, eds. Gynecology and Obstetrics: Reproductive Endocrinology, Infertility, Genetics. Philadelphia: Harper and Row; 1982; 5:1–16.

23. Potts M. History of contraception. In: Sciarra JJ, Walkins TJ, eds. Gynecology and Obstetrics: Fertility Regulation, Psychosomatic Problems, Human Sexuality. Philadelphia: Harper and Row; 1982; 6:1–22.

24. Riddle AF, Sharma V, Mason BA, et al. Two years' experience of ultrasound-directed oocyte retrieval. Fertil Steril. 1987; 48:454–458.

25. Ritchie WG. Sonographic evaluation of normal and induced ovulation. Radiology. 1986; 161:1–10.

26. Schulman H. Second-trimester abortion: Techniques and complications. In: Sciarra JJ, Walkins TJ, eds. Gynecology and Obstetrics: Fertility Regulation, Psychosomatic Problems, Human Sexuality. Philadelphia: Harper and Row; 1982; 6:1–11.

27. Seifer DB, Collins RL, Paushter DM, et al. Follicular aspiration: A comparison of an ultrasonic endovaginal transducer with fixed-needle guide and other retrieval methods. Fertil Steril. 1988; 49:462–467.

28. Senekjian EK, Herbst AL. Update on DES exposure. Contemporary Ob Gyn. 1987; 29:29–46.

29. Stubblefield PG. Surgical techniques for first-trimester abortion. In: Sciarra JJ, Walkins TJ, eds. Gynecology and Obstetrics: Fertility Regulation, Psychosomatic Problems, Human Sexuality. Philadelphia: Harper and Row; 1982; 6:1–15.

30. Stubblefield PG. Induced abortion: Indications, counseling, and services. In: Sciarra JJ, Walkins TJ, eds. Gynecology and Obstetrics: Fertility Regulation, Psychosomatic Problems, Human Sexuality. Philadelphia: Harper and Row; 1982; 6:1–10.

31. Taylor R. Understanding Fertility Problems. Daly City, CA: Krames Communications; 1985:1–16.

32. Thatcher SS, Donachie KM, Glasier A, et al. The effects of clomiphene citrate on the histology of human endometrium in regularly cycling women undergoing in vitro fertilization. Fertil Steril. 1988; 49:296–301.

33. Thickman D, Arger P, Tureck R, et al. Sonographic assessment of the endometrium in patients undergoing in vitro fertilization. J Ultrasound Med. 1986; 5:197–201.

34. Timor-Tritsch IE, Rottem S, Thaler I. Review of transvaginal ultrasonography: A description with clinical application. Ultrasound Quart. 1988; 6:1–34.

35. Vermesh M, Kletzky OA. Follicle-stimulating hormone is the main determinant of follicular recruitment and development in ovulation induction with human menopausal gonadotropin. Am J Obstet Gynecol. 1987; 157:1397–1402.

36. Yuzpe AA, Rioux J-E. Abortion and concomitant sterilization. In: Sciarra JJ, Walkins TJ, eds. Gynecology and Obstetrics: Fertility Regulation, Psychosomatic Problems, Human Sexuality. Philadelphia: Harper and Row; 1982; 6:1–7.

Obstetric Sonography

CHAPTER **12**

Fertilization and Embryology

STEVEN R. GOLDSTEIN, PAULA S. WOLETZ

The goal of obstetric science is to improve reproductive outcome. In the first trimester of pregnancy a very special bridge is formed between obstetrics and gynecology. High-resolution real-time ultrasound has allowed us to view the developing human earlier in its development. Conception and the first stages of development occur outside the uterus and are still beyond the visualizing capabilities of even the most sophisticated ultrasound systems. However, dramatic advances have been made in our ability to evaluate early pregnancy sonographically.

The sonographer is called on by the clinician to confirm or refute clinical impressions by objective assessment using diagnostic ultrasound. Before it is possible to appreciate potentially abnormal situations, a thorough understanding of normal early-pregnancy development is mandatory. The purpose of this chapter is to highlight that process from ovulation through the beginning of the fetal stage.

Ovulation, Fertilization, and Implantation

Ovulation, the release of a mature ovum from a follicle within the ovary, is initiated and controlled by the secretion of hormones from the anterior pituitary gland. Follicle-stimulating hormone (FSH) causes numerous follicles within an ovary to grow. The follicles produce estrogen, which in turn stim-ulates the pituitary to release luteinizing hormone (LH). One follicle reaches maturity, its final growth influenced by the LH. The rest of the follicles undergo atrophy and are replaced by connective tissue. On day 14 of a 28-day cycle, the mature follicle ruptures, releasing a single ovum (Fig. 12-1).

The ovum is picked up by the fimbriated ends of the fallopian tube and begins its course through the tube. Within the ovary, the ruptured follicle becomes a corpus luteum (yellow body) and produces progesterone. Nearby cells within the ovary continue to secrete estrogen. These hormones cause the endometrium of the uterus to grow, as the glands of the endometrium proliferate. If fertilization does not occur, the estrogen and progesterone levels drop, the endometium is shed (menstruation), and the cycle begins anew. When fertilization does occur, the corpus luteum continues to produce its hormones and the endometrium continues to grow. The resultant histologic changes seen in late secretory or early pregnancy stages cause the endometrium to become decidualized and the uterus is thus prepared to receive the fertilized egg.

Fertilization usually occurs in the ampullary portion of the tube, 24 to 36 hours after ovulation, when the outer layer of the ovum (the zona pellucida) is penetrated but not destroyed by the sperm. Upon entering the nucleus of the ovum, the sperm loses its tail and merges its genetic content with

195

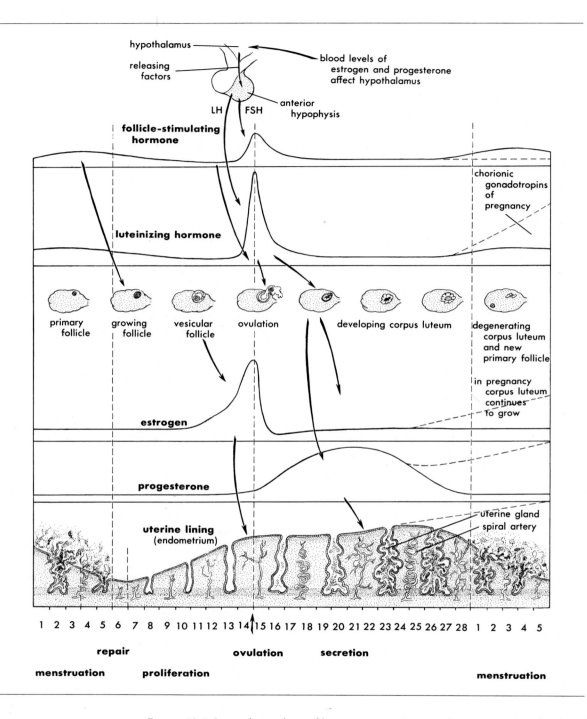

FIGURE 12-1. Interrelationships of hormones to ovarian and uterine activity during the menstrual cycle. The numbers refer to the days of the menstrual cycle. The dashed lines show the level of hormones and height of endometrium in early pregnancy. (From Crouch JE. Functional human anatomy. Philadelphia: Lea & Febiger; 1985:571.)

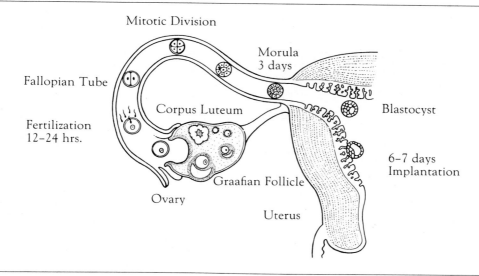

FIGURE 12-2. Schematic illustration of the stages from fertilization of the ovum to implantation of the blastocyst. (Ilustration compliments of the Department of Biomedical Communications, State University of New York, Health Science Center at Brooklyn.)

that of the ovum to form a single cell, the zygote. Initial cell division (mitosis) begins 24 to 30 hours after fertilization, even as the developing zygote moves through the fallopian tube. Cells continue to divide, forming a solid cluster of cells still surrounded and protected by the zona pellucida. This ball of cells, the morula, continues its passage through the fallopian tube and reaches the uterine cavity about 3 days after fertilization (Fig. 12-2).[6]

As the morula takes on an organized form, it becomes known as a blastocyst. The outermost layer of these cells, the trophoblast, surrounds a fluid-filled cavity (the blastocele) and an inner cell mass. Within the uterus, the zona pellucida disappears and the blastocyst receives its nutrients from the secretions of the endometrial glands; however, implantation has not yet occurred.

The trophoblast differentiates into two layers, an inner single layer of cytotrophoblast and an outer multicelled layer of syncytiotrophoblast. An important role of the trophoblast is the production of human chorionic gonadotropin (HCG), a hormone that extends the life of the corpus luteum. Continued secretion of progesterone by the corpus luteum also ensures that the uterus does not shed

its endometrial lining, and with it the rapidly developing products of conception.

Implantation, made possible by the disappearance of the zona pellucida, begins when the trophoblastic cells over the region of the inner cell mass begin to penetrate into the endometrium about 7 days after fertilization. The blastocyst burrows beneath the endometrial surface, and the opening it created is sealed by a blood clot. Decidualized endometrium can be seen to have three distinct layers defined by their relationship to the blastocyst. The decidua capsularis closes over and surrounds the blastocyst. The decidua parietalis, or decidua vera, is the decidua that lines the remainder of the endometrial cavity. The decidua basalis develops at the point of attachment by the blastocyst and will contribute the maternal portion of the placenta (Fig. 12-3).

Development of the Conceptus

The inner cell mass, or embryonic pole, differentiates into two layers: an outer layer of endoderm and an inner layer of ectoderm lying adjacent to the trophoblast. Within the ectoderm the amniotic

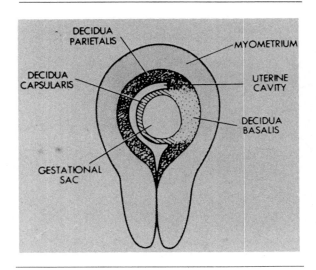

FIGURE 12-3. Schematic drawing of the implantation of an early embryo. The common sonographic term "gestational sac" actually describes the fluid-filled chorionic cavity surrounded by primary villi during a trophoblastic decidual reaction. A gestational sac can be imaged prior to the fusion of decidua capsularis and decidua parietalis.

cavity begins as a small fluid collection. Another fluid-filled structure forms adjacent to the endoderm. This cavity is the primitive yolk sac. Eventually a portion of the primitive yolk sac is pinched off and disappears; the remainder is the secondary yolk sac.

While the inner cell mass is differentiating, the cytotrophoblast multiplies, creating a loose network of cells that fill the rest of the blastocyst's cavity. These cells are the extraembryonic mesoderm. Spaces within the extraembryonic mesoderm form and coalesce. The resultant space, the chorionic cavity or extraembryonic coelom, occupies most of the blastocyst. The extraembryonic mesoderm cells lining the cavity thus enclose the yolk sac, the bilaminar embryonic disc with its small amniotic cavity, and the trophoblast walls (Fig. 12-4). It also forms a stalk connecting the embryonic disc to the trophoblast.

The trophoblast and the lining of mesoderm are now called chorion. Chorionic villi project outward from the walls of the blastocyst into the decidua. As the gestational sac grows, the decidua pa-

rietalis is stretched thin and the chorionic villi that do not proliferate into chorion frondosum disappear, leaving smooth chorion laeve. At the point of implantation, however, villi continue to grow and proliferate, forming the chorion frondosum. This will become the conceptus' contribution to the formation of the placenta.

Within the embryonic ectoderm, a line of cells thickens to form a primitive streak, which migrates to the area between the ectoderm and endoderm. A third layer of cells, the embryonic mesoderm, arises from the primitive streak. The embryonic disc contains the three germ cell layers from which all future tissue is derived. Development of the trilaminar disc (at the end of the third week after fertilization) marks the transition from the preembryonic period to the embryonic stage.

During the embryonic period, the amniotic cavity expands at the expense of the chorionic cavity, and the once flat embryonic disc folds and further differentiates. Eventually the amniotic cavity will completely fill the gestational sac. The cells lining the amniotic cavity (amnion) fuse with the chorion, but this fusion is not complete until at least 12 weeks after the last menstrual period (Fig. 12-5).

All major organs and systems are formed during the remainder of the embryonic stage. By the end of the 8th week after conception (10 menstrual weeks), the embryo has taken on a recognizable body form. Eyes, auricles, and limbs with fingers and toes can be appreciated. The embryonic period is now complete, and the fetal stage, with its rapid growth and maturation of organ systems, commences.

Sonographic Identification of the Early Intrauterine Pregnancy

Most of the early embryonic events previously described are impossible to image even with current high-frequency transvaginal probes. Sonographically, however, one can often see prominent arcuate vessels in the periphery of the myometrium and a thick, lush echogenic endometrial echo (Fig. 12-6).

The first sonographic evidence of an intrauterine pregnancy is the presence of the so-called gestational sac. This is a sonographic term, as anatomically it represents the fluid-filled chorionic cavity

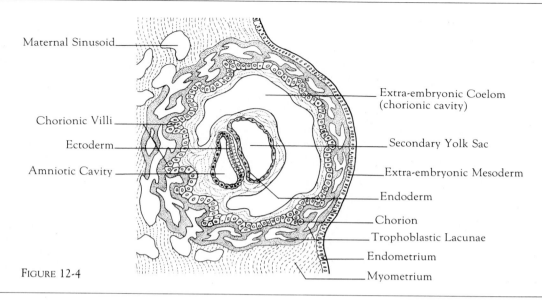

Maternal Sinusoid

Chorionic Villi

Ectoderm

Amniotic Cavity

Extra-embryonic Coelom
(chorionic cavity)

Secondary Yolk Sac

Extra-embryonic Mesoderm

Endoderm

Chorion

Trophoblastic Lacunae

Endometrium

Myometrium

FIGURE 12-4

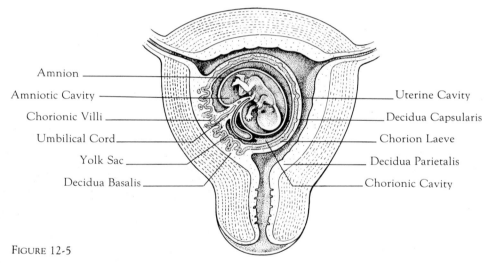

Amnion

Amniotic Cavity

Chorionic Villi

Umbilical Cord

Yolk Sac

Decidua Basalis

Uterine Cavity

Decidua Capsularis

Chorion Laeve

Decidua Parietalis

Chorionic Cavity

FIGURE 12-5

FIGURE 12-4. Drawing of the bilaminar embryonic disc with its associated structures. (Illustration compliments of the Department of Biomedical Communications, State University of New York, Health Science Center at Brooklyn.)

FIGURE 12-5. Drawing illustrating the membranes and cavities surrounding the embryo. (Illustration compliments of the Department of Biomedical Communications, State University of New York, Health Science Center at Brooklyn.)

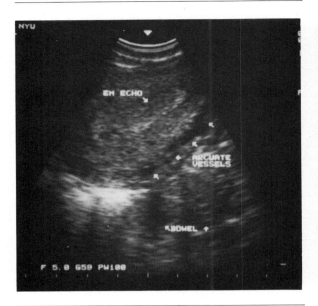

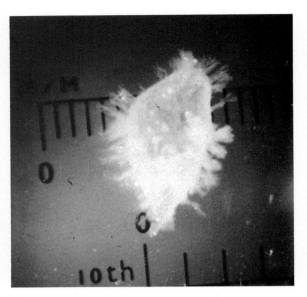

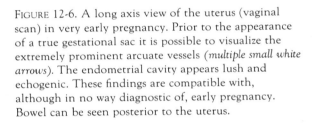

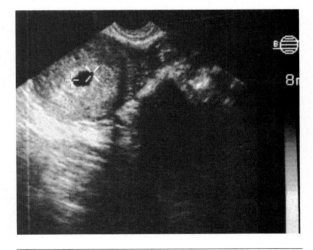

FIGURE 12-6. A long axis view of the uterus (vaginal scan) in very early pregnancy. Prior to the appearance of a true gestational sac it is possible to visualize the extremely prominent arcuate vessels (*multiple small white arrows*). The endometrial cavity appears lush and echogenic. These findings are compatible with, although in no way diagnostic of, early pregnancy. Bowel can be seen posterior to the uterus.

FIGURE 12-7. An entire gestation (of 5.5 weeks LMP) viewed with low-power microscope magnification. Note the chorion with primary villi projecting from it. This is the anatomic basis for the sonographic appearance that we know as the gestational sac.

(containing the amniotic sac, embryonic disc, and yolk sac) surrounded by the primary chorionic villi that are invading maternal decidua (Fig. 12-7). This trophoblastic decidual reaction sonographically appears as a very round, thick, echogenic rind surrounding an anechoic center (Fig. 12-8). Previously the term "double decidual sac" sign was used to describe the decidua capsularis and decidua parietalis before fusion.[8] This sign was used prior to the visualization of structures within the gestational sac, such as yolk sac or fetal pole, to distinguish between an intrauterine gestation and a pseudogestational sac associated with ectopic pregnancy. Such studies were performed using older, conventional transabdominal techniques. Newer transvaginal probes have demonstrated that the gestational sac is recognizable prior to the fusion of the two decidual layers (Fig. 12-9).

FIGURE 12-8. A long axis view of the uterus revealing an 8-mm gestational sac. The thick echogenic rind surrounds (trophoblastic decidual reaction) an anechoic center (chorionic cavity).

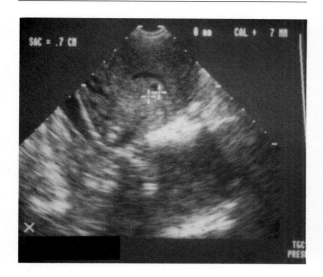

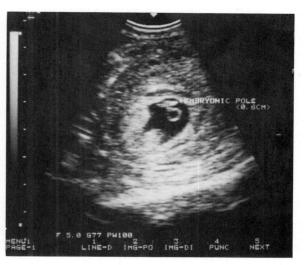

FIGURE 12-9. A 7-mm intrauterine pregnancy. The calipers have been moved so as not to obscure the landmarks of the gestational sac. The crescent-shaped sonolucency adjacent to it represents decidua capsularis not yet fused to decidua parietalis.

FIGURE 12-10. A transvaginal scan demonstrates the 6-mm embryonic pole adjacent to the yolk sac. Cardiac pulsations are visualized virtually as early as one can distinguish the embryonic pole from the yolk sac.

The first structure to be visualized sonographically within the gestational sac is the secondary yolk sac. As mentioned previously, the primary yolk sac, embryonic disc, and amniotic sac have been present but were too small to be imaged. The secondary yolk sac is a round structure approximately 4 mm in diameter. It is very regular and appears as a small sonolucent area surrounded by a highly reflective echogenic ring. It is seen vaginally at about 5 weeks after the last menstrual period (LMP)[8] and transabdominally by 6 to 7 weeks LMP.[9] Using abdominal techniques, Yeh and Rabinowitz described a "double-bleb sign" representing the complex of the sonolucent amniotic sac and yolk sac with the developing embryo between them.[10] Whereas the yolk sac remains fairly constant until about 11 weeks LMP, the embryo grows within the amniotic sac at the expense of the chorionic cavity. It is important not to mistake the yolk sac for an embryonic pole (Fig. 12-10).

Initially the first developing structure within the gestational sac was called a "fetal pole" (Fig. 12-11). Embryonic pole or disc is a more appropriate term. As we have already shown, this development is

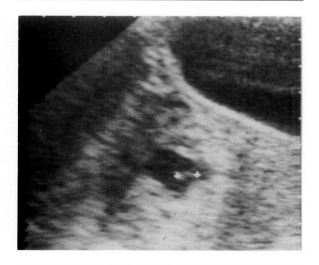

FIGURE 12-11. A transabdominal scan showing fetal pole of 68 mm. Note the relative lack of detail when this view is compared to a similar image obtained with a transvaginal transducer (Fig. 12-10).

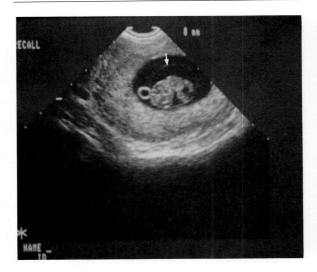

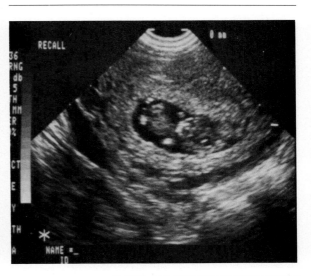

FIGURE 12-12. By 8 weeks LMP the embryo is seen to begin to unfold. The amniotic cavity is enlarging at the expense of the chorionic cavity. The yolk sac is seen to be distinctly extraamniotic. The fetal head is about half the size of the embryo. Arrow points to amnion.

FIGURE 12-13. By 9 weeks LMP limb buds are clearly seen to be developing.

sonographically antedated by the appearance of a yolk sac. The endothelial heart tube folds in on itself and begins pulsating by 21 days after conception. As soon as an embryonic disc can be seen at the periphery of the yolk sac, cardiac pulsations can be visualized and documented with M-mode capability (Fig. 12-10). Without M-mode capability, how early cardiac pulsations can be seen depends on equipment resolution and the visual acuity of the observer.

An embryo grows about 1 mm per day. By 8 weeks LMP it begins to unfold. The head accounts for about one-half of its size (Fig. 12-12). Arm and leg buds begin to develop (Fig. 12-13). Around the time of the 7th or 8th week LMP, some of the embryonic gut may be seen external to the embryo (Fig. 12-14). This represents the normal process of rotation and should not be mistaken as an early indication of an omphalocele. Within the head a posterior sonolucency, the rhombencephalon, is seen (Fig. 12-15). This will develop into the fourth ventricle. The echogenic choroid plexus can be visualized by the 10th week (Fig. 12-16).[2] Fetal spine

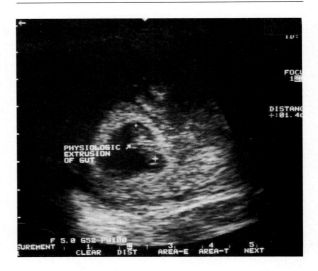

FIGURE 12-14. In this 8-week fetus there is a physiologic herniation of the midgut into the yolk stalk. The bowel will undergo a 270-degree rotation prior to returning to the abdominal cavity. This should not be mistaken for an abdominal wall defect.

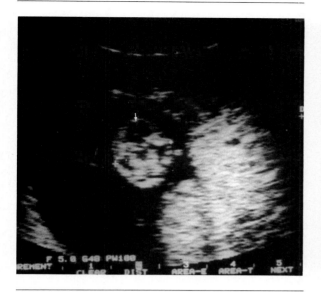

FIGURE 12-15. Sonolucent structure *(arrow)* of the posterior portion of the fetal head is the rhombencephalon, the forerunner of the fourth ventricle.

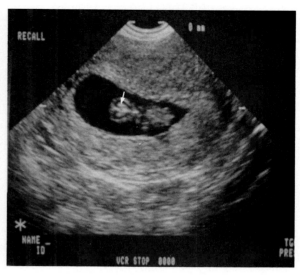

FIGURE 12-16. By 9.5 weeks LMP the echogenic choroid plexus is distinctly seen within the fetal head *(arrow).*

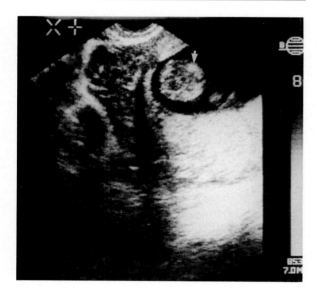

FIGURE 12-17. A cross-section of the fetal abdomen at 10 weeks LMP reveals the echogenic fetal spine *(arrow).* It is insufficiently calcified yet to cause acoustic shadowing.

can be identified, although it is not sufficiently calcified to cause an acoustic shadow (Fig. 12-17). By 10 weeks the umbilical cord and its normal insertion can be seen (Fig. 12-18). By all definitions, the developing organism ceases to be an embryo and becomes a fetus by 10 weeks LMP.

Pregnancy Detection

The use of higher-frequency transvaginal ultrasound has modified expectations of *when* we should be able to see evidence of an intrauterine pregnancy. In 1981, Kadar and colleagues proposed the "discriminatory zone" of HCG.[5] Using a transabdominal sonographic approach, they concluded that when the serum HCG level reached 6000 to 6500 mIU/ml (International Reference Preparation), a normal intrauterine pregnancy should be sonographically visualized. Its absence at those levels would indicate either an ectopic or an abnormal intrauterine pregnancy. Several years later, the discriminatory zone was further refined to 1800 mIU/ml (Second International Standard).[8] It should be noted that the values of the Second International Standard are approximately one-half those of the

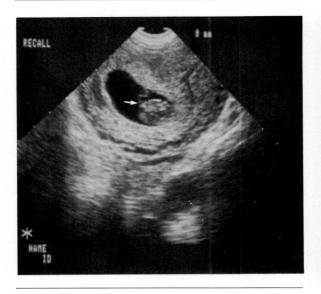

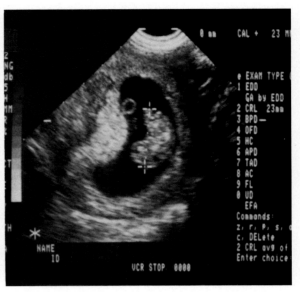

FIGURE 12-18. By 10 weeks the midgut has returned to an intraabdominal position. The normal cord insertion can be demonstrated (arrow).

FIGURE 12-19. A transvaginal sonogram at 9 weeks LMP demonstrates the landmarks for measuring the crown-rump length (CRL). Caution must be exercised not to include the yolk sac, the fetal limbs or a portion of the uterine wall. The transvaginal approach allows for more accurate measurement of CRL than does trans-abdominal scanning, because it clearly defines the yolk sac, limbs, and uterine wall.

International Reference Preparation. Today, using higher-frequency transvaginal probes, the discriminatory HCG zone is in the range of 1025 mIU/ml (IRP)[4] or 300 to 750 mIU/ml (2nd I.S.).[1] With transvaginal ultrasound, most normal gestational sacs can be visualized at 4 weeks plus 1 to 4 days from the LMP.[2] Transabdominally, they should be detectable by 6 weeks LMP.[3] Maternal obesity or significant scarring from previous lower abdominal or pelvic surgery may make visualization difficult with this approach.

Clinicians usually date pregnancy by the woman's last normal menstrual period. Sonographers then try to determine visualization according to the patient's dates. It may be more helpful to the sonographer and the clinician, however, to evaluate the size and contents of the gestational sac. This, correlated with the titer of HCG, provides a much more accurate assessment of normal or abnormal development. To measure the sac, some authors obtain a mean sac diameter by averaging the height, width, and depth of the fluid portion of the sac. This requires measurements in two planes at right angles to each other. Other authors have used maximal sac diameter, as early gestational sacs as

small as 4 mm, corresponding to a menstrual age of 4½ weeks, have been identified. Such sacs are usually uniformly spherical, so a single diameter and a mean diameter would be virtually the same.

The developing and enlarging embryonic pole can be visualized by the 7th week. By measuring the embryo along its longest axis (taking care to exclude the yolk sac), a crown-rump length (CRL) can be obtained. This is the most accurate method of dating the pregnancy (Fig. 12-19).

In summary, the use of high-frequency transvaginal transducers has opened up a new vista for understanding the normal events of early pregnancy. This has given rise to a new application of diagnostic ultrasound, sonoembryology. Only with an improved understanding of "normal" can we expect to expand our understanding and improve our diagnostic acumen in relation to pregnancy failure.

References

1. Bernashek G, Rudelstorfer R, Csaicsich P. Vaginal sonography versus serum human chorionic gonadotropin in early detection of pregnancy. Am J Obstet Gynecol. 1988; 158:608–612.
2. Blumenfeld Z, Rottem S, Elgali S, et al. Transvaginal sonographic assessment of early embryological development. In: Timor-Tritsch IE, Rottem S, eds. Transvaginal Sonography. New York: Elsevier Science Publishing; 1988.
3. Donald I. Sonar as a method of studying prenatal development. J Pediatr. 1969; 75:326.
4. Goldstein SR, Snyder JR, Watson C, et al. Very early pregnancy detection with endovaginal ultrasound. Obstet Gynecol. 1988; 72:200–204.
5. Kadar N, DeVore G, Romero R. Discriminatory HCG zone: Its use in the sonographic evaluation for ectopic pregnancy. Obstet Gynecol. 1981; 58:156–161.
6. Moore KL. The Developing Human. 3rd ed. Philadelphia: WB Saunders, 1982:33.
7. Nyberg DA, Filly RA, Mahony BS, et al. Early gestation: Correlation of hCG levels and sonographic identification. Am J Roentgenol. 1985; 144:451–454.
8. Nyberg DA, Laing FC, Filly RA, et al. Ultrasonographic differentiation of the gestational sac of early intrauterine pregnancy from the pseudogestational sac of ectopic pregnancy. Radiology. 1983; 146:755–759.
9. Nyberg DA, Mack LA, Harvey D, et al. Value of the yolk sac in evaluating early pregnancies. J Ultrasound Med. 1988; 7:129–135.
10. Yeh H, Rabinowitz J. Amniotic sac development: Ultrasound features of early pregnancy—the double bleb sign. Radiology. 1988; 166:97–103.

CHAPTER 13

Sonographic Appearance of Milestones of Pregnancy

CAROL B. BENSON, LISA A. WARNEKE

First Trimester

Sonographic examination during the first trimester can be performed transabdominally utilizing a full bladder or transvaginally. The entire uterus should be imaged, with special attention to the contents of the uterine cavity. Longitudinal and transverse images of the uterus and the gestational sac should be obtained in early first-trimester scans. Measurements, as well as images of fetal anatomy, should be included as soon as they are visible.

In early pregnancy both ovaries should be imaged, because corpus luteum cysts are common. Although corpus luteum cysts are a part of a normal pregnancy, they may become grossly enlarged (to as much as 10 cm) and may cause symptoms.[2]

Approximately 2 weeks after fertilization (4 weeks gestational or menstrual age) the developing embryo and gestational sac implant in the uterine cavity. The first sonographic evidence of an intrauterine pregnancy is the presence of a small anechoic collection within the uterus surrounded by two echogenic rings called the double-sac sign (Fig. 13-1).[3] As the conceptus grows, the placenta forms at the chorionic plate from chorionic villi and the underlying proliferating endometrium. As early as 7 to 8 weeks' gestation the developing placenta is visible sonographically as a thickened area of increased echogenicity along one side of the gestational sac (Fig. 13-2). Placental development may occur on any side of the gestational sac: anterior, posterior, fundal, or lateral. At first, placental lim-

its are poorly defined, making it impossible to determine whether implantation is abnormally low, in which case there is potential for placenta previa. The placenta grows rapidly during the first trimester and in the early part of the second trimester to become a well-defined homogeneously textured crescentic mass adjacent to one surface of the gestational sac (Fig. 13-3). By mid-second trimester (approximately 20 weeks) the now well-defined margins of the placenta permit a better assessment for placenta previa. The placenta continues to grow more slowly into the third trimester.[13]

Within the developing gestational sac the secondary yolk sac becomes visible at approximately 5 to 5.5 weeks' gestational age. Shortly therafter (by 6.5 weeks) a small fetal pole containing a flickering fetal heart can be seen adjacent to or near the yolk sac. The use of transvaginal transducers permits earlier imaging of the developing pregnancy. Additionally, studies are obtained more easily because the mother's bladder need not be full, as it must for abdominal imaging.

The fetal pole develops within an amniotic cavity created by the amniotic membrane. The chorion encloses the entire gestational sac. The yolk sac is located outside the amniotic cavity in the fluid between the chorion lining the uterine cavity and the unfused amnion (Fig. 13-2). A distinct amniotic membrane can be seen sonographically as early as 7 weeks and until as late as 14 to 16 weeks' gestation (Fig. 13-4), by which time the amniotic

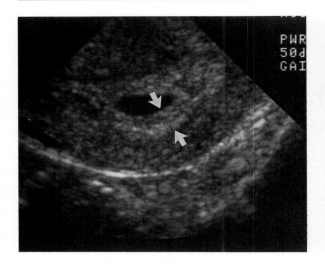

FIGURE 13-1. Double sac sign. Transvaginal demonstration of an intrauterine fluid collection surrounded by two mildly echogenic rings (*arrows*).

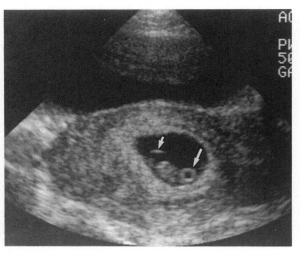

FIGURE 13-2. Transabdominal sonogram at 7 to 8 weeks' gestation with fetal pole adjacent to yolk sac (*long arrow*). A small part of the amnion (*short arrow*) is visible. The echogenic placenta lines the sac posterolaterally to the right.

cavity fills the uterine cavity and the amnion has fused with the chorion.[7,11]

The fetal pole grows rapidly, about 2 mm per day, during the first trimester.[10] As the fetus differentiates, its developing limbs, spine, and head can be recognized sonographically by 9 to 10 weeks' gestation (Fig. 13-5). By the end of the first trimester, much of the fetal anatomy is also visible, including spine, intracranial contents, stomach, and occasionally bladder.

The umbilical cord becomes sonographically visible during the latter half of the first trimester as a tortuous echo-producing band connecting the developing fetus to the placenta (Fig. 13-6). Three vessels, two small spiraling umbilical arteries and a larger umbilical vein, comprise the cord. These vessels increase in size to reach an average diameter of 1 to 2.5 cm.[10] The three components of the umbilical cord should be well-visualized on ultrasound by 16 weeks' gestation (Fig. 13-7).

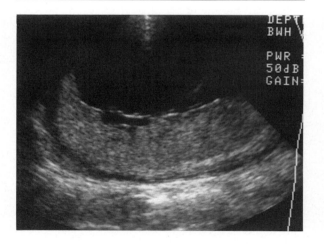

FIGURE 13-3. The well-defined homogeneous placenta lies posterior in the uterine cavity. Anechoic amniotic fluid fills the cavity surrounding the fetus (not seen here).

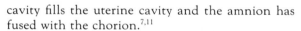

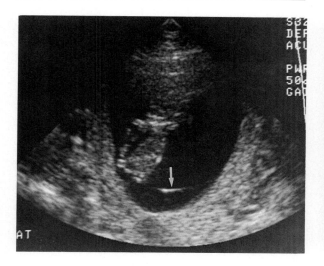

Figure 13-4. The amniotic membrane (*arrow*) can still be seen within the cavity in this 12-week gestation.

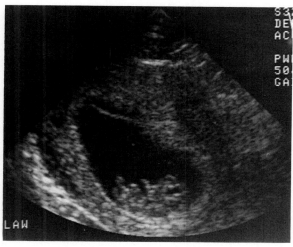

Figure 13-5. Head and limb buds of 9.5-week fetus are visible.

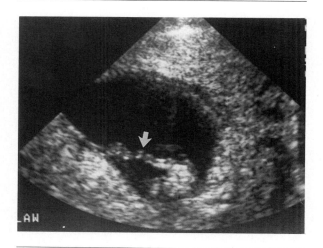

Figure 13-6. The umbilical cord (*arrow*) connects the fetus to the placenta.

Second and Third Trimesters

After the beginning of the second trimester the obstetric sonographic examination should be performed transabdominally and should include a complete assessment of the uterus and its contents. The length of the cervix should be measured, which usually requires a small amount of fluid in the maternal bladder. Caution must be taken not to overfill the bladder, as it might compress the uterus and create the false appearance of placenta previa if the anterior and posterior uterine walls are pressed together. The entire surface of the placenta should be scanned to determine position, extent, and echogenicity. Amniotic fluid volume and its echogenicity should be studied, and both adnexa should be scanned for residual corpus luteum cysts or pathology. After the first trimester the normal ovaries frequently are not visible, as the enlarging uterus obscures them.

Fetal position should be documented and a complete fetal anatomic survey should be performed. The fetus may lie in any position early in the second trimester: cephalic, breech, or transverse with its head to the mother's right or left. At this stage the fetal position may change several times during the course of the sonographic examination. By the

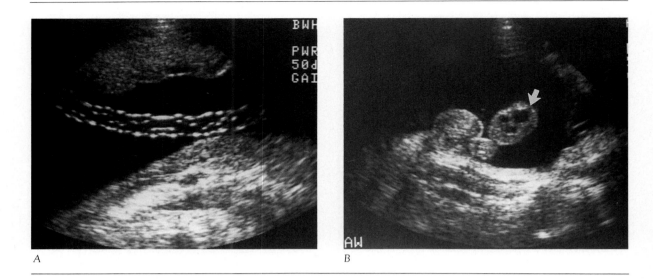

A   B

FIGURE 13-7. (*A*) Longitudinal image of umbilical cord shows tortuous cord with three vessels. (*B*) Transverse image of cord with umbilical vein (*arrow*) and two smaller umbilical arteries.

end of the second trimester, many fetuses have settled into position and will not change orientation again before delivery. As the third trimester progresses, more and more fetuses finally present cephalically. After 36 weeks, change in position is infrequent.[5]

AMNIOTIC FLUID AND MEMBRANES

The fetus lies within the amniotic cavity surrounded by amniotic fluid. As the gestational sac and fetus grow, the volume of amniotic fluid increases to its maximum at 36 to 38 weeks then decreases until delivery. Toward the end of the third trimester, the fluid is less apparent because the fetus occupies so much of the uterine cavity.[2] Amniotic fluid is normally anechoic (see Fig. 13-3) in the first trimester and most of the second. Then, small echogenic particles can be seen floating in the fluid as the gestation progresses (Fig. 13-8). These particles, called vernix, result from sloughing of fetal skin and other debris.[2] If vernix becomes highly concentrated, the amniotic fluid may become diffusely echogenic. Pathologic conditions, such as acute bleeding into the amniotic cavity (Fig. 13-9A)[12] or meconium staining (Fig. 13-9B),[1]

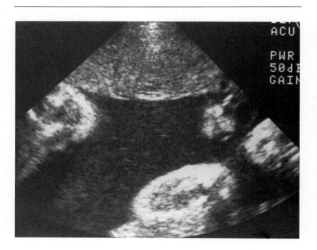

FIGURE 13-8. Scattered echoes of vernix are seen throughout the amniotic fluid in this early–third trimester pregnancy.

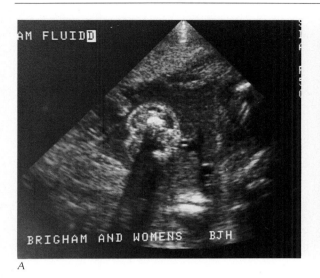
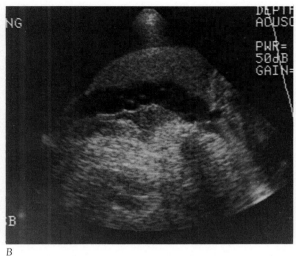

A   *B*

FIGURE 13-9. (*A*) Echogenic amniotic fluid due to an acute bleed surrounds fetal limbs and umbilical cord. (*B*) Echogenic amniotic fluid surrounds length of anechoic umbilical cord. In this case the echoes are produced by meconium. These pathologic conditions cannot be distinguished from normal vernix-filled fluid by ultrasound.

may have similar sonographic appearances; however, it is impossible to differentiate these pathologic states sonographically from normal echogenic vernix-filled amniotic fluid (Fig. 13-9).[2]

Altered amounts of amniotic fluid may be an important indicator of abnormal fetal or maternal conditions, so it is very important to assess fluid volume carefully. Experienced sonographers and sonologists find that subjective determination of the fluid volume is the best and most accurate method. This requires careful sonographic evaluation, as well as knowledge of the gestational age.[2] Quantitative methods for volume assessment, which use measurements of pockets of amniotic fluid, have also proved accurate and would be the best approach for less experienced sonographers (see Chapter 27).[8] The vertical depth of the best pocket of fluid is measured and correlated with gestational age.

The amniotic fluid volume surrounding the fetus is maintained by a delicate balance of many fetal and maternal factors. After 20 weeks' gestation, most of the fluid is produced by the fetal urinary system. Amniotic fluid is recycled by fetal swallowing. Abnormalities of either the genitourinary tract or the gastrointestinal tract can affect the amniotic fluid volume. If the fetus is unable to swallow for any reason, such as a central nervous system lesion or a neck or thoracic mass, or if there is an obstruction of the intestinal tract, the amniotic fluid balance will be disturbed and polyhydramnios will develop (Fig. 13-10). If there is obstruction of the urinary system blocking the production of urine or if renal function is absent, the fetus will not replenish the amniotic fluid and oligohydramnios will develop (Fig. 13-11). Other fetal factors that can alter the amniotic fluid volume include intrauterine growth retardation, which is associated with oligohydramnios, and fetal hydrops of any cause associated with polyhydramnios.[2]

Polyhydramnios is idiopathic in 60% of cases; it is due to fetal factors in 20%, and maternal factors in 20%, the most common being maternal diabetes.

Oligohydramnios is rarely unexplained. The most common cause is premature rupture of membranes. Intrauterine growth retardation and fetal

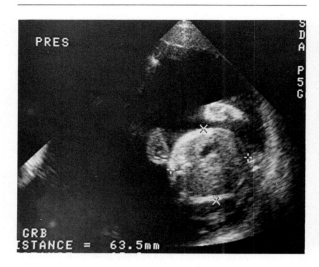

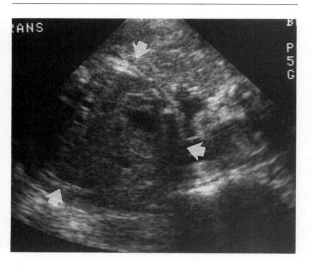

Figure 13-10. Polyhydramnios. Markedly increased anechoic fluid surrounds the fetal abdomen (calipers).

Figure 13-11. Oligohydramnios. Very little amniotic fluid surrounds this fetal abdomen (*arrows*).

genitourinary anomalies account for the others.[2]

Occasionally, after 16 weeks, a membrane may be seen floating in the amniotic cavity or extending across the cavity (Fig. 13-12). Some amniotic membranes may have a free edge and protrude into the amniotic cavity. Amniotic band syndrome results when these sections of amnion involve the fetus, often causing severe fetal deformities[7]; however, these membranes may also be seen within the amniotic cavity without any involvement of the fetus. They are thought to result from reflection of the membranes over a uterine synechia, a scar or adhesion, and are not the result of interruption of the amnion. In these cases, a free edge will be seen within the amniotic cavity, but because the amnion remains intact, the fetus is not involved.[11]

The Uterus

The body of the uterus is made up predominantly of myometrium, a muscular middle layer. The uterine cavity is lined by an inner layer, the endometrium. The perimetrium, or outer layer, surrounds the uterus. The perimetrium may appear very echogenic when it is oriented perpendicular to the ultrasound beam, owing to specular reflection. During pregnancy, the smooth muscle of the myometrium stretches and hypertrophies rapidly. Myometrial vessels also proliferate and enlarge greatly.[10] On sonographic examination, the myometrium appears as a hypoechoic band completely surrounding the gestational sac (Fig. 13-13). It is easiest to identify where it lies in contact with the placenta. The uterine vessels are most abundant along the lateral uterine wall and may alter the echogenic pattern of the myometrium as they enlarge (Fig. 13-14).

Myometrial thickness should be uniform around the gestational sac. Any evidence of thinning at the placental junction may indicate an abnormally adherent placenta, placenta accreta, increta, or percreta (Fig. 13-15).[2,6]

Throughout the pregnancy focal areas of smooth muscle in the uterine wall contract, causing a bulging into the amniotic cavity. These contraction zones should not be confused with fibroids or altered placental patterns. The muscle contractions appear homogeneous in echo texture, do not distort the outer uterine contour, and should disappear within 30 to 45 minutes (Fig. 13-16).[2]

Uterine leiomyomas or fibroids may be located in the wall of the uterus. They tend to be hypoechoic, round, and somewhat heterogeneous. They

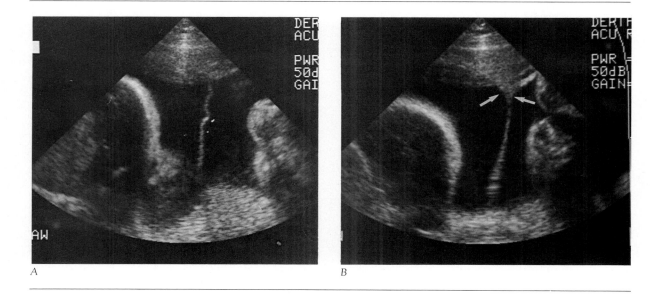

FIGURE 13-12. (A) A membrane (amniotic sheet) is seen crossing a portion of the amniotic cavity. It does not involve the fetus. (B) The leaves of the membrane are reflected over a uterine synechia *(arrows)*.

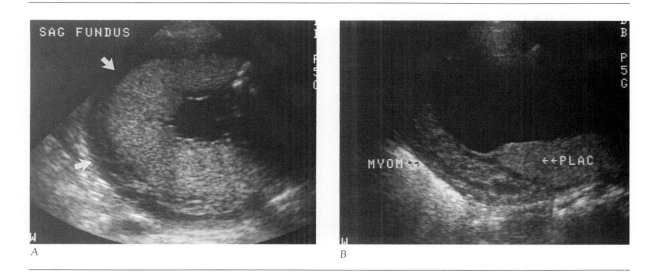

FIGURE 13-13. Myometrium. (A) A hypoechoic band of smooth muscle *(arrows)*, outside the placenta in this image. (B) The myometrium (MYOM, *arrows*) is a thick layer surrounding the entire gestational sac. (PLAC, placenta)

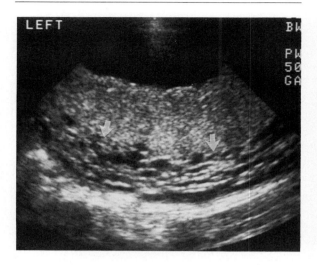

FIGURE 13-14. Many large uterine vessels (*arrows*) are seen along the lateral uterine wall.

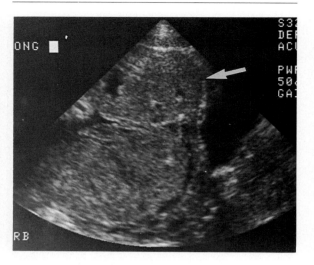

FIGURE 13-15. Absence of hypoechoic band of myometrium (*arrow*) beneath placenta in lower uterine segment is due to abnormally deep invasion by the placenta (placenta percreta).

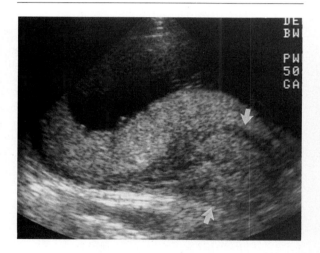

FIGURE 13-16. During contraction, a homogeneous thickening of myometrium (*arrows*) bulges placenta toward amniotic cavity.

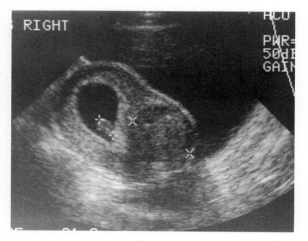

FIGURE 13-17. Fibroid appears as a heterogeneous round mass (x calipers) in anterior uterine wall. Fetal pole (+ calipers) in gestational sac.

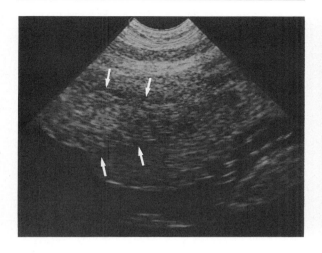

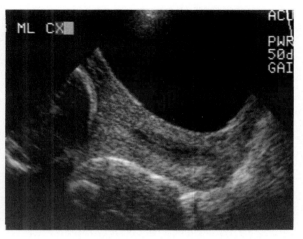

Figure 13-18. Acute subchorionic hematoma (*arrows*) lifts the placenta and mimics a contraction.

Figure 13-19. Longitudinal image of cervix through full bladder. Fetal head lies above internal os in amniotic cavity.

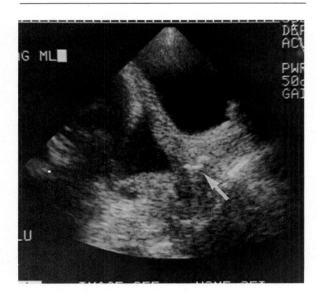

Figure 13-20. Dilated internal cervical os to level of cerclage (*arrow*) represented by bright echoes in distal cervix.

may distort the outer or inner contour of the uterus, but, unlike myometrial contractions, they do not change during the course of a sonographic examination (Fig. 13-17). Fibroids sometimes enlarge during pregnancy and may become symptomatic owing to increased uterine irritability or degeneration. Large fibroids positioned in the lower uterine segment may obstruct delivery.[2,10]

Occasionally a subchorionic hematoma produced by placental abruption may mimic a fibroid or uterine contraction (Fig. 13-18). Within several days this subchorionic collection becomes cystic as the hematoma breaks down and no longer confuses the diagnosis.[2]

The cervix is the most inferior portion of the uterus; in normal pregnancy it remains tightly closed until the time of delivery (Fig. 13-19). Dilatation of the cervix prior to term can lead to second trimester spontaneous aborton or premature delivery. If premature cervical dilatation, called cervical incompetence, is detected before the pregnancy is lost, a cerclage loop can be placed in the cervix to prevent further dilatation and permit the pregnancy to continue. Several sonographic criteria have been proposed for early detection of cervical incompetence. Widening of the cervix at the

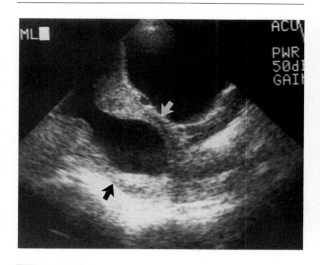

FIGURE 13-21. Membranes and amniotic fluid bulge through dilated cervix (*arrows*).

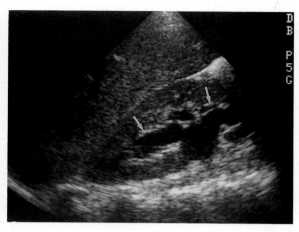

FIGURE 13-22. Moderate hydronephrosis of mother's right kidney (*arrows*) at 22 weeks' gestation.

level of the internal os to more than 20 mm is suggestive of cervical incompetence.[4] In the second trimester if the cervix is shortened (<4 cm) or if the anterior uterine wall in the lower uterine segment is less than 10 mm thick, the diagnosis of cervical incompetence can be raised.[9] Once cerclage is in place it is visible sonographically as several bright echoes within the muscle of the cervix (Fig. 13-20).

Frank dilatation of the cervix with bulging of membranes through the os is a poor prognostic sign (Fig. 13-21). The dilatation may have advanced too far for application of cerclage. Special care should be taken to look at the contents of the fluid and membranes protruding into the cervical canal. The presence of any part of the umbilical cord is a serious threat to the fetus, an obstetric emergency that requires immediate intervention.[2,10]

MATERNAL KIDNEYS AND VESSELS
During pregnancy some degree of hydronephrosis of both kidneys is quite common, especially after the beginning of the second trimester, by which time the uterus has grown out of the pelvis and compresses the ureters (Fig. 13-22). In greater than 80% of cases the right renal collecting system is more dilated than the left.[10] The dilated ureter can

often be followed behind the uterus to the level of the pelvic brim.

The enlarged uterus also compresses the inferior vena cava, particularly when the patient lies supine, as for sonographic examinations. Prolonged compression of the inferior vena cava during a long obstetric ultrasound examination inhibits venous return to the heart and can cause light-headedness and nausea. If symptoms occur during the sonographic examination, the patient should be turned onto her left side.[10]

References
1. Benacerraf BR, Gatter MA, Ginsburg F. Ultrasound diagnosis of meconium—Stained amniotic fluid. Am J Obstet Gynecol. 1981; 139:154.
2. Benson CB, Jones TB, Lavery MJ, et al. Atlas of Obstetrical Ultrasound. Philadelphia: JB Lippincott; 1988.
3. Bradley WG, Fiske CE, Filly RA. The double-sac sign in early intrauterine pregnancy: Use in exclusion of ectopic pregnancy. Radiology. 1982; 148:223.
4. Feingold M, Brook I, Zakut H. Detection of cervical incompetence by ultrasound. Acta Obstet Gynecol Scand. 1984; 63:407–410.
5. Hughey MJ. Fetal position during pregnancy. J Obstet Gynecol. 1985; 153:885.

6. Litwin MS, Loughlin KR, Benson CB, et al. Placenta percreta invading the urinary bladder. Report of three cases and review of the literature. Br J Urol. 1989; 64:283–286.

7. Mahony BS, Filly RA, Callen PW, et al. The amniotic band syndrome: Antenatal sonographic diagnosis and potential pitfalls. Am J Obstet Gynecol. 1984; 152:63–68.

8. Manning FA, Hill LM, Platt LD. Qualitative amniotic fluid volume determination by ultrasound: Antepartum detection of intrauterine growth retardation. Am J Obstet Gynecol. 1981; 139:154.

9. Podobrik M, Bulic M, Smiljanic N, et al. Ultrasonography in the detection of cervical incompetency. J Clin Ultrasound. 1988; 13:383–391.

10. Prichard JA, MacDonald PC, Gant NF. Williams' Obstetrics. 17th ed. Norwalk, CT, Appleton-Century-Crofts; 1985.

11. Randel SB, Filly RA, Callen PW, et al. Amniotic sheets. Radiology. 1988; 166:633–636.

12. Saltzman DH, Benson CB, Barss V, et al. Echogenic amniotic fluid secondary to heparin therapy. J Diagnost Med Sonogr. 1985; 1:555.

13. Spirt BA, Gordon LP. The placenta as an indicator of fetal maturity: Fact and fancy. Semin Ultrasound CT MR. 1984; 5:290.

CHAPTER 14

Normal Anatomy of the Fetal Head, Neck, and Spine

JANE STRELTZOFF, GLENN ISAACSON, FRANK A. CHERVENAK

A systematic approach to sonographic examination of the head, neck, and spine is necessary to reveal the numerous possible abnormalities in this complex region. In this chapter we outline a comprehensive method of examining the neural axis, pausing at various points to describe in detail what can be observed. This subject is important to each sonographer, as a careful evaluation of the fetal head, neck, and spine is now considered to be an integral part of all second- and third-trimester ultrasound examinations.

Head

Historically, serial transverse sonograms have proved very useful in evaluating fetal intracranial anatomy. These transverse planes are, for several reasons, preferred for antenatal ultrasound over the coronal and sagittal ones used by neonatal ultrasonographers and pathologists. When accessible to ultrasound examination, the fetal head is most often in an occiput-transverse position (i.e., the side of the head lies parallel to the mother's abdominal wall). Also, the membranous bones of the fetal cranium do not reflect sound waves to the extent that they do when they are more heavily calcified and rigid, in postnatal life. Finally, a transverse plane produces a large cross section of the brain, in which multiple landmarks may be visualized at one time for orientation (Fig. 14-1).

THE LATERAL VENTRICLE LEVEL

Starting at 16 weeks' gestation, the lateral ventricles can be identified as paired echo-spared areas within the brain substance (Figs. 14-2 to 14-4). The distal ventricle (i.e., the one farthest from the ultrasound transducer) is chosen for study, as reverberation artifacts often obscure the anatomy of the proximal hemisphere. The lateral wall of the ventricle may be visualized consistently as the first echogenic line on the distal edge of the echo-spared ventricle. The medial wall of the ventricle is visualized less consistently. A prominent echogenic area is often seen within the lateral ventricle, which represents the choroid plexus.

In early fetal life, the ventricular system fills a large portion of the developing brain and has the form of two smooth curved tubes joined above the third ventricle. As gestation progresses, the ventricular system develops a conformation that increasingly resembles that in adult life and occupies a decreasing proportion of the brain's volume. Sonographically, this change is manifested by a decrease in the proportion of the brain's cross section occupied by the lateral ventricles. This evolution has been documented by Jeanty,[9] Johnson,[13] and Pretorius,[18] all of whom have generated nomograms comparing the width of the lateral ventricle to the width of the cerebral hemisphere at various gestational ages.

The following technique is necessary to use these

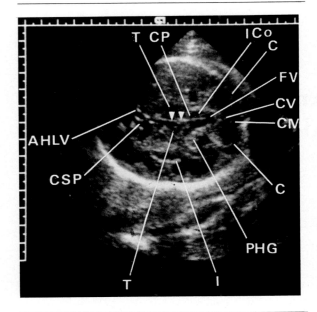

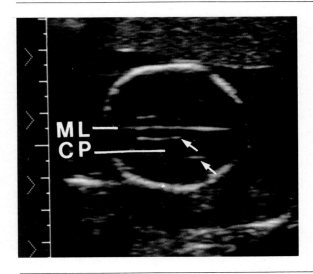

FIGURE 14-1. Transverse sonogram through fetal skull at the level of BPD but angled posteriorly and inferiorly, demonstrates cerebellum (C), cerebellar vermis (CV), cisterna magna (CM), fourth ventricle (FV), inferior colliculus (ICo), cerebellar peduncle (CP), parahippocampal gyrus (PHG), insular cortex (I), thalamus (T), third ventricle (*arrowheads*), cavum septi pellucidi (CSP), anterior horns of lateral ventricles (AHLV).

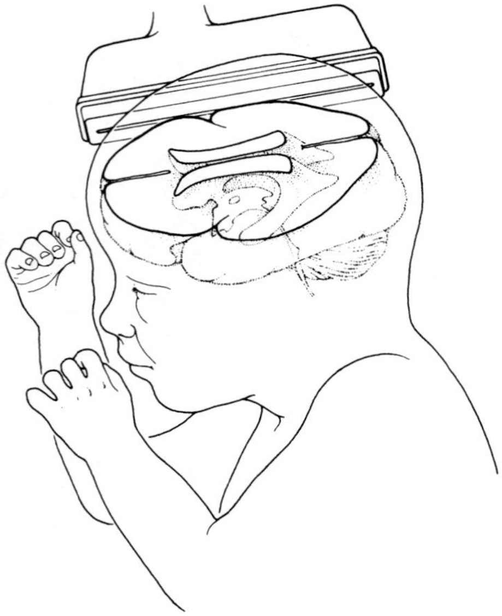

FIGURE 14-2. Diagram demonstrates plane of the lateral ventricular level. (From Chervenak FA, Isaacson F, Lorber J. Anomalies of the Fetal Head, Neck, and Spine: Ultrasound Diagnosis and Management. Philadelphia: WB Saunders; 1988.)

FIGURE 14-3. Transverse sonogram through bodies of lateral ventricles at 18 weeks' gestation demonstrates choroid plexuses (CP) filling the lateral ventricle, with arrows pointing to medial and lateral ventricular walls (ML, midline echo). (From Chervenak FA, Isaacson F, Lorber J. Anomalies of the Fetal Head, Neck, and Spine: Ultrasound Diagnosis and Management. Philadelphia: WB Saunders, 1988.)

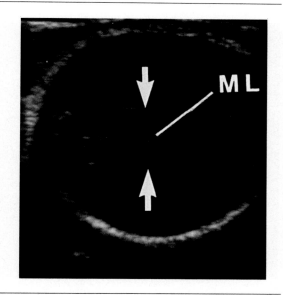

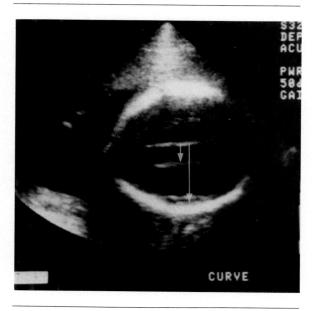

FIGURE 14-4. Transverse sonogram through bodies of lateral ventricles at 34 weeks' gestation with arrows pointing to lateral ventricular walls (ML, midline echo). (From Chervenak FA, Isaacson F, Lorber J. Anomalies of the Fetal Head, Neck, and Spine: Ultrasound Diagnosis and Management. Philadelphia: WB Saunders; 1988.)

FIGURE 14-5. Transverse sonogram through bodies of the lateral ventricles. Arrows demonstrate distance from midline echo to lateral wall of lateral ventricle and distance from midline echo to inner skull table.

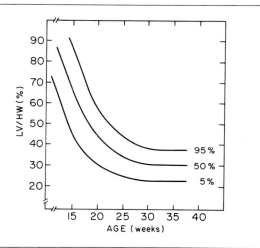

FIGURE 14-6. Lateral ventricle/hemispheric width as a function of gestational age. (Modified from Jeanty P, Dramaix-Wilmet M, Delbeke D, et al. Ultrasound evaluation of fetal ventricular growth. Neuroradiology. 1981;21:127.)

nomograms. The ventricles are explored until the greatest width of the body of the lateral ventricle is found. The lateral ventricular width is measured from the midline echo to the first echo of the lateral wall of the lateral ventricle at the point where the ventricular wall runs parallel to the midline. In the same image, the hemispheric width is measured as the longest distance between the midline and the inner edge of the skull perpendicular to the midline (Fig. 14-5). These values are then expressed as a ratio and compared to a nomogram (Fig. 14-6).

Other methods can be used to assess the normalcy of the ventricular system. Cardoza and colleagues have described the usefulness of measuring the lateral ventricular atrial width. The widest diameter of the atrium is measured through the choroid plexus, and normal measurement should not exceed 10 mm (Fig. 14-7).[4] Mahoney and coworkers have determined that the distance between the medial wall of the lateral ventricle and the medial margin of the choroid plexus should be less than 5 mm at the level of the atrium.[15]

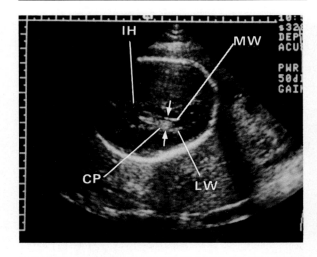

FIGURE 14-7. Transverse sonogram demonstrates distal lateral ventricle with its atrial measurement (*arrows*), lateral wall (LW) and medial wall (MW), choroid plexus (CP), and interhemispheric fissure (IH).

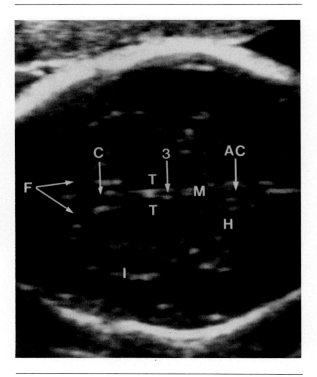

FIGURE 14-8. Transverse sonogram at the level of the BPD demonstrates frontal horn of lateral ventricle (F), cavum septi pellucidi (C), thalamus (T), third ventricle (3), hippocampus (H), midbrain (M), great cerebral vein and ambient cistern (AC), insula (I). (From Chervenak FA, Isaacson F, Lorber J. Anomalies of the Fetal Head, Neck, and Spine: Ultrasound Diagnosis and Management. Philadelphia: WB Saunders; 1988.)

THE BIPARIETAL DIAMETER LEVEL

Perhaps the most intensely studied transverse section of the fetus is at the level of the biparietal diameter (BPD). Several intracranial landmarks are located to define a plane 15 degrees above the canthomeatal line and parallel to the base of the skull. The two landmarks found most consistently are the paired anechoic thalami, which appear somewhat triangular, and the cavum septi pellucidi, which appear as two short anterior lines parallel to the midline. Other structures commonly observed in the same plane and near the midline are from posterior to anterior: the great cerebral vein and its ambient cistern sitting above the cerebellum,[17] the midbrain, the third ventricle between the thalami, and the frontal horns of the lateral ventricles. Laterally placed in the same plane are the spiral hippocampal gyri[14] posteriorly and the bright paired echoes of the insulae with pulsating middle cerebral arteries (Fig. 14-8).

In this plane, the BPD can be reproducibly measured as the distance from the proximal outer table to the distal inner table of the skull.[5,19] In addition, the head perimeter can be determined by direct measurement or calculated by adding the BPD and

occipitofrontal diameter (OFD) measured from the midpoint of frontal and occipital echo complexes and multiplying by 1.62.[11] The ratio of BPD to OFD defines the cephalic index (normal values 75 to 85). A high value determines brachycephaly and a low value, dolichocephaly. With these variants of head shape, BPD may be an inaccurate determinant of gestational age and, rarely, there may be cranial pathology.

There are several sonographic markers that have anatomic correlates that have been a source of confusion. During the second trimester, the echogenic line, once thought to be the sylvian fissure, is a reflection from the insular cortex.[8] The area desig-

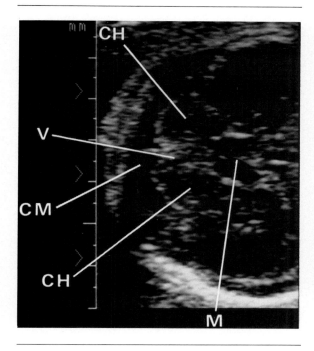

FIGURE 14-9. Transverse sonogram demonstrates cerebellar hemispheres (CH), vermis (V), midbrain (M), and cisterna magna (CM).

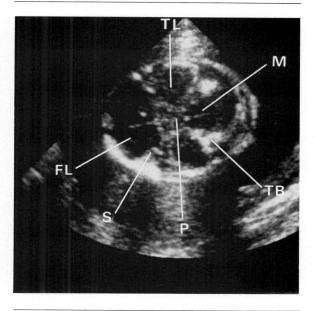

FIGURE 14-10. Sonogram through base of skull showing frontal lobe (FL), temporal lobe (TL), greater wings of sphenoid (S), temporal bone (TB), pituitary stalk (P), and medulla (M).

nated as cerebral peduncles in some texts points to the entire midbrain, of which the crus cerebri or cerebral peduncles form only the most rostral parts. Finally, the echo-spared area caudal to the midbrain, often called the ambient cistern, is in large part composed of the great cerebral vein surrounded by a small amount of cerebrospinal fluid.[7]

THE CEREBELLAR LEVEL
The cerebellum may be visualized in a plane parallel and inferior to the BPD plane. Once located, the cerebellar structures are best studied by rotating the ultrasound transducer 15 degrees inferior from the canthomeatal line. In this plane, the cerebellum (with its brightly echogenic, centrally placed vermis and two relatively nonechogenic hemisperes) may be evaluated and measured (Fig. 14-9). The midbrain may be seen in front of the vermis. The cisterna magna is seen and can be measured between the vermis and the inner table of the occipital bone.[20]

THE BASE OF THE SKULL LEVEL
The base of the skull level may be identified by an echogenic X formed by the lesser wings of the sphenoid bone and the petrous pyramid. These bony ridges demarcate the anterior, middle, and posterior fossae, including frontal lobe anteriorly, pituitary stalk centrally, and medulla posteriorly (Fig. 14-10).

THE SAGITTAL VIEW
Sagittal views of the fetal brain are sometimes helpful to delineate anatomy. The relationship of midline cranial structures can be seen in Figure 14-11.

Face
Unlike the cranium and its contents, which may be studied using an orderly progression of well-defined sonographic planes, characterization of the face requires skill, luck, and ingenuity on the part

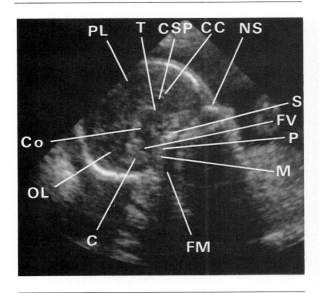

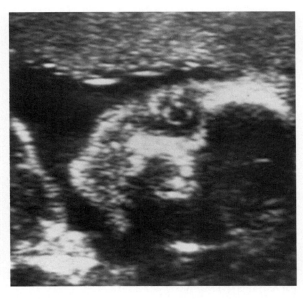

Figure 14-11. Sagittal sonogram which can supply supplemental information for midline cranial anatomy, including nasal septum (NS), body of sphenoid (S), thalamus (T), cavum septi pellucidi (CSP), corpus callosum (CC), parietal lobe (PL), occipital lobe (OL), colliculi (CO), cerebellum (C), fourth ventricle (FV), medulla (M), pons (P), foramen magnum (FM).

Figure 14-12. Coronal view of fetal face. (From Chervenak FA, Isaacson F, Lorber J. Anomalies of the Fetal Head, Neck, and Spine: Ultrasound Diagnosis and Management. Philadelphia: WB Saunders; 1988.)

of the sonographer (Fig. 14-12). We describe approaches to several facial features that have proved successful in visualizing anatomy and detecting anomalies.

Orbits and Eyes

Measurement of the distance between the bony orbits may be useful for determining gestational age and searching for anomalies characterized by hypotelorism or hypertelorism.[10,16] Depending on the position of the fetal head, the inner and outer orbital distances can be measured in coronal or transverse planes (Figs. 14-13, 14-14) and compared to nomograms. The outer orbital distance is the more valuable measurement because it has a greater range of normal variation across gestational age than the inner orbital distance. The technique for obtaining these measurements is illustrated in Figures 14-13 and 14-14.

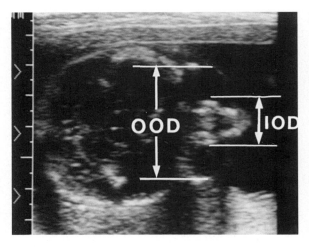

Figure 14-13. Transverse sonogram with outer orbital distance (OOD) and inner orbital distance (IOD) indicated. (From Chervenak FA, Isaacson F, Lorber J. Anomalies of the Fetal Head, Neck, and Spine: Ultrasound Diagnosis and Management. Philadelphia: WB Saunders; 1988.)

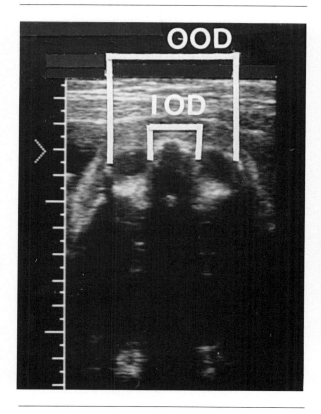

FIGURE 14-14. Demonstration of orbits with fetus facing anteriorly. (From Chervenak FA, Isaacson F, Lorber J. Anomalies of the Fetal Head, Neck, and Spine: Ultrasound Diagnosis and Management. Philadelphia: WB Saunders; 1988.)

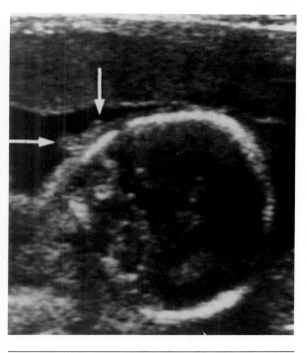

FIGURE 14-15. Smooth fetal pinna at 18 weeks' gestation (arrows). (From Chervenak FA, Isaacson F, Lorber J. Anomalies of the Fetal Head, Neck, and Spine: Ultrasound Diagnosis and Management. Philadelphia: WB Saunders; 1988.)

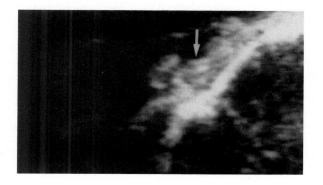

FIGURE 14-16. Mature, ridged fetal ear at 36 weeks' gestation (arrow). (From Chervenak FA, Isaacson F, Lorber J. Anomalies of the Fetal Head, Neck, and Spine: Ultrasound Diagnosis and Management. Philadelphia: WB Saunders; 1988.)

The lens of the fetal eye may be visualized as a circular area on the front of the globe (Fig. 14-12). On occasion, the aqueous and vitreous humor, extraocular muscles, and ophthalmic artery may be recognized.[12]

EARS

The pinna of the ear and the development of its cartilages have been observed sonographically.[2] The pinna is initially smooth but becomes increasingly ridged as gestation progresses (Figs. 14-15, 14-16). Occasionally, even the basal turn of the cochlea or superior semicircular canal may be visualized within the petrous portion of the temporal bone.[6]

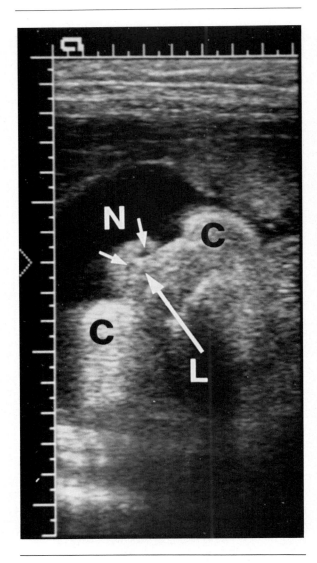

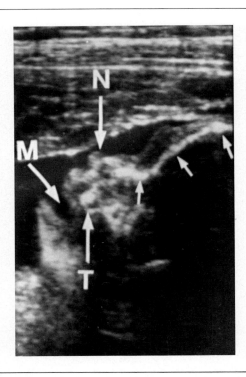

FIGURE 14-18. Fetal profile demonstrates bones of face (*small arrows*), tooth (T), nose (N), and mouth and lips (M). (From Chervenak FA, Isaacson F, Lorber J. Anomalies of the Fetal Head, Neck, and Spine: Ultrasound Diagnosis and Management. Philadelphia: WB Saunders; 1988.)

the midline sagittal view) is useful for verifying the position of the nose, the contour of the chin, and the shape of the facial midline (Fig. 14-18).

Neck

The neck should be examined with particular attention to its surface contours, as a variety of lesions may protrude from this area. The trachea and carotid bifurcation may be seen within the substance of the neck (Fig. 14-19). Measurement of skin thickness behind the occipital bone, termed nuchal fold (Fig. 14-20), has been reported to predict Down's syndrome.[1] If the measurement is greater than 5 mm, the sonographer should check whether the neck is extended, as that might increase the nuchal fold thickness.

FIGURE 14-17. Oblique coronal sonogram looking up at fetal upper lip (L), cheeks (C), and nares (N). (From Chervenak FA, Isaacson F, Lorber J. Anomalies of the Fetal Head, Neck, and Spine: Ultrasound Diagnosis and Management. Philadelphia: WB Saunders; 1988.)

LOWER FACE

The nares and upper lip can be visualized in an oblique transverse scan (Fig. 14-17). This plane may be used to search for cleft lip and palate. The tongue and its motion may be observed and the act of swallowing may be studied. The fetal profile (i.e.,

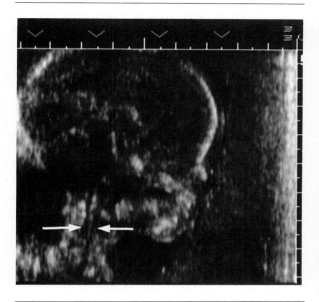

FIGURE 14-19. Sagittal sonogram demonstrating anterior contour of neck and carotid bifurcation (*arrows*). (From Chervenak FA, Isaacson F, Lorber J. Anomalies of the Fetal Head, Neck, and Spine: Ultrasound Diagnosis and Management. Philadelphia: WB Saunders; 1988.)

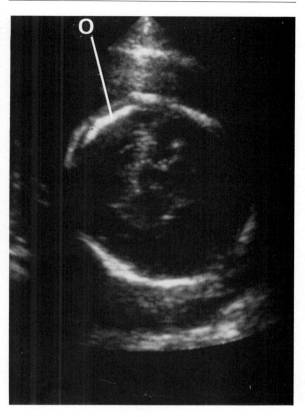

FIGURE 14-20. Transverse sonogram of fetal skull demonstrates level at which skin thickening is measured, behind occipital bone (O).

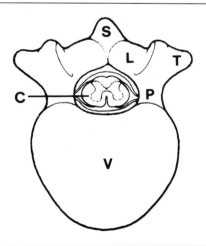

FIGURE 14-21. Transverse view of fetal vertebra (V, vertebral body; P, pedicle; L, lamina; T, transverse process; S, spinous processes; C, spinal cord). (From Chervenak FA, Isaacson F, Lorber J. Anomalies of the Fetal Head, Neck, and Spine: Ultrasound Diagnosis and Management. Philadelphia: WB Saunders; 1988.)

Spine

An appreciation of the variability in the shapes of the vertebral bodies and the changing sonographic appearance of the spine during gestation is necessary to differentiate small defects in the spine from normal anatomy (Figs. 14-21 to 14-23).[3]

By 16 weeks' gestation, individual vertebrae may be identified by the observation of three echogenic ossification centers in the transverse plane. Two of these ossification centers are posterior to the spinal canal in the laminae and one is anterior, representing the vertebral body (Fig. 14-24). If the spine is scanned sagitally, a line of vertebral bodies and a line of posterior elements may be seen on either side of the anechoic spinal canal. In the coronal plane, the two echogenic posterior ossification cen-

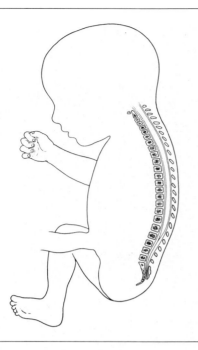

FIGURE 14-22. Sagittal view of fetal spine demonstrates vertebral bodies and varying angles of spinous processes. (From Chervenak FA, Isaacson F, Lorber J. Anomalies of the Fetal Head, Neck, and Spine: Ultrasound Diagnosis and Management. Philadelphia: WB Saunders; 1988.)

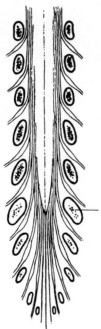

FIGURE 14-23. Coronal view of lumbosacral fetal spine through vertebral pedicles demonstrates spinal cord ending at S1. (From Chervenak FA, Isaacson F, Lorber J. Anomalies of the Fetal Head, Neck, and Spine: Ultrasound Diagnosis and Management. Philadelphia: WB Saunders; 1988.)

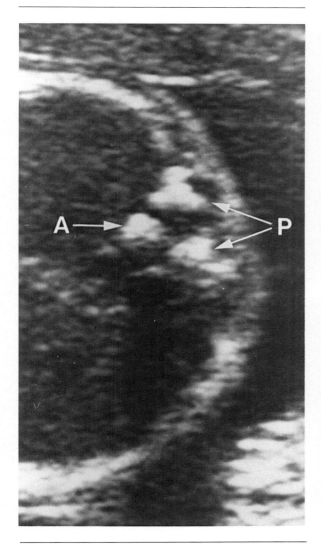

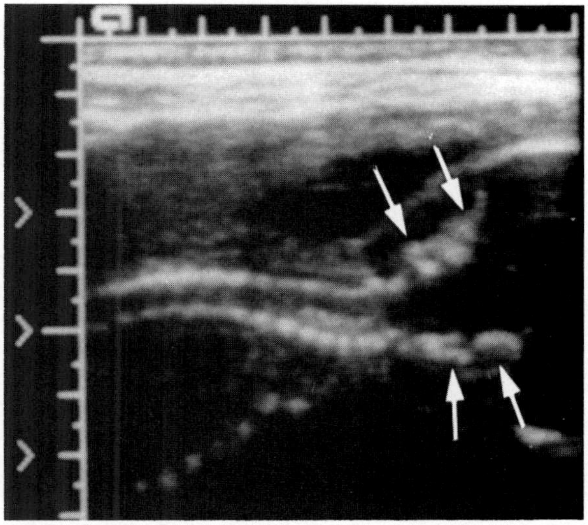

FIGURE 14-25

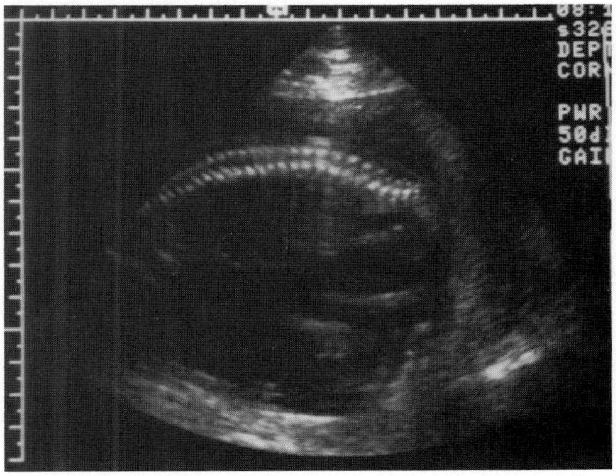

FIGURE 14-26

FIGURE 14-24. Transverse sonogram of thoracic fetal spine at 18 weeks' gestation demonstrates two posterior (P) and one anterior (A) ossification centers. (From Chervenak FA, Isaacson F, Lorber J. Anomalies of the Fetal Head, Neck, and Spine: Ultrasound Diagnosis and Management. Philadelphia: WB Saunders; 1988.)

FIGURE 14-25. Coronal sonogram of fetal spine demonstrates a cervical spine widening (arrows) toward the base of the skull (S).

FIGURE 14-26. Coronal sonogram of fetal spine demonstrates normal tapering of sacral spine.

ters are seen to diverge progressively in the cervical region as one moves closer to the base of the skull (Fig. 14-25). In contrast, the ossification centers converge as one follows them from the lumbar to the sacral regions (Fig. 14-26).

During the third trimester, much more detail may be seen. The vertebral body, pedicles, transverse processes, posterior laminae, and spinous process all may be identified as echogenic structures in transverse scans (Fig. 14-27). In addition, the spinal

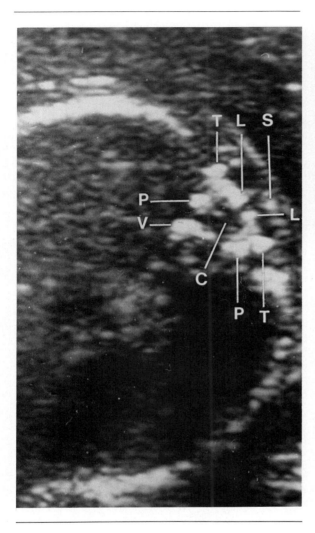

Figure 14-27. Transverse sonogram of mature fetal spine shows vertebral body (V), pedicles (P), transverse processes (T), lamina (L), spinous process (S), and spinal canal (C). (From Chervenak FA, Isaacson F, Lorber J. Anomalies of the Fetal Head, Neck, and Spine: Ultrasound Diagnosis and Management. Philadelphia: WB Saunders; 1988.)

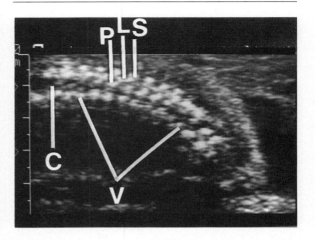

Figure 14-28. Sagittal sonogram of lumbosacral spine shows vertebral bodies (V), spinal cord (C), pedicle (P), lamina (L), and spinous process (S). Note how the spinal canal moves posteriorly in the sacral region. (From Chervenak FA, Isaacson F, Lorber J. Anomalies of the Fetal Head, Neck, and Spine: Ultrasound Diagnosis and Management. Philadelphia: WB Saunders; 1988.)

canal and intervertebral foramina may be seen as anechoic areas. In the sagittal plane, a line of vertebral bodies is still seen, but the posterior echoes are more complex, with spinous processes seen jutting from the line of other posterior elements (Fig. 14-28).

References

1. Benecerraf BR, Barss VA, Laboda LA. A sonographic sign for the detection in the second trimester of the fetus with Down's syndrome. Am J Obstet Gynecol. 1985; 153:49.
2. Birnholz JC. The fetal external ear. Radiology. 1983; 147:819.
3. Birnholz JC. Fetal lumber spine: Measuring axial growth with ultrasound. Radiology. 1986; 158:805.
4. Cardoza JD, Goldstein RB, Filly RA. Exclusion of fetal ventriculomegaly with a single measurement: The width of the lateral ventricular atrium. Radiology. 1988; 169:711–717.
5. Hadlock FP, Deter RL, Harrist RB, et al. Fetal biparietal diameter: Rational choice of plane of section for sonographic measurement. Am J Roentgenol. 1982; 138:871.
6. Isaacson G, Mintz MC. Prenatal sonographic visualization of the inner ear. J Ultrasound Med. 1986; 5:409.
7. Isaacson G, Mintz MC, Crelin ES. Fetal Sectional Anatomy: With Ultrasound and Magnetic Resonance Imaging. New York: Springer-Verlag; 1986.
8. Jeanty P, Chervenak FA, Romero R, et al. The syl-

vian fissure: A commonly mislabeled cranial landmark. J Ultrasound Med. 1984; 3:15.

9. Jeanty P, Dramaix-Wilmet M, Delbeke D, et al. Ultrasonic evaluation of fetal ventricular growth. Neuroradiology. 1981; 21:127.

10. Jeanty P, Dramaix-Wilmet M, Delbeke D, et al. Fetal ocular biometry by ultrasound. Radiology. 1982; 143:513.

11. Jeanty P, Romero R. Obstetrical Ultrasound. New York: McGraw-Hill; 1984; 87–90.

12. Jeanty P, Romero R, Staudach A, et al. Facial anatomy of the fetus. J Ultrasound Med. 1986; 5:607.

13. Johnson ML, Dunne MG, Mack LA, et al. Evaluation of fetal intracranial anatomy by static and real-time ultrasound. J Clin Ultrasound. 1980; 8:311.

14. McGahan JP, Phillips HE, Ellis WG. The fetal hippocampus. Radiology. 1983; 147:201.

15. Mahony BS, Nyberg DA, Hirsch JH, et al. Mild idiopathic lateral cerebral ventricular dilatation in utero: Sonographic evaluation. Radiology. 1988; 169:715–721.

16. Mayden KL, Tortora M, Berkowitz RL, et al. Orbital diameters: A new parameter for prenatal diagnosis and dating. Am J Obstet Gynecol. 1982; 144:289.

17. Pilu G, DePalma L, Romero R, et al. The fetal subarachnoid cisterns: An ultrasound study with report of a case of congenital communicating hydrocephalus. J Ultrasound Med. 1986; 5:365.

18. Pretorius DH, Drose JA, Marco-Johnson ML. Fetal lateral ventricular ratio determination during the second trimester. J Ultrasound Med. 1986; 5:121.

19. Shepard M, Filly RA. A standardized plane for biparietal diameter measurement. J Ultrasound Med. 1982; 1:145.

20. Smith PA, Johansson D, Tzannatos C, et al. Prenatal measurement of the fetal cerebellum and cisterna cerebellomedullaris by ultrasound. Prenat Diag. 1986; 6:133.

CHAPTER 15

Ultrasound of the Normal Fetal Chest, Abdomen, and Pelvis

HARRIS L. COHEN, RAYMOND ATWOOD, MARTHA NEWELT

Ultrasound is the dominant technique for visualizing the fetus in utero. In the early 1970s, the diagnosis of gross abnormality such as hydrocephalus was at the leading edge of sonographic accomplishment. Today, real-time ultrasound examination allows rapid changes in transducer angulation and enhanced imaging of areas of concern. Improved contrast resolution has allowed visualization of small differences in fetal soft tissue structures, and better spatial resolution has allowed definition of smaller fetal structures.[26] The identification of fetal abnormalities allows critical decisions to be made with regard to the continuation of a pregnancy or the preparation by parents and the perinatal team for a difficult delivery or during neonatal life.

Knowledge of the normal allows for recognition of variations in normal as well as diagnosis of the abnormal. In this chapter we concentrate on the normal fetal chest, abdomen, and pelvis.

Scanning Technique and Principles

Principles for the sonographic evaluation of the fetus are to a large extent similar to those used in evaluating newborn infants. Transverse (transaxial), sagittal (longitudinal), and coronal views enhance the three-dimensional image that can be envisioned (Table 15-1).

There are difficulties that are peculiar to imaging a fetus:

Amniotic Fluid Levels. An adequate amount of surrounding amniotic fluid must separate the fetus from the adjacent uterine wall, especially in the evaluation of the anterior and posterior skin surfaces of the thorax and abdomen. The fluid acts as a window for ultrasonic evaluation of internal fetal anatomy.

Fetal Motion. Fetal position varies from moment to moment due to movement of the fetus. The fetus is flexed within a compartment (the uterus) that is smaller than its length.

Fetal Lie. The examiner must be aware of the fetus' orientation with respect to the uterus. Various organs present different screen images depending on the fetal position and presentation.[51]

Shadowing deep to bony elements makes the evaluation of some structures such as the spine easier in one position (e.g., spine up, or prone) than another (e.g., spine down, or supine). Structures deep to the transducer's focal point are seen less well than structures that fall within it.

Technique must be rigorous; the operator must maintain a constant vigil on fetal position and transducer position. Special techniques may be necessary to adequately visualize the fetus. These range from subtle corrections of transducer angulation to broad shifting of transducer position, shifting the mother's position on the table, having the mother walk about the department, or, in un-

Table 15-1. Areas to be imaged in routine obstetric sonographic examinations

Head and Neck
   Transverse view at level of frontal horns for BPD, thalami, calvarium
   Transverse view at level of atrium of lateral ventricles for ventricular size
   Transverse view at level of cerebellar hemispheres for cerebellar shape and cisterna magna identification
   Transverse view of orbits for OOD, orbital size
   Face in coronal, transverse or profile
   Transverse neck for posterior masses, completeness of posterior elements and skin

Thorax
   Four-chamber view of heart (transverse oblique view)
   Transverse and longitudinal view of thoracic spine
   Coronal or longitudinal view for diaphragm
   Transverse high thorax for clavicles
   Transverse at IV septum level for thoracic circumference, evaluation of lungs and heart for anatomy and rhythm,
      to rule out pleural and pericardial effusion

Abdomen
   Transverse and sagittal abdomen to rule out anterior wall defect, note umbilical vessel entry
   Transverse upper abdomen for AC determination (biometry) and stomach, intrahepatic portion of umbilical vein
      and spine and sometimes gallbladder, spleen evaluation
   Longitudinal and transverse spine views
   Transverse and longitudinal views through kidneys to rule out obstruction, evaluate size, rule out cystic disease

Pelvis
   Transverse or coronal views to visualize urinary bladder
   Sacral spine transverse and longitudinal
   Genitalia
   Femur

---

usual circumstances, postponing evaluation to another day.

The Thorax

The routine examination includes the thorax and its contents from the thoracic inlet at the base of the neck (the level of the clavicles) to the diaphragms separating the lung base from the abdominal contents. Transverse and longitudinal views are taken through the thorax. Points to be noted are the symmetry of the bony elements of the thorax; chest size in relationship to the fetus, the fetal abdomen, and the heart; pulmonary echo texture and symmetry and presence of the diaphragms.[19] With varying degrees of effort, smaller structures such as the fetal trachea, thyroid, and esophagus have been noted.

Bony Elements of the Thorax

The bony thorax consists of the clavicles, ribs, scapulae, vertebral bodies, and sternum that surround the lungs, heart, and mediastinum. In the early stages of pregnancy, only ossified portions of the fetal skeleton are imaged directly as areas of increased echogenicity. With time, more echopenic, purely cartilaginous structures are also visualized. Knowledge of the timing of ossification center development may help in determining gestational age. Clavicular ossification is noted as early as 8 to 9 weeks, the ribs and scapulae at 10 to 11 weeks, and the sternum between 21 and 27 weeks.[50]

The clavicles are seen as bright echoes at the junction of the fetal neck and thorax. Their absence may be noted as part of several clinical syndromes (e.g., cleidocranial dysostosis).[53] In a true transverse section they should be symmetric. Owing to their natural curvature it is difficult to image them in their entirety,[3] especially in older fetuses. Clavicular growth is directly related to gestational age.[58]

Ribs appear as echogenic bands projecting in a fanlike pattern from the spine.[50] Their curvilinear shape makes it difficult to image large portions of several adjacent ribs (Fig. 15-1).[3] Ribs may be assessed for symmetry, and their symmetry may be

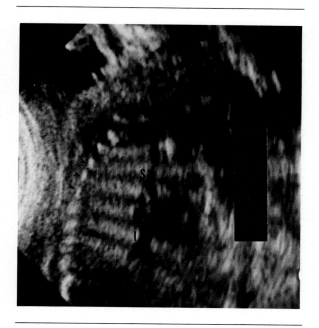

FIGURE 15-1. Oblique right parasagittal plane shows portions of the posterior right ribs (*arrowheads*) as echogenic densities between the heart and the thoracic periphery. Incidentally noted are the superior (S) and inferior (I) venae cavae.

used as an indication that the plane of the scan is suitable for biometric measurement. Particularly thick or thin ribs suggest an abnormality.

The scapula is seen external to the ribs and surrounded by hypoechoic muscles.[3] The scapular echo, which like that of other bones, does not correspond to the true size of the bone, is typically **Y**- or **V**-shaped, depending on the angle of insonation.[3,50]

The typical single anterior and paired posterior echoes of the ossification centers of the developing vertebral body are assessed for convergence of the posterior elements toward the nonossified spinous process. The posterior skin surface is evaluated to rule out a skin break associated with myelomeningocele.

The sternum is highly variable with respect to the development of its ossification centers. It is unusual to note the typical radiographic "string of beads" appearance of the normal sternal ossification centers, since this requires a coronal or coro-

nal oblique view of the most anterior portion of the thoracic wall. Transverse sections show single anterior circular echoes.[50]

SOFT TISSUE STRUCTURES OF THE CHEST

The muscles of the chest wall are hypoechoic and thin. They become somewhat more evident as the pregnancy progresses through the third trimester. The soft tissues may appear thick in general anasarca of the fetus or because of subcutaneous fat deposits in infants of diabetic mothers. Anterior chest wall masses consistent with fetal breasts under the influence of maternal hormone stimulation may be seen in fetuses of either sex.[16,20]

CHEST BIOMETRY

Various investigators have taken different thoracic measurements in attempts to see whether such information can be used to assess gestational age or to rule out pulmonary hypoplasia. Thoracic diameter measurements are obtained from outer edge to outer edge on a true transverse view at the level of cardiac motion or just above the diaphragm.[31,42] Thoracic circumference measurements are taken along the outer limits of the thoracic cage at the level of the atrioventricular valve during fetal diastole. Both measurements increase with progression of the pregnancy. Kurtz believes the usefulness of thoracic diameter measurements is limited because of the great standard deviations in the accumulated studies.[29] Nimrod and colleagues found a 0.87 correlation of thoracic circumference measurements with gestational age. Although this correlation is not as high as the 0.93, 0.92, and 0.95 correlations obtained with biparietal diameter, abdominal circumference, and femur length, respectively, the necessity for a useful measurement to avoid missing pulmonary hypoplasia makes this data essential.[39]

Since the major components of the thorax are the heart and lungs, a significant decrease in lung volume, as would be found with pulmonary hypoplasia, should be reflected by a small-for-gestational-age thoracic circumference and a smaller ratio of thoracic circumference to abdominal circumference.[39] Chitkara noted little change throughout pregnancy in the 0.89 ratio of thoracic to abdominal circumference. Decreasing ratios are suspicious for a small thorax and possible pulmo-

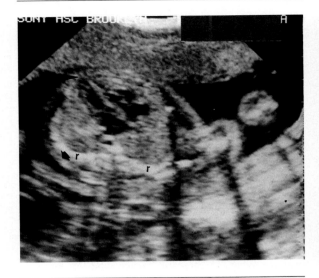

FIGURE 15-2. Transverse plane of normal chest. Symmetric homogeneous echogenicity of the lungs surrounds the echo-free cardiac chambers. The cardiac apex (*arrowhead*) points to the left side of this fetus in vertex presentation. Note the relatively symmetric posterior ribs (r) and the hypoechoic thoracic muscles (*arrows*).

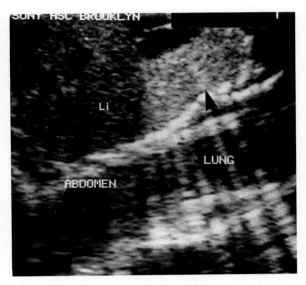

FIGURE 15-3. Coronal plane, right-side view of the normal chest and abdomen. The right lung is highly echogenic (*arrowhead*) compared to the subdiaphragmatic liver (Li).

nary hypoplasia. The heart occupies about one-third of the cross-sectional area of the thorax.[3] In the transverse view, if the heart appears too large pulmonary hypoplasia must be considered as well as the more obvious possibility, cardiomegaly.

LUNG

During fetal life, the deflated lungs appear as solid, space-occupying masses between the heart and ribs.[43] On a transverse view of the thorax the lungs typically are granular, with few breaks in the homogeneity of this pattern (Fig. 15-2). Each lung may be compared to its counterpart. Longitudinal or coronal views allow the echogenicity of the lungs to be compared with that of the liver or spleen. The lungs are separated from these abdominal organs by the smooth, hypoechoic diaphragm.[3,19] Early in gestation lung echogenicity is equal to or slightly less than that of the liver. As the gestation progresses, lung echogenicity increases until it is greater than that of the liver (Fig.

15-3).[19] Some investigators claim that the lungs are always more echogenic than the liver.[51] Several authors have debated the use of fetal lung echogenicity patterns and the lungs' acoustic transmission and compressibility to assess lung maturity and thereby avoid amniocentesis for biochemical analysis of fetal lung maturity. Theoretically, enhanced acoustic transmission and increased echogenicity may be based on the known increase in lung fluid and the significant increase in the number of alveolar and terminal lung units as well as the transformation of the alveolar cell lining from columnar to cuboidal as the pregnancy progresses, most particularly between weeks 32 and 40.[7] The determination of fetal lung maturity is a crucial consideration in managing certain difficult pregnancies.[17] With currently available diagnostic sonography units, biochemical measurements of the lecithin-sphingomyelin ratio (ratios of 2.0 or greater are considered indicative of pulmonary maturity) and the presence of phosphatidyl glycerol remain the gold standard for evaluation of fetal lung matu-

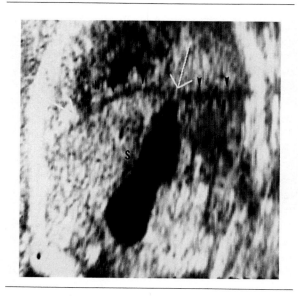

FIGURE 15-4. Left parasagittal view of chest, abdomen, and diaphragm. Arrowheads point to the hypoechoic band separating the thorax from the abdomen. Anteriorly is the heart (H) and posteriorly, the echo-free fluid-filled stomach (S).

rity.[6,7,17] Biparietal diameter (BPD) measurements and placental grading have proven unreliable for determining fetal lung maturity.[24]

DIAPHRAGM

The diaphragm (Fig. 15-4), noted as a hypoechoic band, was seen in only 3% of a group of normal 14-week fetuses evaluated in a study by Zador and colleagues. This increased to 43% at 20 weeks, with a high of 81% at 35 weeks.[59] Its presence can help differentiate cystic intrathoracic masses of pulmonary origin from those that are intraabdominal in origin. However, as with all curved structures, even when the fetus is positioned optimally the entire structure may not be visualized and small defects may be imagined or missed.

The Abdomen

By the beginning of the second trimester, the abdominal organs have attained their normal adult position and structure.[19] The liver, kidneys, and adrenal glands are readily identifiable. The echo-

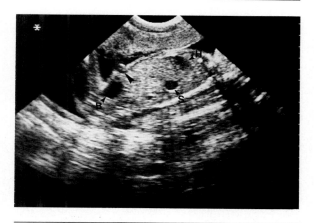

FIGURE 15-5. Left parasagittal plane view of normal anterior abdominal wall. The fetus is facing toward the left of the page. Evident are the echo-free heart (H), stomach (S), and bladder (B). Umbilical vessel entry is noted in the lower anterior abdominal wall (*large arrowhead*).

free fluid filling the gallbladder and stomach and the echo-free blood filling large vessels make them readily distinguishable. Visualization of the spleen is more variable, and the pancreas is seen far less often. Collapsed small bowel—and in the third trimester fluid-filled colon—are often seen.

Examination of the abdomen is performed by transverse, coronal, and sagittal imaging of the fetus as a unit and, with proper angulation, its individual organs. Transverse views throughout the spine are evaluated for posterior elements that are parallel to each other or that meet centrally instead of diverging. The presence of an intact skin surface overlying the individual vertebral bodies is a helpful secondary sign to rule out myelomeningocele. Images are recorded of a transverse view of the upper abdomen for abdominal circumference measurements and visualization of the stomach and liver. A lower transverse view is obtained to confirm the presence of two kidneys and to evaluate their anatomy. A sagittal view of thorax, abdomen, and (usually) pelvis allows evaluation of the relative size of thorax and abdomen as well as the relationship of umbilical vessel entry to the anterior abdominal wall (Fig. 15-5). Umbilical vessel entry can also be readily noted on a transverse section of

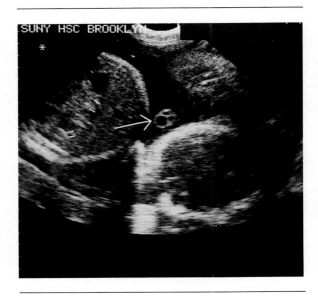

FIGURE 15-6. On transverse section, an arrow points to a normal umbilical cord. The two smaller umbilical arteries and the larger umbilical vein assume a masklike or "Mr. Bill" configuration.

the abdomen taken at the level of the umbilicus. On both transverse and longitudinal-coronal views the abdomen is checked for defects.

An optimal study should include three sagittal planes for evaluating fetal body surface and for general orientation: right paramedian through thorax and trunk to evaluate lung and liver, left parasagittal to include the stomach, and midsagittal for evaluation of umbilical vein through its course to the ductus venosus.[49] Adequate fluid must surround the skin surface of concern. General views allow the operator to determine abdominal situs and to readily rule out the clinically significant possibility of cardiac apex and stomach being on opposite sides of the body.

As with the thorax, anatomic evaluation of the abdomen depends on fetal position, fetal flexion, and an adequate amount of surrounding amniotic fluid.[26] Significant maternal body fat limits evaluation.

Soft Tissues

Abdominal wall muscles are hypoechoic. Occasionally thin echogenic lines may be seen that represent fascial planes between the three main muscle groups, the internal oblique, transverse abdominal, and external oblique.[3] The echogenic skin line, highlighted by good sound transmission through surrounding amniotic fluid and the deeper hypoechoic muscle, may result in what Rosenthal and colleagues have described as the "pseudoascites sign."[45]

Umbilical Cord and Abdominal Vasculature

A major difference between fetal and adult abdominal anatomy is the presence of patent umbilical vessels and ductus venosus acting as a conduit between the portal and systemic veins.[19]

The allantois, a caudal outpouching of the yolk sac that is not visible sonographically, is involved in early blood production. Its blood vessels become the umbilical artery and veins.[19,37] The umbilical cord (Fig. 15-6) consists of two umbilical arteries with a mean width of 2.4 mm and one umbilical vein with a mean width of 8 mm. In 1% of pregnancies, the right umbilical artery regresses or does not form and there is a single umbilical artery. Usually this is not significant, but it has been associated by various authors with an increased incidence of trisomy, low birth weight, twins, offspring of diabetic mothers, and stillborns.[27,38]

The thin-walled single umbilical vein enters the anterior abdomen, taking a cephalad oblique course, without branching, and enters the left portal vein (LPV) (Fig. 15-7). Blood flows from the LPV either into the narrow channel of the ductus venosus, bypassing the liver and entering the systemic venous system via the left hepatic vein or inferior vena cava, or medially into the right portal vein, perfusing the liver. Within 2 weeks before birth, the ductus venosus closes and is seen as an echogenic line in the fissure of the ligamentum venosum between the left and the caudate lobes.[8,19]

The two umbilical arteries, which carry most of the fetal aortic blood to the placenta, can be followed caudad from the anterior abdominal wall cord insertion site to the internal iliac arteries, which are just lateral to the bladder. The vessels can be followed to their origin at the iliac artery bifurcation. The abdominal aorta can often be seen throughout its course and is often an aid in noting the expected position of the kidneys on coronal views.[8,19,46,49]

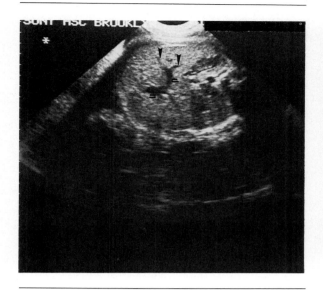

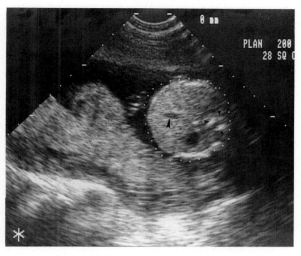

FIGURE 15-7. Transverse oblique plane view of umbilical vein entry into left portal vein. The intrahepatic portion of the umbilical vein (U) is seen in its antero-posterior course to the portal venous system (P), running in a medial-lateral direction. The right portal vein bifurcation is marked by arrowheads.

FIGURE 15-8. Abdominal circumference is imaged in the transverse plane. A short segment of the intrahepatic portion of the umbilical vein (*large arrowhead*), the echo-free stomach, and the vertebral body ossification centers (*small arrowheads*) are seen. The ribs are equidistant.

Biometry

The abdominal circumference (AC) has proved to be a key and accurate measurement in the evaluation of gestational age and fetal weight and in ruling out asymmetric growth retardation with its associated liver glycogen depletion and decreased liver size.[13,23,29] Its importance requires correct measurement. A true axial view of the abdomen is obtained at the level of umbilical cord entry into the LPV. Measurements are made along the outer perimeter of the abdomen. Indications of proper positioning include a circular abdominal outline, equidistant left and right side rib echoes, and visualization of the three ossification centers of the vertebral body (Fig. 15-8). A long segment of the intrahepatic portion of the umbilical vein, especially if it extends anteriorly, suggests an oblique rather than a true axial view. Angulated views that include lung are not acceptable. Shadowing from long bones, elliptical outlines due to myometrial contraction, and decreased amniotic fluid levels limit measurement.[3,29,49] Abdominal circumference

measurements are known to vary according to gender (males larger than females) and racial group (Europeans 30% larger than Asian Indians) and among offspring of diabetics, who have greater amounts of abdominal wall soft tissue.[36,41] To properly assess AC measurements, therefore, the clinician must know his or her own clinical population.

Liver, Gallbladder, Pancreas, and Spleen

The fetal liver is a large homogenously echogenic organ occupying the right upper quadrant and crossing midline to the left. It represents 10% of a fetus' weight at 11 weeks' gestation and represents 5% of the weight of the fetus at term.[19] Whereas in an adult the right lobe is much larger than the left lobe (ratio 6:1), in the fetus the left lobe is as large as—and in fact slightly larger than—the right, possibly because it receives a greater percentage of oxygenated blood.[27] This may make it difficult to determine which side of the body is being imaged unless the fluid-filled left-sided stomach is visible. The liver grows throughout pregnancy. Gross and coworkers describe a transverse ratio of the portion

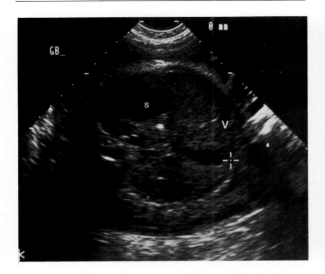

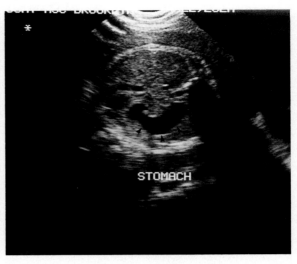

Figure 15-9. Transverse oblique plane shows the teardrop-shaped gallbladder to the right of the midline intrahepatic umbilical vein (V), stomach (S).

Figure 15-10. A more longitudinal view of the fluid-filled stomach is seen in this transverse plane of a normal fetus (*arrowheads*).

of the fetal liver that lies to the left of the umbilical part of the LPV to the portion that lies to the right as 1.04 (range 0.78 to 1.3). This ratio remains unchanged throughout gestation, even in the presence of intrauterine growth retardation.[22,29,55]

The gallbladder (Fig. 15-9), in its position to the right of midline, separates the right lobe from the medial left lobe, as does the middle hepatic vein. The fluid-filled gallbladder may appear similar to the tubular intrahepatic portion of the umbilical vein. Key differentiating points are the gallbladder's teardrop shape, its extrahepatic location (posteroinferior to the liver), and the lack of communication between the gallbladder and vessels of the umbilical cord. Unlike the umbilical vein, the gallbladder does not reach the anterior abdominal wall.[3] The gallbladder is passive in fetal life and does not respond to fat ingested by the mother.[19]

The pancreas is rarely visualized. Occasionally the fluid-filled stomach and its location anterior to the splenic vein may aid in identifying it. Its echogenicity is slightly greater than that of the liver.[27]

The spleen is a well-circumscribed homogeneous mass in the left upper abdomen. It can be seen at 18 weeks' gestation and thereafter.[19] We agree with

Kurtz that it may be difficult to delineate in the absence of ascites. Landmarks used to identify it are the left hemidiaphragm and spine; the fluid-filled, usually anterior, stomach is the most consistent.[29] Best seen on transverse scans, the spleen is similar in echogenicity to the kidney and slightly less echogenic than the liver. Its size increases during gestation: Mean length at 20 weeks is 1.8 cm; at 30 weeks, 3.4 cm; and at 40 weeks, 6.2 cm. During this time spleen volume increases approximately 18-fold.[47]

Stomach and Bowel

The stomach (Fig. 15-10) should be seen in the second trimester. Occasionally, it is not visualized in normal fetuses in the early weeks of the trimester. Typically, the stomach is filled with variable amounts of echo-free fluid.[3] Wladimiroff and colleagues have reported filling times of up to 45 minutes and emptying times that vary from a few minutes to (rarely) 30 minutes.[57] The stomach, if present, should therefore be seen at some point during a 60-minute examination. Filling volumes increase during the pregnancy: 1 ml is the mean at 20 weeks, 5 ml at 30 weeks, and 8 ml at 35 weeks.

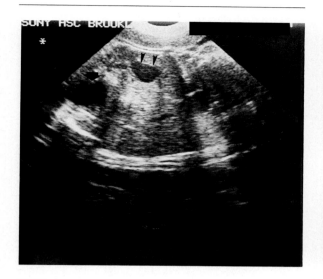

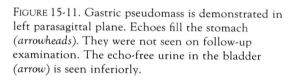

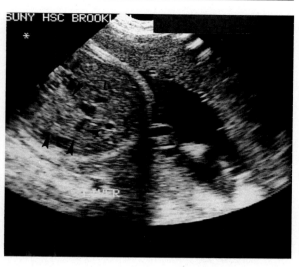

FIGURE 15-11. Gastric pseudomass is demonstrated in left parasagittal plane. Echoes fill the stomach (*arrowheads*). They were not seen on follow-up examination. The echo-free urine in the bladder (*arrow*) is seen inferiorly.

FIGURE 15-12. Transverse oblique plane view shows an echogenic pseudomass of collapsed small bowel (*arrowheads*) posterior and inferior to the liver (L).

Volumes as great as 22 ml have been noted in a normal nonobstructed stomach of a 35-week fetus.[54]

Echogenicity within the stomach fluid has been seen in cases of third-trimester placental abruption; this represents swallowed blood.[56] We have often seen what Fakhry and coworkers have labeled a fetal gastric pseudomass (Fig. 15-11). Seen in 1% of a series of their cases, this idiopathic echogenicity within the stomach fluid, which is commonly seen in the second trimester and disappears on follow-up examination, may be due to aggregates of swallowed cells and cell fragments. This seems logical, in that particles can be seen in normal amniotic fluid as early as week 16.[15] The stomach grows linearly during gestation in transverse, longitudinal, and anteroposterior planes.[18]

Early in gestation, small bowel normally herniates into the base of the umbilical cord as the bowel grows beyond abdominal capacity and undergoes part of its normal rotation about the superior mesenteric artery. By week 14, this normal herniation has been reduced, and it is from 14 weeks on that

abdominal wall defects may be diagnosed.[12] Before significant amounts of fluid enter the small bowel it appears as an echogenic pseudomass (Fig. 15-12), without shadowing, occupying a substantial portion of the abdomen. By 26 weeks this mass becomes less echogenic and sharply defined. By 29 to 30 weeks, the rate of fetal swallowing has overcome the resorptive capacity of stomach and proximal duodenum, allowing filling of distal small bowel and disappearance of the pseudomass.[35] Peristalsis may be seen in the small bowel that occupies the central abdomen. Nyberg reports that no normal segment should be noted that is greater than 7 mm in diameter or 15 mm long.[40]

The colon is a long continuous tubular structure at the abdominal periphery (Fig. 15-13). Although it may be seen as early as 22 weeks, it is typically seen at 28 weeks and later. Nyberg and coworkers examined the colons of 130 fetuses and found linear increases in diameter throughout the third trimester. There is a maximal diameter of 18 mm at term for normal colon. No peristalsis is seen. Meconium, which is less echogenic than bowel wall, may be routinely noted in discrete portions of colon. Transverse colon (Fig. 15-14) is seen most

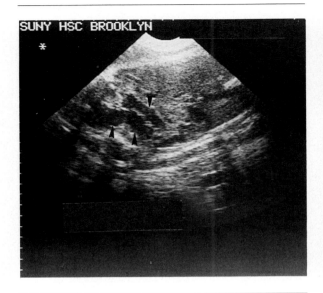

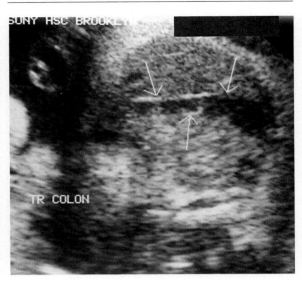

FIGURE 15-13. Coronal oblique plane shows fluid-filled normal colon (*arrowheads*), representing descending colon and sigmoid, at the abdominal periphery.

FIGURE 15-14. On this transverse oblique plane arrows point to the fluid-filled transverse colon inferior to the liver.

easily just caudad to the liver.[40] By the third trimester, normal bowel was seen in at least 80% of Zador and colleagues' 2389 examinations.[59]

KIDNEYS AND ADRENALS

The fetal kidneys can be seen as early as the 15th week after LMP. The vast majority may be routinely imaged between weeks 17 and 22. Identification of the kidneys early in gestation is limited by the lack of significant contrast between the kidneys and the nearby soft tissues. This situation improves with the deposition of echogenic perirenal fat by the third trimester.[11,44]

On transverse images (Fig. 15-15) the kidneys are hypoechoic ovoid masses on either side of the spine. The echogenic center of renal sinus fat is noted more consistently later in pregnancy. Grannum has noted that the ratio of kidney circumference to abdominal circumference remains approximately 0.3 throughout pregnancy.[21,30]

Parasagittal views of each kidney show them to be paraspinous and bean-shaped. As in neonates, the normal hypoechoic renal pyramids (Fig. 15-16) may be seen arranged in anterior and posterior

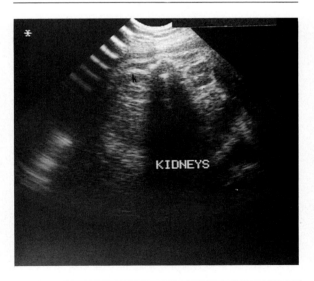

FIGURE 15-15. Echopenic normal kidneys (k, right kidney) flank the spine of this prone fetus (transverse plane view). Echogenicity at the center of the kidney is consistent with renal sinus fat. The echogenicity at the kidney periphery is consistent with perirenal fat.

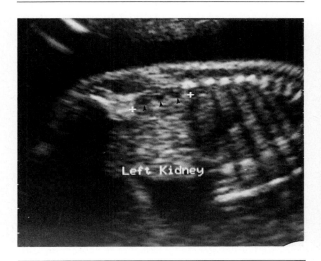

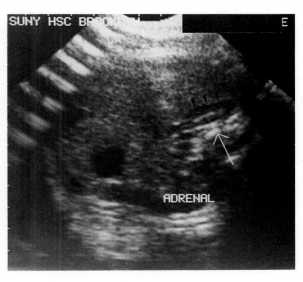

Figure 15-16. Crosses mark the superior and inferior extent of the kidney viewed in the left parasagittal plane. Echopenic pyramids (*arrowheads*) are noted along the posterior aspect of the kidney, the side closest to the transducer. In many cases, both the anterior and posterior row of pyramids can be visualized.

Figure 15-17. A normal right adrenal (*arrowheads*) is seen to the side of the spine in a transverse oblique plane view. Note the echogenic central medulla and the hypoechoic periphery. (White arrow points to area of adrenal.)

rows around the renal pelvis. They should not be mistaken for renal cysts. Bertagnoli and colleagues have noted average renal lengths of 3.0 cm at 32 weeks and 3.8 cm at 40 weeks. Our own measurements are somewhat greater.[1,33] The renal pelvis is typically collapsed (i.e., not urine-filled) and therefore is not imaged. If filled with urine, an echo-free renal pelvis, less than 1 cm (and certainly less than 8 mm) in anteroposterior diameter, is considered normal and the dilatation physiologic. This may be related to transient fetal urinary reflux or obstruction of pelvic urine outflow due to a filled fetal bladder. This slight pelvic dilatation seen in fetal life is rarely noted as significant dilatation in the kidneys of these infants after birth.[11]

Ureters normally are not visualized unless there is significant genitourinary system reflux or obstruction.[11]

The adrenals are ovoid, triangular, or heart-shaped masses that are often imaged in the suprarenal area in fetuses that are 30 weeks or older. Lewis and colleagues claim ready visual separation from adjacent renal parenchyma, although if the fetus is positioned side up, evaluation of the side that is more distant from the transducer is more difficult.[32]

On transverse view the adrenals may appear reniform. This is particularly true in association with ipsilateral renal agenesis. There is an echogenic central medulla and a hypoechoic thick outer cortex. Histopathologically the cortex is composed of a thick inner "fetal zone" and a thin outer permanent cortex (Fig. 15-17). The "fetal" portion of the adrenal is the portion that may be involved in adrenal hemorrhage. The fetal zone contributes to the adrenal gland being proportionately 20 times the size of the adult adrenal. This fetal zone atrophies within the first 3 to 12 months of life.[44]

While typically suprarenal in fetal life, by childhood the adrenal attains its more anterior and medial position in relation to the kidney.[10] The high retroperitoneal position of the adrenals can limit their imaging, owing to obscuration from rib shadowing. Ratios of adrenal length to renal length are between 0.48 and 0.66.[29] The adrenals increase in

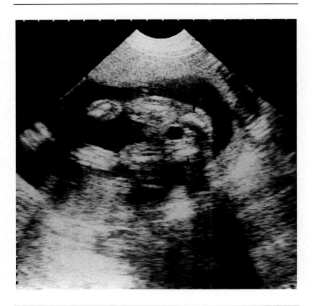

Figure 15-18. A circular bladder is seen medial to the echogenic iliac bones (*arrowheads*) of the pelvis in this coronal view.

size during pregnancy.[25,32] Human chorionic gonadotropin contributes to adrenal growth in the first half of pregnancy; thereafter adrenocorticotropic hormone controls its growth.[33]

The Pelvis

The pelvis is a small structure in the fetus. Its sonographic image is made up predominantly of the bones of the pelvis, the pelvic muscles, and the bladder.

The bony pelvis consists of echogenic iliac crests separated from the echogenic sacrum by the echopenic sacroiliac joint. Three ossification centers are noted along the sacrum. Although, as in the craniocervical region, there is some soft tissue prominence noted as hypoechoic density between skin and spine in the lumbosacral region, masses should not be seen. The hypoechoic gluteal muscles may be separated by thin fascial lines. The ischium and pubis are noted as echogenic anterior densities, and often the echogenic nonossified femoral head can be seen at the acetabular area.[3]

The bladder (Fig. 15-18) is seen as an echo-free intrapelvic mass by 15 weeks' gestational age. It is circular to oblong in shape. Wall thickness cannot be appreciated in the normal bladder without the presence of ascites. It is a dynamic structure whose size varies with the degree of filling. At 32 weeks the bladder's capacity is 10 ml, filling at the rate of 10 to 12 ml per hour. By week 40, capacity increases to 40 ml, filling at 27 ml per hour. The fetus voids about once per hour.[5] If the bladder fills at least one functioning kidney is present. If no bladder is seen on examination, a repeat examination is performed. If necessary, the fetus may be challenged by injecting the mother intravenously with furosemide, which should induce diuresis within 15 to 45 minutes.[34] Occasionally the bladder may appear distended when there is no pathology. Waiting will allow one to prove when the bladder empties. When distended, normally or pathologically, the bladder rises out of the narrow pelvis and into the upper abdomen.[11]

Genitals

The identification of fetal genitalia requires adequate visualization of the perineum. A crossed thigh can readily hide a scrotum. Differences in genitalia are not very prominent before week 16.[11] In Elejalde and colleagues' work and literature review, the reported 3% error rate in gender identification occurred when gender assignment was made before the 24th week. His group identified the genitalia in 100% of cases after 20 weeks. This is not the universal experience. Of 3891 examinations reported in the literature, genitalia could not be visualized in 30%.[14] Birnholz reported a 3.3% error rate in gender assignment in fetuses before 24 weeks and an overall error rate of 1.7%.[2]

Gender identification is of key clinical interest in diagnosing males affected by severe X-linked inherited disorders such as hemophilia or Duchenne's muscular dystrophy. Proof of different genitalia in twins can help prove dizygosity and rule out twin-to-twin transfusion syndrome and other problems associated with monozygotic twins. Rare intersex problems may be diagnosed if there is a discrepancy in karyotype gender from visualized genitals (e.g., testicular feminization syndrome, in which a fetus has a male karyotype and female genitalia).[11,33,52]

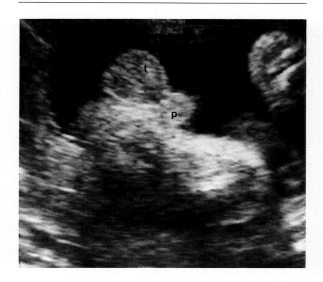

FIGURE 15-19. Coronal view of male genitalia. The penis (p) is seen in cross section. Echogenicity within the scrotum represents testes (t).

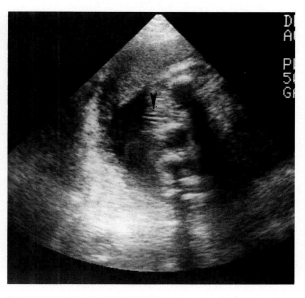

FIGURE 15-20. Coronal view of female genitalia. A central echogenic line represents the labia minora. To their side are the labia majora (*arrowhead*, right labia majora). The thighs are seen to a small extent, laterally.

In the male, the penis and scrotum (Fig. 15-19) are readily visualized between the thighs. Often noted on coronal or transverse views of the pelvis, one must be aware of the possibility of a nearby umbilical cord simulating a penis. One may see voiding into the amniotic fluid. Erections are not unusual. After 32 weeks, 93% of testicles have descended into the scrotum and are noted as echogenic masses.[2,11,48]

In females (Fig. 15-20) the labia majora are noted as masses of moderate echogenicity off the perineum. A central linear echogenicity between them represents the labia minora. The normal ovaries, uterus, and vagina typically are not visualized in a normal fetus.[11,14]

References

1. Bertagnoli L, Lalatta F, Gallicchio R, et al. Quantitative characterization of the growth of the fetal kidney. J Clin Ultrasound. 1983; 11:349–356.
2. Birnholz J. Determination of fetal sex. N Engl J Med. 1983; 309:942–944.
3. Bowerman R. Thorax. In: Bowerman R. Atlas of Normal Fetal Ultrasonographic Anatomy. Chicago: Year Book Medical Publishers; 1986.
4. Bowie J, Rosenberg E, Andreotti R, et al. The changing sonographic appearance of fetal kidneys during pregnancy. J Ultrasound Med 1983; 2:505–507.
5. Campbell S, Wladimoroff J, Dewhurst C. The antenatal measurement of urine production. J Obstet Gynaecol Br Commonw. 1973; 80:680–686.
6. Carson P, Meyer C, Bowerman R. Prediction of fetal lung maturity with ultrasound. Radiology. 1985; 155:533.
7. Cayea P, Grant D, Doubilet P, et al. Prediction of fetal lung maturity: Inaccuracies of study using conventional ultrasound instruments. Radiology. 1985; 155:473–475.
8. Chinn D, Filly R, Callen P. Ultrasonic evaluation of fetal umbilical and hepatic vascular anatomy. Radiology. 1982; 44:153–157.
9. Chitkara U, Rosenberg J, Chervenak F, et al. Prenatal sonographic assessment of the fetal thorax: Normal values. Am J Obstet Gynecol. 1987; 156:1069–1074.
10. Co C, Filly R. Normal fetal adrenal gland location (letter to the editor). J. Ultrasound Med. 1986; 5:117.

11. Cohen H, Haller J. Diagnostic sonography of the fetal genitourinary tract. Urol Radiol. 1987; 9:88–98.

12. Cyr D, Mack L, Schoenecker SA, et al. Bowel migration in the normal fetus: US detection. Radiology. 1986; 161:119–121.

13. Deter R, Harrist R, Hadlock F, et al. Fetal head and abdominal circumferences. I. Evaluation of measurement errors. J. Clin Ultrasound. 1982; 10:357–363.

14. Elejalde, B, de Elejalde M, Heitman T. Visualization of the fetal genitalia by ultrasonography: A review of the literature and analysis of its accuracy and ethical implications. J Ultrasound Med. 1985; 4:633–639.

15. Fakhry J, Shapiro L, Schechter A. Fetal gastric pseudomass. J Ultrasound Med. 1987; 6:177–180.

16. Fleischer A, Killam A, Boehm F, et al. Hydrops fetalis: Sonographic evaluations and clinical implications. Radiology. 1981; 141:163–168.

17. Fried, A, Loh F, Umer M, et al. Echogenicity of fetal lung: Relation to fetal age and maturity. AJR. 1985; 145:591–594.

18. Goldstein I, Reece E, Yarkoni S, et al. Growth of the fetal stomach in normal pregnancies. Obstet Gynecol. 1987; 70:641–644.

19. Goldstein R, Callen P. Ultrasound evaluation of the fetal thorax and abdomen. In: Callen P. Ultrasonography in Obstetrics and Gynecology. 2nd ed. Philadelphia: W B Saunders; 1988.

20. Graham D, Sanders R. Sonographic evaluation of the fetal chest. In: Sanders R, James A Jr, eds. The Principles and Practice of Ultrasonography in Obstetrics and Gynecology. 3rd ed. East Norwalk, CT: Appleton-Century-Crofts; 1985.

21. Grannum P, Bracken M, Silverman R, et al. Assessment of fetal kidney size in normal gestation by comparison of ratio of kidney circumference to abdominal circumference. Am J Obstet Gynecol. 1980; 136:249–254.

22. Gross B, Harter L, Filly R. Disproportionate left hepatic lobe size in the fetus. J Ultrasound Med. 1982; 1:79–81.

23. Hadlock F, Deter R, Harrist R, et al. Fetal abdominal circumference as a predictor of menstrual age. AJR. 1982; 1339:367–370.

24. Hadlock F, Irwin J, Roecker E. Ultrasound prediction of fetal lung maturity. Radiology. 1985; 155:469–472.

25. Hata K, Hata T, Kitao M. Ultrasonographic identification and measurement of the human fetal adrenal gland in utero. Int J Gynaecol Obstet. 1985; 23:355–359.

26. Hatta R, Rees G, Johnson M. Normal fetal anatomy. Rad Clin North Am. 1982; 20:271–284.

27. Hill L. Sonographic detection of fetal gastrointestinal anomalies. Ultrasound Quart. 1988; 6:35–67.

28. Hill L, Kislak S, Runco C. An ultrasonic view of the umbilical cord. Obstet Gynecol Surv. 1987; 42:82–88.

29. Kurtz A, Goldberg B. Fetal body measurements. In: Kurtz A, Goldberg B. Obstetrical Measurements in Ultrasound. A Reference Manual. Chicago: Year Book Medical Publishers; 1988.

30. Lawson T, Foley W, Berland L, et al. Ultrasonic evaluation of fetal kidneys: Analysis of normal size and frequency of visualization as related to stage of pregnancy. Radiology 1981; 138:153–156.

31. Levi S, Erbsman F. Antenatal fetal growth from the nineteenth week: Ultrasonic study of 12 head and chest dimensions. Am J Obstet Gynecol. 1975; 121:262–268.

32. Lewis E, Kurtz A, Dubbins P, et al. Real-time ultrasonographic evaluation of normal fetal adrenal gland. J Ultrasound Med. 1982; 1:205–207.

33. Mahony B. The genitourinary system. In: Callen P, ed. Ultrasonography in Obstetrics and Gynecology. 2nd ed. Philadelphia: WB Saunders; 1988.

34. Mahony B, Filly R. The genitourinary system in utero. In: Hricak H, ed. Genitourinary Ultrasound. New York: Churchill Livingstone; 1986.

35. Manco L, Nunan F, Sohnen H, et al. Fetal small bowel simulating abdominal mass at sonography. J Clin Ultrasound. 1986; 14:404–407.

36. Meire H, Farrant P. Ultrasound demonstration of an unusual growth pattern in Indians. Br J Obstet Gynaecol. 1981; 88:260–263.

37. Moore K. The fetal membranes and placenta. In: Moore K. The Developing Human. 3rd ed. Philadelphia: WB Saunders; 1982.

38. Morin F, Winsberg F. The ultrasonic appearance of the umbilical cord. J Clin Ultrasound. 1978; 6:324–326.

39. Nimrod C, Davies D, Iwanicki S, et al. Ultrasound prediction of pulmonary hypoplasia. Obstet Gynecol. 1986; 68:495–498.

40. Nyberg D, Mack L, Patten R, et al. Fetal bowel. Normal sonographic findings. J Ultrasound Med. 1987; 6:3–6.

41. Ogada E, Sabbagha R, Metzger B, et al. Serial ultrasonography to assess fetal macrosomia: Studies in 23 pregnancy diabetic women. JAMA. 1980; 243:2405–2408.

42. Pap G, Szoke J, Pap L. Intrauterine growth retardation: Ultrasonic diagnosis. Acta Paediatr Hung. 1983; 24:7–15.

43. Romero R, Pilu G, Jeanty P, et al. The lungs. In: Romero R, Pilu G, Jeanty P, et al., eds. Prenatal Diagnosis of Congenital Anomalies. East Norwalk, CT: Appleton & Lange; 1988.

44. Rosenberg E, Bowie J, Andreotti R, et al. Sono-

graphic evaluation of fetal adrenal glands. AJR. 1982; 139:1145–1147.

45. Rosenthal S, Filly R, Callen P, et al. Fetal pseudoascites. Radiology. 1979; 131:195–197.

46. Sanders R, Miner N, Martin J. Fetal anatomy. In: Sanders R, James A Jr. The Principles and Practice of Ultrasonography in Obstetrics and Gynecology. 3rd ed. East Norwalk, CT: Appleton-Century-Crofts; 1985.

47. Schmidt W, Yarkoni S, Jeanty P, et al. Sonographic measurement of the fetal spleen: Clinical implications. J Ultrasound Med. 1985; 4:667–672.

48. Seeds J. Antenatal sonographic assessment of the genitourinary tract. In: Sanders R, Hill M, eds. Ultrasound Annual. New York: Raven Press; 1986.

49. Staudach A. Abdomen. In: Staudach A. Sectional Fetal Anatomy in Ultrasonography. Berlin: Springer Verlag; 1987.

50. Staudach A. Skeleton. In: Staudach A. Sectional Fetal Anatomy in Ultrasonography. Berlin: Springer Verlag; 1987.

51. Staudach A. Thorax (heart, lung, great vessels). In: Staudach A. Sectional Fetal Anatomy in Ultrasonography. Berlin: Springer Verlag; 1987.

52. Stephens J. Prenatal diagnosis of testicular feminization. Lancet. 1984; 2:1038.

53. Taybi H. Radiology of Syndromes. Chicago: Year Book Medical Publishers; 1975.

54. Vandeberghe K, DeWolf F. Ultrasonic assessment of fetal stomach function. Physiology and clinic. In: Kurjak A, ed. Recent Advances in Ultrasound Diagnosis 2. Excerpta Medica International Congress Series 498; Amsterdam: Elsevier; 1980.

55. Vintzileos A, Neckles S, Campbell W, et al. Fetal liver ultrasound measurements during normal pregnancy. Obstet Gynecol. 1985; 66:477–480.

56. Walker J, Ferguson D. The sonographic appearance of blood in the fetal stomach and its association with placental abruption. J Ultrasound Med. 1988; 7:155–161.

57. Wladimiroff J, Legis R, Smith B. Human fetal stomach profile. In: Kurjak A, ed. Recent Advances in Ultrasound Diagnosis. 2. Excerpta Medica International Congress Series 498, 1980.

58. Yarkoni S, Schmitt W, Jeanty P, et al. Clavicular measurements: A new biometric parameter for fetal evaluation. J Ultrasound Med. 1985; 4:467–470.

59. Zador I, Bottoms S, Tse G, et al. Nomograms for ultrasound visualization of fetal organs. J Ultrasound Med. 1988; 7:197–201.

CHAPTER 16

Fetal Echocardiography

DALE R. CYR, WARREN G. GUNTHEROTH, LAURENCE A. MACK

As ultrasonography has developed, the ability to improve image resolution has been the basis for a multitude of sonographic advances. No ultrasound technique has been affected more by equipment advances than fetal echocardiography.[2−4,6,14] The use of ultrasound to evaluate the fetal heart has evolved beyond obtaining anatomic information for diagnosing congenital heart disease; by using other modalities such as M-mode and Doppler, cardiac hemodynamic information can be obtained as well.[2−4,19,20,49,59,61] In this chapter we discuss the diagnostic spectrum of fetal echocardiography as well as the basic knowledge needed to obtain and perform this subspecialty technique.

Normal Development and Anatomy

It is helpful for fetal echocardiographers to have a basic understanding of normal and abnormal cardiogenesis so that sonographic examination of the fetal heart can be more comprehensive and conclusive. In the first weeks of embryonic development the cardiovascular system is one of the first to function. This development progresses as blood begins to circulate through the embryo at the end of the third postconception week.[44] With high-resolution transvaginal transducers, sonographers may visualize the fetal heart beating at this time, 3 to 4 weeks after conception, 5 to 6 weeks after the last menstrual period (LMP). At this time the primitive heart tube is formed by partial fusion of the cardiogenic cords (Fig. 16-1). Once fusion occurs, the primitive heart tube thickens to form the myoepicardial mantle, which will give rise to the myocardium and epicardium. The inner portion of the heart tube will go on to form the endocardium.[1,44]

During the 4th and 5th weeks of gestation, the heart tube elongates and begins to divide and forms three primary areas: the bulbus cordis, ventricle, and atria. The truncus arteriosus, which also developed during this period, is contiguous with the bulbus cordis and supplies blood to the multiple aortic arches that exist at this time in gestation (Fig. 16-2).

The atrioventricular (AV) canal is created by thickening of the ventral and dorsal walls of the bulboventricular loop, better known as endocardial cushions.[1,25,44] The endocardial cushions continue to grow inward and fuse to form the septum of the AV canal, dividing the canal into right and left sides. The atrium is divided into the left and right atria by the formation of the septum secundum and septum primum, which is fused with the septum of the AV canal. The venae cavae and pulmonary veins communicate with the right and left atria, respectively. The partitioning of the ventricle begins at the apex, and moves superiorly toward the endocardial cushions (AV canal), where it eventually fuses by the end of the 7th week. The cardiac valves form from subendocardial tissue at the orifices of the great vessels and AV canals.[1,25]

At the end of the 5th week (LMP), ridges form

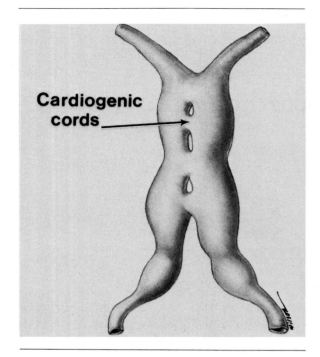

FIGURE 16-1. Schematic diagram of cardiogenic cords at approximately 5 weeks' gestation.

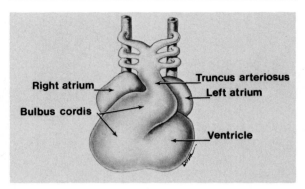

FIGURE 16-2. Schematic diagram of the fetal heart during the 5½ to 6th weeks of gestation demonstrating bulbus cordis, truncus arteriosus, ventricle, atria, and multiple aortic arches.

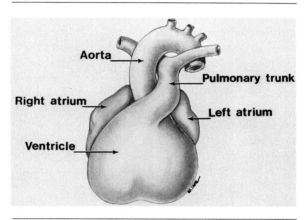

FIGURE 16-3. Schematic diagram of the fetal heart after approximately 8 weeks' gestation. At this point the heart has conformed to traditional anatomy and is considered fully developed.

within the wall of the bulbus cordis and the truncus arteriosus. Both sets of ridges are in communication with each other and eventually fuse to form the aorticopulmonary septum. This newly formed septum divides the bulbus cordis and truncus arteriosus into two channels: the aorta and pulmonary trunk. Because the aorticopulmonary septum has a spiral orientation, the pulmonary trunk is formed twisting around the aorta. The bulbus cordis then becomes incorporated into the ventricular walls.[1]

Around the 40th day of gestation the embryonic heart has completed its complex formation. The last developmental transformation allows the multiple aortic arches to conform to the normal aortic arch and cranial branches with which we are familiar. The embryonic heart can now be considered fully developed and will function and circulate in the same way throughout the rest of gestation (Fig. 16-3). Most congenital heart anomalies, which are in essence mishaps of cardiac embryogenesis, are also complete.[1,44]

FETAL CIRCULATION

The fetal circulation is fully developed after final embryogenesis, which is approximately 8 weeks LMP.[44] It is also at this point in gestation that the fetal heart rate is slowest, averaging 100 beats per minute. This can be easily visualized using commercially available high-resolution real-time units, by either transabdominal or transvaginal tech-

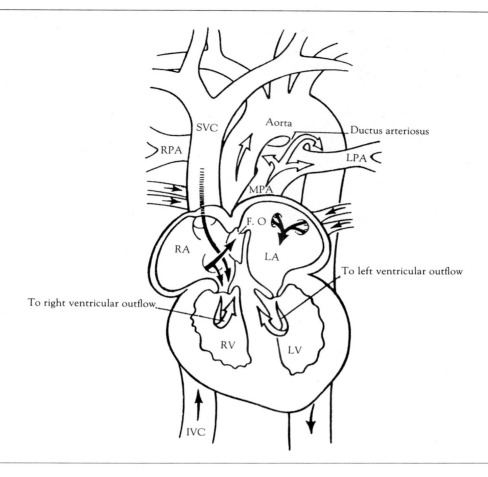

FIGURE 16-4. Schematic diagram of intracardiac fetal circulation (IVC, inferior vena cava; RV, right ventricle; LV, left ventricle; LA, left atrium; RA, right atrium; FO, foramen ovale; MPA, main pulmonary artery; RPA, right pulmonary artery; LPA, left pulmonary artery; SVC, superior vena cava).

niques. Fetal heart rate reaches a plateau after 9 weeks (ranging from 137 to 144 beats per minute).[31]

The fetus receives blood from the placenta via the umbilical vein. The umbilical vein then traverses the fetal abdomen and enters the liver, where it forms an anastomosis with the portal sinus (left portal vein) where blood may take two routes. The majority of blood will pass through the fetal liver and enter the inferior cava (IVC) through the hepatic veins. The remaining volume of blood enters the ductus venosus (between 10 and 50% of umbilical vein volume), which bypasses the liver circulation by entering the hepatic veins draining into the IVC, or entering the IVC directly.

Blood then enters the right atrium from the IVC and is channeled by the eustachian valve toward the foramen ovale and the left atrium; this valve also reduces regurgitant flow during ventricular systole. Approximately 60% of the highly oxygenated IVC blood volume is directed toward the atrial septum by the eustachian valve, which is in direct communication with the lower edge of the septum secundum of the interatrial septum, called the crista dividens. A small percentage of highly oxygenated blood remains in the right atrium and mixes with the blood volume from the superior vena cava.[52]

This blood then traverses the tricuspid valve and

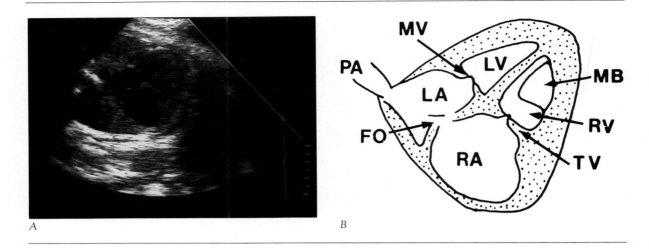

FIGURE 16-5. (A) Sonogram of the four-chamber view. (B) Schematic demonstrating the four-chamber view. (PV, pulmonary veins; LA, left atrium; MV, mitral valve; LV, left ventricle; MB, moderator band; RV, right ventricle; TV, tricuspid valve; RA, right atrium). (Modified from Cyr DR, Guntheroth WG, Mack LA, et al. J Ultrasound Med 1986;5:343-350).

enters the main pulmonary artery through the right ventricular outflow tract and pulmonary valve. The majority of blood flow (90%) continues down the ductus arteriosus and directly enters the descending aorta for systemic circulation. The ductus arteriosus acts to bypass the largely nonfunctioning fetal lungs, which require only 10% of the right ventricular output. After birth the ductus arteriosus constricts to form the ligamentum arteriosum and ceases to function.

The left atrium receives its blood from the inferior vena cava via the foramen ovale and the small amount of blood returning from the fetal lungs. The left atrial blood volume then traverses the mitral valve and exits the left ventricle through the left ventricular outflow tract and aortic valve, and is mainly distributed to the cranial half of the fetus via brachiocephalic vessels arising from the aortic arch (Fig. 16-4).[1,35,44,52]

Sonographic Technique and Anatomy

When performing fetal echocardiography, the most important step is to identify the anatomic orientation of the fetal heart. This is accomplished by determining the fetal lie and fetal spine location.

This information allows the sonographer to ascertain the left, right, cranial, caudal, dorsal, and ventral aspects of the fetal heart.[10]

The most important fetal echocardiographic view is the four-chamber view (Fig. 16-5).[8,10] This view allows the two atria, ventricles, AV valves (mitral and tricuspid), and the interatrial and interventricular septa to be visualized. This view is obtained by imaging the fetal thorax in a transverse plane. One must remember that in utero the apex of the heart lies perpendicular to the fetal spine.

In this imaging plane it is important to distinguish left and right sides of the heart. This may be accomplished by visualizing the foramen ovale flap moving in and out of the left atrium, caused by atrial shunting of blood from the right atrium to the left during systole.[1,44] Occasionally, the foramen ovale cannot be recognized because of poor fetal position, so identification of the moderator band in the apex of the right ventricle can assist in left/right orientation. The moderator band, which runs from the interventricular septum to the lower free wall of the right ventricle, should not be mistaken for an intraventricular tumor.[10,13] Once left-right orientation has been determined, the appro-

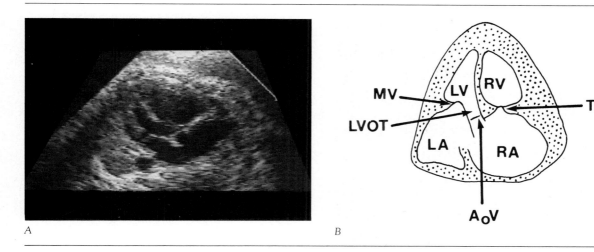

FIGURE 16-6. (A) Sonogram demonstrating the five-chamber view. (B) Schematic demonstrating the five-chamber view. (LA, left atrium; LVOT, left ventricular outflow tract; MV, mitral valve; LV, left ventricle; RV, right ventricle; TV, tricuspid valve; RA, right atrium; AoV, aortic valve.) (Modified from Cyr DR, Guntheroth WG, Mack LA, et al. A systematic approach to fetal echocardiography using real-time/two-dimensional sonography. J Ultrasound Med 1986;5:343-350.)

priate atrioventricular valves and cardiac chambers can be identified.

Additional cardiac anatomy may be sought by subtle anterior transducer angulation from the four-chamber view, producing the five-chamber view (Fig. 16-6), which demonstrates the left ventricular outflow tract as well as the proximal aortic root. The anatomic relationship between the interventricular septum and aorta is also appreciated in the five-chamber view. Further anterior movement of the transducer will bring the main pulmonary artery into view. The pulmonary valve may be seen within the pulmonary artery, arising from the right side of the fetal heart. Thus, all major parts of fetal intracardiac anatomy, as well as the great vessels, may be imaged, starting from the four-chamber view. Fortunately the four-chamber view can be obtained 99% of the time in any fetal position. It has also been shown that most abnormalities can initially be detected from this very important echocardiographic plane.[6,8]

Another important view for fetal echocardiography is the long axis view (Fig. 16-7). To image this anatomy, the transducer should be positioned so the fetus is being imaged in a transverse plane. The transducer also must be angulated slightly lateral and cephalad, to visualize the left ventricular outflow tract in relationship to the interventricular septum. The left ventricle, left atrium, interatrial septum, right ventricle, and part of the right atrium may also be evaluated in this view. With further cranial angulation of the transducer the aortic arch may be imaged (Fig. 16-8), including the left carotid, left subclavian, and brachiocephalic artery. With subtle lateral transducer adjustment, the ductus arteriosus may be seen entering the descending aorta. From the long axis view one may image the right ventricular inflow view (Fig. 16-9). This is accomplished by angling the transducer toward the right lateral aspect of the fetus. The right ventricular inflow view is an excellent plane to evaluate the right atrium, tricuspid valve, right ventricle, and right ventricular outflow tract (RVOT). Further lateral movement of the transducer with slight obliquity will demonstrate the right atrial inflow view (Fig. 16-10). This plane allows the superior and inferior venae cavae to be seen entering the right atrium. The eustachian valve may also be seen at the junction of the inferior vena cava and the right atrium.[10]

The short axis view is probably the second most important fetal echocardiographic plane. To ob-

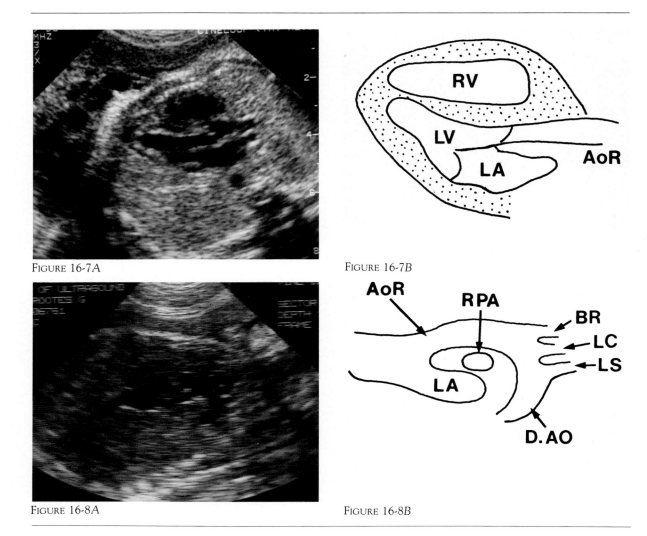

FIGURE 16-7A

FIGURE 16-7B

FIGURE 16-8A

FIGURE 16-8B

FIGURE 16-7. (A) Sonogram demonstrating the long axis view. (B) Schematic of the long axis view. (LV, left ventricle; LA, left atrium; AoR, aortic root; RV, right ventricle.) (Modified from Cyr DR, Guntheroth WG, Mack LA, et al. A systematic approach to fetal echocardiography using real-time/two-dimensional sonography. J Ultrasound Med 1986;5:343-350.)

FIGURE 16-8. (A) Sonogram demonstrating the aortic arch. (B) Schematic diagram of aortic arch. (LA, left atrium; AoR, aortic root; RPA, right pulmonary artery; BR, brachiocephalic artery; LC, left carotid artery; LS, left subclavian; D.AO, descending aorta.) (Modified from Cyr DR, Guntheroth WG, Mack LA, et al. A systematic approach to fetal echocardiography using real-time/two-dimensional sonography. J Ultrasound Med. 1986;5:343-350.)

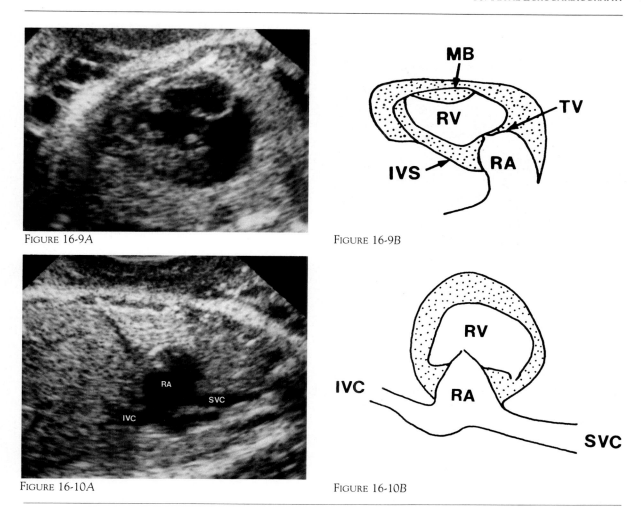

FIGURE 16-9A

FIGURE 16-9B

FIGURE 16-10A

FIGURE 16-10B

FIGURE 16-9. (A) Sonogram demonstrating the right ventricular inflow view. (B) Schematic diagram of right ventricular inflow view. (IVS, interventricular septum; RV, right ventricle; MB, moderator band; TV, tricuspid valve; RA, right atrium.) (Modified from Cyr DR, Guntheroth WG, Mack LA, et al. A systematic approach to fetal echocardiography using real-time/two-dimensional sonography. J Ultrasound Med. 1986;5:343-350.)

FIGURE 16-10. (A) Sonogram demonstrating right atrial inflow (SVC, superior vena cava; RA, right atrium; IVC, inferior vena cava). (B) Correlating schematic drawing demonstrating right atrial inflow view (IVC, inferior vena cava; RA, right atrium; RV, right ventricle; SVC, superior vena cava). (Modified from Cyr DR, Guntheroth WG, Mack LA, et al. A systematic approach to fetal echocardiography using real-time/two-dimensional sonography. J. Ultrasound Med. 1986;5:343-350.)

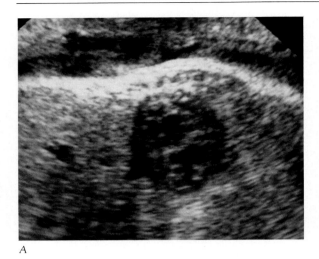

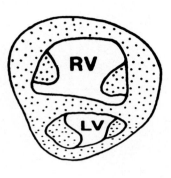

A

B

Figure 16-11. (A) Sonogram demonstrating short axis view at ventricular level. (B) Correlating schematic of short axis view at ventricular level (RV, right ventricle; LV, left ventricle).

tain this view, one must image the fetus in a sagittal plane, remembering that the apex of the heart lies horizontally within the thorax. Having imaged the fetal heart in cross section, the sonographer may sweep the heart from the apex to its superior aspect. Three distinct levels are described in the short axis view. The first level is at the ventricular apices, demonstrating both ventricles and the inferior aspect of the muscular ventricular septum (Fig. 16-11). Further transducer movement toward the left lateral aspect of the fetus (superior within the fetal heart) allows the aortic root to be imaged in a transverse plane with the pulmonary artery wrapping around the aortic root (Fig. 16-12). The pulmonary valve, as well as the pulmonary bifurcation, can be seen at this level. Slight transducer movement superiorly may image the ductus arteriosus arising from the main pulmonary artery and entering the descending aorta, demonstrating great vessel orientation. Although this view can be imaged in a large percentage of patients, it is best seen when the fetus is in a spine-posterior or spine-left lie.[12]

The views described above allow a very detailed anatomic examination of the fetal heart.[5,10,17,32,56] The extent to which one may be able to visualize the fetal heart depends on the position of the fetus and its gestational age.[12] Ideal gestational ages in which to image the fetal heart are from 20 through 34 weeks' gestation. Before 20 weeks the fetal heart is very small and creates sound beam artifacts such as "partial voluming," which may falsely project specific anatomy to be associated with nontraditional anatomic sites. Fetuses less than 20 weeks in gestation are also extremely mobile, making it a difficult task to image the heart for detailed study. After 34 weeks' gestation the fetal skeletal system has more calcium, giving rise to severe shadowing artifacts and reducing the ability to utilize fetal intercostal sonographic windows.

Fetal position has been shown to be the most important factor in imaging the fetal heart. The ability to image specific cardiac anatomy directly depends on what acoustic windows are available, which correlates to fetal spine position. Table 16-1 demonstrates the difference in four-chamber, five-chamber, and short axis views in relation to fetal spine position.[2,8,12]

If the fetus is not in a suitable position for specific anatomic surveillance, gently jostling the maternal abdomen with the transducer to induce fetal movement may help the fetus move into a favor-

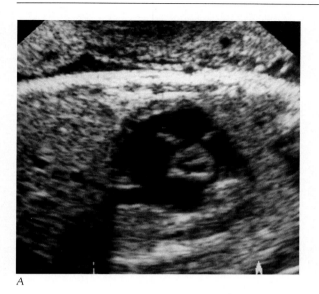

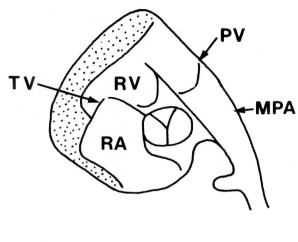

A   *B*

FIGURE 16-12. (*A*) Sonogram of short axis view at aortic-pulmonic level. (*B*) Schematic of short axis view at aortic/pulmonic level. (RA, right atrium; TV, tricuspid valve; RV, right ventricle; PV, pulmonary valve; MPA, main pulmonary artery.) Note cross section of aortic valve in center. (Modified from Cyr DR, Guntheroth WG, Mack LA, et al. A systematic approach to fetal echocardiography using real-time/two-dimensional sonography. J. Ultrasound Med. 1986;5:343-350.)

able position. If this technique fails, having the mother go for a walk may also induce fetal movement. A last resort is to reschedule the examination for another time when the fetus might be in a more favorable position. Table 16-2 demonstrates basic fetal echocardiographic views that should be incorporated into every obstetric examination. Advanced fetal echocardiographic views that should be used for further evaluation of the fetal heart are also outlined.

M-MODE

The use of M-mode sonography in conjunction with two-dimensional imaging is essential to performing modern fetal echocardiography.[4,17] The information that can be derived from fetal M-mode images allows individual chamber sizes and wall thickness to be evaluated in relation to gestational age or in comparison to other cardiac chambers; nomograms for sizes of fetal cardiac structures are shown in Figure 16-13.

TABLE 16-1. Visualization of fetal cardiac views in relation to spine position

	PREVALENCE		
POSITION	FOUR-CHAMBER (%)	FIVE-CHAMBER (%)	SHORT AXIS (%)
Spine up	100	82	55
Spine down	100	100	100
Spine left	98	67	93
Spine right	100	85	100

(Modified from Cyr DR, Komarniski CA, Guntheroth WG, et al. The prevalence of imaging fetal cardiac anatomy. J Diagn Med Sonogr. 1988;6:299–304.)

From the M-mode study many measurements may be made that give pertinent diagnostic and physiologic information.[59] The ability to detect rate of atrial and ventricular contractions gives the fetal echocardiographer the opportunity to diagnose a variety of arrhythmias and congenital heart block, as well as certain morphologic abnormalities. DeVore and colleagues have recently reported that aortic root dimensions in relation to left atrial size may be an accurate indicator of tetralogy of Fallot.[23]

Ideally, the best position of the fetal heart for M-mode investigation is a four-chamber view with the fetal spine toward either side of the mother.[20] This allows the M-line to be placed through both atria and, by repositioning, through both ventricles. Both systolic and diastolic ventricular measurements should be made on all M-mode studies. Most equations for calculating ventricular function need both systolic and diastolic components (see below). These measurements can be made from hard copy images with hand-held calipers or with calibrators accessible on the ultrasound screen. During maximal ventricular contraction (systole), measurements should be made from the anterior wall of the ventricle to the coexisting contraction on the interventricular septum. The same process is repeated during the diastolic cycle, measuring from the anterior ventricular wall to its corresponding diastolic septal component. Caution should be observed not to include the chordae tendinae in either measurement. Atrial measurements generally are performed to determine size, not function, so only one measurement is required. Measuring from either the left or the right atrial wall, depending on which atrium one is investigating, to the atrial septum is all that is required. Because atrial walls do not have significant contractions, measurements made during systole and during diastole are not significantly different. Figure 16-14 A and B demonstrate typical M-mode appearances through ventricles and atria. Figure 16-14C demonstrates M-mode sites of measurement during systole and diastole.

When performing fetal M-mode studies it is important to note what sweep speed is being used and in what time frame the time markers are being projected on the screen. Multiple cardiac cycles must be demonstrated on one monitor sweep for accurate contraction times and chamber measurements to be made. Usually the time markers seen on a monitor are at 1-second intervals. If so, simply counting the number of contractions over a 2-sec-

ond period and multiplying by 30 yields a fetal heart rate for a 1-minute interval.

Fetal cardiac arrhythmias can be diagnosed most reliably with M-mode technology. The ability to look at atrial and ventricular wall contractions

TABLE 16-2. Routine views for evaluating the fetal heart

VIEW	STRUCTURES VISUALIZED
Four-chamber	All four chambers AV valves AV septum
Five-chamber (anterior movement from four-chamber)	Left ventricular outflow, aortic root; aorta-left ventricle continuity
Pulmonary artery view (anterior movement from five-chamber view)	Right ventricular outflow in continuity with right ventricle; main pulmonary artery
Advanced Imaging Four-chamber	Same as above
Five-chamber (anterior movement from four-chamber)	Same as above
Pulmonary artery view from four-chamber (anterior transducer movement from five-chamber view)	Same as above
Long axis view	Left ventricular outflow tract (LVOT), left atrium, left ventricle, aortic root, ventricular septum; aorta-LVOT continuity
Aortic arch view	Ascending aorta, aortic arch, descending aorta with cephalic vessels
Right ventricular inflow view	Right atrium, tricuspid valve, right ventricle and ventricular septum
Right atrial inflow view	Inferior and superior venae cavae, right atrium
Short axis view, apical level	Right and left ventricle in transverse plane; ventricular septum and papillary muscles
Pulmonary/aortic level	Aorta in cross section with main pulmonary artery lying anterior to aorta; right ventricle

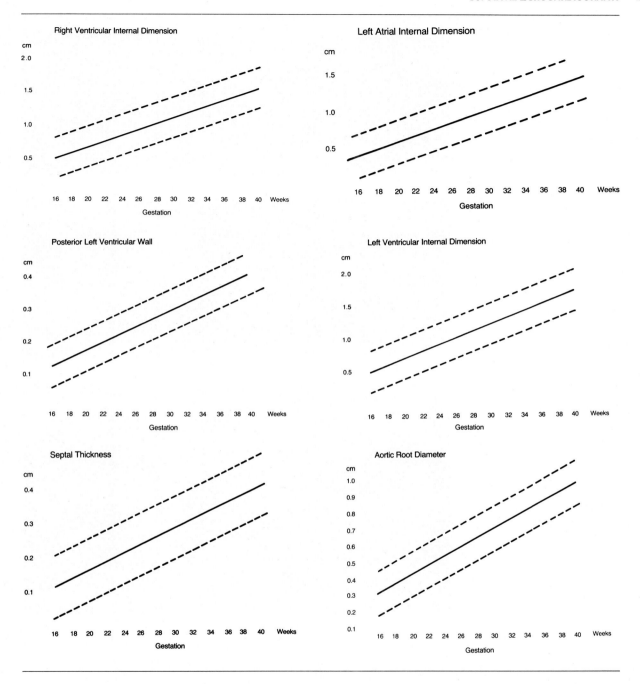

FIGURE 16-13. Nomograms of left atrial, left ventricular, right ventricular, and aortic root diameters. Also interventricular septal thickness and posterior left ventricular wall thickness. (Modified from Allan LD, Joseph MC, Boyd EG, et al. Echocardiography in the developing human fetus. Br Heart J. 1982;47:573.)

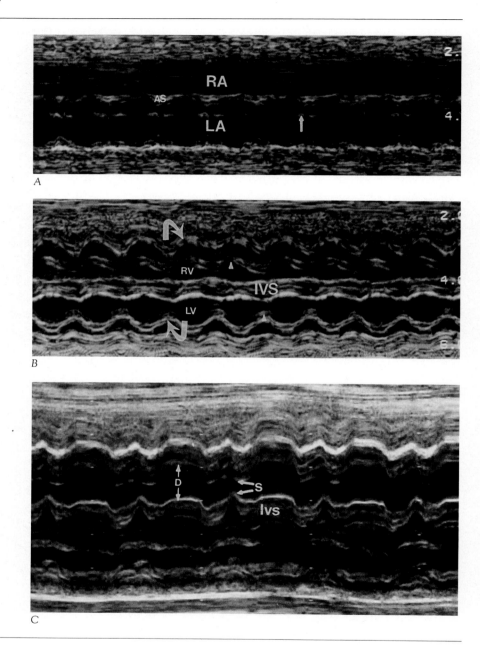

FIGURE 16-14. (A) M-mode scan through both fetal atria (RA, right atrium; LA, left atrium; AS, atrial septum; *arrow*, foramen ovale flap). (B) M-mode scan through both fetal ventricles (RV, right ventricle; LV, left ventricle; IVS, interventricular septum). Curved arrows point at left and right ventricular posterior walls; arrowheads demonstrate chordae tendineae. (C) Fetal ventricular M-mode scan demonstrates caliper placement during systole (S), and diastole (D) (IVS, interventricular septum).

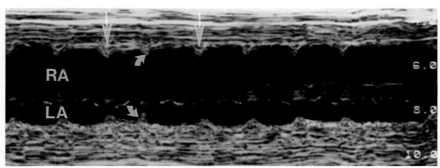

FIGURE 16-15

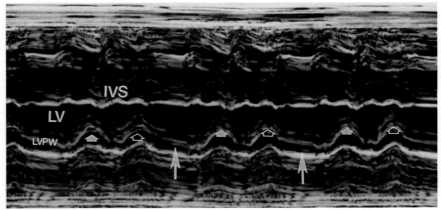

FIGURE 16-16

FIGURE 16-15. M-mode view through both atria of a 34-week fetus with premature atrial contractions (RA, right atrium; LA, left atrium). Curved arrows point to premature atrial contractions in relation to regular atrial contractions (*straight arrows*).

FIGURE 16-16. M-mode sonogram demonstrates premature ventricular contractions with compensatory pause (LV, left ventricle; IVS, interventricular septum; LVPW, left ventricular posterior wall). The regular ventricular contractions are demonstrated by arrows; the premature ventricular contractions, by open arrows. The compensatory pause is demonstrated by a large arrow.

over time allows diagnosis of premature atrial or ventricular contractions and life-threatening supraventricular tachyarrhythmias.[4,17,18,21,30,37,42,58,60]

The most prevalent arrhythmias identified in fetuses are premature atrial contractions (PACs). They are benign and are usually seen between the gestational ages of 25 and 35 weeks (Fig. 16-15).[4,14,20] PACs may or may not conduct to the ventricle.

Premature ventricular contractions are also common in utero, and are also benign in healthy fetuses. These arrhythmias usually show a classic compensatory pause caused by the AV node refractory period (Fig. 16-16). It is not uncommon for PACs and PVCs to be concurrent.[20,30] Supraventricular tachyarrhythmias (SVTs) are of great concern to the clinician if they persist, as they can

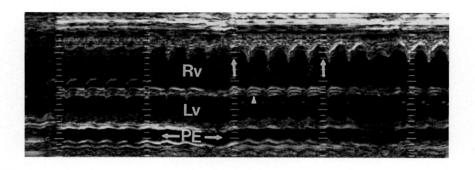

FIGURE 16-17. M-mode sonogram through 26-week fetal ventricles demonstrates supraventricular tachycardia (RV, right ventricle; LV, left ventricle). The ventricular rate is calculated at 270 beats per minute (4.5 beats per second × 60). The white hatch marks are 1-cm markers; arrowhead, interventricular septum. Also note pericardial effusion (PE).

cause fetal death from in utero heart failure (Fig. 16-17).[37] Treatment and conversion of SVTs have been well-documented in the literature using digoxin, verapamil, and quinidine.[30,36-38] Atrial and ventricular rates during SVT may approach 300 beats per minute (bpm). Because of inevitable heart failure, fetal hydrops is a common finding with persistent SVT.[30,36]

Information derived from M-mode examination that is particularly important when heart disease is suspected is the shortening fraction (SF). This equation gives an index of ventricular systolic function (contractility) and is calculated from the following formula using ventricular dimensions:

$$\frac{(\text{Diastolic ventricular dimension} - \text{systolic ventricular dimension})}{\text{Diastolic ventricular dimension} \times 100\%}$$

= Percentile systolic ventricular function

Normal fractional shortening of the fetal heart is greater than 25%.[21]

M-mode also allows pericardial effusions to be visualized, and followed with precision.[3,14] Contracting myocardium must be seen moving away from the pericardial fluid for a definitive diagnosis to be made. Normally, the fetal pericardium appears to have sonolucent areas that have been reported to represent small effusions.[34] Strict ana-

tomic investigation of the sonolucent pericardium has not been done to substantiate that it is indeed fluid.

DOPPLER ECHOCARDIOGRAPHY

Pulsed Doppler has become another diagnostic tool in studies of the fetal heart.[2,14,15,33,50,62] Recent improvements in equipment—namely smaller sample volumes and higher pulsed repetition frequencies—have allowed fetal echocardiographers to interrogate specific areas of the fetal heart to analyze flow characteristics. The most common use is to see whether valve regurgitation is occurring and to evaluate flow through septal defects and even to detect no flow, as in atresia of valves or vessels.[14,15] Ventricular inflow as well as great vessel investigation may provide further information.[50,51,62] It is important to keep in mind that the pressures and pressure gradients that help determine flow velocities and turbulence are quite different in fetuses. The two fetal ventricles have pressures that are approximately equal; consequently, ventricular septal defects in utero may not demonstrate the typical high-velocity jets on Doppler.[52]

Although using Doppler in the fetal heart is a special application, it must be emphasized that traditional Doppler principles still apply. The fetal echocardiographer must be aware of exactly which area of the heart is being imaged at all times. The

TABLE 16-3. Intracardiac Doppler velocities in the normal fetus

PARAMETER	AORTA	MAIN PULMONARY ARTERY	MITRAL VALVE	TRICUSPID VALVE
Maximum velocity (cm/sec)	70 ± 3	60 ± 4	47 ± 4	51 ± 4
Mean velocity (cm/sec)	18 ± 2	16 ± 2	11 ± 1	12 ± 1

(Modified from Reed KL, Meijboom EJ, Sahn DJ, et al. Cardiac Doppler flow velocities in human fetuses. Circulation. 1986;73:41–46.)

rapid heart rate and fetal movement change the sample volume position constantly. It is also important to realize how big the sample volume is in relation to the structure that is being interrogated. Typical chamber and great vessel sizes are routinely under 1 cm, and caution should be used to rule out partial voluming artifacts. It is also important to be aware constantly of the velocity scale (Nyquist limit), to avoid mistaking normal velocity and abnormal flow. Doppler filters, which affect sensitivity, should be used cautiously to avoid "flooding" the spectral analysis with excess noise that may give a false impression of turbulence, which may indicate stenosis. On the other hand, too much Doppler filter may eliminate turbulence or regurgitant jets, giving a false-negative impression. It is essential to understand how each piece of equipment displays and processes these important variables.

Reed and co-workers performed fetal intracardiac studies to derive normal ranges of velocities and volume flows through all cardiac valves (mitral, tricuspid, pulmonic, aortic).[50] These values seem to be consistent throughout gestation (Table 16-3). Velocities may be displayed as meters per second or centimeters per second, and volume flows (Q) may be calculated using the formula $Q =$ Velocity $\times$ Area. Calculation of the area of valve orifices is subject to very high intra- and interobserver variation, and small measurement differences make significant errors in these calculations because the area formula uses the square of the diameter. Ratios using peak velocities during systole and diastole have also been formulated, in hopes of determining abnormal intracardiac blood flow.[14,16,18,33,35,50,51]

The role of Doppler color flow mapping in fetal echocardiography is rapidly expanding. Early reports have focused on visualizing septal defects and regurgitant jets.[19] Color flow Doppler has a slower pulse repetition rate than standard pulsed Doppler, which may cause unique artifacts, especially with the rapid flow rates seen in fetal hearts. In addition, the threshold for "turbulence" is relatively low, and normal high-velocity flow may be confused with disturbed flow. The sonographer must also beware of fusion of two flow paths that may suggest defects where they do not exist.

The Abnormal Fetal Heart

Given state-of-the-art equipment, an experienced examiner can identify most congenital heart lesions in utero. When imaging the fetal heart, the fetal echocardiographer must evaluate several conditions. The first and most important is whether the two sides of the heart are symmetric. Given that the right side of the fetal heart is only slightly larger than the left side, the two should appear nearly the same size. Actual measurement and comparison with norms for size is important, since the apparently small chamber might be normal and the apparently normal ventricle might be enlarged. Cardiac rate and rhythm should also be documented. When imaging the great vessels, it is extremely important to ensure that they originate from the proper side of the heart. Thus, using the previously described fetal echocardiographic planes in relation to the specific cardiac anatomy demonstrated by each view, normal versus abnormal cardiac morphology can be ascertained.

Beam width artifact may give a false impression of abnormal vessel origin, but multiple views will usually resolve any question of anomalies. Finally, observing both the ventricular and atrial septa and both AV valves will allow the fetal echocardiographer to verify endocardial continuity and integrity of both septa.

When abnormalities are seen in any of these sys-

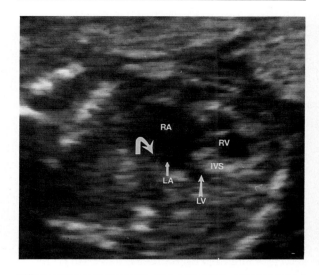

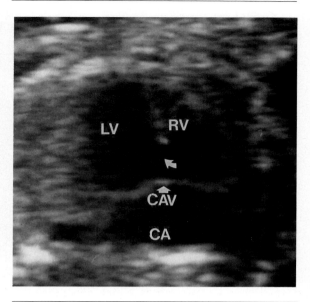

Figure 16-18. Four-chamber view in a 23-week fetus demonstrates hypoplastic left heart syndrome (RA, right atrium; RV, right ventricle; IVS, interventricular septum). Note the right-sided enlargement in relation to left ventricle (LV) and left atrium (LA). Curved arrow demonstrates the interatrial septum. On further examination, the aorta and mitral valve were also found to be hypoplastic.

Figure 16-19. Four-chamber view in a 28-week fetus demonstrates complete atrioventricular canal (LV, left ventricle; RV, right ventricle; CAV, common atrioventricular valve, CA, common atrium). Also note the rather large VSD (*curved arrow*).

tematic observations, congenital heart disease must be considered. (Diseases of the myocardium should be considered as should arrhythmias and their effects.) We will describe the most common forms of fetal congenital defects and their sonographic appearances.

Hypoplastic Heart Syndrome

Hypoplastic heart syndrome is a lethal lesion that most often affects the left side, although hypoplastic right ventricles also occur. It is characterized by hypoplasia of the ventricle, atrium, AV valve, and great vessel of the affected side. The unaffected side is enlarged, and the fetus may or may not have hydrops, depending on the severity of the hypoplasia, whether it is obstructive to pulmonary venous return, and whether the other ventricle can assume the function of pump for both the systemic and pulmonic circulation.[3,26,39,45] When only one side of the heart can be visualized in the four-chamber view, hypoplastic heart must be considered. It is

imperative that the affected side be imaged in detail. The ventricle, atrium, and most importantly the AV valve and great vessel are usually hypoplastic. It is not uncommon for the unaffected AV valve to have valvular insufficiency, as the enlargement of that side stretches the annulus.[54] Figure 16-18 demonstrates a classic appearance of hypoplastic left heart.

Endocardial Cushion Defects

Failure of the common AV orifice to separate into the mitral and tricuspid valves and failure of both septa to close give rise to a broad range of endocardial cushion defects (ECD).[1,44,47] Two major forms of ECD are classified as complete and partial AV canals. Other terms in current use for ECD are AV septal defect and AV communis.[25]

Complete AV canal has a large combined AV defect with a common septal leaflet of the AV valves. There may be absence of the interatrial septum and a large ventricle that has an incomplete

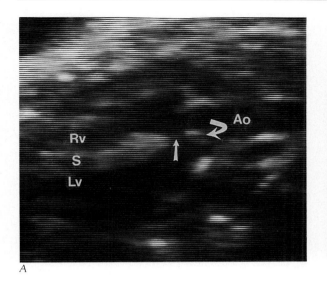
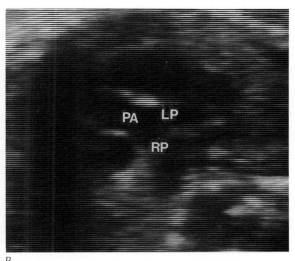

A   *B*

FIGURE 16-20. Four-chamber view and short axis view demonstrate an overriding aorta with ventricular septal defect (*straight arrow*) consistent with tetralogy of Fallot. (*A*) Four-chamber view (RV, right ventricle; S, interventricular septum; LV, left ventricle; AO, aorta; aortic valve {curved arrow}). (*B*) Short axis view demonstrates normal-looking pulmonary artery (PA) and bifurcation (LP, left pulmonary artery; RP, right pulmonary artery). After birth, the newborn was found to have moderate infundibular pulmonary stenosis. (Courtesy of John Denny, M.D.)

septum. There may be mitral and tricuspid regurgitation.[8,14,15] This defect is commonly associated with Down's syndrome. Figure 16-19 demonstrates an example of a complete endocardial cushion defect.

Partial AV canal invariably has a low, primum atrial-septal defect and there may be a small ventricular septal defect (VSD); the complete form has a large VSD. Both forms demonstrate a cleft in the septal leaflet of the mitral valve, which may or may not cause mitral regurgitation.[25]

Tetralogy of Fallot

The features of this lesion may vary in severity. Large VSDs occur with varying degrees of overriding aorta. Some form of pulmonary stenosis is present; infundibular, pulmonary atresia may also occur.[24] The most common initial sonographic appearance is the overriding aorta and visualization of the VSD.[29] Even using Doppler, the pulmonary

stenosis may not be apparent early in gestation. The chambers may or may not be symmetric, depending on the severity of the pulmonary stenosis and the size of the septal defect, and the problem may be overlooked unless great care is taken at the time of the initial scan. Figure 16-20 shows a fetus that was diagnosed with tetralogy of Fallot.

Ebstein's Anomaly

Ebstein's anomaly is defined as inferior displacement of the tricuspid valve causing atrialization of the right ventricle. The valve is incompetent, and right ventricular function may be impaired; however, the degree of valvular compromise varies considerably, and the prognosis depends on the severity.[55,61] The sonographic appearance shows variable asymmetry of the chambers on the four-chamber view.[15] The right atrium appears larger than the left one; how much so depends on the severity of the valvular disease. Doppler examination of the tricuspid valve is essential to determine the extent of regurgitation (see Fig. 16-21).

TRANSPOSITION OF THE GREAT ARTERIES

Transposition of the great arteries (TGA) may be seen as an isolated entity or associated with other cardiac defects. Because of "partial voluming" artifacts and the unique angles permitted by fetal heart imaging, the false-positive and false-negative diagnosis rates may be high, even in the most experienced hands.

It is of the utmost importance to be certain of the fetal heart orientation (left, right) when considering this diagnosis. Since both arteries are of similar size in the fetus and have almost identical Doppler signals, careful two-dimensional imaging proves or disproves this particular diagnosis.

The classic appearance of dextrotransposition of the great arteries (d-TGA) or complete TGA is when the aorta arises from the right of the pulmonary artery, as usual, but anteriorly instead of posteriorly; the pulmonary artery arises from the left ventricle and is to the left and posterior (Fig. 16-22). In corrected transposition, or levotransposition, of the great arteries (l-TGA) the arteries arise from the functionally correct ventricle, but the ventricles are morphologically reversed. The aorta is to the *left* of the pulmonary artery. Using the parallel arteries sign (aorta and pulmonary arteries appear to be exiting the heart in parallel) may be helpful in diagnosing TGA. More views would be needed to confirm this suspicion. Another helpful scanning technique is to image the aortic arch and trace it back to the originating artery. If these signs cannot be demonstrated and these techniques cannot be performed, this diagnosis cannot be ruled in or out. Septal defects are relatively common in transpositions.[49]

TRUNCUS ARTERIOSUS

Truncus arteriosus occurs when the embryonic truncus arteriosus fails to partition to separate the aorta and pulmonary artery and some degree of continuity between these vessels remains. Three major types of truncus occur, ranging from a common conduit that functions as both aorta and pulmonary arteries, from which the left and right pulmonary arteries arise, to almost complete cleavage of the two arteries. (A fourth type, in which there

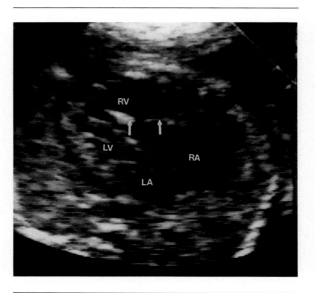

FIGURE 16-21. Four-chamber view in a 24-week fetus demonstrates atrialization of the right ventricle and inferior displacement of tricuspid valve (*arrows*) consistent with Epstein's anomaly. RA, right atrium; LA, left atrium; LV, left ventricle; RV, right ventricle.

are no identifiable pulmonary arteries, is now considered a form of pulmonary atresia.[43]) Sonographically, the demonstration of continuity between the two great vessels should arouse suspicion of this lesion. A ventricular septal defect is almost always present. Using Doppler, there may or may not be turbulence or high velocity within the common vessel or at the roots of the aorta or pulmonary arteries.[56] This is a subtle lesion that may not be diagnosable because of limitations of fetal position, age, and size (Fig. 16-23).

ISOLATED SEPTAL DEFECTS

Visualization of isolated VSDs depends on the size of the defect. Obviously, the larger the defect the better the chance of visualizing it. Since VSDs are the most common form of congenital heart disease, every echocardiographer eventually images one (Fig. 16-24). Atrial septal defects (ASDs) are very difficult to diagnose as the foramen ovale is normally patent throughout gestation. In our experi-

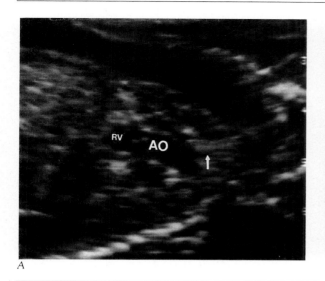
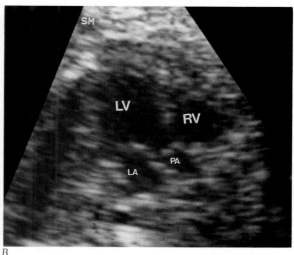

FIGURE 16-22. Sonograms demonstrate dextrotransposition of the great arteries. The pulmonary artery arises from the left ventricle, while the aorta arises from the right ventricle. (A) Oblique view demonstrates an anteriorly placed aorta (AO) arising from the right ventricle (RV). Also note a cephalic vessel demonstrated by small arrow. (B) Four-chamber view demonstrating the posterior pulmonary artery arising from the left ventricle. (PA, pulmonary artery; LV, left ventricle; LA, left atrium; RV, right ventricle.)

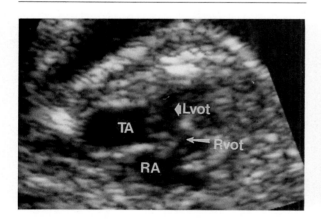
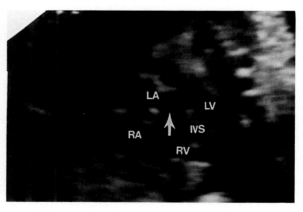

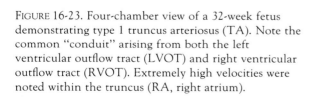

FIGURE 16-23. Four-chamber view of a 32-week fetus demonstrating type 1 truncus arteriosus (TA). Note the common "conduit" arising from both the left ventricular outflow tract (LVOT) and right ventricular outflow tract (RVOT). Extremely high velocities were noted within the truncus (RA, right atrium).

FIGURE 16-24. Four-chamber view in a 30-week fetus demonstrates a rather large ventricular septal defect (arrow). LA, left atrium; LV, left ventricle; RA, right atrium; RV, right ventricle; IVS, interventricular septum.

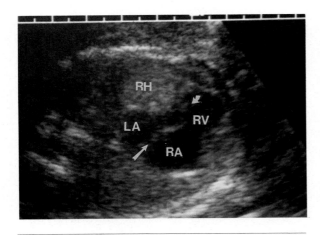

Figure 16-25. Four-chamber view demonstrates a large echogenic left ventricular mass consistent with rhabdomyoma or rhabdomyosarcoma (RH). Note the mass effect on the interventricular septum (*curved arrow*) (LA, left atrium; RA, right atrium; RV, right ventricle; interatrial septum {*arrow*}). After birth, this patient was also diagnosed as having tuberous sclerosis.

ence only large defects or complete septal agenesis have been diagnosed reliably.[28]

Ventricular Hypertrophy

In utero ventricular hypertrophy is most commonly associated with severe outlet stenosis or obstruction, but it may indicate a cardiomyopathy, including the type associated with a maternal history of diabetes. With M-mode the ventricles and the myocardial thickness can be measured.[4,21,37]

Cardiac Tumors

Although they are rare, congenital cardiac tumors and masses have been diagnosed in fetuses. The most common tumors reported are rhabdomyomas and rhabdosarcomas, which cannot be distinguished from one another sonographically (Fig. 16-25).[11,13,18] They appear as echogenic masses in any or all of the cardiac chambers. They are commonly associated with tuberous sclerosis. Other possible fetal intracardiac tumors are fibromas, myxomas, and teratomas, the last of which often are pericardial in origin but may appear intracardiac.[11]

It is important for the fetal echocardiographer to

Table 16-4. Sonographic appearance of fetal congenital heart defects

Heart Defect	Sonographic Appearance
Univentricular heart	Left-right heart asymmetry. Normal-sized great vessels. VSD or ASD may be present.
Pulmonary atresia	Right side of heart enlarged if no VSD present. Pulmonary artery not visualized in specific views (anterior four-chamber, short axis). Careful duplex scanning may help diagnose no right ventricular outflow.
Double-outlet right ventricle	Both great arteries arise from right ventricle. Septal defects may be present.
Total anomalous pulmonary venous return	Several forms exist; diagnosis in utero very difficult. Important to follow pulmonary veins that may empty into right atrium or ventricle. Chamber asymmetry may not be seen. Both great vessels appear normal.
Situs inversus	Important to be absolutely sure of left-right orientation of fetal heart in relation to fetal position. Fetal heart itself appears normal. Abdominal structures may also be transposed.
Ectopia cordis	Fetal heart is partially or totally outside fetal thorax, usually through sternal defect. Important to look for congenital heart disease and other fetal abnormalities.
Valvular atresia	Chamber dilatation proximal to atretic valve. Contralateral dilatation if no VSD is present to decompress volume overload.
Interrupted aortic arch	Slight enlargement of right ventricle. Abnormally small ascending aorta.
Coarctation of the aorta	Possibly slight right ventricular enlargement. Possibly turbulent descending aortic flow distal to ductus arteriosus entrance.

determine that these masses are located within the heart. Congenital lung masses such as cystic adenomatoid malformation and pulmonary sequestration may also give the false impression of cardiac masses, as they may displace and indent the cardiac space. Fetal hydrops may or may not occur, depending on how large these masses are and whether blood flow is obstructed (Fig. 16-24). Other congenital heart anomalies that are diagnosable in utero and their probable echocardiographic appearances are outlined in Table 16-4.

Summary

Sonographic imaging of the fetal heart has gained sophistication over the last few years. It is a very difficult and time-consuming examination, but performed expertly it can yield information to aid the perinatologist in caring for mother and fetus. It is imperative that the sonographer be very familiar with the equipment: every imaginable sonographic artifact is magnified in fetal echocardiography. It is also imperative to have a full understanding of fetal development and congenital heart disease so that proper interrogation of the fetal heart can be made.

References

1. Adams FH. Fetal and neonatal circulations. In: Adams FH, Emmanouilides GC, eds. Heart Disease in Infants, Children and Adolescents. 3rd ed. Baltimore: Williams & Wilkins; 1983; 11–17.

2. Allan LD, Chita SK, Al-Ghazali, et al. Doppler echocardiographic evaluation of the normal human fetal heart. Br Heart J. 1987; 57:528–533.

3. Allan LD, Little D, Campbell S, et al. Fetal ascites associated with congenital heart disease. Br J Obstet Gynecol. 1981; 88:453–455.

4. Allan LD, Joseph MC, Boyd EGCA, et al. M-mode echocardiography in the developing human fetus. Br Heart J. 1982; 47:573–583.

5. Allan LD, Tynan MJ, Campbell S, et al. Echocardiographic and anatomical correlates in the fetus. Br Heart J. 1980; 44:444–451.

6. Benacerraf BR, Pober BR, Sanders SP. Accuracy of fetal echocardiography. Radiology. 1987; 165:847–849.

7. Copel JA, Kleinman CS. The impact of fetal echocardiography on perinatal outcome. Ultrasound Med and Biol. 1986; 12:327–335.

8. Copel JA, Pilu G, Green J, et al. Fetal echocardiographic screening for congenital heart disease: The importance of the four-chamber view. Am J Obstet Gynecol. 1987; 157:648–655.

9. Crawford DC, Drake DP, Kwaitkowski D, et al. Prenatal diagnosis of reversible cardiac hypoplasia associated with congenital diaphragmatic hernia: Implications for postnatal management. J Clin Ultrasound. 1986; 14:718–721.

10. Cyr DR, Guntheroth WG, Mack LA, et al. A systematic approach to fetal echocardiography using real-time/two-dimensional sonography. J Ultrasound Med. 1986; 5:343–350.

11. Cyr DR, Guntheroth SG, Nyberg DA, et al. Prenatal diagnosis of an intrapericardial teratoma. A cause for nonimmune hydrops. J Ultrasound Med. 1988; 7:87–90.

12. Cyr DR, Komarniski CA, Guntheroth WG, et al. The prevalence of imaging fetal cardiac anatomy. J Diag Med Sonogr. 1988; 6:299–304.

13. Dennis MA, Appareti K, Manco-Johnson ML. The echocardiographic diagnosis of multiple fetal cardiac tumors. J Ultrasound Med. 1985; 4:327–329.

14. DeVore GR: Fetal echocardiography—A new frontier. Clin Obstet Gynecol. 1984; 27:359–377.

15. ———. The prenatal diagnosis of congenital heart disease: A practical approach for the fetal sonographer. J Clin Ultrasound. 1985; 13:229–245.

16. DeVore GR, Platt LD. The random measurement of the transverse diameter of the fetal heart: A potential source of error. J Ultrasound Med. 1985; 4:335–341.

17. DeVore GR, Donnerstein RL, Kleinman CS, et al. Fetal echocardiography. I. Normal anatomy as determined by real-time–directed M-mode ultrasound. Am J Obstet Gynecol. 1982; 144:249.

18. DeVore GR, Hakim S, Kleinman CS, et al. The in utero diagnosis of an interventricular septal cardiac rhabdomyoma by means of real-time–directed, M-mode echocardiography. Am J Obstet Gynecol. 1982; 143:967–969.

19. DeVore GR, Horenstein J, Siassi B, et al. Fetal echocardiography. VII. Doppler color flow mapping: A new technique for the diagnosis of congenital heart disease. Am J Obstet Gynecol. 1987; 156:1054–1064.

20. DeVore GR, Siassi B, Platt D. Fetal echocardiography. III. The diagnosis of cardiac arrhythmias using real-time–directed M-mode ultrasound. Am J Obstet Gynecol. 1983; 146:792.

21. ———. Fetal echocardiography. IV. M-mode assessment of ventricular size and contractility during the second and third trimesters of pregnancy in the normal fetus. Am J Obstet Gynecol. 1984; 150:981–988.

22. DeVore GR, Siassi B, Platt LD. Fetal echocardiogra-

phy: The prenatal diagnosis of tricuspid atresia (Type lc) during the second trimester of pregnancy. J Clin Ultrasound. 1987; 15:317–324.

23. ———. Fetal echocardiography. VIII. Aortic root dilatation—A marker for tetralogy of Fallot. Am J Obstet Gynecol. 1988; 159:129–136.

24. Emmanouilides GC, Baylen BG, Nelson RJ. Pulmonary atresia with intact ventricular septum. In: Adams FH, Emmanouilides GC, eds. Heart Disease in Infants, Children and Adolescents. 3rd ed. Baltimore: Williams & Wilkins; 1983; 263–270.

25. Feldt RH, Edwards WD, Puga FJ, et al. Atrial septal defects and atrioventricular canal. In: Adams FH, Emmanouilides GC, eds. Heart Disease in Infants, Children and Adolescents. 3rd ed. Baltimore: Williams & Wilkins; 1983; 118–133.

26. Freedom RM. Hypoplastic left heart syndrome. In: Adams FH, Emmanouilides GC, eds. Heart Disease in Infants, Children and Adolescents. 3rd ed. Baltimore: Williams & Wilkins; 1983; 411–421.

27. Gersony WM. Coarctation of the aorta. In: Adams FH, Emmanouilides GC, eds. Heart Disease in Infants, Children and Adolescents. 3rd ed. Baltimore: Williams & Wilkins; 1983; 188–198.

28. Graham TP, Bender HW, Spach MS. Ventricular septal defect. In: Adams FH, Emmanouilides GC, eds. Heart Disease in Infants, Children and Adolescents. 3rd ed. Baltimore: Williams & Wilkins; 1983; 134–153.

29. Guntheroth WG, Kawabori I, Baum D. Tetralogy of Fallot. In: Adams FH, Emmanouilides GC, eds. Heart Disease in Infants, Children and Adolescents. 3rd ed. Baltimore: Williams & Wilkins, 1983; 215–227.

30. Guntheroth WG, Cyr DR, Mack LA, et al. Hydrops from reciprocating AV tachycardia in a 27-week fetus requiring quinidine for conversion. Obstet Gynecol. 1985; 66:295–300.

31. Hertzberg BS, Mahoney BS, Bowie JD. First-trimester fetal cardiac activity. Sonographic documentation of a progressive early rise in heart rate. J Ultrasound Med. 1988; 7:573–575.

32. Huhta JC, Hagler DJ, Hill LM. Two-dimensional echocardiographic assessment of normal fetal cardiac anatomy. J Reprod Med. 1984; 29:162–167.

33. Huhta JC, Strasburger JF, Carpenter RJ, et al. Pulsed Doppler fetal echocardiography. J Clin Ultrasound. 1985; 13:247–254.

34. Jeanty P, Romero R, Hobbins JC. Fetal pericardial fluid: A normal finding of the second half of gestation. Am J Obstet Gynecol. 1984; 149:529–532.

35. Kenny JF, Plappert T, Doubilet P. Changes in intracardiac blood flow velocities and right- and left ventricular stroke volumes with gestational age in the normal human fetus: A prospective Doppler echocardiographic study. Circulation. 1986; 74:1208–1216.

36. Kleinman CS, Copel JA, Weinstein EM, et al. Treatment of fetal supraventricular tachyarrhythmias. J Clin Ultrasound. 1985; 13:265–273.

37. Kleinman CS, Donnerstein RL, DeVore GR, et al. Fetal echocardiography for evaluation of in utero congestive heart failure. N Engl J Med. 1982; 306:568–575.

38. Kleinman CS, Weinstein EM, Talner NS, et al. Fetal echocardiography—Applications and limitations. Ultrasound Med Biol. 1984; 10:747–755.

39. Lang P, Norwood WI. Hemodynamic assessment after palliative surgery for hypoplastic left heart syndrome. Circulation. 1983; 68:104–108.

40. Lange LW, Sahn DJ, Allen HD, et al. Qualitative real-time cross-sectional echocardiographic imaging of the human fetus during the second half of pregnancy. Circulation. 1980; 62:799–806.

41. Leithiser RE, Fyfe D, Weatherby III E, et al. Prenatal sonographic diagnosis of atrial hemangioma. AJR. 1986; 147:1207–1208.

42. Lingman G, Lundstrom N, Marsal K, et al. Fetal cardiac arrhythmia. Acta Obstet Gynecol Scand. 1986; 65:263–267.

43. Mair DD, Edwards WD, Fuster V, et al. Truncus arteriosus. In: Adams FH, Emmanouilides GC, eds. Heart Disease in Infants, Children and Adolescents. 3rd ed. Baltimore: Williams & Wilkins; 1983; 400–410.

44. Moore KL. The Developing Human: Clinically Oriented Embryology. 3rd ed. Philadelphia: WB Saunders, 1982.

45. Neill CA, Ursell P. Endocardial fibroelastosis and left heart hypopasia revisited. Int. J Cardiol. 1984; 5:547–550.

46. Nimrod C, Nicholson S, Machin G. In utero evaluation of fetal cardiac structure: A preliminary report. Am J Obstet Gynecol. 1984; 148:516.

47. Nora JJ. Etiologic aspects of heart disease. In: Adams FH, Emmanouilides GC, eds. Heart Disease in Infants, Children and Adolescents. 3rd ed. Baltimore: Williams & Wilkins; 1983; 2–10.

48. Norwood WI, Lang P, Hansen DD. Physiologic repair of aortic atresia: Hypoplastic left heart syndrome. N Engl J Med. 1983; 308:23–30.

49. Paul MH. Transposition of the great arteries. In: Adams FH, Emmanouilides GC, eds. Heart Disease in Infants, Children and Adolescents. 3rd ed. Baltimore: Williams & Wilkins; 1983; 296–332.

50. Reed KL, Meijboom EJ, Sahn DJ, et al. Cardiac Doppler flow velocities in human fetuses. Circulation. 1986; 73:41–46.

51. Reed KL, Sahn DJ, Scagnelli S, et al. Doppler echo-

cardiographic studies of diastolic function in the human fetal heart: Changes during gestation. J Am Coll Cardiol. 1986; 8:391–395.

52. Rudolph AM. Distribution and regulation of blood flow in the fetal and neonatal lamb. Circulation Res. 1985; 57:811–821.

53. Sahn DJ, Lange LW, Allen HD, et al. Quantitative real-time cross-sectional echocardiography in the developing normal human fetus and newborn. Circulation. 1980; 62:588–597.

54. Sahn DJ, Shenker L, Reed KL, et al. Prenatal ultrasound diagnosis of hypoplastic left heart syndrome in utero associated with hydrops fetalis. Am Heart J. 1982; 104:1368–1372.

55. Sharf M, Abinader EG, Shapiro I, et al. Prenatal echocardiographic diagnosis of Ebstein's anomaly with pulmonary atresia. Am J Obstet Gynecol. 1983; 147:300–303.

56. Silverman NH, Golbus MS. Echocardiographic techniques for assessing normal and abnormal fetal cardiac anatomy. J Am Coll Cardiol. 1985; 5:20S–29S.

57. Silverman NH, Enderlein MA, Golbus MS. Ultra- sonic recognition of aortic valve atresia in utero. Am J Cardiol. 1984; 53:391–392.

58. Silverman NH, Enderlein MA, Stanger P, et al. Recognition of fetal arrhythmias by echocardiography. J Clin Ultrasound. 1985; 13:255–263.

59. Sutton M, Raichlen JS, Reichek N, et al. Quantitative assessment of right and left ventricular growth in the human fetal heart: A pathoanatomic study. Circulation. 1984; 70:935–941.

60. Tonge HM, Wladimiroff JW, Noordam MJ. Fetal cardiac arrhythmias and their effect on volume blood flow in descending aorta of human fetus. J Clin Ultrasound. 1986; 14:607–612.

61. van Mierop LHS, Schiebler GL, Victoria BE. Ebstein's anomaly. In: Adams FH, Emmanouilides GC, eds. Heart Disease in Infants, Children and Adolescents. 3rd ed. Baltimore: Williams & Wilkins, 1983:283–295.

62. Wilson N, Reed K, Allen HD, et al. Doppler echocardiographic observations of pulmonary and transvalvular velocity changes after birth and during the early neonatal period. Am Heart J. 1987; 113:750–758.

C H A P T E R **17**

Assessment of Fetal Age and Size: Techniques and Criteria

Terry J. DuBose

A large portion of any obstetric sonographic examination involves measuring various parameters of the pregnancy. These measurements have two objectives: to determine the size and development of the fetus and to date the pregnancy. Both objectives are interrelated. Fetal size can be an indicator of the dates of the pregnancy, assuming the fetus is growing normally.

The estimated date of confinement (EDC) is the term generally used to indicate the expected birth date, and it is important for planning delivery, cesarean section, or termination, gauging growth, and suggesting whether or not the pregnancy is progressing normally. Fetal size is also an important indicator of fetal health. In general, reasonably large babies are considered healthier than relatively smaller babies of the same gestational age. Fetal measurements also provide information about the normalcy of fetal proportions. Performing multiple fetal measurements routinely establishes a method of fetal observation that reduces the possibility of omitting any important part of a normal examination.

This chapter provides an overview of fetal sizing and dating by sonographic measurements. A nomogram for estimating fetal size and age by multiple parameters is given on pages 280 to 281. The parameters discussed were selected because they are relatively accurate and easy to obtain. Several different measurements are presented because there

does not appear to be one magic parameter that is consistently accurate in all fetuses. (If there were one, variations in fetal position would often make it difficult to obtain.) Using more than one or two fetal parameters also improves the accuracy in assessing dates and fetal size.[30,39,51,76]

The earliest work in fetal sonographic biometry was reported by Dr. Ian Donald, of Glasgow, Scotland. In the late 1950s and early 1960s Dr. Donald used a borrowed A-mode scanner to measure gestational sacs and the biparietal diameters (BPDs) of fetal heads.[42,44] From this modest beginning it is now possible to find published reports of the sonographic measurement of virtually every major fetal organ, from head volume to the length from great toe to heel.

This chapter on sonographic fetal biometry describes the commonly used and most accurate fetal parameters. The physical principles and instrumentation that influence the measurement of these dimensions are also explained and advice is offered on how to obtain the most accurate measurements.

General Scanning Methodology and Use of Fetal Age Charts

All normal fetuses originate from a single fertilized egg and grow to a birth size that varies from infant to infant. The most accurate measurements of fetal age are those made early in the pregnancy, before individual growth patterns have had much effect on the fetus. Such individuation takes place later in gestation.

Although earlier measurements tend to produce the most accurate date, there has been some discussion in the literature of the efficacy of sonographic examinations during the first trimester for the sole purpose of dating when there is no other indication for the examination. This position was stated well by Dr. Roy Filly:

That a pregnancy can be more accurately dated, by any set of observations, in the first than in the early second trimester does not mean that it *should*. Too high a price is paid to gain a small advantage in age estimation. At 18 weeks, one can characterize a large number of important features of a pregnancy that cannot be judged at all in early pregnancy. . . . Despite the slightly improved accuracy of pregnancy dating in the first trimester, one is poorly advised to pursue pregnancy dating early unless there are other mitigating circumstances besides an uncertain menstrual history.[21]

Another point to be made about fetal size-age charts in general is that normal human fetuses tend to be uniform in morphology regardless of gene pool.[29,73,78] While there may be some differences in various normal growth parameters due to altitude, race, and other influences, any differences are small in most cases. This is especially true of the average fetus early in gestation. Variations in any single parameter's prediction of age will usually be less than ±4 weeks at term. This means that virtually any published chart derived from valid scientific methods can be used to estimate fetal age but it is very important that the user know how the measurements were generated to compose the chart. If, for example, the chart was created using BPD measurements that were taken from the outer edge to the inner edge of the skull, it will produce valid age estimates only if the BPD for the fetus being examined is measured the same way. In other words, if the sonographer does not know how the author of a particular chart made the measurements to produce that chart, then that chart is virtually useless.

There is some disagreement among experts in the field as to whether a parameter should be measured several times and averaged for the measurement of record[5] or whether the sonographer should make a single "correct" measurement.[45] The former of these two methods is preferred. Multiple measurements (three, four, or more) are made of any given parameter and are observed for a "cluster" with a range of less than 2 or 3 mm. Any measurements that fall outside the cluster range are discarded and the remaining measurements are averaged for the measurement of record.

There are generally two ways of listing age in fetal age charts. One is to list the estimated age in weeks and days; the other is to use weeks and tenths of weeks. Either method is valid. In this chapter the latter method is used because it is easier to compute average ages and to determine the number of weeks for serial studies using weeks and tenths. Also, using weeks and days implies an accuracy that sonography does not possess. In reality few sonographic parameters have an accuracy better than ±1 week. Fetal age is usually computed in "menstrual weeks" because of the historical precedent of using the date of the last menstrual period (LMP) for calculating the dates of the pregnancy. Normally conception takes place about 2 weeks after the LMP. Birth normally occurs 40 weeks from the LMP (a 38-week gestation ± 2 to 3 weeks). In this chapter embryonic and fetal ages are given as the number of weeks since the LMP, unless otherwise stated (i.e., 28 weeks LMP means the pregnancy is in the 28th week after the LMP).

Accuracy of Sonographic Measurements

The sonographer must understand that two resolution components govern a sonographic beam.[50,65,83] Axial resolution is one aspect of image resolution and the beam width is the other (Fig. 17-1). The image resolution determines the accuracy of measurements that can be achieved in any sonogram. Axial resolution governs any dimension that is measured along the axis or path of the beam; lateral resolution governs any dimension measured transversely, or across the path of the beam. The focal range of a sonographic transducer is the depth at which the sound beam width (lateral resolution) is narrowest or best focused.

Axial resolution is related directly to the frequency of the sound and the pulse length and re-

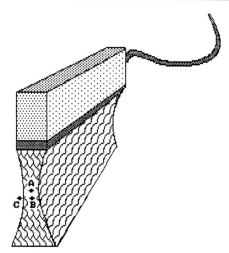

Points A and B are resolved AXIALLY.

Points C and B are resolved LATERALLY.

FIGURE 17-1. Sonographic beam resolution. An oblique view of a focused, linear-array, real-time sonographic beam. The two horizontal dots (B, C) represent echoes imaged with lateral resolution; the two vertical dots (A, B) represent echoes imaged with axial resolution. Note that dots A and C are about equal in distance from B. A and B will be resolved as separate echoes in the axial plane, but dots B and C may not be resolved as separate echoes, as the distance between them is equal to or less than the beam width.

production rate of those pulses producing the sonographic beam. Short and frequent pulses yield the greatest axial resolution. An ultrasound system cannot distinguish the echoes from two different structures separated by less than the length of a single pulse. This explains why transducers that produce higher-frequency sound usually produce shorter pulses, and therefore better axial resolution.[77] Accordingly, a sonographer should use the highest-frequency transducer that produces adequate penetration and diagnostic-quality images.

Lateral resolution is related to beam width. In general, it may be said that the wider the beam of sound is, the wider a single echo in the image will appear. It can also be said that an ultrasound system cannot separate echoes that are closer together than the width of the beam. A beam-width artifact tends to make measurement points a bit fuzzy.[80,87] Cursors should be placed at the edge of the most definite echo observed but should not include the beam width artifact (see Fig. 17-1).

It is important for the sonographer to understand how axial and lateral resolution affect fetal measurements with respect to the orientation of the fetal structure to the beam. Sonographers must be aware of whether the measurement being taken is in axial resolution or lateral resolution. In general, it is true that axial resolution produces the least measurement error while measurements taken transversely to the beam, or using lateral resolution, show the greatest errors. Usually only BPD and the diameters of the gestational sac and abdomen that are parallel to the beam can be easily obtained using axial resolution. Almost all other parameters are measured using lateral resolution and exhibit some indistinctness at the edges owing to beam width artifact. The sonographer must exercise judgment and skill when selecting the appropriate transducer, obtaining the images, and placing cursors if the greatest accuracy is to be obtained.

While any modern real-time transducer can be used effectively for fetal measurements, linear-array transducers, with their larger near field of view, make measurements easier to obtain in advanced pregnancy.[31] In early pregnancy (before 8 to 9 weeks LMP) transvaginal transducers provide much clearer images, especially in cases of ectopic pregnancy. Measurements can also be taken directly from the film, after the examination is completed, using a straightedge or dividers to compare the parameter or object of interest to the scale along the edges of the image.

Regardless which type of transducer is used to obtain measurements, it should be tested for accuracy. Sonographers can test for proper equipment function using an AIUM Standard Test Object or other acceptable sonographic phantoms. If measurements on the test object appear inaccurate, the machine should be recalibrated by an authorized service person. Generally, sonographic measurement errors in the range of 1 to 2% (1 or 2 mm/10 cm) can be expected.[64] Standard errors may be due to beam width, machine calibration, and interoperator cursor placement variation.[11,86]

Multiple Fetal Parameters Technique

Because all fetuses are proportioned differently, it must be recognized that any single fetal parameter, used alone, may not be as specific an indicator of fetal age as is desired, especially later in pregnancy. This can be important in serial studies for fetal growth and development, because in subsequent examinations fetal position or other changing conditions may preclude exact replication of fetal measurements used in earlier examinations. It has been found that in cases of premature rupture of the membranes, the external uterine pressure on the fetal skull can produce errors in the BPD and the transverse cephalic index 45% of the time.[53,69]

Other problems may occur in progressive diseases such as hydrocephalus or maternal diabetes. Figure 17-2 is a computer analysis of fetal parameters for a diabetic mother which illustrates the advantage of using multiple fetal parameters. If only one or two parameters are measured in routine examinations, then in the event of progressive diseases or changing conditions one may have difficulty making growth comparisons with subsequent examinations. For this reason it is recommended that the following measurements be obtained routinely as a minimum: head measurements, AC, and the length of at least one extremity long bone, preferably the femur. As a general rule, the more measurements that are taken, the more accurate the fetal age estimate will be.

In 1981, Bovicelli and coworkers suggested that using the combined crown-rump length (CRL) and BPD improved on the estimation of fetal age early in gestation. This study considered only the first trimester.[6] In 1983, Hadlock et al found that an average of the sonographically determined ages of multiple fetal parameters yielded a more accurate estimation of fetal age throughout gestation than any single parameter used alone. Hadlock's group used the average of four fetal parameters: BPD, transverse head circumference (THC), AC, and the femoral diaphysis length (FEM). They referred to this average age as the multiple fetal parameter (MFP) average age.[34,35] This research was replicated and confirmed in 1986 by Ott.[71]

There are two obvious reasons why an average of multiple fetal parameters is a more accurate indicator of fetal age than a single parameter. The first is that early in the gestation the fetal parameters are so small that any error in measurement due to the limits of resolution in the sonographic instrument used or to operator error will be relatively larger. The second reason is that late in gestation there is more molding of the fetal skull and individuation of fetal proportions (i.e., late in pregnancy some fetuses become relatively dolichocephalic and others more brachycephalic, some fatter, some thinner, some longer, and some shorter). Using multiple parameters tends to minimize the errors and average out normal individual variations.[12]

Inherent in the concept of estimating age from an average of MFPs is the idea that no single parameter is a perfect indicator of fetal age.[13,75] Since all people have slightly different proportions, it is unlikely that any single parameter is an absolutely correct predictor for all individual fetuses.

By using several parameters and determining the average age, sonographers can increase the accuracy of the fetal age estimate and avoid basing their complete judgment of how the fetus is developing on a single parameter that may turn out to be difficult to obtain or abnormal in subsequent examinations. Because all fetal parameters cannot be measured throughout pregnancy, the following chart (Table 17-1) can be used to determine which parameters are best used during progressive weeks of the pregnancy. While it may be possible to obtain many of these measurements earlier or later than this chart illustrates, the recommended times of parameter measurement are based on both the ease of obtaining the measurement and its relative accuracy. The use of transvaginal transducers may allow measurements 1 to 4 weeks earlier than the recommended weeks in this chart. The sonographer measures and calculates the age suggested by each parameter (Table 17-2).[16]

Measurement Techniques in the First Trimester

Gestational Sac Diameter (GSD)

The earliest measurement of the GSD for dating pregnancy was made by Ian Donald, using an average of three diameters.[42] The shape of the early gestational sac can vary greatly, depending on many factors such as presence of uterine fibroids, shape of the uterus (degree of retroflexion or anom-

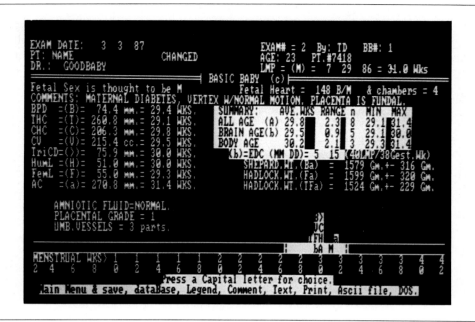

FIGURE 17-2. MFP and BBII. Computer-generated analysis of the fetus of a diabetic mother (names were changed). This case emphasizes the importance of using multiple fetal parameters (MFP). Age as determined by AC is ahead of age as determined by average brain size (cranial) by +1.9 weeks, which indicates a relatively fat fetus, but it is not greater than +2SD (see discussion of ARA). This discrepancy of size and age is easily observed in the time-series distribution plot of symbols at the bottom of the image. This diabetic patient delivered, by cesarean section, a 10-lb 5-oz, 22-inch boy on 5-7-87; EDC, 5-15-87 via average brain age (b). (BPD, biparietal diameter; THC, transverse head circumference; CHC, coronal head circumference; CV, cranial volume; TriCD, coronal head triangle circumference diameter; HumL, humeral length; FemL, femoral length; AC, abdominal circumference; LMP, last menstrual period weeks; EDC, estimated date of confinement; ave.wks, average ages of parameters; brain age, average ages of cranial parameters; range, difference between maximum and minimum age; n, number of parameter ages used in ave.wks and range; white bar above week line shows ± 2SD for age range analysis.)

alies), presence of pelvic pathology, and pressure from a full urinary bladder. Using transvaginal transducers avoids the latter problem but does not alleviate the effects of the other problems.

For these reasons the GSD measurements are seldom used routinely, and a more subjective approach to the early pregnancy is preferred.[54] If one can observe an intrauterine sac with a "double ring" sign (Fig. 17-3A), and if the human chorionic gonadotropin (HCG) titer is appropriate, an intrauterine gestation is presumed to exist. The pregnancy can be dated using the largest GSD diameter or the average of three diameters. It would seem that the average of three perpendicular diameters should improve the accuracy of the GSD measurement, but this is not necessarily the case.[8] GSD shape and interoperator variation in cursor placement are often problems.[60,86] More accurate dating can be done a few weeks later, when direct fetal measurements can be obtained.

When a single diameter is used, the longest inside GSD is measured. For a three-diameter aver-

Table 17-1. Measurements timetable

Name	Advantages	Disadvantages	Use	Accuracy*
Gestational sac diameter (GSD)	Can be obtained easily early in gestation	High variability of measurements; low accuracy	Before 12 wk LMP	± 2 wk
Crown-rump length (CRL)	Highest accuracy early in gestation; relatively easy to obtain	Not available after 1st trimester	7–15 wk LMP	± 3–5 days
Cranial three-dimensional average (3-D)	High accuracy in 2nd and 3rd trimester; encourages closer neurologic observation	Requires three measurements	10 wk LMP to term	± 1 wk
Cranial volume (CV)	Highest accuracy in 3rd trimester; encourages closer neurologic observation	Requires three measurements and complex calculations	10 wk LMP to term	± 1 wk
Transverse head circumference (THC)	Requires only two measurements; accepted as standard	Does not reflect vertical cranial diameter	10 wk LMP to term	± 1 wk
Biparietal diameter (BPD)	Easy to obtain; low interoperator variability	Affected by skull molding after 34 weeks LMP	9–33 wk LMP	± 2 wk
Abdominal circumference (AC)	Important for fetal weight estimates	Interoperator variability and fetal position may affect accuracy	12 wk LMP to term	± 2–2.5 wk
Femoral length (FEM)	Relatively easy to obtain	Fetal motion may make measurements difficult	14 wk LMP to term	± 2.2 wk
Humeral length (HUM)	Relatively easy to obtain	Fetal motion may cause difficulty; moderate to low accuracy	14 wk LMP to term	± 2.8 wk
Binocular distance (BiOD)	Occasionally easy to obtain when fetus faces up and BPD is difficult	Low accuracy; fetal position can make measurements impossible	15–30 wk LMP	± 3.3 wk

*The accuracy of fetal measurements varies inversely with fetal age. The stated accuracy is ± 2 standard deviations for older fetuses; deviations will be smaller for earlier gestations and should be used only as general rules of thumb.

age, three inside perpendicular diameters are used.

A rule of thumb is that the GSD, in centimeters, plus 4 nearly equals the age in menstrual weeks. Some authors use the GSD plus 3 cm.[60]

Crown-Rump Length (CRL)
Once the embryo is clearly visible in the gestational sac, its CRL can be measured. The CRL has been called "the single most accurate method of assessing fetal age because of its minimal biologic variation in size in the first trimester and the rapid growth of this measurement at this stage of pregnancy."[25] This measurement usually is considered accurate to within 3 to 5 days if it is properly taken in the first trimester.[88]

There are several different published CRL age charts. One of the most recent, by MacGregor and colleagues, was computed from known ovulation dates from fertility studies.[63] This study indicated that the best CRL charts underestimate fetal age by about 3 to 3.5 days. The authors of this new CRL chart proposed several theories to explain these differences: biologic differences, use of longitudinal data rather than cross-sectional data (one study), and variations in the length of the preovulatory phases. As more and more fetal parameters are reevaluated using known dates of ovulation or conception in fertility studies, more accurate charts should be developed. Another report has shown that the CRL age charts derived from transabdominal images are also valid for transvaginal measurements.[9]

Methods of Measuring Crown-Rump Length. The fetal CRL is measured from the top of the head to the bottom of the rump, excluding the legs (Figs. 17-3, 17-4). When measuring early in the first trimester (6 to 8 weeks LMP) the yolk sac (which will usually be very close to the fetal or embryonic pole) should not be included. The embryonic period of development lasts until the 8th gestational (10th menstrual) week. From that time until term the baby is a fetus, although the terms embryo and fetus are often used interchangeably.[66]

Identification of the body can easily be made if cardiac motion can be observed with real-time ultrasonography. In that case, simply take the longest diameter observed, excluding the yolk sac. If cardiac motion is not observed by the 7th or 8th week after the LMP, then viability of the pregnancy is questionable. A good rule of thumb is that the fetal pole should be visible when the gestational sac reaches 2.5 cm or greater as measured with modern real-time equipment.[56,67,68]

More accurate measurements can be made by enlarging the image as much as possible while keeping the entire CRL in view. This will make cursor placement easier and more uniform. The CRL is less accurate beyond the first trimester because of variations in fetal position and flexion. In addition, after 15 weeks the CRL exceeds the field of view of most transducers.

Measurement Techniques in the Second and Third Trimester

FETAL HEAD MEASUREMENTS

Biparietal Diameter (BPD). The fetal BPD has long been a primary sonographic indicator of fetal age and no doubt is written about more than any other single fetal parameter. This is because the BPD is usually easy to obtain, has a distinctive appearance, and provides a relatively accurate measurement.

The BPD measurement carries a small interobserver variance or error (usually less than 2 mm), but molding and normal morphologic variations of the fetal head also affect the BPD's accuracy as an indicator of fetal age. These effects tend to be greatest after the 33rd menstrual week of the pregnancy because this is the time of greatest extrinsic pressure on the fetal skull. It is the resulting fetal skull molding that makes the BPD a less accurate parameter for fetal age after that time. The BPD can also be affected by oligohydramnios, which can cause molding of the skull.[53,69,79]

A large number of BPD-age charts have been published. Two of the most notable were published by Sabbagha and Hughey (1978)[74] and by Kurtz and associates (1980).[55] The first study developed a composite BPD-age chart from four previously published ones. The second study by Kurtz's group was a historical review of 25 BPD charts published worldwide. By studying the methods used to produce each chart the investigators found that 17 were devised by sound scientific methods. They then used the data from the 17 studies to produce a single chart, which they estimated was valid for approximately 90% of the world's population. Both of these BPD charts produce virtually identical results, although Sabbagha and coworkers' gives a mean age result and Kurtz's gives a weeks' variation result. These two charts are probably the most widely used indicators of sonographic fetal age throughout the world today.

Most of the published BPD charts, including the ones discussed above, were created using leading edge measurements (outer to inner edges) of the skull obtained in a transverse view with a lateral approach (Figs. 17-5 to 17-7). The plane of this transverse view has been widely described. It produces very accurate measurements, because the leading edges of the parietal bones reflect very sharp, specular echoes enhanced by the axial resolution of the sound beam. As a result, the measurements are not only accurate but easy to obtain.

Measurement methods. The BPD can be measured routinely from 12 weeks' gestation, and occasionally earlier. The sonographer must first identify the fetal lie. Beginning at the base of the fetal cranium the sonographer locates the base X formed by the

TABLE 17-2. Correlation of fetal parameters with age

LMP Weeks	GSD (MM)	CRL (MM)	BPD (MM)	THC (MM)	CHC (MM)	CV (CC)	AC (MM)	FSL (MM)	FEM (MM)	HUM (MM)	BiOD (MM)	LMP Weeks
3	3											3
4	10	2										4
5	16	4										5
6	23	5.9										6
7	30	10	5.7	17	12	0.06						7
8	37	16	8	26	20	0.17	25					8
9	46	25	11	36	28	0.62	31		3	3	6	9
10	56	36	14	47	36	1.3	38		4	4	9	10
11	68	45	17	58	44	2	46		5	5	11	11
12	80	58	20	69	53	4	55	11	7	6	13	12
13	89	71	24	81	63	7	67	13	10	9	15	13
14	97	80	27	93	74	11	78	15	13	12	18	14
15	104	93	31	106	85	15	89	17	16	16	20	15
16	110	102	34	119	95	21	100	20	19	19	23	16
17	117	113	38	131	105	28	113	22	23	22	25	17
18	125	123	41	144	114	36	124	25	26	26	27	18
19		132	44	155	123	45	136	28	29	29	29	19
20		138	47	165	130	55	146	30	32	31	31	20
21		146	50	176	138	67	158	32	34	33	33	21
22			53	189	147	81	168	34	37	36	35	22
23			57	201	156	99	180	37	39	38	37	23
24			61	212	165	117	192	39	42	40	39	24
25			64	223	173	134	203	41	45	42	41	25
26			66	234	181	151	213	43	47	44	42	26
27			69	243	188	170	221	45	50	45	44	27
28			72	251	195	189	230	47	52	47	45	28
29			74	259	201	207	240	49	54	49	47	29
30			76	268	208	227	250	52	56	50	48	30
31			79	277	214	250	261	54	58	52	49	31
32			81	286	221	271	273	56	61	55	51	32
33			83	293	226	292	284	59	64	57	53	33
34			85	300	231	313	296	61	66	58	54	34
35			87	306	236	336	308	63	68	61	56	35
36			89	313	241	358	322	65	71	62	57	36
37			91	321	247	379	336	67	73	64	59	37
38			93	327	252	401	350	69	75	65	60	38
39			95	336	257	424	361	71	77	66	62	39
40			97	343	263	454	370	73	78	68	64	40
41			100	351	269	481	376	74	80	70	66	41
42			102	358	275	509	382	75	82	71	67	42

Summary:

PARAMETER	GSD	CRL	BPD	THC	CHC	CV	AC	FSL	FEM	HUM	BiOD	3D BPD
LMP AGE)	|	|	|	|	|	|	|	|	|	|	|	|

Total of *all* ages = _____ Total of *cranial* ages = _____
Divide by *n* measurements: *n* = _____ Divide by *n* (cranial) = _____
Average of all ages = _____ Average cranial age = _____
Range: Maximum age — minimum age = Range of ages = _____
Relative fetal weight estimation: Location in normal distribution.
AC age — Cranial age = _____ dist. location ($\pm$ 2SD $\simeq$ 10% cranial age)

(DuBose T. J. Basic Baby Fetal Age Database: BASIC BABY: Instruction Manual. Austin, TX: (Mind's Eye Images; 1987) BBII Fetal Age Table 1987. Used with permission.

Table 17-2. *(continued)*

Instructions: Take measurements and calculate the values.
Circle the values and enter ages below the columns.

Calculations:
All circumferences are calculated from two diameters: Circ. $= (d_1 + d_2) \times 1.57$. The CV requires three diameters:
BPD, FOD, & VCD (in mm) to obtain approximate volume (in cc) from one of two formulas below:
1. $CV \simeq (\{([FOD + BPD + VCD]/60)^3\} \times 4.189)$
   or, to use the more standard volume formula (mm to cc):
2. $CV \simeq 0.5236 \times (BPD \times FOD \times VCD) \times 0.00106 \simeq 0.000555 \times BPD \times FOD \times VCD$.
   For 3-D BPD correction: Average FOD, BPD, & VCD = BPD age = 3-D age.

Age Range Analysis (ARA):
Sum ages and divide by the number of ages for *average age* (AA). *Cranial age* may be substituted for AA in order to
exclude comparative parameter.

Age range = Maximum age − Minimum age.

Relative fetal parameter age (PA) location in normal distribution:
$(PA - AA)/(AA \times 0.05) \simeq$ Standard deviations location (2SD $\simeq$ 20% age, i.e., $\pm$10%).

If AC age is equal to the *cranial average age* then AC age − cranial average age will equal 0, which puts the relative
weight at the mean of the normal distribution. If the difference is >10% of the cranial average age then the weight
estimate will be above +2SD; if the difference is <10% of the cranial average age then the weight estimate is below
−2SD. $\pm$1SD will be approximately 5% of the cranial average age or AA. ARA for fetal length: The same concept
will work when comparing the FEM age to the cranial average age to estimate relative fetal length.

Following are descriptions of each of the measurements in Table 17-2.

GSD	Gestation sac diameter (mm)	= largest single inside diameter
CRL	Crown-rump length (mm)	= Crown-to-rump length; do not include legs
BPD	Biparietal diameter (mm)	= Leading edge to leading edge (outer to inner)
THC	Transverse head circumference	= (BPD + FOD) × 1.57; BPD as above + longest skull diameter (FOD, mid-edge to mid-edge)
CHC	Coronal head circumference	= (BPD + VCD) × 1.57; BPD as above + vertical skull diameter (mid-HBL to midvertex)
CV	Cranial volume (cc)	= $(\{([BPD + FOD + VCD]/60)^3\} \times 4.189)$
3-D BPD	3-D BPD correction	= (BPD + FOD + VCD)/3 = BPD
AC	Abdominal circumference (mm)	= (Transverse abdominal diameter + AP abdominal diameter) × 1.57
FSL	Fractional spine length	= Fractional spine length (mm) (7 thoracolumbar vertebral bodies & spaces)
FEM	Femur length (mm)	= Diaphysis (osseous shaft)
HUM	Humerus length (mm)	= Diaphysis (osseous shaft)
BiOD	Binocular distance (mm)	= Distance between outer edges of the ocular globes

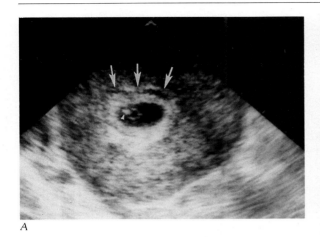

A

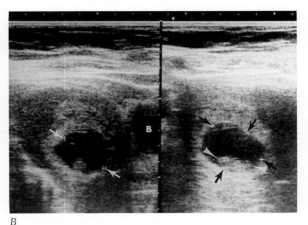

B

Figure 17-3. GSD. (A) Transvaginal scan of a normal 5.1-week (LMP) gestational sac with a double-ring sign (*arrows*). The small, circular yolk sac can be seen adjacent to the embryonic pole (*small arrowhead*). The largest diameter of the sac is 15.7 mm; and the CRL of the embryonic pole is 4.0 mm, both of which are the equivalent of 5.1 weeks. The embryonic heart rate (FHR) was measured at 97 beats per minute by motion mode using the transvaginal transducer. The FHR correlates with 5.0 weeks LMP. (B) Linear array split image demonstrating the three-dimensional measurement of a gestational sac (GS). The left side image, a midsagittal plane view, shows the uterus, maternal urinary bladder (B), and one dimension of the GS (*white arrows*). The right side image is a transverse plane with cephalic angulation making it perpendicular to the measurement on the sagittal (left) image. Two dimensions of the GS are measured in the right image (*black arrows*); a valid CRL was also obtained from the right image (*white arrowheads*). The three GSD measurements resulted in a mean GSD of 30 mm, or 7.0 weeks LMP. The single largest GSD was 39 mm, or 7.8 weeks. The CRL was 18.0 mm, or 8.1 weeks; BPD was 7.3 mm, or 8.3 weeks; the CV was 0.2 cc, or 8.1 weeks; the FHR was 169 beats per minute, or 8.2 weeks; and the average age for five cranial and for all eight parameters was 8.2 weeks LMP, with a range of ages from 7.8 to 8.7 weeks.

sphenoid bones (bilateral anteriorly) and petrous bones (bilateral posteriorly) (see Fig. 17-6A). The proper plane for the BPD lies parallel to and above this base X.[1,7,23] From the base X scans are made progressively higher in the head, always parallel to the plane of the base X and keeping the midline of the hemispheres equidistant from the parietal bones, until the thalamus and cavum septi pellucidi are located.[1,7,12,23,53] For an optimal measurement, the entire calvarium should be seen as a complete oval. A transverse plane that includes the top of the cerebellum is too low in the posterior portion of the image (Figs. 17-6B,C).[64]

The BPD is measured using *outer to inner* or *leading edge to leading edge* of the fetal parietal bones which form the lateral walls of the skull (Figs. 17-5 to 17-7). The BPD is measured at the widest transverse diameter of the skull, just above the ears. The view for the BPD measurement should be made perpendicular to the interhemispheric fissure (midline) in either the transverse or coronal plane and should include the thalamus (see Figs. 17-5 to 17-7).[1,7,12,22,23] When measuring from the leading edge of the parietal bone the soft tissue of the scalp should be excluded (see Figs. 17-6, 17-7). Lowering the system gain helps distinguish soft tissue from (*Text continues on page 287.*)

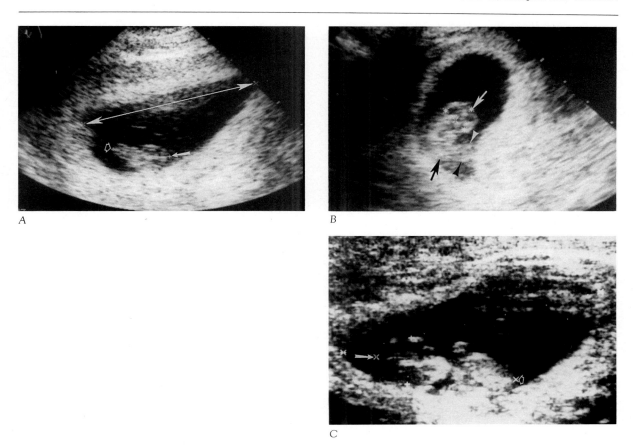

FIGURE 17-4. CRL. (A) Transabdominal, real-time, sector image of a gestational sac containing an 8.3-week embryo. The largest GSD (X's at each end of long, double arrow) and CRL were taken from this image (crown, *small, white arrow;* rump, *open white arrow*). The coronal head and interhemispheric fissure are well-demonstrated. The average age of seven parameters was 8.3 weeks LMP, with a range of 8.0 (CRL) to 8.7 (GSD); the FHR was 159 beats per minute, which correlated to 7.7 weeks LMP. The cranial volume (CV) was approximately 0.2 cc, or 8.1 weeks LMP. (B) Transvaginal scan of an 8.2-week LMP embryo in a coronal view. The CRL (*arrows*) measured 18.7 mm, which indicates 8.2 weeks LMP. The electronic calipers are marking the coronal triangle and vertical cranial diameter (VCD). The umbilical cord (*arrowheads*) is relatively large at this early age. Seven fetal parameters were evaluated for age during this examination as follows in weeks LMP: GSD, 8.1; CRL, 8.2; BPD, 8.6; THC, 8.4; CHC, 8.2; CV, 8.2; TriCD, 8.6; and FHR 177 beats per minute, 8.4 weeks. The average age of all seven parameters and the five head parameters were 8.3 and 8.4 weeks, respectively; age range was 0.4 weeks between the minimum and maximum parameter ages. The reported LMP was 8.4 weeks prior to the examination. (C) Transabdominal, linear-array image of the CRL (*arrows*) of a 9.7-week LMP embryo; the CRL was 32 mm or 9.9 weeks LMP. The white arrow points to the fetal head, in which the midline can be seen. The open arrow marks the rump. The crosshatches measure this BPD as 12.2 mm, or 9.6 weeks. The CRL was 32.0 mm, or 9.9 weeks. The average age using nine parameters was 9.7 weeks LMP, with an overall range from 9.1 weeks (THC) to 10.2 weeks (GSD). The CV was 1.1 cc, or 10.0 weeks.

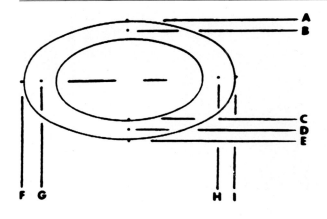

FIGURE 17-5. Transverse head. Line drawing demonstrates the sites that have been used by various authors for fetal head measurements.[17,71] This stylized rendering of a transverse section of the fetal skull shows the points that can be used for BPD and FOD measurements. Middle of frontal calvariam echo to middle of accipital calvariam echo FOD measurements are indicated by points G to H; leading edge–to–leading edge BPDs are indicated by A to C. The transverse cephalic index (ratio BPD:FOD) of these measurements is similar to that ratio using *all* outer edge–to–outer edge measurements. Algebraically, this is stated: AE/FI = BD/GH, and AC = BD; therefore, AE/FI = AC/GH. (From DuBose TJ. Fetal biometry: Vertical calvarial diameter and calvarial volume. J Diagn Med Sonogr. 1985;1:205–217.)

FIGURE 17-6. Various transverse heads. (A) Scan of the base of the fetal skull shows the base **X** formed by the bilateral sphenoid bones (S) anteriorly and the bilateral petrous (P) bones posteriorly. This plane is parallel to the plane of the transverse head circumference (THC) but is much too low for a BPD measurement. The plane is perpendicular to the plane of the coronal head circumference (CHC).[1,6,7,17] The optic chiasm (hypoechoic **X**) and pons can be observed at the center of the image. (B) A scan taken slightly higher in the fetal skull but still too low in the posterior skull for a BPD measurement. The cerebellum (*white arrows*) can be seen in the posterior portion of the skull between the petrous bones (P). (C) The anterior aspect of the image is too low for a valid BPD measurement. This can be determined because the sphenoid bone over the orbit of the eye (O) is visualized. The top of the cerebellum is between the arrows. (D) The correct plane for a BPD measurement. This is confirmed by the central midline and the visualization of the thalamus (*white arrows inside skull*) and the cavum septi pellucidi (S). Note that in this image the frontal bone is on the right near the cavum septi pellucidi (*white arrowhead*). The BPD leading edge–to–leading edge measurement is indicated by the wide, black arrows. The FOD, taken from the middle of the echo from the edge of the frontal bone (*solid white, wide arrow*) to the middle of the echo from the edge of the occipital bone (*open wide arrow*) is also shown. The very narrow "double midline" of the third ventricle (*white arrowhead*) lies at the exact center of the thalamus. (E) Scan is too high in the skull for a BPD measurement, as demonstrated by the long, continuous midline and absence of the midbrain structures.

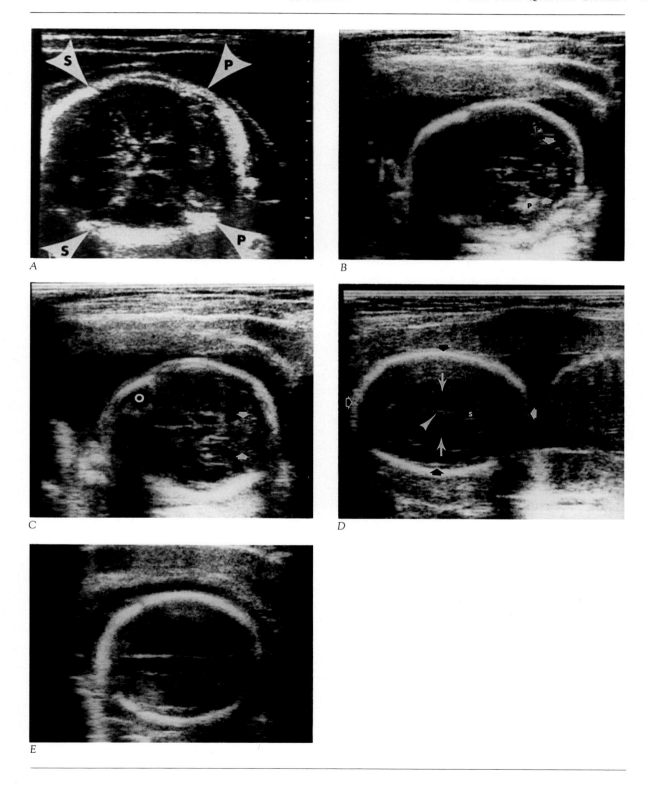

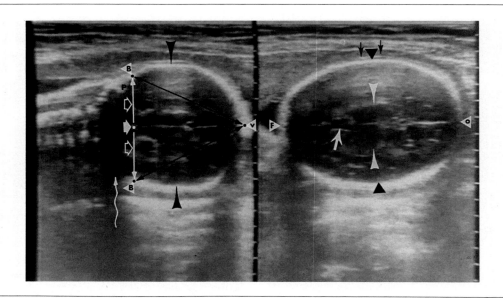

FIGURE 17-7. 3-D cranial measurement. A split linear-array image of the coronal view of the head on the left and the transverse view on the right. The right image shows the correct plane for the BPD; thalamus *(white arrowheads inside skull)* and the cavum septi pellucidi *(white arrow)*. The BPD is measured from leading edge-to-leading edge (black triangles) of the parietal bones. The two small, black arrows mark the scalp. The FOD is measured between the white triangles (F, frontal; O, occipital). The left image is a coronal image showing the measurement of the vertical cranial diameter (VCD), which is between the vertex of the skull (white triangle with v) and the base of the skull *(wide, white arrow)*. The VCD is the height of a triangle described by the white triangles (B-B-V). The base of the triangle is an imaginary line (B-B) (hippocampal baseline, HBL), which is tangential to the circles around the bilateral hippocampal gyri *(open arrows)* and the tops of the petrous bones (P), which cause the acoustic shadow *(wavy arrow)*. The VCD is measured from the midpoint of the HBL along the interhemispheric fissure to the vertex of the skull.[17] The coronal circumference around the triangle (B-B-V) will be a nearly perfect circle in normally shaped heads, and its diameter (TriCD) will be equal to the BPD *(black arrowheads)*.[16-18] The computation for the circumference around the triangle and its diameter is a complex mensuration formula that is best left to computers.[3] The anechoic bodies of the lateral cerebral ventricles can be seen fitting snugly in the apex of the coronal triangle. The average of the BPD, FOD, and VCD is equal to the BPD in normally shaped heads. This three-dimensional average has been called the three-dimensional BPD correction and will yield more accurate dates near term than the BPD or THC used alone.[18] The three-dimensional average can be used in a standard BPD fetal age table for fetal ages near term, regardless of the skull shape or molding.

bone; the bone echoes persist at lower gain settings.

If the fetus' face is turned directly toward or away from the maternal spine or if the fetus' head is low in the pelvis, behind the maternal pubic bone, measurement of the BPD may be difficult. When the fetus' head is low in the pelvis a slight Trendelenburg position (maternal pelvis elevated, head lowered) sometimes helps to bring the head out of the mother's pelvis. The fetus may move to a more convenient position in response to the mother's changing position or if the sonographer proceeds with other parts of the examination and returns later to try the measurement again. As uncooperative as fetuses may be, an experienced sonographer should be able to obtain accurate measurements at least 95% of the time and satisfactory measurements 100% of the time. In the rare event of an extremely uncooperative fetus, the sonographer is fortunate that there are several other fetal parameters that also serve as adequate indicators of fetal age. If the fetal head is very low in the pelvis transvaginal transducers may allow BPD measurements; however, in these cases molding of the fetal skull is more likely to make the BPD inaccurate for age.

The accuracy of the predictive value of the BPD has been reported by some authors as ±3 weeks from 29 weeks LMP to term[79]; however, many consider the BPD accurate (±2 weeks) until about 33 weeks LMP.[53] Consequently, if the BPD is going to be used to estimate fetal age, the measurement should be performed before 33 weeks LMP.[53]

A good rule of thumb for determining fetal age from the BPD is as follows[85]: When BPD is less than 75 mm, fetal age in weeks after LMP is equal to (BPD + 15)/3; when BPD is more than 75 mm, fetal age is equal to (BPD − 15)/2. These rule-of-thumb formulas are generally accurate to within ±1 week for a menstrual age when compared to measurements provided by nomograms.

Transverse Head Circumference. The transverse head circumference (THC) was first suggested as an indicator of fetal age by Levi and Erbsman in 1975.[57] Many authors have suggested that the BPD may be inaccurate owing to normal variations in head shape and molding.[32,43,57] The rationale for more accurate measurements using the THC rather than a single diameter, such as the BPD, exists because the fetal skull and its contents are fluids and solids. The consistency of the fetal head has been referred to as plastic.[20] Normally there are no compressible free gases in the fetal body. Since, for our purposes, fluids and solids do not compress, when external pressure is placed upon one axis of the fetal head it must be displaced and exaggerated along another axis. If pressure against the external lateral wall(s) of the skull shortens the BPD, then the long and/or vertical axis will be displaced and lengthened. Likewise, if the long and/or vertical axis is compressed, the width (BPD) of the skull will be enlarged to compensate. Therefore, two-dimensional circumferences of the fetal skull are more accurate than one-dimensional diameters, and three-dimensional measurements are more accurate than two-dimensional ones.[53]

The long axis diameter of the fetal skull has been called by various names: frontooccipital diameter (FOD),[1,23,33,53] occipitofrontal diameter (OFD),[40,79] longitudinal dimension,[32] and long skull diameter (LSD).[12,13]

Hadlock and colleagues[38] found that using the two diameters in the formula for the circumference resulted in essentially the same measurement as direct outlining methods, if the BPD and FOD are measured outer edge–to–outer edge. Because many outlining methods are tedious and slow, the use of the two diameters to calculate the circumference is generally recommended. Whatever method is employed, a chart that was generated using the same method and formula for estimating fetal age should also be used (see Table 17-2). If one wishes to measure the THC using the perimeter tracing method, the measurement should be made around the outer edge of the calvarium. Table 17-2 is not recommended for fetal age determination with the tracing method, because the THC there was generated from leading edge–to–leading edge BPDs and mid-edge–to–mid-edge FODs.[24] The same anatomic landmarks should be seen in the transverse section where the FOD is measured as in the BPD section. This transverse view should include the cavum septi pellucidi, interhemispheric fissure (midline), and thalamus. The greatest source of error in measuring the THC is selection of an improper plane; this produces a measurement that is less than the greatest THC. A shortened THC measurement can result if the proper transverse plane is not used (see Fig. 17-6).

Measurement methods. The THC can be measured directly from the photographed image using a map measurer (planimeter) or by using a track ball or joy stick to trace the outline of the skull on the display screen. If these direct circumference outlining methods are inconvenient or unavailable, the BPD and long axis diameter or FOD can be measured and used to calculate the circumference. The average of two diameters of the fetal skull, the BPD and long axis, is used in the following formula for the circumference of a circle:

$$\text{Circumference} = (d_1 + d_2)/2 \times \pi$$
$$= (d_1 + d_2) \times 1.57,$$

where d_1 and d_2 represent the two diameters and the constant, π, is 3.14159.

The FOD has been measured two ways, outer edge–to–outer edge or middle of frontal calvariam echo to middle of accipital calvariam echo (Fig. 17-5).[12,79] Because the use of outer edge–to–outer edge FOD measurements results in a slightly larger variance than the use of the middle of echo to middle of echo FOD, the latter method is recommended.[12] This larger variance in the outer to outer measurements is thought to be due to the inclusion of the beam width artifact or lateral resolution of the beam, which causes a bit of fuzziness to the echoes from the edges of the frontal and occipital bones.[38]

Cephalic Index. The cephalic index (CI = BPD/ FOD × 100) is used to determine the shape of the fetal skull and the reliability of the BPD; however, the CI does not address the variation of the vertical axis of the head.[13] Usually the CI is approximately 80% (±10%) in about 95% of fetuses. These percentages vary somewhat from investigator to investigator, depending on how the head measurements are taken.[12,32,48,53]

A fetus whose CI is below normal (<70%) is called dolichocephalic; the head is relatively long and narrow. A fetus whose BPD is relatively wide and whose FOD is short is called brachycephalic; the CI is greater than normal (>90%). Other fetal head dysmorphisms are acrocephaly, turricephaly, and oxycephaly, in all of which the vertical diam-

eter of the cranium is greater than normal.[14] Oxycephaly can be associated with various forms of craniostosis in which the various calvarium bones prematurely fuse (ossification) at the sutures[70] and with premature rupture of membranes.[53,69] An apparent reverse oxycephaly is called platycephaly. It may occur late in pregnancy or when crowding of the fetus puts pressure on the vertex of the skull, causing shortening of the vertical dimension of the skull and widening of the transverse diameters, which may not affect the CI.

Three-Dimensional Head Measurements and Calculations. By using the BPD, FOD, and vertical cranial diameter (VCD) in a formula for the volume of a sphere, an approximate cranial volume (CV) can be obtained that is more closely correlated with the fetal age than BPD or THC, but this formula is more difficult to calculate and is less desirable for routine use without a computer (see Figs. 17-2, 17-7, and Table 17-2).[3,12,53]

A new method that is easier to calculate than the CV and is as accurate is the simple average of the three diameters of the skull[12,14] (see Fig. 17-7):

$$\text{3-D} = (\text{BPD} + \text{FOD} + \text{VCD})/3$$

It is coincidental that this three-dimensional average of the fetal skull (3-D) is equal to the BPD in normally shaped heads (ratio of BPD/3-D = 0.99, ±2SD = 0.08).[14] This means that if the head is abnormally shaped due to morphologic variation or normal molding the 3-D average will be equal to a "corrected BPD" for that fetus, regardless of degree of brachycephaly, dolichocephaly, oxycephaly, or platycephaly.[10,12,14,43,49,53,65,69,70] This assumes, of course, that the head is simply abnormally shaped and not microcephalic or megalocephalic. The 3-D average can be used to correlate with the estimated fetal age on a standard BPD chart.[14]

The average 3-D BPD correction is more accurate than the BPD or the THC for estimating fetal age but not significantly more accurate if the fetus has a normally shaped head. This method is most useful for obviously abnormal head shapes and is particularly useful after about 33 to 35 weeks LMP or with premature rupture of membranes, when the head is more likely to be molded. If accuracy of fetal dates and growth are important in serial studies then this method is recommended for routine use.

Measurement methods. The coronal view of the fetal skull used for the VCD measurement is perpendicular to the transverse plane used for the BPD and FOD. The VCD is measured from the middle of the echo from the edge of the vertex of the skull to the midpoint of an imaginary line that is tangential to the bases of the circles around the bilateral hippocampal gyri (hippocampal baseline or HBL; see Fig. 17-7). This imaginary line is also in the plane of the base X (see Fig. 17-6A).[1,7,12,23]

The anatomic structures that are often visualized with this view are the interhemispheric fissure (falx cerebri), the body of the corpus callosum, the bodies and temporal horns of the lateral ventricles, the third ventricle, the thalamus, the petrous and squamous portions of the temporal bones, the midbrain and superior brain stem, the pons, the hippocampus, amygdala, both parietal bones, and the cervical spine. This coronal plane may be used to obtain five different dimensions of the fetal skull (see Fig. 17-7). The coronal view is obtained simply by rotating the transducer from the transverse view of the fetal skull to the vertical view.

FETAL BODY MEASUREMENTS

Abdominal Circumference. AC is a valuable indicator of fetal growth, because it reflects the development of abdominal organs such as the liver and spleen. Few other fetal parameters are so often mismeasured, however, as is the AC. Since most modern formulas for estimating fetal weight rely heavily on this measurement, its importance cannot be overemphasized. Abdominal measurements can also be affected by the degree of spinal flexion, fetal breathing motions, technique, and accurate visualization of the skin line.

The measurement of the AC at the standard cross-sectional level of the confluence of the umbilical and portal veins is usually the largest transverse section of the abdomen and is also reflective of the size of the liver and spleen, which are indicators of fetal health and well-being. The liver is proportionally larger in the fetus than in the adult.[26,28] The AC also reflects the subcutaneous fat, which has a large influence on fetal weight. For these reasons the AC is more important as an in-

dicator of fetal weight and health than as an indicator of fetal age.[72]

Measurement methods. The standard view for obtaining the AC is at the level of the umbilical vein junction with the portal vein and perpendicular to the spine.[41] The AC should also be circular in shape. If the plane used to measure the AC is oblique to the spine, one axis will be elongated, erroneously resulting in a measurement that is too large.

A successful measuring technique for obtaining the fetal AC is to first visualize the long axis of the fetal spine. After the lie of the spine is observed, the transducer field of view is turned perpendicular to the midportion of the spine; the fetal stomach and umbilical vein are then located. The favored view will demonstrate the confluence of the umbilical and portal veins in the fetal liver, called the "hockey stick" view by some authorities because the configuration of the veins form a curved shape similar to that of a hockey stick (see Fig. 17-8). If these veins cannot be visualized owing to fetal position or obesity, then a section demonstrating the fluid-filled fetal stomach is acceptable. It is important, however, when using the stomach as a landmark, to not mistake fluid in the lower gastrointestinal tract for the stomach. Measurements above or below the standard hockey stick view may produce an erroneously small AC.[41] Visualization of the fetal kidneys is an indication that the section is too low for accurate AC measurement.[58] The lower ribs may be observed bilaterally and, if seen, should be symmetric.

After the view is obtained and the image frozen, two perpendicular abdominal diameters are obtained. Both are measured from the outer skin lines. The transverse abdominal diameter (TAD) is measured from side to side and the anteroposterior abdominal diameter (AAD) is taken from the skin line above the umbilical cord insertion to the skin line just behind the spine. Care must be taken to measure to the skin line so that the resulting circumference is not underestimated. Acoustic shadowing from extremities or the spine can also make the skin line difficult to see in some segments of the AC. It often helps to look at the "full circle" of the abdomen rather than to focus attention on a single area. Measurements should be taken several times and observed for a cluster range, eliminating any

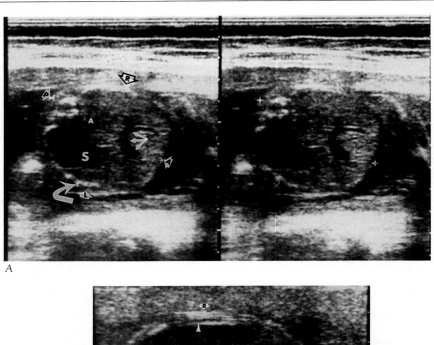

A

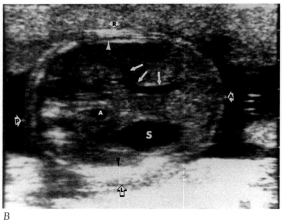

B

FIGURE 17-8. AC. (A) The abdomens seen in Figure 17-8A are nearly perfect circles. The anteroposterior abdominal diameter (AAD) is indicated by the wide white arrows with A and P. The transverse abdominal diameter (TAD, left) is actually measured incorrectly to the edge of a rib *(curved arrow)* rather than to the more appropriate skin line *(white arrows* L and R). The fluid-filled stomach (S) lies just distal to the fetal spine. The umbilical-portal vein confluence is marked by the three white arrows. (B) The AC appears slightly elongated front to back, owing to compression between the placenta and the maternal spine. Good judgment had to be exercised to be sure that the plane of section in Figure 17-8B was appropriate and not simply an oblique plane. The confluence of the umbilical and portal veins is marked by three white arrows. The AC measurement in this image was 177.4 mm, or 22.2 weeks LMP, which is −0.1 week less than the average brain (cranial) age. This would place the approximate fetal weight very near the 50th percentile of normal weights for a 22.3-week LMP fetus and was well within −1 SD of fetal weights.

measurements falling outside of the "best" cluster. The best measurements are then averaged for the measurements of record.

While ACs have been measured and calculated using the same techniques as the THC, some trace the circumference directly on the image and others use two diameters and the formula for the circumference of a circle. The two-diameter calculation of the circle circumference method is recommended here for the same reasons as for the THC: The results are similar and tracing the circumference is tedious, time consuming, and subject to operator error. The formula is:

$$AC = 1.57 \times (d_1 + d_2),$$

where d_1 and d_2 are the two diameters of the abdomen. The resulting AC will be in the same units as the diameters (i.e., diameters measured in millimeters will yield an AC in millimeters).

Sonographers should be sure that the measurements extend to the outer abdominal wall and not just to the peritoneum. This error is most common when a lateral approach to the abdomen is used and when positioning the caliper for the distal abdominal wall. The peritoneal cavity wall and ribs often generate very strong specular echoes. Errors of this type result in underestimation of the AC by excluding the hypoechoic skin, muscle, and baby fat from the measurement (see Fig. 17-8).

FETAL EXTREMITIES MEASUREMENTS

Long Bones. The fetal long bones are also good indicators of fetal growth. Although the head and abdomen may be subject to changes in shape due to molding or position, the long bones are not. A limiting factor in using long bones for measurements is that they are affected by the genetic pool; tall parents tend to have long babies. The accuracy of the humerus, tibia, and ulna measurements in predicting fetal age are considered to be approximately ± 3 weeks at term, and for the femur, about ± 2.2 weeks near term, and less earlier in gestation.[47] Fetal femur length has been shown to correlate both with fetal age and crown-heel length at birth.[36]

Visualization and measurement of any fetal long bone or other linear structure with sonography requires some mental gymnastics involving eye-hand coordination. The greatest source of error in measuring any long bone occurs when the transducer is positioned slightly oblique rather than along the axis of the bone and does not include both ends of the bone. An attempt to exclude the effects of beam width artifacts at the ends of linear structures must be made whenever measurements are being taken.

Femoral Length (FemL). The femur is among the most commonly used parameters for estimating fetal age and may be more accurate than the BPD late in pregnancy.[47,84] It is usually called a femur length measurement (FemL), but this is a misnomer. The femoral measurement generally used in obstetric sonography is actually the length of the osseous femoral diaphysis, or shaft, of the bone. This measurement does not include the femoral head or the condyles. In Figure 17-9 a small but distinct echo is visible continuing from the shaft toward the distal end of the femoral condyles. This echo is not a beam width artifact. It is a specular echo reflected from the edge of the epiphyseal cartilage, which Goldstein, Filly, and Simpson have called the distal femur point (DFP).[27] The DFP is always seen on the side of the condyles nearest the transducer and should not be included in the diaphysis measurements.

Measurement methods. To locate the femur, it is first necessary to determine the fetal position (head, spine, and rump). The sonographer can locate the femurs by scanning transversely along the spine until the echogenic, obliquely oriented iliac bones are visible. Then the transducer is moved along the iliac bone until the echogenic linear echo produced by the femur is seen. Once the femur's general location is identified, it becomes necessary to angle the transducer until a symmetric linear echo with a clean acoustic shadow is generated. The femur may have a slightly curved or bowed appearance, but this does not normally affect its size.[27] In Figure 17-9 the correct measurement does not include the DFP and is between the wavy arrows, which also demarcate the acoustic shadow. For more detailed instruction see Chapter 25.

Humeral Length. The humerus nearest to the transducer is usually easy to find in relationship to the head and spine, but the humerus away from the transducer is often obscured by the fetal ribs or spine. The humerus has similar measurements to

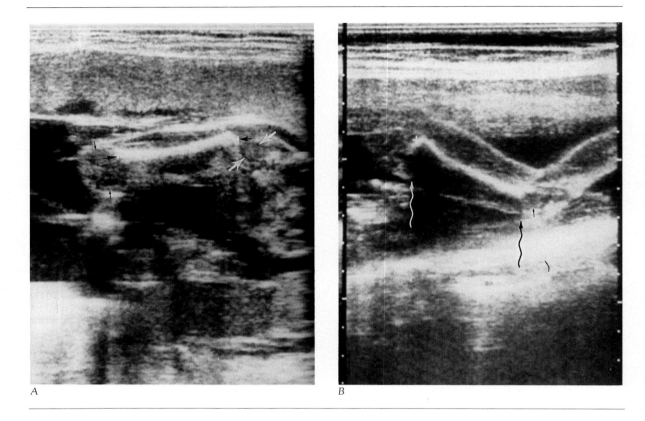

A   *B*

FIGURE 17-9. FemL. Coronal (A) and sagittal (B) images of the femur. (A) The ossified portion of the femoral diaphysis is measured between the large black arrows. The hypoechoic condyles of the distal femur are shown between the small black arrows and the echopenic femoral head is circular (*white arrows*). (B) The fetal thigh, calf, and slightly bent knee are imaged from a posterior view. The diaphysis of the femur creates an acoustic shadow (*wavy arrows*); the length of the diaphysis is commonly referred to sonographically as the femur length (FemL). The distal, hypoechoic femoral condyle is marked by the small arrow at the knee.

the femur, the more common parameter for fetal age.[47]

Measurement methods. The humerus is best located by first imaging the fetal head and spine in order to assess the fetal lie. The transducer is then moved caudad from the head until the neck region is located. As the transducer is moved farther caudad, the shoulder will appear. At this point the transducer should be rotated until a well-defined linear echo is reflected from the shoulder to the elbow. To make sure that this is the single bone of the humerus, the transducer should be rocked

from side to side to rule out the existence of two linear bone echoes, which would represent the radius and ulna.

In some projections the distal end of the humerus appears to have a split or relatively echo-free, central Y-shaped portion (Fig. 17-10). The **Y** shape is caused by scanning coronally through the humerus, showing the coronoid fossa between the lateral and medial epicondyles. The recommended measurement includes the entire ossified portion of the humerus. In the case of a coronal **Y**-shaped distal humerus the recommended measurement is to

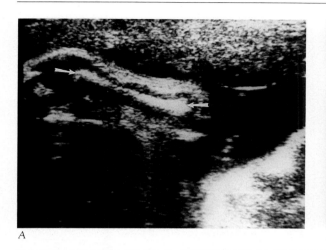
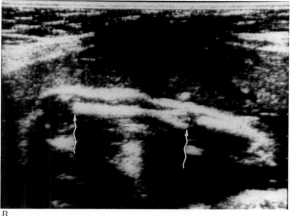

A   B

FIGURE 17-10. HumL. (A) The humeral length shown is from a sagittal scan plane. White arrows mark either end of the humerus measurement. (B) A coronal projection with a **Y**-shaped distal humerus. The white arrows here show the acoustic shadow marking the ends of the humeral shaft. Measurement is made to the midportion of the split end, or the **Y** of the epicondyles.

the middle of an imaginary line across the ends of the epicondyles. (see Fig. 17-10).

Distal Extremity Bones. The distal long bones of the arms and legs can be difficult to measure because the fetus moves them frequently and one cannot reliably predict where they may be in relationship to the spine or the head. Once the bone is located, measuring it is not difficult. If one encounters a fetus with a disparity of the more common parameters, the distal bones can help resolve the conflict in age estimates. Routine measurements of the distal long bones are not necessary for most sonographic examinations, but the bones should be observed for normal morphology.

Ulna. In order to measure the ulna the sonographer should do a survey scan of the fetus to locate the head, spine, and humerus. The sonographer follows the humerus out to the elbow. There it can be determined whether the elbow is flexed or extended, and the ulna can be followed out to the hand. The sonographer should be aware that there are two bones in the forearm, the ulna and radius. The ulna is the larger of the two and is anatomically medial in location. The increased length of

the ulna over the length of the radius is most obvious at the proximal or elbow end of the bones (Fig. 17-11). If the fetal wrist and hand are rotated, the ulna and radius will be crossed rather than parallel.[47]

Tibia. The tibia, like the ulna, can be positioned anywhere in the uterus, depending on the fetus' position and activity. To locate the tibia, the sonographer follows the femur from the hip out to the knee and determines whether the knee is flexed or extended. The tibia is the larger of the two bones in the lower leg and is located medially (Fig. 17-12).[47]

OTHER MEASUREMENTS

Fetal Weight

Calculation from measurement parameters. Weight is one of the most often sought parameters of fetal growth in obstetrics. This is because low birth weight, or intrauterine growth retardation (IUGR), has been associated with higher incidences of neonatal morbidity and death, whereas normal to slightly higher birth weights are usually associated with healthy babies. Therefore, an estimate of the

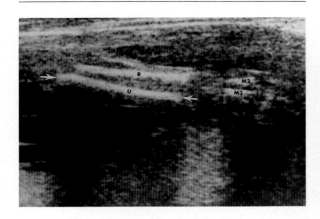

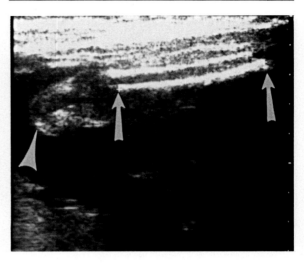

FIGURE 17-11. Ulna. The parallel bones of the ulna (U) and radius (R) and a portion of the hand. The two hand bones are the second and third metacarpals (M2, M3); the fourth and fifth metacarpals lie in the acoustic shadow of the second and third metacarpals. The first metacarpal, or thumb, is not in the plane of the image. The ulna is the larger of the two bones in the forearm, and its measurement is indicated by the arrows.

FIGURE 17-12. Tibia. The tibia is the larger of the two bones, the shin bone, in the lower leg of the fetus. This measurement is not difficult to make once the tibia is located (arrows). Location is often varied owing to fetal motion. The large, white arrowhead marks the fetal heel.

relative fetal weight is important to alert the obstetrician to developing problems and to assist in subsequent management of the pregnancy. An indication of the importance of this parameter is the fact that over 19 different studies of sonographic fetal weight estimates had been published by 1986.[31,72]

Fetal weight estimates have been based on many fetal parameters, mainly the BPD, THC, AC, and the length of the femur. The most accurate of the estimates have been based on combinations of parameters used in regression analysis formulas. These formulas require a solid understanding of algebra and can be difficult to compute using a simple calculator. Computers are ideal for these complex calculations, and several available computer programs include fetal weight estimations in their algorithms (see Chapter 35).[31,37,81,82]

Most of the multiple-parameter fetal weight estimation formulas are a variation of a theme that uses parameters of the fetal head or abdomen or other somatic parameters to estimate the relative fat content, as well as the size of the head and liver and the fetus' length. This works because the brain is the most uniform organ of human growth, whereas the size of the abdomen indicates fat content and liver size, and the femur length is usually proportional to fetal length.[36] The caveat for these methods is that they cannot detect "symmetric IUGR" in a single examination. The sonographer should be particularly careful when taking measurements to be used in weight estimates, particularly those involving abdominal diameter and AC. It is very easy to err on the small side and underestimate fetal weight. A detailed discussion and charts for estimating fetal weight can be found in Chapter 27.

Fetal Heart Rate (FHR). Early in the first trimester, before 8 weeks LMP, the gestational sac is often the only measurement that can be used for dating the pregnancy. During this early time (before 9.5 weeks LMP) the embryonic or fetal heart rate (FHR) can also be used to estimate the embryo's age.[16,17,19,24] From approximately 5.5 weeks LMP, the FHR accelerates from about 85 beats per minute (bpm) to a peak of about 170 bpm during the 9th and 10th

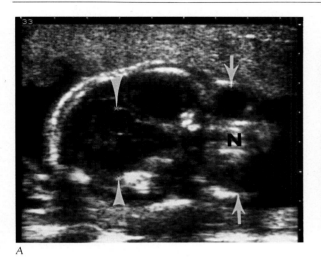

A

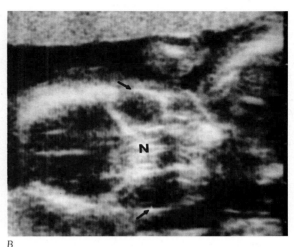

B

FIGURE 17-13. BiOD, the binocular distance between the outsides of the ocular globes is demonstrated *(arrows)*. (A) The cerebellum can often be observed from the same transverse image as the BiOD (between the white arrowheads). (B) In a coronal plane view through the fetal facial bones and orbits *(black arrows)* the interhemispheric fissure of the frontal lobes of the brain can also be observed. In both images the echogenic nasal bones (N) are seen between the orbits. The zygomatic bones form the major portion of the lateral echoes of the orbits, and the BiOD is measured to the inside of the bilateral zygomas *(arrows)*.

weeks LMP. This is a rate of acceleration of just over 3 bpm per day. Until recently the FHR has not been used for dating, and it is not as accurate as the CRL, but it is more accurate than the GSD and can be especially helpful to corroborate the early dates when using a vaginal transducer.[16,17]

The estimation of embryonic age from the FHR uses a simple linear regression formula:

Age in gestational days ($\pm$8) = (FHR $\times$ 0.3) $-$ 8

or

Age in menstrual days ($\pm$8) = (FHR $\times$ 0.3) + 6

This formula is accurate within $\pm$8 days if an accurate FHR is used before 9.5 weeks LMP.[15,16] The FHR should be determined using M-mode sonography for greater accuracy. Attempting to count an embryonic heart rate that may approach 170 bpm during the 9th and 10th weeks LMP, while watching a clock, can yield large errors.

Binocular Measurement. The distance from the outer edges of the left and right fetal eyes is called the binocular distance (BiOD).[46] The BiOD is useful when fetal position makes the BPD or other measurements difficult to obtain. To measure the BiOD, both orbits must be imaged at their greatest diameter. The outer orbit-to-outer orbit distance is measured from the outside of the globes or the insides of the skeletal orbit (Fig. 17-13). It must be pointed out that this measurement may also be difficult to obtain at times owing to the fetus' position. Late in gestation, fetal nasal bones tend to shadow the detail of the eye farthest from the transducer during lateral scans. These shadowing effects of the nasal bones may cause the observer to measure to the inside of the lateral retina at times or to the inner surface of the zygoma at other times.

The diameters of the individual globes of the eyes and the interocular (between the eyes) distance have also been used to estimate fetal growth.[40] Because these measurements are relatively small, any error in cursor placement will cause a relatively large percentage error. For this reason, the larger BiOD is favored.

Fractional Spine Length. The fractional spine length (FSL) is a little-used fetal parameter; however, if the fetus is lying prone with its extremities underneath its body, out of easy reach of the sonographic beam, the spine can be a convenient additional measurement. It is not very accurate owing to the effects of flexion and position. The FSL should include seven thoracolumbar vertebral bodies and seven vertebral spaces.[4,59] Table 17-2 contains an FSL nomogram.

Fetal Kidneys. Fetal kidney size has also been used by some[52,58] for estimating fetal age, but this is not recommended because the kidneys are often difficult to measure consistently. Simple observation of the fetal urinary tract and gastrointestinal tract should be a routine part of any obstetric sonographic examination. In the case of an anomaly, such as obstruction causing obvious fluid build-up within the renal pelvis, measurements of each kidney should be obtained and recorded in order to permit serial follow-up.[52,58] As a general rule, kidney diameters should be about 30% of the corresponding abdominal diameter (i.e., with transverse or anteroposterior[52] {kidney diameter/abdominal diameter} $\times$ 100 = 26% to 31%).

Summary

Factors of which the sonographer should be particularly aware are listed below:

1. To use any fetal parameter size–age chart the user must know how the measurements were taken and must take measurements by the methods used by the author to construct the chart.
2. The use of a single parameter for estimating age from size will be misleading in dating the pregnancy if the parameter is abnormal or "off normal" but still within a normal range or if a measurement error is made.
3. The use of MFP average ages and the range of the ages will produce more accurate dates and will be more likely to expose abnormal parameters or erroneous measurements than will the use of single fetal parameters.
4. AC is easily underestimated because the skin line is often difficult to visualize. This failure can lead to an erroneous diagnosis of asymmetric IUGR. The AC can also be overestimated if an oblique plane is used for the measurements.
5. Long bone (femur, humerus) sonographic measurements should include only the osseous portions of the bone diaphysis (shaft). The sonographer should be careful not to include beam width artifacts in the measurement.

References

1. Athey PA, Hadlock FP. Ultrasound in Obstetrics and Gynecology. St. Louis: CV Mosby; 1981:23–36.
2. Bartrum RJ, Crow HC. Real-Time Ultrasound: A Manual for Physicians and Technical Personnel. 2nd ed. Philadelphia: WB Saunders; 1983:147.
3. Beyer WH, ed. CRC Standard Mathematical Tables. 28th ed. Boca Raton, FL: CRC Press; 1987:122.
4. Birnholz JC. Fetal lumbar spine: Measuring axial growth with US. Radiology. 1986; 158:805–807.
5. Birnholz JC. Ultrasonic Measurements. In: Deter RL, Harrist RB, Birnholz JC, et al., eds. Quantitative Obstetrical Ultrasonography. New York: John Wiley & Sons; 1986; 1:10.
6. Bovicelli L, Orsins LF, Rizzo N, et al. Estimation of gestational age during the first trimester by real-time measurement of fetal crown-rump length and biparietal diameter. Clin Ultrasound. 1981; 9:71–75.
7. Bowie JD. Real-time ultrasonography in the diagnosis of fetal anomalies. In: Winsburg F, Cooperberg PL, eds. Clinics in Diagnostic Ultrasound. New York: Churchill, Livingstone; 1982; 10:228.
8. Chilcote WS, Asokan S. Evaluation of first-trimester pregnancy by ultrasound. Clin Obstet Gynecol. 1977; 20:253–263.
9. Cullinan JA, Wilson S, Toi A, et al. Validation of transvaginal crown-rump length measurements. J Ultrasound Med. 1988:7:S108. (abstr).
10. Deter RL, Harrist RB, Hadlock FP, et al. Longitudinal studies of fetal growth using volume parameters determined with ultrasound. J Clin Ultrasound. 1984; 12:313–324.
11. DuBose TJ. A simple test of excessive B scanner transducer ring. Med Ultrasound. 1983; 7:169–172.
12. DuBose TJ. Fetal biometry: Vertical calvarial diameter and calvarial volume. J Diagn Med Ultrasound. 1985; 1:205–217.
13. DuBose TJ. Basic Baby II Instruction Manual. Austin, TX: Mind's Eye Images; 1987:24–25.

14. DuBose TJ. 3-D BPD Correction. J Ultrasound Med. 1988; 7:S97.

15. DuBose TJ, Cunyus JA, Johnson L. Embryonic heart rate and age. J Diag Med Sonography. 1990. (in press)

16. DuBose TJ, Cunyus JA, Dickey DK, et al. Fetal gestational days = (fetal heart rate × 0.3) + 7. J Diag Med Ultrasound. 1989; 4:198.

17. DuBose, TJ, Dickey DK, Butschek CM, et al. Fetal heart rate communication. J Ultrasound Med. 1988; 7:237–238.

18. DuBose TJ, Poole E, Butschek CM, et al. Range of multiple fetal parameters. J Ultrasound Med. 1988; 7:S205.

19. DuBose TJ, Porter L, Dickey DK, et al. Sonographic correlation of fetal heart rate and gender. J Diagn Med Sonogr. 1989; 5:49–53.

20. Eastman NJ, Hellman LM. Williams' Obstetrics. New York: Appleton-Century-Crofts; 1961:416–417.

21. Filly R. Editorial. Radiology. 1988; 166:274–275.

22. Finberg HJ. Fetus power (lecture). Radiol Today. 1987; 1.

23. Fiske CE, Filly RA. Ultrasound evaluation of the normal and abnormal fetal neural axis. In: Callen PW, ed. Ultrasonography in Obstetrics and Gynecology. Philadelphia: WB Saunders; 1983; 6:100.

24. Fine C, Cartier M, Doubilet P. Fetal heart rates: Values throughout gestation. J Ultrasound Med. 1988; 7:S105.

25. Goldberg BB, Wells PNT. Ultrasonics in Clinical Diagnosis. 3rd ed. New York: Churchill Livingstone; 1983:32.

26. Goldstein RB, Callen PW. Ultrasound evaluation of the fetal thorax and abdomen. In: Callen PW, ed. Ultrasonography in Obstetrics and Gynecology. 2nd ed. Philadelphia: WB Saunders; 1988; 9:222–223.

27. Goldstein RB, Filly RA, Simpson G. Pitfalls in femur length measurements. J. Ultrasound Med. 1987; 6:203–207.

28. Gross BH, Harter P, Filly RA. Disproportionate left hepatic lobe size in the fetus: Ultrasonic demonstration. J Ultrasound Med. 1982; 1:79–81.

29. Hadlock FP. Evaluation of fetal dating studies. In: Deter RL, Harrist RB, Birnholz JC, et al., eds. Quantitative Obstetrical Ultrasonography. New York: John Wiley & Sons; 1986; 3:39.

30. Hadlock FP. Evaluation of fetal dating studies. In: Deter RL, Harrist RB, Birnholz JC, et al., eds. Quantitative Obstetrical Ultrasonography. New York: John Wiley & Sons; 1986; 3:42–43.

31. Hadlock FP. Evaluation of fetal weight estimating procedures. In: Deter RL, Harrist RB, Birnholz JC, et al., eds. Quantitative Obstetrical Ultrasonography. New York: John Wiley & Sons; 1986; 6:115–117.

32. Hadlock FP, Deter RL, Carpenter RJ, et al. Estimating fetal age: Effect of head shape on BPD. AJR. 1981; 137:83–85.

33. Hadlock FP, Deter RL, Harrist RB, et al. Fetal head circumference: relation to menstrual age. AJR. 1982; 138:649–653.

34. Hadlock FP, Deter RL, Harrist RB, et al. Computer-assisted analysis of fetal age in the third trimester using multiple growth parameters. J Clin Ultrasound. 1983; 11:313–316.

35. Hadlock FP, Deter RL, Harrist RB, et al. Estimating fetal age: Computer-assisted analysis of multiple fetal growth parameters. Radiology. 1984; 152:497–501.

36. Hadlock FP, Deter RL, Roecker E, et al. Relation of fetal femur length to neonatal crown-heel length. J Ultrasound Med. 1984; 3:1–3.

37. Hadlock FP, Harrist RB, Sharman RS, et al. Estimation of fetal weight with the use of head, body, and femur measurements—A prospective study. Am J Obstet Gynecol. 1985; 151:333–337.

38. Hadlock FP, Kent WR, Loyd JL, et al. An evaluation of two methods for measuring fetal head and body circumferences. J Ultrasound Med. 1982; 1:359–360.

39. Hansmann M, Hackeloer BJ, Staudach A. Normal fetal anatomy in the second and third trimester. In: Hansmann M, Hackeloer BJ, Staudach A, eds. Ultrasound Diagnosis in Obstetrics and Gynecology. Berlin: Springer-Verlag; 1985; 7:113.

40. Hansmann M, Hackeloer BJ, Staudach A. Normal fetal anatomy in the second and third trimester. In: Hansmann M, Hackeloer BJ, Staudach A, eds. Ultrasound Diagnosis in Obstetrics and Gynecology. Berlin: Springer-Verlag; 1985:169–175.

41. Hansmann M, Hackeloer BJ, Staudach A. Normal fetal anatomy in the second and third trimester. In: Hansmann M, Hackeloer BJ, Staudach A, eds. Ultrasound Diagnosis in Obstetrics and Gynecology. Berlin: Springer-Verlag; 1985:124–130.

42. Hellman LM, Kobayashi M, Fillisti L, et al. Growth and development of the human fetus prior to the twentieth week of gestation. Am J Obstet Gynecol. 1969; 103:789–800.

43. Hill LM, Breckle R, Gehrking WC. The variable effects of oligohydramnios on the biparietal diameter and the cephalic index. J Clin Ultrasound. 1984; 3:93–95.

44. Holmes JH. Diagnostic ultrasound during the early years of A.I.U.M. J Ultrasound Med. 1980; 8:299–308.

45. Jeanty P. Basic Baby II. J Ultrasound Med. 1987; 6:548.

46. Jeanty P, Cantraine F, Cousaert E, et al. The binocular distance: A new way to estimate fetal age. J Ultrasound Med. 1984; 3:241–243.

47. Jeanty P, Rodesch F, Delbekd D, et al. Estimation of gestational age from measurements of fetal long bones. J Ultrasound Med. 1984; 3:75–79.

48. Jordaan HVF. The differential enlargement of the neurocranium in the full-term fetus. S Afr Med J. 1976; 50:1978–1981.

49. Jordaan HVF, Dunn LJ. A new method of evaluating fetal growth. Obstet Gynecol. 1978; 51:659–665.

50. Kremkau FW. Diagnostic Ultrasound: Physical Principles & Exercises. Orlando, FL: Grune & Stratton; 1980:47–50.

51. Kurtz AB, Goldberg BB. Combined fetal head and body measurements. In: Kurtz AB, Goldberg BB, eds. Obstetrical Measurements in Ultrasound: A Reference Manual. Chicago: Year Book Medical Publishers; 1988; 7:137.

52. Kurtz AB, Goldberg BB. Fetal body measurements. In: Kurtz AB, Goldberg BB, eds. Obstetrical Measurements in Ultrasound: A Reference Manual. Chicago: Year Book Medical Publishers; 1988; 6:91.

53. Kurtz AB, Goldberg BB. Fetal head measurements. In: Kurtz AB, Goldberg BB, eds. Obstetrical Measurements in Ultrasound: A Reference Manual. Year Book Medical Publishers; 1988; 5:22–35.

54. Kurtz AB, Shaw W, Wapner RJ, et al. The inaccuracy of total intrauterine volume: Sources of errors and proposed solution (abstr.). J Ultrasound Med. 1983; 2:101.

55. Kurtz AB, Wapner RJ, Kurtz RH, et al. Analysis of biparietal diameter as an accurate indicator of gestational age. J Ultrasound Med. 1980; 8:319–326.

56. Laing FC. First trimester bleeding: The role of ultrasound (lecture). SDMS Spring Symposium, Orlando FL: 1986.

57. Law RG, MacRae KD. Head circumference as an index of fetal age. J Ultrasound Med. 1982; 1:281–288.

58. Lawson TL, Foley WD, Berland LL, et al. Ultrasonic evaluation of fetal kidneys. Radiology. 1981; 138:156.

59. Li DFH, Woo JSK. Fractional spine length: A new parameter for assessing fetal growth. J Ultrasound Med. 1986; 5:379–383.

60. Lyons EA, Levi CS. Ultrasound in the first trimester of pregnancy. Radiol Clin North Am. 1982; 20:261.

61. McDicken WN. Diagnostic Ultrasound: Principles and Use of Instruments. 2nd ed. New York: John Wiley & Sons; 1981:31–32.

62. McDicken WN. Diagnostic Ultrasound: Principles and Use of Instruments. 2nd ed. New York: John Wiley & Sons; 1981:34.

63. MacGregor SN, Tamura RK, Sabbagha RE, et al. Underestimation of gestational age by conventional crown-rump length dating curves. Obstet Gynecol. 1987; 70:344–348.

64. McLeary RD, Kuhns LR, Barr M. Ultrasonography of the fetal cerebellum. Radiology. 1984; 151:439–442.

65. Martinez DA, Barton JL. Estimation of fetal body and fetal head volumes: Description of technique and nomograms for 18 to 41 weeks of gestation. Am J Obstet Gynecol. 1980; 137:78–84.

66. Moore KL. The Developing Human. 3rd ed. Philadelphia: WB Saunders; 1982:70–92.

67. Nyberg DA, Laing FC, Filly RA. Threatened abortion: Sonographic distinction of normal and abnormal gestation sacs. Radiology. 1986; 158:397–400.

68. Nyberg DA, Mack LA, Laing FC, et al. Distinguishing normal from abnormal gestational sac growth in early pregnancy. J Ultrasound Med. 1987; 6:23–27.

69. O'Keeffe DF, Garite TJ, Elliott JP, et al. The accuracy of estimated gestational age based on ultrasound measurements of biparietal diameter in preterm premature rupture of the membranes. Am J Obstet Gynecol. 1985:151:309–312.

70. Olmstead WW, Smirniotopoulos JG. Congenital dysplasias primarily involving the skull. In: Putnam CE, Ravin CE, eds. Textbook of Diagnostic Imaging. Philadelphia: WB Saunders; 1988; 1:110.

71. Ott WJ. Accurate gestational dating. Obstet Gynecol. 1985; 66:311.

72. Rose BI. Abbreviated tables for estimating fetal weight with ultrasound. J Reprod Med. 1988; 33:298–300.

73. Ruvolo KA, Filly RA, Callen PW. Evaluation of fetal femur length for prediction of gestational age in a racially mixed obstetric population. J Ultrasound Med. 1987; 6:417.

74. Sabbagha RE. Gestational age. In: Sabbagha RE, ed. Diagnostic Ultrasound, Applied to Obstetrics and Gynecology. 2nd ed. Philadelphia: JB Lippincott; 1987; 8:94.

75. Sabbagha RE. Gestational age. In: Sabbagha RE, ed. Diagnostic Ultrasound, Applied to Obstetrics and Gynecology. 2nd ed. Philadelphia: JB Lippincott; 1987; 8:96–107.

76. Sabbagha RE. Gestational age. In: Sabbagha RE, ed. Diagnostic Ultrasound, Applied to Obstetrics and Gynecology. 2nd ed. Philadelphia: JB Lippincott; 1987; 8:109.

77. Sabbagha RE. Gestational age. In: Sabbagha RE, ed. Diagnostic Ultrasound, Applied to Obstetrics and Gynecology. 2nd ed. Philadelphia: JB Lippincott; 1987; 8:109–110.

78. Sabbagha RE, Hughey M. Standardization of sonar

cephalometry and gestational age. Obstet Gynecol. 1978; 52:402–406.

79. Sabbagha RE, Barton FB, Barton BA. Sonar biparietal diameter I. Analysis of percentile growth differences in two normal populations using same methodology. Am J Obstet Gynecol. 1976; 126:479–484.

80. Sarti DA. Diagnostic Ultrasound. 2nd ed. Chicago: Year Book Medical Publishers: 1987; 1:14–15.

81. Shepard MJ, Richards VA, Berkowitz RL, et al. An evaluation of two equations of predicting fetal weight by ultrasound. Am J Obstet Gynecol. 1982; 142:47.

82. Warsof SL, Gohari P, Berkowitz RL, et al. The estimation of fetal weight by computer-assisted analysis. Am J Obstet Gynecol. 1977; 128:881.

83. Winter J, Kimme-Smith C, King W III. Measurement accuracy of sonographic sector scanners. AJR. 1985; 144:645–648.

84. Wolfson RN, Peisner DB, Chik LL, et al. Comparison of biparietal diameter and femur length in the third trimester: Effects of gestational age and variation in fetal growth. J Ultrasound Med. 1986; 5:145.

85. Yaghoobian J. Simplified method for estimation of fetal age by biparietal measurement. J Diagn Med Sonogr. 1987; 3:33–35.

86. Zador IE, Sokol RJ, Chik L. Interobserver variability: A source of error in obstetric ultrasound. J Ultrasound Med. 1988; 7:245–249.

87. Zagzebski JA. Basic Physics. In: Sabbagha RE, ed. Diagnostic Ultrasound, Applied to Obstetrics and Gynecology. 2nd ed. Philadelphia: JB Lippincott; 1987; 1:12–13.

88. Zagzebski JA. Basic Physics. In: Sabbagha RE, ed. Diagnostic Ultrasound, Applied to Obstetrics and Gynecology. 2nd ed. Philadelphia: JB Lippincott; 1987; 1:26.

CHAPTER **18**

The Placenta and Umbilical Cord

LINDA M. CHASE, PAUL D. CAYEA

Sonography of the placenta was first described in 1966.[21] Since that time, extensive research and technologic advances have given sonographers a powerful diagnostic tool. The placenta can now be localized with virtually 100% accuracy, and its texture can be analyzed better than ever before. As a result, detection of pathologic conditions affecting the placenta and umbilical cord has improved tremendously. Accurate assessment of these structures is both a challenge to the sonographer and a necessity. Any changes in these vascular organs, such as umbilical cord compression or placental tumor, may produce subsequent changes in vascular resistance and severely compromise the fetus. Moreover, the condition of these organs may indicate the presence of coincident fetal anomalies.

A further benefit of technologic advance has been to render established techniques such as amniocentesis quicker, safer, and easier to perform. In addition, a variety of new invasive procedures such as umbilical vein aspiration, chorionic villus sampling, and placental biopsy have added to the fetal diagnostic repertoire.

Placenta

PLACENTAL STRUCTURE AND FUNCTION

Size, Shape, Location. The placenta is a flat, discoid (circular), vascular organ that weighs about 500 to 600 gm at term (one-sixth to one-seventh of fetal weight). It may be located anywhere in the uterine cavity. At the fetal side is a fused layer of amnion and chorion (choroid plate), whereas at the maternal side are about 20 functional lobes, or cotyledons, composed of central maternal sinusoids and peripheral villous lacunae (Fig. 18-1).[42] It is a relatively homogeneous organ that may exhibit varying degrees of calcification late in its development.

The final shape of the placenta is attained by the end of the 4th month of gestation; it is almost always discoid. The cord usually inserts centrally, but it may insert eccentrically near the margins (battledore placenta) or into membranes (velamentous insertion) (Fig. 18-2).[8] In general, the wider the base of attachment, the thinner the placenta. Normally the placenta is between 1.5 and 5 cm thick,[19] although any placenta thicker than 4 cm is considered by some to be abnormal.[9,18] Placental volume increases linearly throughout pregnancy, reaching a maximum well before term.[50]

Placental Circulation. Oxygenated maternal blood is pumped through spiral arterioles terminating at the base of the placenta. The blood enters the intervillous space around the villous capillaries, where gases and nutrients are exchanged. It is here, at the level of gas exchange, that nutrition, respiration, and waste removal take place. The resulting oxygenated blood enters the fetus through the umbilical vein.[22,43] Returning deoxygenated fetal blood enters the placenta through the umbilical arteries (Fig. 18-1).

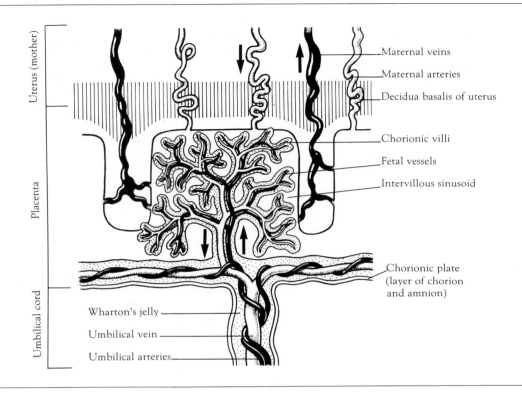

Uterus (mother)

Maternal veins
Maternal arteries
Decidua basalis of uterus

Chorionic villi
Fetal vessels
Intervillous sinusoid

Placenta

Chorionic plate
(layer of chorion
and amnion)

Wharton's jelly
Umbilical vein
Umbilical arteries

Umbilical cord

FIGURE 18-1. Diagram of placental and umbilical cord structure showing fetoplacental circulation. Note that the darker-looking vessels in the diagram contain deoxygenated blood.

NORMAL SONOGRAPHY OF THE PLACENTA

Morphology. The early placenta is usually visualized by 8 to 10 weeks as focal thickening of the decidual reaction surrounding the gestational sac (Fig. 18-3). By 12 weeks, the placenta is clearly visualized as a discoid structure with a homogeneous granular texture. The sharp, linear acoustic interface of the chorionic plate on the fetal side of the placenta can usually be identified also at this stage (Fig. 18-4).[8,42]

Intraplacental Texture. The mature placenta generally retains its granular, homogeneous texture; however, in the second and third trimesters intraplacental and subchorionic vascular spaces may sometimes be seen and usually have no clinical significance (Fig. 18-5A). When very large, they have been seen in association with increased maternal serum α-fetoprotein (AFP). A very mature placenta may exhibit cystic areas located centrally within clearly delineated lobes. These are not vascular and are thought to represent areas of necrosis (Fig. 18-5B).

The Retroplacental Complex. No assessment of the placenta is complete without evaluation of the retroplacental complex. This zone is composed of decidua basalis and portions of the myometrium, including maternal veins draining the placenta. It is consistently imaged after 18 weeks regardless of placental position[12,13,22,32] and measures on average approximately 9.5 mm (Fig. 18-6).[32] Proper identification of this area is quite important. A prominent anterior retroplacental complex can produce excessive bleeding during invasive procedures such as amniocentesis or cesarean section.[15] In addition, the retroplacental complex can mimic abruptio placentae, degenerating fibroids, or hydatidiform

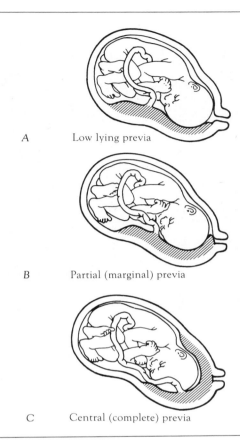

A   Low lying previa

B   Partial (marginal) previa

C   Central (complete) previa

FIGURE 18-2. Diagram of three types of placenta previa. (A) In complete previa placental tissue completely covers the internal os and is attached to the uterine wall on both sides of the os. (B) In marginal or partial previa placental tissue may cover the os but is not attached to the wall at the other side. (C) In low-lying placenta the edge of the placenta is visualized near the os.

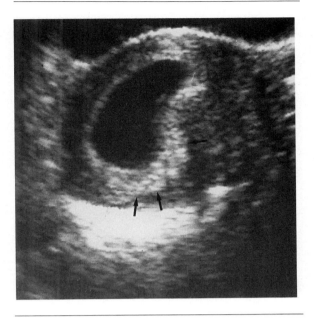

FIGURE 18-3. Real-time linear scan of 8 or 9 weeks' gestation shows focal thickening along one side of gestational sac (*arrows*), representing early placental formation.

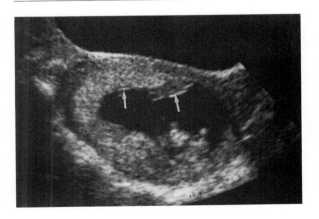

FIGURE 18-4. The chorionic plate is already visible as bright, linear echoes on this sector scan of an early placenta (*arrows*). A smaller portion of this membrane can be appreciated in a sector scan than in a static or linear scan (see Fig. 18-12B), since the beam is perpendicular to less of this specular reflector at any point in the sector scan.

mole. Real-time visualization of blood flow in this area will help distinguish the normal complex from these pathologic conditions.[13,22]

Sonographically the complex appears as a sonolucent subplacental region containing many horizontal linear echoes.[22,24,43] Large venous channels may be visualized within the complex, most commonly in posteriorly located placentas, where the effects of gravity-induced pressure can overdistend the veins.[22,42,43] This may also occur when the beam

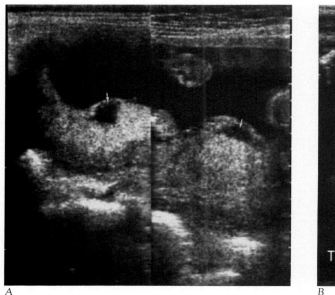
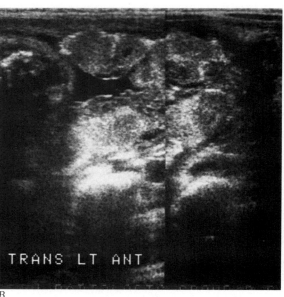

A   B

FIGURE 18-5. (A) Dual-format linear scan shows two views of a large subchorionic venous lake (arrows). (B) Dual format linear scan of a mature placenta demonstrates calcifically delineated cotyledons with centrally located sonolucent areas.

strikes tangentially, as with a fundal or lateral placenta.[9,43]

Normal Placental Calcification. Placental calcium deposition is a normal physiologic process occurring throughout pregnancy, with more than 50% of placentas showing some degree of macroscopic calcification after 33 weeks.[40,43] Although the degree of normal calcification is quite variable, it generally increases throughout pregnancy, becoming more prominent as first the basal area and then the interlobar septa calcify (Fig. 18-7).[8] Calcium may also be found in the villous, perivillous, and subchorionic spaces.[8,43] Intraplacental calcifications are visualized sonographically as strong acoustic echoes without significant acoustic shadowing.[43]

SCANNING TECHNIQUES AND HELPFUL HINTS
Real-Time and Static Scanners, Transvaginal Probes and Doppler. The image quality of both static and real-time units is comparable, so both can do an adequate job. This leaves personal preference to

determine which type of equipment is used. Static scanners do afford a more global view of the placenta; however, a similar result can be achieved using a linear real-time probe (particularly if a dual image mode is available; Fig. 18-8).

The advent of transvaginal transducers has added a new dimension to obstetric ultrasound. Using this method, visualization of the placenta and umbilical cord (as well as the fetus) is obtained with great clarity at a much earlier phase of gestation than with transabdominal scanning. In addition, since the transducer is placed within the vagina, directly adjacent to the uterus, there is no need for a full bladder. Figure 18-9 shows the difference in visualization obtained with the two methods at an early phase of pregnancy.

In the past few years valuable information has been obtained from Doppler studies of the umbilical cord and placenta. It should be noted that use of pulsed-wave Doppler may expose the fetus to higher intensities than are consistent with safety. This fact has caused the FDA to set strict guidelines

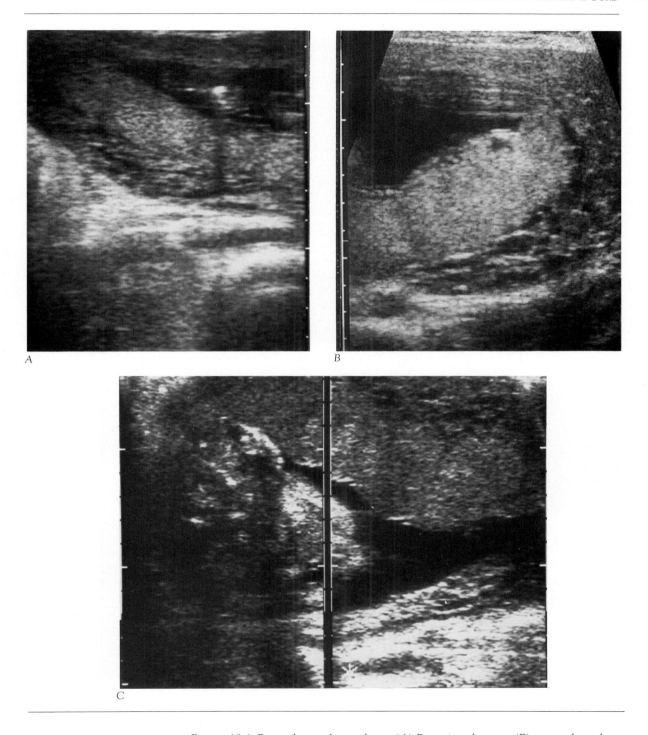

FIGURE 18-6. Retroplacental complexes. (A) Posterior placenta, (B) posterolateral placenta, and (C) anterior placenta showing the convoluted, tubular maternal draining veins that are part of the retroplacental complex.

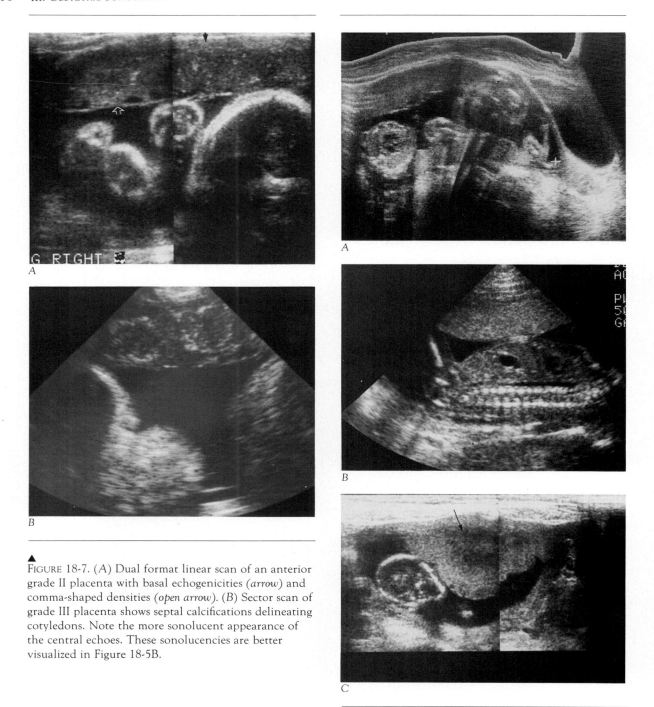

▲
Figure 18-7. (A) Dual format linear scan of an anterior grade II placenta with basal echogenicities (*arrow*) and comma-shaped densities (*open arrow*). (B) Sector scan of grade III placenta shows septal calcifications delineating cotyledons. Note the more sonolucent appearance of the central echoes. These sonolucencies are better visualized in Figure 18-5B.

on the use of Doppler ultrasound in fetal evaluation. It is suggested that Doppler be used on the fetus only when that study is clinically indicated, and that power output and examination time be minimized. This is discussed fully in Chapter 19.

Is a Full Bladder Important? Unfortunately for the patient, the answer is still a qualified yes. Cervical length is a good indicator of whether or not a bladder is adequately full. A cervical measurement of 3 to 5 cm is considered optimal. A properly full bladder enhances placental visualization in early pregnancy and improves imaging of the lower uterine segment later in gestation (Fig. 18-10). This latter point is particularly relevant when one is considering a diagnosis of placenta previa, since an over-distended bladder can cause a false appearance of previa (Fig. 18-11). This happens when a very full bladder causes close apposition of the anterior and posterior walls of the lower uterine segment, causing apparent superior migration of the internal cervical os. The sonographer can improve patient acceptance and reduce the false-positive rate for diagnosing placenta previa by varying the degree of bladder distention during the examination (i.e., start with full bladder, then have the patient pass 1 cup at a time).[23]

The use of transvaginal probes has decreased the need for a full bladder, because examinations can be performed routinely with the bladder empty in the first and second trimester and when evaluating the lower uterine segment for placenta previa in the third trimester.[46] It should be noted, however, that in some laboratories vaginal scanning is prohibited if vaginal bleeding has occurred during the pregnancy.

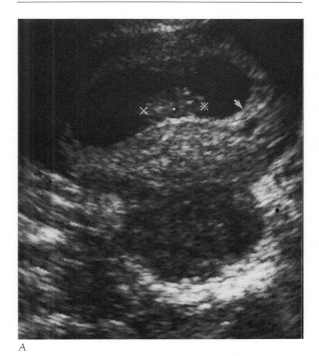

A

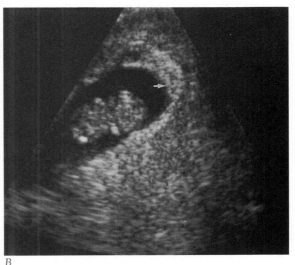

B

◄ FIGURE 18-8. Comparison of static scan of the placenta to real-time sector and linear scans. (*A*) Static scan of twin pregnancy with anterior and posterior placentas demonstrates the large field of view obtained. (*B*) In real-time sector scan of anterior placenta only a small portion of placenta is visualized, owing to small field of view provided by sector shape. (*C*) Dual-format linear scan of anterior placenta shows a wide field of view similar to that of the static scan. Note the subplacental uterine contraction (*arrow*).

FIGURE 18-9. Comparison of transabdominal and transvaginal scans. (*A*) Transabdominal scan of an early pregnancy (about 8 weeks). The placental tissue is poorly defined (*arrow*). Note the fibroid located posterior to the uterus. (*B*) Transvaginal scan of the same gestation clearly defines focal thickening of the early placenta (*arrow*).

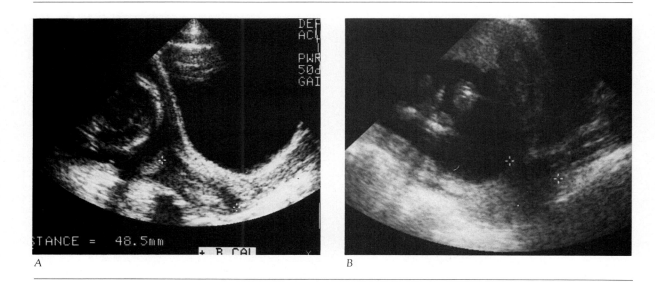

A *B*

FIGURE 18-10. (A) Sector scan of the lower uterine segment shows an adequately full bladder. The cervix measured 4.8 cm, which is within normal limits. (B) Sector scan of the lower uterine segment with an inadequately full bladder. The entire lower segment, including the cervix, is difficult to visualize.

Transducer, Angle, Frequency, and Gain Settings. A 3- or 3.5-MHz medium-focused transducer is adequate for most routine imaging of the placenta. A lower-frequency, longer-focused transducer may be needed to improve visualization in large patients, late in the third trimester, or when the fetus lies over a posterior placenta. On the other hand, the retroplacental complex of an anteriorly located placenta may be obscured by ring-down or near-field artifacts. Changing to a higher-frequency, shorter focused transducer, or even using a water path can be helpful in these cases. Most newer generation, real-time units allow the user to electronically vary the focal zone of the probe.

When scanning the placenta, the beam should be perpendicular to the chorionic plate, especially when measuring thickness, and the gains should be adjusted so that the placenta has a uniform and homogeneous granular texture. Both the sharp, linear acoustic interface of the chorionic plate and the sonolucent retroplacental zone should be seen clearly (Fig. 18-12). Differentiation of placental tissue from that of a uterine contraction or myoma is dependent on clear visualization of these structures.[9,13,43] The gains may have to be reduced with posterior placentas to offset enhanced acoustic transmission from the overlying amniotic fluid. Increasing the gain in order to visualize flowing blood during real-time observation can be useful in distinguishing placental lakes from other sonolucent placental masses.

Patient Positioning. It is usually sufficient to perform the examination with the patient in the supine position; however, rotating the patient from side to side may be necessary to improve the visualization of a posterior placenta. The Trendelenburg position can displace a low-lying fetal head that obscures the inferior placental margin.

Measurement of Placental Thickness. The sonographer should first identify the placental-myometrium interface in a midpoint position that is as free of fetal shadowing as possible. The measurement should exclude the myometrium and retroplacental complex, and the transducer should be perpendicular

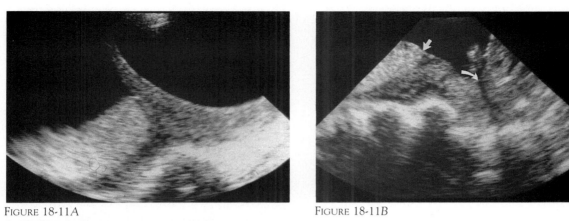

FIGURE 18-11A

FIGURE 18-11B

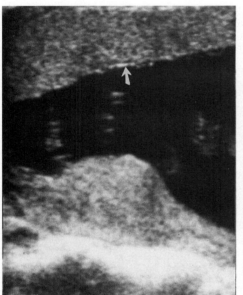

FIGURE 18-12A

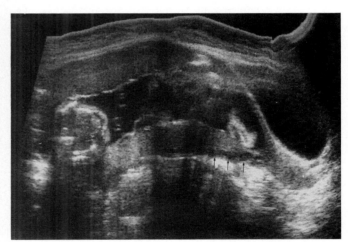

FIGURE 18-12B

FIGURE 18-11. (A) Sector scan of overdistended bladder. The cervix is not easily measured and the position of the internal os is unclear. Due to compression of the lower uterine segment, the edge of the placenta appears to cover the internal os. (B) Postvoiding scan of same patient. The internal os (*curved arrow*) is now seen to be clearly separate from the edge of the placenta (*straight arrow*).

FIGURE 18-12. (A) Real-time linear scan of anterior placenta shows distinct chorionic plate (*arrow*). Note increased echogenicity of posterior uterine contraction due to the transsonicity of the amniotic fluid. (B) Static scan of twin gestation demonstrates the bright, linear echoes of chorionic plate along the length of both anterior and posterior placentas. The chorionic plate is visualized well, because the transducer in a static scanner can be kept perpendicular to the structure throughout its length. Part of the posterior retroplacental complex can be appreciated (*arrows*).

to the myometrium, lest the resultant measurement be falsely high (Fig. 18-13).[18] Evaluation of this measurement should take into consideration the shape of the placenta. For example, a broad-based placenta may be thinner and a narrow-based placenta thicker, without indicating the presence of any pathology. The amount of amniotic fluid present may also affect apparent placental thickness.[18]

Helpful Hints for Placental Scanning

Visualization of both the sharp, linear interface of the chorionic plate and the hypoechoic retroplacental zone helps to differentiate placental tissue from that of a uterine contraction or myoma, particularly since posterior contractions (see Fig. 18-7) may appear as echogenic as placental tissue. In these cases, the only way to prove that a particular tissue is placental is to demonstrate areas of placental demarcation.

Other than the site of cord insertion, the subchorionic area usually appears smooth and uninterrupted; however, subchorionic and intraplacental lucencies are sometimes seen that are generally vascular and represent venous lakes. Turning the transducer 90 degrees to demonstrate the tubular nature of the structure helps to prove its vascularity (Fig. 18-14). Vascular structures may also be differentiated from other, pathologic, entities by scanning at increased gain settings, demonstrating red blood cell movement.[8,19,30,40] Occasionally, an area of the chorionic plate may be seen that appears separated from the placenta. This could represent an area of prior placental hemorrhage and may be correlated with a previous episode of vaginal bleeding.

Within the placental tissue itself, any area that does not demonstrate the normal granular, echogenic appearance should be assessed carefully. Areas of varied echogenicity; a multiple cystic or vesicular appearance; irregular, hypoechoic areas; or highly echogenic areas with hypoechoic margins should be carefully documented.

Placental thickness should be measured and correlated with clinical data (see Table 18-1), the location of the placenta should be noted, and, most importantly, the retroplacental area should be studied for possible areas of elevation.

PLACENTAL GRADING

A grading system based on the degree of placental calcification (Table 18-2) has been used as an in-

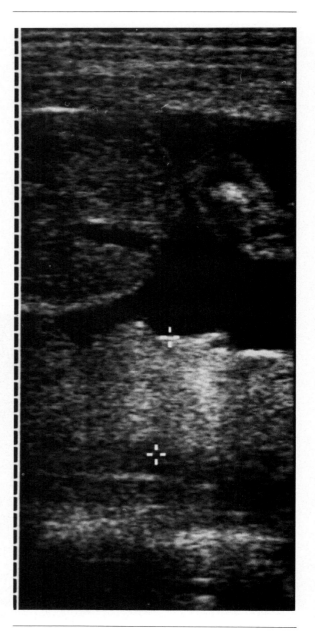

FIGURE 18-13. Real-time linear scan of posterior placenta shows placement of cursors for measurement of placental thickness. Beam is perpendicular to the midpoint of the placenta, and the retroplacental complex is not included in the measurement.

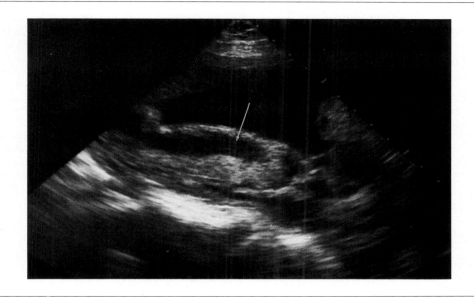

FIGURE 18-14. Sector scan of subchorionic tubular, lucent space in posterior placenta *(arrow)*. Real-time scanning, showing movement of red blood cells, confirmed its vascular nature.

TABLE 18-1. Disease states in relation to placental appearance[8,14,37,43]

INCREASED PLACENTAL THICKNESS (>5 cm)	DECREASED PLACENTAL THICKNESS (<1.5 cm)	EARLY PLACENTAL MATURATION	DELAYED PLACENTAL MATURATION
Diabetes (nonvascular types)	Preeclampsia	IUGR	Gestational diabetes
Rh disease (hydropic changes)	IUGR	HTN	Rh Disease
CMV infection	Juvenile diabetes		
Abruption*	(vascular forms)		
Chorioangioma			
Multiple gestation			

*Apparent thickening due to retroplacental clot, isoechoic with placenta[8]

dicator of fetal pulmonary maturity. Initial studies indicated that heavily calcified (grade III) placentas had a 100% correlation with fetal lung maturity,[13,39,41] thus obviating amniocentesis. Subsequently, there were multiple reported cases in which fetuses with grade III placentas had immature lungs, as determined by lecithin-sphingomyelin ratios.[13] Furthermore, only 10 to 20% of pregnancies attain a grade III placenta by term.[8,34,41] It is now known that multiple factors, including smoking, low maternal age, parity, and even season of the year can affect the degree of placental calcification.[3,13,14,19,27,34,42,43]

TABLE 18-2. Placental grading based on placental calcifications

1. Placental Grading[8,9]

Grade 0	No calcifications	to about 31 weeks
I	Scattered calcifications	31–36 weeks
II	Basal calcifications	36–38 weeks
III	Basal and interlobar septal calcifications	38 weeks+

2. The placenta matures considerably after the 40th week.
3. Two parts of the placenta may have different grades[9] in which case the highest grade is assigned.
4. Most term pregnancies have grade I or II placenta.
5. Only about 10 to 15% of term placentas are grade III.

Table 18-3. Sonographic characteristics of placental abnormalities

Abnormality	Description	Sonographic Characteristics	Differential Diagnosis
Placenta previa	Placental tissue obstructing internal os; most common cause of bleed in 2nd & 3rd trimester	Placental tissue seen to cover internal os, whether completely, partially, or marginally	Uterine contraction, fibroid, overdistended bladder may mimic placenta previa
Abruption	Premature separation of all or part of placenta	Elevated portion of placenta or extramembraneous[9]; retroplacental, sub-chorionic, or intraplacental[40]; sonolucent or complex, transsonic mass of varying echogenicity[24]; may appear as normal placenta; may appear as thickened placenta[24]	Retroplacental thrombosis, normal placenta, abnormally thick placenta, normal retroplacental complex
Placenta accreta	Decidual formation defect with abnormal placental penetration and attachment to uterine wall[37]	Normal retroplacental sonolucent area not visualized	Myometrial scar
Sonolucent Lesions			
Fibrin deposits	Secondary to vascular thrombosis and cystic degeneration of fibrin	Anechoic areas in intervillous spaces beneath chorion; lack real-time evidence of blood flow[8,40]	Venous lake, hematoma
Hematoma	Area of retroplacental or intraplacental clot	May be sonolucent or of varying echogenicity depending upon age of clot; lack real-time evidence of blood flow	Venous lake, fibrin deposition
Intervillous thrombi	Interplacental areas of hemorrhage and pooling of blood; increased in Rh isoimmunity[8,43]	Echo-poor areas of varying size throughout placenta	Hematoma
Breus' mole	Massive subchorionic thrombosis (rare) secondary to extreme venous obstruction, leads to PMD; unrelated to fibrin deposition[8,43]	Extensive sonolucent hematoma without evidence of venous flow[43]	Placental tumor fibroid hematoma[9,43]

TABLE 18-3. (continued)

ABNORMALITY	DESCRIPTION	SONOGRAPHIC CHARACTERISTICS	DIFFERENTIAL DIAGNOSIS
Neoplastic Lesions			
Chorioangioma	Tumor resulting from vascular malformation[43]; most common placental tumor; benign, may be multiple, small, or single large; associated with fetal edema[33,42,49]	Usually isoechoic with placenta; may show as placental thickening without discrete mass[8,33]; large mass may extend from fetal surface of placenta; associated with hydramnios; may see vascular channels within mass	Fibroid
Teratoma	Rare-benign to highly malignant germ cell tumor	Complex, heterogeneous mass may have calcifications	Fibroid

More to the point, assessment of placental calcification is important in certain serious maternal and fetal conditions. For example, premature placental calcification can occur in maternal hypertensive states and in association with intrauterine growth retardation[9,28,37]; other conditions such as maternal diabetes or fetal cardiopulmonary disorders can retard the rate of placental calcification. Therefore, evaluating placental maturity in relation to the age of gestation can give additional, important input to the entire clinical picture.

ABNORMALITIES OF THE PLACENTA (Table 18-3)
Abnormal Shape and Configuration

Bilobed placenta; succenturiate placenta. Although it is usually one mass, the placenta may be bilobed or have a smaller accessory (succenturiate) lobe (0.14 to 3.0% of cases) (Fig. 18-15).[43] The accessory lobe is connected to the main placental mass, either by vessels within a membrane or by a bridge of chorionic tissue.[43] Identification of an accessory lobe is clinically relevant, owing to the high risk of postpartum hemorrhage associated with retained accessory lobes.[8,40] There is also a risk of massive intrapartum fetal bleeding secondary to rupture of connecting vessels.[42] Therefore, sonographic delineation of placental tissue in two parts of the uterus (not to be confused with a fold in the placenta), and if possible the connecting bridge, especially if it overlies the os, is a valuable contribution to the management of the patient.[8,19]

Annular placenta; placenta membranacea. Annular placenta refers to a ring-shaped placenta that attaches circumferentially to the myometrium. Placenta membranacea refers to a condition in which the placenta covers all or most of the surface of the gestational sac. Both types have been associated with antepartum and postpartum hemorrhage. Neither has been detected sonographically,[26,42] but there is no reason why antenatal visualization may not be possible in the future, keeping in mind our ability to identify placental tissue in various aspects of the uterus.

Abnormal Placental Size. Variation in placental size may be indicative of several important fetal and maternal conditions (Table 18-1). Therefore, much research has been conducted to determine the best sonographic means of assessing placental size in relation to gestational age. Although surface area and volumetric measurements show this relationship best, they are extremely time consuming, cumbersome, and impractical,[8,40] requiring serial scans at least every 2 cm and the application of complicated equations.[8,9,40,50] Thickness is more variable and less accurate than volume, being a function of gestational age, placental location, and transducer angle; however, since it is easier to measure, thickness is used routinely.

As a general rule, after 23 weeks the placenta should be no thinner than 1.5 cm or thicker than 5.0 cm. An abnormally thick placenta can be seen

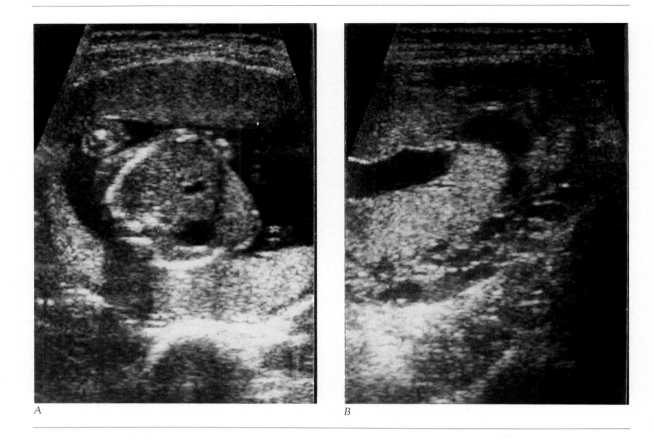

A   B

FIGURE 18-15. (*A*) A bilobed placenta shows both anterior and posterior components. The connecting membrane is not visible. (*B*) Posterior placenta with anterior accessory lobe. The connecting membrane is well-visualized.

in association with maternal diabetes (due to villous edema) or in any case of placental hydrops. A thin placenta (<1.5 cm) may be seen in pregnancies with intrauterine growth retardation and placental infarction (the result of coagulation necrosis of the villi) and in pregnancies complicated by essential hypertension and preeclampsia.[43]

Placental Hydrops. The abnormal thickness of a hydropic placenta is due to fluid overload, usually secondary to high-output cardiac failure in the fetus. This can occur in erythroblastosis fetalis (immune hydrops; Fig. 18-16), fetomaternal and twin-to-twin transfusion syndromes, chorioangioma (in which fetal blood is shunted through the placental circulation), and vascular obstruction such as umbilical vein thrombosis.[4,5] Sonography of the hydropic placenta shows it to be abnormally thick (usually >5.0 cm) with an abnormally echogenic acoustical texture.[35]

Abnormal Location—Placenta Previa. When the placenta partially or completely covers the internal cervical os, the patient is said to have placenta previa. Clinically, three forms of previa are described—total, which occurs when implantation of the placenta crosses the internal os, partial (marginal), and low-lying. Sonographically, complete

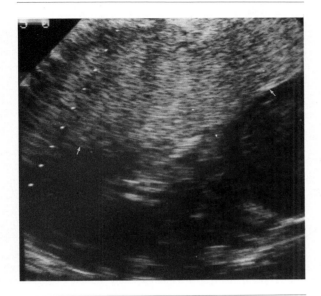

FIGURE 18-16. Sector scan of an enlarged anterior placenta (arrows) in a confirmed Rh immunosensitive pregnancy. The perpendicular thickness measurement is over 5 cm. Note the increased echogenicity of the placental tissue.

placenta previa is detected when the body of the placenta completely covers the os (Fig. 18-17). When just the edge of the placenta is seen to abut or cover the os, it is a marginal, or partial, placenta previa (Fig. 18-18). In these cases, implantation does not cross the os. If the edge of the placenta is near the os it is considered to be a low-lying placenta (Fig. 18-19).

Although clinically uncommon, placenta previa is frequently seen in the sonography laboratory, as up to 93% of these patients experience significant painless, vaginal bleeding that requires sonographic evaluation.[21] Indeed, placenta previa is said to be the cause of most third-trimester bleeding.[13] Most authorities agree (although there is some dissention[17]) that placenta previa is the result of an abnormally low implantation of the conceptus and is more common in patients with previous lower uterine incisional scars for cesarean section or myomectomy, in older women, and in multiparas. This scarring leads to the development of a poorly vascularized, thinner placenta, which occupies a greater uterine surface area or increasing the probability of cervical os encroachment.[21]

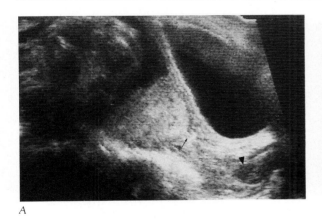

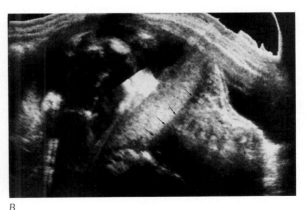

A   B

FIGURE 18-17. Static scans of complete placenta previa. (A) Scan showing placenta covering entire internal os (arrow). Placental tissue is attached to uterine wall on both sides of the os. Note the presence of a vaginal hematoma (arrowhead). (B) In this scan of a complete previa the location of the internal os is somewhat obscured by the presence of a large cervical myoma (arrows) that grew throughout the pregnancy and measured close to 12 cm at term.

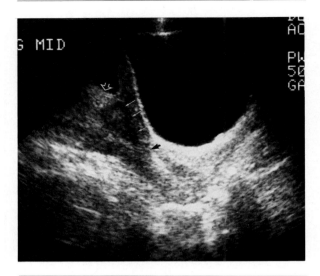

FIGURE 18-18. Sector scan of a marginal placenta previa. Note that the placenta (*open arrow*) covers the area of the os (*closed arrow*) but is not attached to the uterine wall on the other side. The edge of the placenta has been elevated by a marginal hematoma (*small arrows*).

Although a sonographic diagnosis of placenta previa can be made with considerable accuracy,[13] it is important that the sonographer keep several things in mind. First, this diagnosis cannot be made prior to 34 to 36 weeks, unless more than one-third of the placenta covers the internal os.[19] The reason for this is that in many suspected second-trimester placenta previa cases apparent "placental migration" (caused by late second and early third trimester differential growth of the lower uterine segment) will result in most patients (63 to 91%) having a normal implantation at term.[19,20,21,47] On the other hand, a persistent placenta previa can present as early as 20 weeks, if the placenta completely covers the internal os.

Second, since the clinical course and outcome of placenta previa is related to the degree of cervical os encroachment, it is important for the sonographer to try and establish the degree of previa that is present.

Third, the sonographer should always use the technique of varying the degree of bladder distention to decrease the rate of false-positive diagnosis.

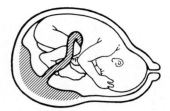

A   Central insertion

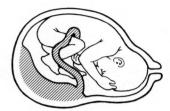

B   Battledore placenta (marginal insertion)

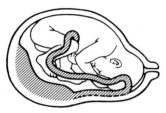

C   Velamentous insertion

FIGURE 18-19. Diagram of umbilical cord insertions. (A) Central insertion of cord into placenta. (B) Battledore insertion; cord is inserted near the margin or edge of the placenta. (C) Velamentous insertion; cord is inserted into chorioamniotic membranes, which extend beyond the placental parenchyma and lie along the uterine wall. This type of insertion near the lower uterine segment can lead to complications such as vasa previa.

This can also help to determine the type of previa. In late pregnancy, it may be necessary to scan through a fairly empty bladder, making visualization of the cervical area difficult; however, as a rule of thumb, if a third-trimester placenta is shown to cover the fundus, chances of a previa are slim[19] unless the placenta is thin and flat, covering a greater area of the intrauterine surface, or an accessory lobe is present covering the lower segment.

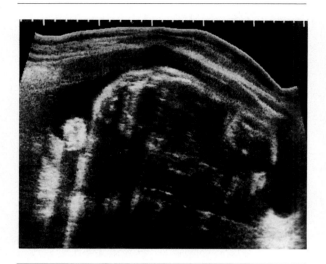

FIGURE 18-20. Static scan of placenta previa. In the later stages of pregnancy, especially with a posterior placenta, it is not always easy to visualize the cervical area. In those cases, the sonographer should measure the distance from the presenting part (in this case, the fetal back) to the bright echoes of the maternal sacrum. A measurement of over 1.5 cm will indicate the possibility of intervening placental tissue. The measurement here is about 4 cm.

Last, a focal, symmetric, lower uterine segment contraction can be mistaken for placenta previa.[21] Repeat scanning after a half hour has elapsed should show that the contraction has subsided.

When in doubt, it is most important to err on the side of assuming the presence of placenta previa. A false-positive diagnosis does not harm the mother or fetus, whereas a missed diagnosis is potentially catastrophic. The usual causes of missed diagnosis are poor technique and poor visualization of a posterior placenta obscured by an overlying fetal head. It has been suggested that a measurement of less than 1.5 cm between the fetal head and the maternal sacrum rules out placenta previa (Fig. 18-20). In the case of a questionable anterior placenta previa, the measurement of less than 1.5 cm between the presenting area and the maternal bladder will rule out previa.[9] But if the placenta is compressed or lateral in location, this distance can be less and placenta previa is still not excluded.

Retroplacental Hemorrhage—Placental Abruption. Placental abruption is the premature separation of all or part of the placenta from the underlying myometrium. It is not entirely clear why this happens, but abruption has been associated with, among other things, maternal vascular disease, maternal hypertension, trauma, short umbilical cord, and maternal age.[42] Abruption may manifest itself in three ways: as external bleeding without significant intrauterine hematoma, as formation of a retroplacental or marginal hematoma with or without external bleeding, and as formation of a submembranous clot at a distance from the placenta, with or without external bleeding.[43,44] It is important to recognize that the bleeding associated with abruption is usually painful (especially when retroplacental in location), and although it is classically described as a cause for third-trimester bleeding (in up to 32% of cases), it can occur early in pregnancy as well.[43,48]

The sonographic appearance of retroplacental hemorrhage is varied, depending on the location, size, and age of the hemorrhage.[13,14,24,43] The hematoma usually is hypoechoic or of mixed echogenicity; echogenicity increases as the clot becomes more organized.[8,9,13,14,24,31,33,42,43,48] As the hematoma matures its echogenicity increases so it may appear isoechoic with the placenta. In such cases, at first glance the placenta may appear to be abnormally thick; however, closer scrutiny usually demonstrates the underlying clot (Fig. 18-21).[24]

An interesting example of a secondary finding in one case was the report of an echogenic mass within the fetal stomach (thought to represent ingested blood clot) in association with retroplacental hemorrhage.[48] Presumably some intraamniotic bleeding must have occurred in association with the abruption, suggesting that the presence of such a finding might alert the sonographer to the underlying cause.

Sonography does not represent the gold standard for diagnosing retroplacental abruption. Clinical assessment (abnormal bleeding, fetal distress, acute abdominal pain, tense and tender uterus) is far better. Sonography is useful only if a clot or elevation of part of the placenta is visualized.[22,39] It should be emphasized that sonography cannot be relied upon to exclude the diagnosis if no hematoma is seen,[5,8,33] as in some cases of abrup-

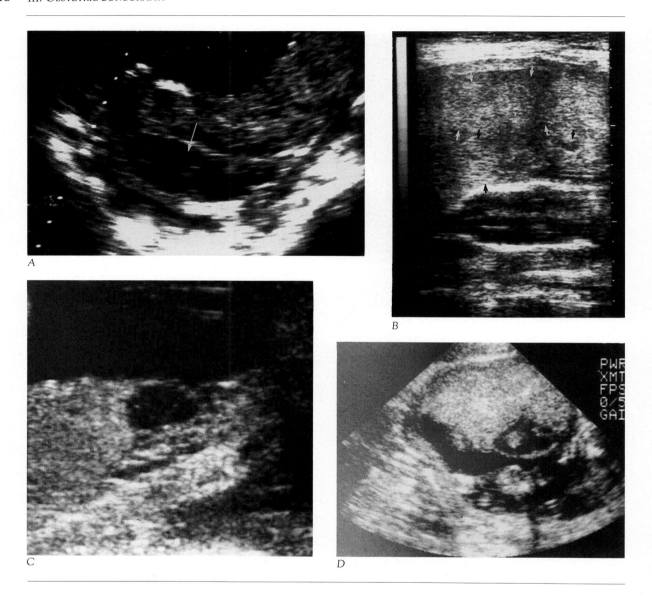

FIGURE 18-21. Placental abruption. (A) Subplacental abruption (*arrow*) in which a large portion of placental tissue has lifted away from the subjacent myometrium. The sonolucent appearance of the hematoma would indicate that the damage was very recent, although the presence of a few internal echoes might indicate that some clotting has taken place. (B) Linear scan of placental abruption, which has the appearance of a hydropic placenta because the acoustic texture of the subplacental hematoma (*white arrows*) is isodense with that of the placental tissue (*black arrows*). The echogenic appearance of the hematoma indicates a clot of several days' standing. (C) Linear scan of marginal hematoma shows an area of recent bleeding. (D) Sector scan of a subchorionic hematoma that was noted to be a postamniocentesis bleed.

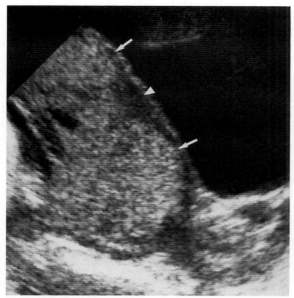

FIGURE 18-21.1

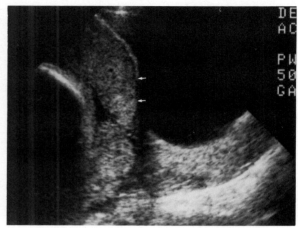

FIGURE 18-21.2

FIGURE 18-21.1. Sector scan of a full placenta previa with coincident placenta percreta. Placental tissue appears to extend right to the external portion of the uterine wall in several places (*arrows*), with small patches of intervening myometrium (*arrowhead*). At delivery, placental tissue was actually found to have invaded the maternal urinary bladder.

FIGURE 18-21.2. Sector scan of a low anterior placenta with focal placenta accreta. Note the gradual thinning of the basal plate (*arrows*).

tion the placenta may look normal, especially late in pregnancy.[22,35,42]

Differential diagnosis of retroplacental hemorrhage includes normal maternal veins in the retroplacental complex, hydatidiform mole, and chorioangioma.[33] Clinical outcome depends upon the size of the abruption and its location. For example, a paraplacental (marginal) clot has much less clinical importance than a large retroplacental hematoma associated with placental separation, which could lead to premature delivery or miscarriage.

Abnormal Placental Attachment—Placenta Accreta, Increta, Percreta. Some relatively uncommon conditions result from defective decidual formation causing abnormal attachment of the placenta to the uterine wall. As with placenta previa, the presence of uterine scarring seems to predispose patients to the development of this condition. In fact, up to two-thirds of cases occur in association with placenta previa, and in patients with a history of prior cesarean section.[45] In placenta accreta, the chorionic villi are in direct contact with the uterine muscle. Placenta increta and -percreta are more severe forms in which the placental villi invade or penetrate the uterine wall, respectively.[8,21,45]

Sonography reveals obliteration of the normal retroplacental sonolucent complex (Figs. 18-21.1,2).[8,19,21,45] As previously described, visualization of the retroplacental complex can be difficult in an anteriorly located placenta owing to the presence of superimposed transducer reverberation artifact.[8,22] In this event, visualization might be enhanced by using a standoff device. It can also be

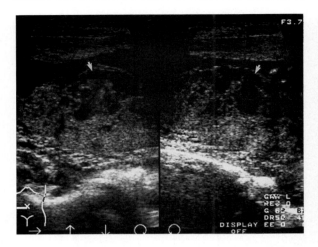

FIGURE 18-22. Dual image linear scan of posterior placenta shows two views of an area of large, abnormal vascular spaces (*arrows*). This was thought to be a Breus' mole, but histologic confirmation was not available.

difficult to diagnose this condition in a posterior placenta, particularly late in gestation, when the overlying fetus may obscure visualization of the retroplacental complex.[21] Antenatal detection of this condition is difficult but extremely important; if it is not treated (usually by hysterectomy) it can lead to maternal exsanguination.[19,21]

Placental Lesions

Intervillous thrombosis. Intervillous thromboses represent intraplacental areas of hemorrhage and clot, occurring in up to 50% of term pregnancies. They are probably the result of a tear in the villi causing leakage of fetal red blood cells, which stimulates maternal coagulation.[43] These appear sonographically as hypoechoic lesions of varying sizes. More extensive sonolucencies may represent massive subchorionic thrombosis (Breus' mole), a rare occurrence secondary to venous obstruction (Fig. 18-22).[8,43]

Fibrin deposition. Fibrin deposition is apparently clinically insignificant; probably the end-result of intervillous and subchorionic thrombosis,[40] which, in turn, is the result of pooling and stasis of maternal blood in the perivillous and subchorionic

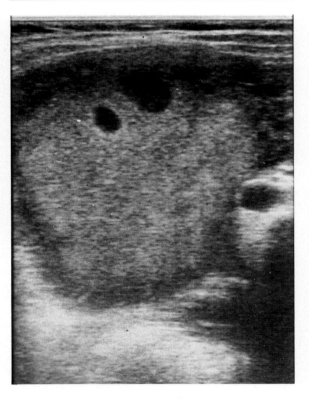

FIGURE 18-23. Linear scan of a placenta with two areas of fibrin deposition.

spaces.[8,43] Fibrin deposits also appear sonographically as sonolucencies in the subchorionic area or within the placental mass (Fig. 18-23).[43]

Placental infarction. Placental infarcts are also thought to result from intervillous thrombosis and may occur in up to 25% of term placentas. Although generally they are found to have no clinical significance, they appear to be more common in association with intrauterine growth retardation and preeclampsia.[43] There has been no documented sonographic visualization of placental infarcts,[1] but demonstration of areas of placental thinning might point a finger to this condition.

Placental Tumors

Chorioangioma. Chorioangioma and teratoma represent the two primary nontrophoblastic tumors of the placenta. Chorioangioma is a vascular malfor-

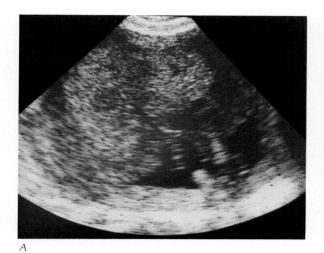
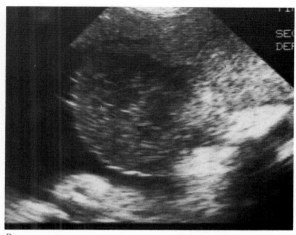

A   B

FIGURE 18-24. Sector scans of placental hemangiomas. Both show heterogeneous texture caused by numerous vascular channels and stroma. Vascular channels are seen in B.

mation and is by far the more common. Large chorioangiomas may cause significant vascular shunting,[13,40] leading to the development of fetal hydrops, low birth weight, premature labor, or fetal demise.[43]

Chorioangiomas are usually composed of clusters of small tumors and so may appear sonographically only as areas of focal thickening of the placenta.[8,10,33,49] If large, the tumor is usually single and may appear as a well-circumscribed, complex mass on the fetal surface of the placenta, adjacent to the cord insertion[49] or protruding into the amniotic cavity (Fig. 18-24).[33,42,43] Vascular channels may be seen within the mass.[42]

Teratoma. Teratomas of the placenta are very rare. They are usually benign but can be highly malignant.[8,42,43] Sonographically, they appear as a complex mass.

The Umbilical Cord
STRUCTURE AND FUNCTION
The umbilical cord normally contains two arteries and one vein surrounded by a mucoid connective tissue (Wharton's jelly), all enclosed in a layer of amnion.[29] The arteries carry deoxygenated blood

from the fetus to the placenta and the vein brings fresh, oxygenated blood to the fetus. The umbilical arteries are longer than the vein, causing them to wind around it. All are longer than the cord itself, resulting in twisting and bending of the cord and vessels (see fig. 18-1).[7,29] The arteries have a thicker wall and a smaller cross-sectional area (4 mm) than the vein (1.0 cm).[7,38] At term the mean length of the cord is about 55 cm (range 30 to 120), with a mean circumference of 3.6 cm.[2,11,35]

SCANNING TECHNIQUE
The umbilical cord is best visualized in the late second and early third trimester, when amniotic fluid volume is at its peak. Owing to the extreme length of the cord it is impossible, on a routine basis, to scan it in its entirety to rule out abnormalities. If such a lesion is suspected, every effort must be made to view as much of the cord as possible. Changing the mother's position from side to side may help by shifting the position of the fetus. The cord insertion site on the placenta as well as on the fetus (to rule out hernia or omphalocele) should be imaged and documented routinely, as should the presence of three vessels within the cord. Visualization of a three-vessel cord may be difficult in the

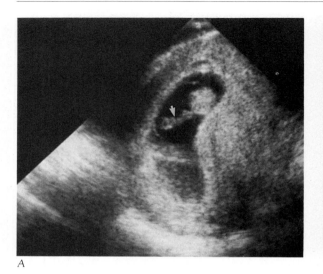
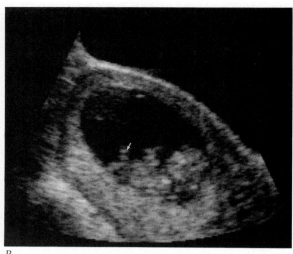

A

B

Figure 18-25. (A) Transvaginal scan of early gestation showing the umbilical cord extending from the fetus (*large arrow*). The twisted configuration of the cord is evident. (B) Transabdominal scan at about the same age shows less definition. The cord appears as a series of short, linear echogenicities (*small arrow*).

third trimester owing to relative lack of fluid and the presence of potentially obstructing fetal parts. Any change in diameter along the length of the cord should be noted.

Normal Sonographic Appearance

In early pregnancy, the umbilical cord may appear as a series of short, linear echoes extending from the fetus to the placenta (Fig. 18-25). As pregnancy progresses, transverse images through the cord reveal the three-circle, or "Mickey Mouse" sign, confirming the presence of three vessels (the largest circle representing the vein). Longitudinal images at this stage reveal a series of parallel linear echoes within the amniotic fluid (Fig. 18-26). The "stack of coins" appearance refers to visualization of several portions of cord folded on each other (Fig. 18-27).[11] Real-time scanning demonstrates arterial pulsations within the umbilical arteries.[30] The insertion of the umbilical cord into the placenta appears as a V- or U-shaped sonolucent area just beneath the chorionic plate (Fig. 18-28).[7,38]

Abnormalities of the Umbilical Cord (Table 18-4)

Abnormalities of Cord Insertion. The umbilical cord usually inserts in the center of the placenta; however, it may be marginal or velamentous (Fig. 18-2). In the latter case, vessels are found lying on the surface of the chorioamniotic membranes, a condition associated with various fetal anomalies and umbilical malpresentation.[7,11,38] For this reason, careful examination of the placental insertion site is important.

True and False Knots. As previously described, the differential in umbilical vein, umbilical artery, and cord stromal length gives rise to bending and twisting of the umbilical cord. Sometimes this twisting may appear as a false knot, which has no clinical significance.[7] It can, however, be sonographically confused with a true knot of the cord, when the fetus actually passes through a loop of cord. This potentially hazardous situation occurs in about 1% of deliveries[38] but is difficult to detect sonographically.

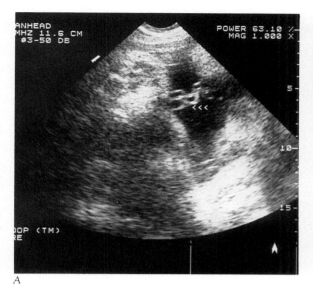

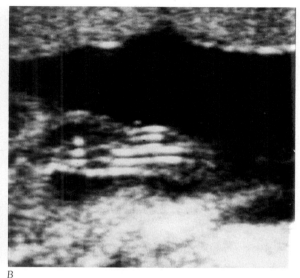

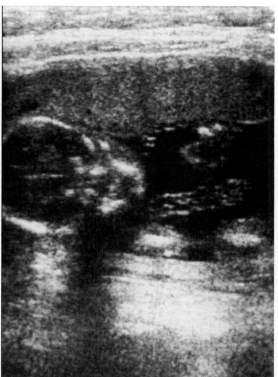

A

B

C

FIGURE 18-26. (A) Linear scan of umbilical cord in transverse plane shows the large vein and two smaller arteries. This is commonly called the Mickey Mouse sign. (B) The cord in longitudinal section commonly appears as parallel bright linear echoes. (C) In this scan the twisting of the vessels within the cord is apparent.

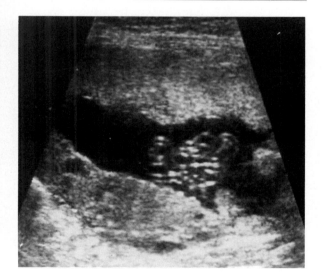

FIGURE 18-27. When several portions of the cord are folded on top of one another, this "stack of coins" appearance is seen.

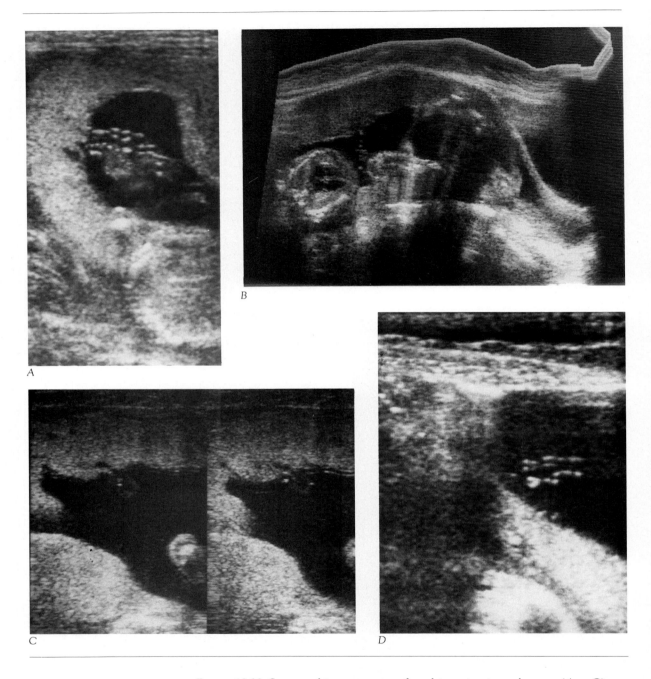

FIGURE 18-28. Sonographic appearance of cord insertion into placenta. (*A* to *C*) Static and linear scans of centrally located cord insertions. Note that the "typical" **V**-shaped sonolucent area is more evident on the static scan. (*D*) Linear scan of marginal (battledore) insertion into placenta.

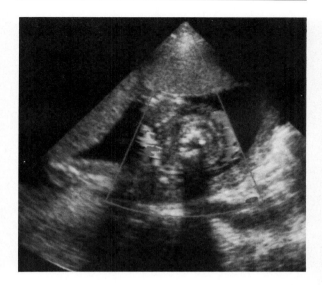

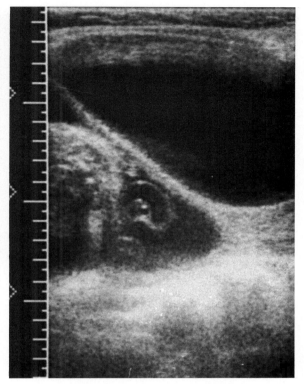

FIGURE 18-28.1 Transverse image of cord wrapped around the fetal neck (Nuchal Cord). This image was produced with a color flow Doppler transducer (the color could not be reproduced here). The visualization of flow in red and blue greatly enhanced the ability to clearly see this structure.

FIGURE 18-29. Linear scan of vasa previa. Loops of cord are visualized between the cervix and the presenting fetal part. This situation can present grave complications during delivery.

Abnormal Cord Position

Nuchal cord. In about one fifth of all deliveries, the umbilical cord is looped around the neck of the fetus[29] and has been so demonstrated during routine sonography (Fig. 18-28.1).[7] This diagnosis should be considered whenever umbilical cord is imaged around or near the fetal neck.

Cord prolapse. Umbilical cord prolapse occurs in several forms. Occult prolapse refers to loops of cord adjacent to the fetal presenting parts; vasa previa refers to a segment of umbilical cord located between presenting fetal parts and the lower pole of intact membranes (Fig. 18-29); and frank prolapse refers to cord protrusion into the cervix, usually through ruptured membranes.[6,16,38] Velamentous insertion of the umbilical cord or a low-lying placenta may be noted in some cases.[6] Sonographic detection of this condition is clinically important, as it may lead to cord compression compromising the fetal circulation, a potentially fatal situation. Predisposing factors to the development of umbilical cord prolapse are fetal malpresentation, prematurity, polyhydromnios, premature rupture of membranes, excessive cord length, multiple gestation, and cephalopelvic disproportion.[16]

Single Umbilical Artery. A two-vessel cord is seen in 0.5 to 1.0% of all pregnancies, caused either by primary agenesis of one of the embryonic umbilical arteries or by atrophy of a previously normal umbilical artery.[9,38,40] Ten percent of these have associated fetal anomalies of a more or less serious nature, such as renal agenesis, IUGR, and central nervous system and cardiovascular anomalies. On sonographic investigation, the cord will have lost its braided appearance[38] and only two vessels will be viewed transversely (Fig. 18-30).

TABLE 18-4. Sonographic characteristics of umbilical abnormalities

ABNORMALITY	DESCRIPTION	SONOGRAPHIC CHARACTERISTIC	DIFFERENTIAL DIAGNOSIS
Excessive Wharton's jelly	Diffuse or focal deposits of excess Wharton's jelly[2,36]; may liquefy and get very large[7]	Variably echogenic soft tissue mass w/three vessels visible within, usually near fetal abdomen; may be cystic if liquefied[7]	Hernia, tumor, hematoma, cysts
Omphalocele	Protrusion of abdominal structures (liver, bowel) into base of cord covered by peritoneum[7]; high incidence of associated congenital abnormalities	Mass adjacent to anterior abdominal wall, covered by membrane, into apex of which cord appears to insert; sac may be distended by ascites	Gastroschisis, cord hematoma
False knot	Folding of vessels which are longer than covering membrane[2] or simple dilatation of vessels	Irregular protrusion from cord[2]	True knot
True knot	Results from excessive fetal movement, especially with a long cord, or polyhydramnios[38]; may become tightened and occlude umbilical vessels[2]; associated with increased incidence of congenital anomalies[38]	Irregular protrusion from cord[38]	False knot
Stricture	Localized narrowing of cord, disappearance of Wharton's jelly, torsion of cord or thickening of vessel walls with narrowing of lumen	Narrowing of cord close to fetus with edematous area distal[38]	Transient constriction of cord
Umbilical vein thrombosis	Occlusion of umbilical vein secondary to localized increase of resistance in umbilical circulation; associated with maternal diabetes, arthritis, nonimmune hydrops[1,3,7]	Increased echogenicity of umbilical vessels or echogenic material within lumen	Artifact

Enlargement of the Umbilical Cord. Enlargement of the cord is very rare. It may be a normal variant, associated with tumors or cysts, or an indicator of possible isoimmune sensitivity. In the later case, intraabdominal umbilical vein dilatation generally precedes dilatation in the cord.[7,11,35] When any mass on the cord is visualized, careful examination of the anterior abdominal wall of the fetus should be made to rule out any associated fetal abdominal wall malformation. The sonographer should also examine the mass for the presence of vessels within.

Diffuse enlargement of the cord may be due to edema, hypoosmolarity,[2] or excessive deposits of Wharton's jelly.[2,36] Focal enlargement may be due to hernia, omphalocele, false or true knot, and various cystic and solid lesions.

Umbilical Cord Masses

Cystic. Cystic masses of the cord are usually related to vestigial patency of an embryonic structure,[7,36,38] or rarely, to an aneurysm of an umbilical artery. Excessive deposits of Wharton's jelly may liquefy and present as a large, cystic mass.[7]

TABLE 18-4. (continued)

ABNORMALITY	DESCRIPTION	SONOGRAPHIC CHARACTERISTIC	DIFFERENTIAL DIAGNOSIS
Cystic Masses			
Allantoic cyst (developmental urachal cyst)	Fluid-filled remnant of allantoid duct[7,36,38] associated with patent urachus and lower tract obstructions	Usually small, mild, focal dilatation of cord, namely of persistent patent urachus in fetal abdomen	Omphalomesenteric cyst
Omphalomesenteric cyst	Vestigial patency and dilatation of duct seen after 16 weeks[36,38]	Cystic dilatation up to 6 cm, usually located close to fetus	Hematoma, liquefied Wharton's jelly
Solid Masses			
Hemangioma	Benign tumor of vessels or Wharton's jelly, if large, can cause vascular obstruction[36]; may be associated with increased amniotic fluid and α-fetoprotein[7] and nonimmune hydrops[38]	Varied appearance: hyperechoic mass with smooth lobulated contours, up to 15 cm; may have small ovoid lucencies or numerous small highly echogenic reflectors; surrounding cord may appear edematous, usually located near placental margin[7,25,38]	Hematoma, teratoma
Hematoma	Rare. Result from extravasation of blood into Wharton's jelly[38] from rupture of umbilical vein[2,7,36]; may be due to congenital weakness of vessel wall or iatrogenic; associated w/perinatal fetal loss[7]	May be septate, hyper- or hypoechoic, depending on age of clot; may be more irregular than other cystic lesions; may appear as enlargement of cord with constriction of vessels[36]; has been reported as large, sonolucent, septate mass adjacent to fetal abdomen[2,7,38]	Tumors, cysts
Teratoma	Rare germ cell tumor	Disorganized, heterogeneous mass, up to 9 cm in diameter; may have calcifications, found at any point along the cord[38]	Hemangioma, hematoma[38]

Hematomas may also appear cystic or sonolucent, depending on their age. Differentiation may be difficult, but hematomas may be more irregular than other cystic lesions and may be septate. If a cyst is discovered, serial examinations should be performed to verify normal fetal growth and to note any change in the size of the cyst, as an expanding cyst may compress blood vessels. Doppler evaluation may be helpful in such cases.[7]

Solid. Solid masses of the umbilical cord include hemangiomas, angiomyxomas, dermoids, and teratomas.[7] Although precise sonographic diagnosis of hemangioma is not possible, the presence of a heterogeneous, solid umbilical cord mass near the placental end of the cord should suggest the diagnosis (Fig. 18-31). As with any mass of the cord, mechanical impairment of circulation is a possible consequence, especially as these tumors arise from the vascular tissue itself.[7,25,38]

The presence of calcifications in a disorganized, heterogeneous mass anywhere along the length of the cord is suggestive of teratoma. Again, the fetus should be evaluated for possible vascular compromise or hydrops.[38]

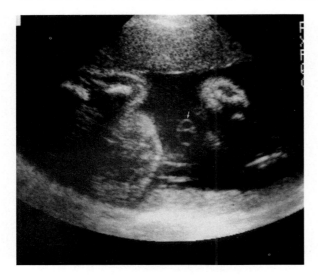

FIGURE 18-30. Sector scan shows a two-vessel cord best visualized transversely. The arrow points to the single artery, which is slightly smaller than the vein although somewhat larger than an artery in a three-vessel cord. The two vessels may also appear to be the same size.

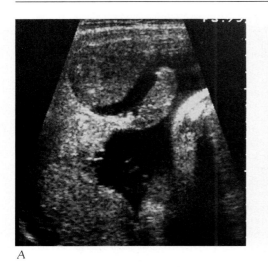

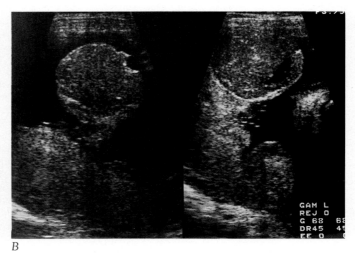

A   B

FIGURE 18-31. Umbilical cord hemangioma. In A and on the right side of B it is difficult to determine whether the hemangioma is of placental or umbilical cord origin. In the left-hand image of B, however, the entire hemangioma is visualized separate from the placenta, and the tubular lucency in the other frames was determined to represent the umbilical vein.

Strictures of the Umbilical Cord. Although no sonographic visualizations of this abnormality have been recorded to date, it should be possible to see one or more areas of narrowing of the cord, usually close to the fetus, associated with distal cord swelling. Once again, this finding should alert the sonographer to carefully assess the fetus for congenital anomalies or vascular compromise.[38]

Umbilical Vein and Arterial Thrombosis. Umbilical vein thrombosis and occlusion is a serious condition associated with nonimmune fetal hydrops and a high degree of prenatal mortality. Thrombosis may also occur in the umbilical arteries, with associated aneurysmic dilatation.[38] The thrombosis may be primary (the incidence of this condition increases in diabetic mothers[1]), or it may occur secondary to a mechanical cord impairment such as torsion, knotting, compression, or hematoma. Sonographically, the thrombus may present as increased echogenicity of the umbilical vessels.[1,38]

Conclusion

As we have seen, improved technology and enhanced resolution of ultrasound equipment have enabled sonographers to evaluate the placenta and umbilical cord with amazing accuracy. Currently, the use of Doppler for evaluating umbilical and placental blood flow is finding its proper place in the clinical setting. It is now recognized that, when used judiciously in medically indicated cases, valuable information can be gained from Doppler analysis. It is expected that the research now being performed in this area will clarify even further the parameters of umbilical Doppler ultrasound.

References

1. Abrams SL, Callen PW, Filly RA. Umbilical vein thrombosis: Sonographic detection in utero. J Ultrasound Med. 1985; 4:283–285.
2. Allen M. Diagnostic challenge I: Excessive amount of Wharton's jelly. J Diagn Med Sonogr. 1987; 3:27, 29, 30.
3. Clair MR, Rosenberg E, Tempkin D, et al. Placental grading in the complicated or high-risk frequency. J Ultrasound Med. 1983; 2:297–301.
4. Crane JP. Sonographic evaluation of multiple frequency. Semin Ultrasound CT MRI. 1984; 5:144–156.
5. Cyr D. Fetal umbilical Doppler. In: SDMS 5th Annual Conference Proceedings. Dallas. 1988.
6. Gianopoulos J, Carver T, Tomich PG, et al. Diagnosis of vasa previa with ultrasonography. Obstet Gynecol. 1987; 69:488–491.
7. Graham D, Campbell T, Litchfield KL. Sonography of the umbilical cord. In: Sanders RC, James AE Jr, eds. The Principles and Practice of Ultrasonography in Obstetrics and Gynecology. 3rd ed. Norwalk, CT: Appleton-Century-Crofts; 1985.
8. Graham D, Guidi S, Sanders RC. Sonography of the placenta. In: Sanders RC, Hill MC, eds. Ultrasound Annual. New York: Raven Press; 1984.
9. Grannum P, Hobbins JC. The placenta. In: Callen PW, ed. Ultrasonography in Obstetrics and Gynecology. Philadelphia: WB Saunders; 1983.
10. Grundy HO, Byers L, Walton S, et al. Antepartum ultrasonographic evaluation and management of placental chorioangioma. A case report. J Reprod Med. 1986; 31:520–522.
11. Hadlock FP. The amniotic fluid and umbilical cord. In: Athey PA, Hadlock FP, eds. Ultrasound in Obstetrics and Gynecology. St. Louis: CV Mosby; 1981.
12. Hadlock FP. The placenta. In: Athey PA, Hadlock FP, eds. Ultrasound in Obstetrics and Gynecology. St. Louis: CV Mosby; 1981.
13. Hadlock FP. The placenta. In: Athey PA, Hadlock FP, eds. Ultrasound in Obstetrics and Gynecology. 2nd ed. St. Louis: CV Mosby; 1985.
14. Hadlock FP, Rothchild S. Use of ultrasound in invasive procedures. In: Athey PA, Hadlock FP, eds. Ultrasound in Obstetrics and Gynecology. St. Louis: CV Mosby; 1981.
15. Hadlock FP, Deter RL, et al. Hypervascularity of the uterine wall during pregnancy: Incidence, sonographic appearance, and obstetric implications. J Clin Ultrasound. 1980; 8:399–404.
16. Hales ED, Westney LS. Sonography of occult cord prolapse. J Clin Ultrasound. 1984; 12:283–285.
17. Hisley JC, Mangum C. Placental location in pregnancies following cesarean section. J Clin Ultrasound. 1982; 10:427–428.
18. Hoddick WK, Mahony BS, Callen PW, et al. Placental thickness. J Ultrasound Med. 1985; 4:479–482.
19. Jeanty P, Romero R. Obstetrical Ultrasound. New York: McGraw-Hill; 1984.
20. Khan AT, Stewart KS. Ultrasound placental localization in early pregnancy. Scot Med J. 1987; 32:19–21.
21. Laing FC. Ultrasound evaluation of obstetric problems relating to the lower uterine segment and cervix. In: Sanders RC, James AE Jr, eds. The Principles and Practice of Ultrasonography in Obstetrics and Gynecology. 3rd ed. Norwalk, CT: Appleton-Century-Crofts; 1985.
22. Marx M, Casola G, Scheible W, et al. The subplacental complex: Further sonographic observations. J Ultrasound Med. 1985; 4:459–461.
23. de Mendonia LK. Sonographic diagnosis of placenta accreta: Presentation of six cases. J Ultrasound Med. 1988; 7:211–215.
24. Mintz MC, Kurtz AB, Arenson R, et al. Abruptio placentae: Apparent thickening of the placenta caused by hyperechoic retroplacental clot. J Ultrasound Med. 1986; 5:411–413.
25. Mishriki YY, Vanyshelbaum Y, Epstein H, et al. Hemangioma of the umbilical cord. Pediatr Pathol. 1987; 7:43–49.

26. Molloy CE, McDowell W, Armour T, et al. Ultrasonic diagnosis of placenta membranacea in utero. J Ultrasound Med. 1983; 2:377–379.

27. Monaghan J, O'Herlihy C, Boylan P. Ultrasound placental grading and amniotic fluid quantitation in prolonged pregnancy. Obstet Gynecol. 1987; 70:349–352.

28. Montan S, Jorgensen C, Svalenius E, et al. Placental grading with ultrasound in hypertensive and normotensive pregnancies. A prospective, consecutive study. Acta Obstet Gynecol Scand. 1986; 65:477–480.

29. Moore KL. Fetal membranes and placenta. In: Moore KL. The Developing Human. 3rd ed. Philadelphia: WB Saunders, 1982.

30. Morin F, Winsberg F. Real-time identification of blood flow in the placenta and umbilical cord. J Clin Ultrasound. 1982; 10:21–24.

31. Nyberg DA, Mack LA, Benedetti TJ, et al. Placental abruption and placental hemorrhage: Correlation of sonographic findings with fetal outcome. Radiology. 1987; 164:357–361.

32. Persutte WH, Lenke RR. Maternal urinary bladder filling for middle- and late-trimester ultrasound: Is it really necessary? J Ultrasound Med. 1988; 7:203–206.

33. Price SA. Ultrasound visualization of abruptio placentae with massive hemorrhage protruding into the amniotic cavity. J Diagn Ultrasound. 1986; 2:161–163.

34. Proud J, Grant AM. Third-trimester placental grading by ultrasonography as a test of fetal wellbeing. Br Medical J (Clin Res). 1987; 294:1641–1644.

35. Queenan JT, O'Brien GD. Diagnostic ultrasound in erythroblastosis fetalis. In: Sanders RC and James AE Jr, eds. The Principles and Practice of Ultrasonography in Obstetrics and Gynecology. 3rd ed. Norwalk, CT: Appleton-Century-Crofts; 1985.

36. Ramanathan K, Epstein S, Yaghoobian J. Localized deposition of Wharton's jelly: Sonographic findings. J Ultrasound Med. 1986; 5:339–340.

37. Reece EA, Hobbins JC. Ultrasonography and diabetes mellitus in pregnancy. In: Sanders RC, James AE Jr, eds. The Principles and Practice of Ultrasonography in Obstetrics and Gynecology. 3rd ed. Norwalk, CT: Appleton-Century-Crofts; 1985.

38. Romero R, Pilu G, Jeanty P, et al. The umbilical cord. In: Prenatal Diagnosis of Congenital Anomalies. Norwalk, CT: Appleton & Lange; 1988.

39. Sauerbrei EE, Pham DII. Placental abruption and subchorionic hemorrhage in the first half of pregnancy: Ultrasound appearance and clinical outcome. Radiology. 1986; 160:109–112.

40. Sauerbrei EE, Nguyen KT, Nolan RL. A Practical Guide to Ultrasound in Obstetrics and Gynecology. New York: Raven Press; 1987.

41. Shah YG, Graham D. Relationship of placental grade to fetal pulmonary maturity and respiratory distress syndrome. Am J Perinatol. 1986; 3:53–55.

42. Spirt BA, Kagen EH. Sonography of the placenta. (Obstetrical Ultrasound Update). Semin Ultrasound 1980; 1:293–310.

43. Spirt BA, Gordon LP, Kagen EH. Sonography of the placenta. In: Sanders RC, James AE Jr, eds. The Principles and Practice of Ultrasonography in Obstetrics and Gynecology. 3rd ed. Norwalk, CT: Appleton-Century-Crofts; 1985.

44. Spirt BA, Kagan EH, et al. Clinically silent retroplacental hematoma: Sonographic and pathologic correlation. J Clin Ultrasound. 1981; 9:203–205.

45. Tabsh KMA, Brinkman CR III, King W. Ultrasound diagnosis of placenta increta. J Clin Ultrasound. 1982; 10:288–290.

46. Timor-Tritsch IE, Retten S, et al. How transvaginal sonography is done. In: Timor-Tritsch IE, Rottem S, eds. Transvaginal Sonography. New York: Elsevier; 1988.

47. Townsend RR, Laing FC, Nyberg DA, et al. Technical factors responsible for "placental migration": Sonographic assessment. Radiology. 1986; 160:105–108.

48. Walker JM, Ferguson DD. The sonographic appearance of blood in the fetal stomach and its association with placental abruption. J Ultrasound Med. 1988; 7:155–161.

49. Willard DA, Moeschler JB. Placental chorioangioma: A rare cause of elevated amniotic fluid alpha-fetoprotein. J Ultrasound Med. 1986; 5:221–222.

50. Wolf H, Oosting H, Treffers PE. Placental volume measurement by ultrasonography: Evaluation of the method. Am J Obstet Gynecol. 1987; 156:1191–1194.

CHAPTER **19**

Doppler Ultrasound in the Assessment of Fetal Status

JOANNE ROSENBERG

History of Doppler Ultrasound Technique

In 1842 an Austrian professor of mathematics and geometry, Dr. Christian Johann Doppler, first described in detail the effect that now bears his name.[13] Dr. Doppler did not observe the effect on sound but on shifts in light frequencies emitted from double stars.

In the 1930s Barcroft and associates performed radiographic studies on fetal lambs and goats to establish the circulatory pathways.[3] Lind and Wegelius[30] in 1954 employed cardiographic techniques to describe the arterial and venous circulation in human fetuses and found it was similar to that of fetal sheep. Numerous other investigators reported on highly invasive procedures on preabortive fetuses.

Satomura first described the clinical application of Doppler ultrasound technology in 1959.[44] Early continuous-wave (CW) transducers were not very specific, as they were unable to distinguish whether flow moved toward or away from the transducer. This deficit was overcome with the addition of spectrum analyzers and audible signals, which allowed estimation of the frequency of the Doppler shift and the direction of flow.

Pulsed-wave (PW) Doppler was introduced in the late 1960s almost simultaneously by two independent laboratories. Baker in Washington studied transcutanous blood flow measurements in humans,[1,2] while Peronneau in France used his system initially on animals.[39,40] PW emits short bursts of ultrasound energy into the body, allowing detection of a moving target at a given depth. Duplex Doppler imaging—PW Doppler used in conjunction with two-dimensional ultrasound imaging—allows us to obtain a Doppler sample from almost any vessel visualized.

Bioeffects

To date, Doppler and real-time ultrasound have not been associated with any ill effects to fetus or mother. This assessment has been arrived at independently by every consensus group that has reviewed the literature and research findings in this area.[31]

The U.S. FDA guidelines state that there are no known risks associated with use of Doppler ultrasound at the recommended power levels. There are specific FDA guidelines for fetal ultrasound, including that the Doppler spatial peak-temporal average intensity (SPTA) be less than 94 mW/cm^2 in situ. SPTA is a unit used to measure ultrasound energy intensity. Most commercial equipment employs variable acoustic power outputs between 1 and 46 mW/cm^2. The power output of a given Doppler unit should be known before it is used on a fetus.

Physics

Continuous-Wave Doppler Ultrasound

The Doppler effect is a change in frequency resulting from motion of the sound source or scatter (Fig. 19-1). The Doppler effect has applications in everyday life ranging from home burglar alarms to police radar detectors. In medicine, Doppler ultrasound is used to detect and measure blood velocity and flow.

Reflections of blood flow can be studied with two basic Doppler techniques. The simplest technique is CW Doppler; the other, PW, will be discussed later. With CW Doppler a single transducer has two separate piezoelectric crystals, one that continuously emits sound and another that simultaneously receives it (Fig. 19-2). The frequency of the received echo is compared to the frequency of the transmitted echo to derive the Doppler shift.

Since the crystals are either emitting sound or receiving it, CW Doppler measures no range or depth resolution. No imaging is available with this system, but it may be used in conjunction with real-time imaging to locate or confirm the vessel sampling site.

CW is limited to the study of superficial vessels because it cannot discriminate between signals arising from different structures along the beam path, but it is inexpensive, portable, and simple to operate.

Pulsed-Wave Doppler

In PW Doppler, short bursts of ultrasound energy are emitted at regular intervals (see Fig. 19-2). The same piezoelectric crystal both sends and receives the signals. This allows for range or depth discrimination. The depth of the target is calculated from the elapsed time between transmission of the pulse and reception of its echos, assuming a constant speed of sound in tissues. With PW a sample volume can be electronically steered by manipulating the joystick on the Doppler keyboard. Steering allows the operator to obtain a reading of a vessel at a certain depth. This is done by adjusting the depth of the gate. The area inside the opened gate is the sample volume site (Fig. 19-3). The gate can also be adjusted between 1 and 15 mm, to adjust the size of the sample volume.

Duplex Doppler sonography combines PW Doppler with real-time imaging. This allows us to

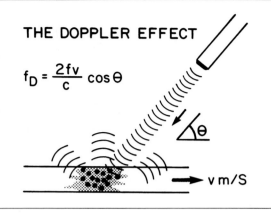

THE DOPPLER EFFECT

$$f_D = \frac{2fv}{c} \cos \theta$$

Figure 19-1. An incident ultrasound beam of frequency (f) is scattered by moving red blood cells. As a result of the Doppler effect, the back-scattered echo has a center of frequency which is higher by f_D. $f_D = 2fv \cos \theta/c$, where f_D is the change in ultrasound frequency, also known as the Doppler shift frequency; f is the frequency of the incident ultrasound; v is the relative velocity between the target and the transducer; θ is the angle between the beam and the direction of the movement of the target; and c is the velocity of sound in the medium. (Used with permission.[8])

sample vessels at specific anatomic locations. With direct visualization, the direction of the insonating Doppler beam can be adjusted in order to obtain optimal waveforms with maximum velocities. The gate depth and width can also be selected under direct visualization. Direct visualization of the vessels provides accuracy in the sampling, helping to identify normal versus abnormal waveform ratios. For example, an abnormal uterine artery waveform can produce the same Doppler signal as a normal common iliac artery waveform.

The angle of insonation is the angle at which the Doppler beam encounters or intersects the vessel to be sampled. Mirror imaging or artifacts can occur when the angle of insonation is close to 90 degrees. If this happens, the system cannot distinguish direction of flow and produces the same waveform above and below the baseline. The optimal angle for PW Doppler is 30 to 60 degrees.

Aliasing is a phenomenon that occurs in PW systems when the pulse repetition frequency (PRF) is less than two times the correct Doppler shift fre-

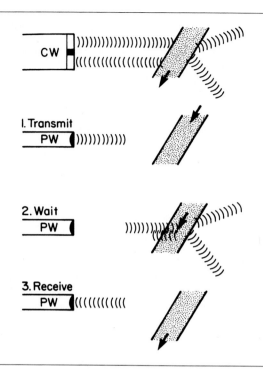

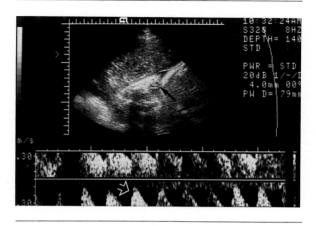

FIGURE 19-3. Duplex Doppler sonogram demonstrates aliasing. Note the wraparound of the peak systolic peaks (*open arrow*). The area inside the opened gate is the sample volume site (*arrow*).

FIGURE 19-2. (*A*) CW Doppler transducer that continually transmits and receives reflections to and from the target. (*B*) PW Doppler transducer (1) transmits a single pulse, and (2) waits for it to return. (3) The time it takes to return is determined by the depth of the target.

quency (Fig. 19-3). This occurs during attempts to sample high-velocity blood flow. PRF is the number of pulses sent out by the transducer per second. The Nyquist limit is the minimum PRF required to register a frequency without aliasing.[38] This proves to be one-half the frequency. For example, to detect a frequency of 10 kHz, the PRF must be 20 kHz. It is the speed of sound that basically limits the PRF as a function of depth. Aliasing can be avoided by increasing the PRF, increasing the angle of insonation, using a lower-frequency transducer, or switching to CW (CW Doppler has no range resolution).

In a study by Mehalek and colleagues,[34] CW and PW flow velocity waveforms were compared using the patient as the control. The systolic-to-diastolic (S/D or A/B) ratios obtained with CW and PW Doppler systems were found to be comparable. Therefore, a laboratory can use either a CW or PW Doppler system effectively.

Analysis of the Doppler Signal

Doppler ultrasound has many uses in examining the maternal-fetal circulation. Qualitative Doppler allows us to identify the direction of blood flow and detect flow disturbances such as stenosis or turbulences. More importantly, Doppler allows us to identify abnormal flow patterns that help to identify pregnancies at risk of poor fetal outcome. Quantitative flow measurements include blood velocity and flow. Qualitative measurements look at characteristics of the waveforms, which indirectly give an approximation of flow and resistance to flow. These include the S/D ratio,[45] the resistance index (RI),[41] and the pulsatility index (PI)[21] (Fig. 19-4).[21]

Waveform analysis is affected by cardiac contractility, blood viscosity, elasticity of the vessel wall, the peripheral resistance in the circulation, the distance of the sampling site from the heart, and the presence or absence of turbulence.[22]

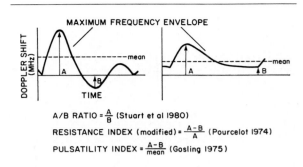

A/B RATIO = $\frac{A}{B}$ (Stuart et al 1980)

RESISTANCE INDEX (modified) = $\frac{A-B}{A}$ (Pourcelot 1974)

PULSATILITY INDEX = $\frac{A-B}{mean}$ (Gosling 1975)

FIGURE 19-4. Diagram of Doppler waveform and the indices used to describe them. (A indicates systole; B indicates diastole.)

QUANTITATIVE DOPPLER INDICES

Quantitative Doppler can quantify flow disturbances, estimate absolute blood flow, assess vascular impedance, and help characterize tissue. Quantitative Doppler indices include velocity and flow measurements. Velocity is defined as the maximum Doppler shift over a cardiac cycle. Flow is defined as the average velocity times the lumen area of a vessel. If the vessel is circular, the area can be determined from one diameter, whereas if it is an ellipse two diameters are required.

Several potential errors are inherent in measuring fetal blood flow volume. One source of error is the inaccurate measurement of the angle of the vessel to the insonating ultrasonic beam. The estimate of velocity is strongly dependent on the magnitude of the angle. A linear-array transducer with a Doppler offset at a fixed angle will give an accurate measurement of the angle. If the insonating beam angle is 30 degrees there is a 3 to 4% error in the Doppler velocity measurement; a 60-degree angle produces a 15% error; but an 80-degree angle produces a 50% error. (Error rates given include a 5% error in measuring the angle.[19]) The need to measure the angle of insonation limits this method to vessels whose axis lies in the same plane for a few centimeters of their course. The intraabdominal umbilical vein or the fetal descending aorta is suitable. Yet another error in estimating flow volume comes in measuring the vessel diameter. Small measurement errors in vessels of small diameter create huge errors. For example, a 1-mm error in the measurement of an 8-mm vessel produces a 25% error

variation in the flow calculation.[8] The diameter of vessels—especially the fetal aorta—may vary 20% over the cardiac cycle. The sample volume must embrace the entire lumen, to ensure that it is uniformly insonated (Fig. 19-5).

In a study by Gill and Kosoff,[20] low venous flow values were detectable an average of 1 week before sonography could detect intrauterine growth retardation (IUGR) and antenatal hypoxia. With Doppler technique investigators found increased umbilical vein blood flow with Rh isoimmunization, antepartum hemorrhage, and placental pathology.

QUALITATIVE DOPPLER INDICES

Qualitative measurements of flow velocity waveforms are angle independent and are therefore easier to obtain. The A/B or S/D ratio was first described by Stuart and colleagues[45] in 1980. This is the ratio of the peak systolic velocity to the end-diastolic velocity. In 1974, Pourcelot[41] first described the RI as a mathematical derivative of the simple S/D ratio. RI is the difference between systolic and diastolic pressure divided by the systolic pressure. Gosling and King[21] in 1975 showed that, analyzed in a certain way, time velocity waveforms are sensitive to changes in impedance. They proposed the PI, the difference between peak systolic pressure and end-diastolic pressure divided by the mean maximum frequency over the entire cardiac cycle. A microcomputer is required to outline the maximum envelope of the waveform.

In 1983, Campbell and colleagues[10] developed a new index for waveform analysis, the frequency index profile (FIP). Developed specifically for the uteroplacental arteries, the FIP consists of a complicated computerized analysis of the standard waveform. The maximum Doppler shift (f_D) is measured every 0.04 seconds throughout the cardiac cycle. Each value of f_D is divided by the mean of all the measured frequencies throughout the cardiac cycle. This is expressed as a percentage of the mean f_D. The FIP was designed to detect subtle changes in waveforms.

The qualitative ratios do not measure blood flow, but generally these indices are inversely related to it. Constant perfusion pressure and all other parameters remaining constant, the flow increases as the impedance to flow decreases.

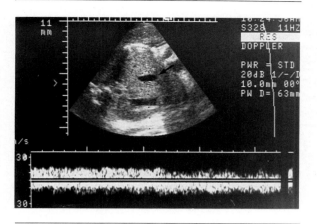

FIGURE 19-5. Umbilical vein flow is demonstrated. The gate (*arrow*) is opened wider than the vein to ensure even insonation.

TABLE 19-1. Indication for fetal Doppler examination

Maternal disease
  Hypertension (chronic or pregnancy-induced)
  Collagen vascular disease
  Renal disease
  Diabetes (classes B,C,R,F)
  Malnutrition
  Rh or Kell sensitization
  Anemia
Suspected IUGR
  Estimated fetal weight $\leq$10th percentile
  Incorrect dates versus IUGR
  Unexplained oligohydramnios
Risk Factors for IUGR
  Previous IUGR infant
  Smoker $>$1 pack/day cigarettes
  Drug or alcohol ingestion
  Elevated maternal serum α_2-fetoprotein
  Discordant growth of multiple gestations
Other
  Umbilical cord anomaly
  Previous fetal demise
  Fetal chromosomal anomaly
  Inadequate placentation

Clinical Applications

PLACENTAL CIRCULATION

Pregnancy places tremendous stress on the maternal circulation. Cardiac output increases in early pregnancy, reaching a peak of 30 to 50% above nonpregnant values at 20 to 24 weeks' gestation.[24] This increase in the maternal cardiac output is caused by the dramatic increase in uterine blood flow needed to satisfy the metabolic demands of the fetus. The maternal blood volume normally expands by approximately 40% to compensate for the slight drop in the mean arterial pressure.

In the placental circulation, blood enters the placenta from the fetus via the paired umbilical arteries. The blood is distributed throughout the chorionic plate to the chorionic villi, where it passes through villous capillaries and drains into a network of veins that are parallel to the arteries. Exchange of oxygen, carbon dioxide, nutrients, and waste products occurs across the villous capillaries. The blood is then returned to the fetus via the umbilical vein.

UMBILICAL CORD

The umbilical cord is the crucial intrauterine link between the fetal and the placental circulation. It is normally composed of two arteries and a single large vein ensheathed in Wharton's jelly for protection.

The umbilical arteries are a single-layered intima of endothelial cells resting on a medium of smooth muscle cells. Fine elastic fibrils are scattered throughout the arterial walls. The umbilical vein consists of a thin intima and a well-defined internal elastic lamina. The medial subintimal smooth muscle fibers are arranged longitudinally.[12] The vessels are arranged spirally to reduce torsion and knots that would occur if they were floating free. Doppler ultrasound can be used to determine adequacy of umbilical cord blood flow (Table 19-1).

UTERINE VASCULATURE

The blood supply to the pregnant uterus is derived chiefly from the uterine arteries. The ovarian arteries also contribute, but to a lesser degree. The main uterine artery derived from the internal iliac artery branches off once it reaches the uterus to form the arcuate arteries. The arteries circle the anterior and posterior surfaces, forming anastomoses with the arcuate arteries on the opposite side. The radial arteries branch off the arcuates and are directed into the uterine lumen to form the spiral arteries, which pass into the uterine decidua to feed the intervillous space (Fig. 19-6).

Early in pregnancy the trophoblast invades the

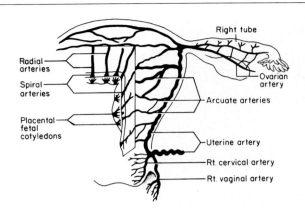

FIGURE 19-6. The uterine circulation. (Used with permission.[49])

spiral artery in the decidua to form lakes of maternal blood. At 16 to 24 weeks the placental cytotrophoblasts invade the spiral arteries in the myometrium, eroding their walls and producing dilated vessels with low resistance. If this does not occur the vessels remain constricted and exhibit increased resistance. This may place the patient at risk for preeclampsia and IUGR. Early changes in uterine- and arcuate artery blood flow can be detected and followed by serial Doppler flow studies.

Scanning Technique

CONTINUOUS-WAVE STUDY OF THE UMBILICAL ARTERY

Since CW Doppler systems are blind to the exact location of the Doppler signal, they may be used in conjunction with a real-time ultrasound system to aid in vessel identification. Real-time ultrasound may be useful for determining the origin of an abnormal signal, but each vessel has its own unique waveform and sound and can often be identified without real-time imaging.

The fetal umbilical artery and the maternal uterine and arcuate arteries are the vessels studied most commonly with CW Doppler. While the blood vessels are examined the patient lies in a semirecumbent position, to prevent supine hypotension.[33] To reduce Doppler scanning time the umbilical cord

can be identified with real-time sonography to guide the placement of the beam for Doppler scanning. It has been documented that arterial resistance is greater at the insertion of the umbilical cord into the fetal abdomen than at the placental cord insertion.[35] If the placental cord insertion cannot be identified, a free loop midcord is sampled. The angle of the transducer is manipulated slightly, until a strong signal is obtained.

The signal should be sharp and easily distinguished (Fig. 19-7). If the borders of the peak and troughs are not clear, the gain is raised or lowered until a distinguishable signal is obtained. Wall filters should be set as low as possible. If the gain is lowered too much the end-diastolic velocity may be obliterated. The arterial signal should be visualized on one side of the baseline, with the steady nonpulsatile venous flow in the opposite direction. Because fetal breathing activity can alter flow ratios, it is good practice to wait until breathing stops.[33] Breathing can be identified either by an undulating venous Doppler signal or by fetal chest wall movements. Once three or four waveforms of equal height are obtained, the image is frozen while the necessary measurements are taken. A single waveform should never be used for quantitative assessment; rather a number of sequential waveforms should be averaged to minimize beat-to-beat variation.[33]

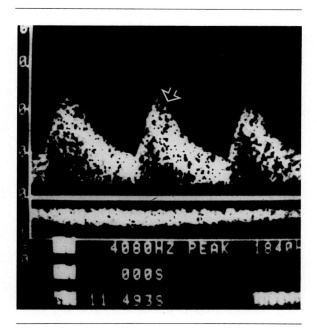

FIGURE 19-7. CW umbilical Doppler waveform. Open arrow demonstrates peak-systole.

UTERINE ARTERY

To evaluate the maternal uterine or arcuate artery with CW Doppler the transducer should be placed parauterine in the maternal iliac fossa. Slight medial and caudal angulation may be necessary to obtain the correct signal. Slight moves are made with the transducer until the much slower maternal pulse is audible. The normal uterine arterial waveform is distinct and should have sufficient diastolic blood flow (Fig. 19-8A), whereas the iliac arteries will have reversed end-diastolic flow or none. Reversal of flow is defined as flow that extends under the Doppler baseline. Absent end-diastolic flow is described as the absence of flow during the diastolic part of the cardiac cycle. Abnormal uterine arteries can give a similar waveform to the internal iliac artery, so care must be exercised.

Arcuate arteries are located between the umbilicus and the iliac crest on the lateral side of the uterine fundus, although the exact location varies with gestational age. Having the patient lie in the semirecumbent position makes obtaining the signal quicker and easier. The transducer can be angled medially until the proper signal is obtained (Fig. 19-8B).

PULSED-WAVE DOPPLER

Umbilical Waveforms. To image the umbilical artery with a duplex system is fairly easy. The cord is located with the real-time transducer; a loop is identified at midcord or at the placental umbilical cord insertion,[35] and the Doppler cursor is dropped into the umbilical vessels. Since S/D, PI, and RI are angle-independent measurements, it is not necessary to correct for the angle of insonation. The umbilical waveform (UWF) should demonstrate clean peaks of equal height, and umbilical vein flow should be visible in the opposite direction.

As discussed previously, flow cannot be measured correctly with conventional scanners. The umbilical artery is tortuous; the angle of insonation is difficult to measure; and flow studies seldom are done. The umbilical vein flow, however, can be measured with the proper equipment, such as a water-path scanner.

Uterine Waveforms. To image the uterine artery with PW Doppler, the external iliac artery is first visualized with real-time equipment. The external iliac artery most commonly appears in the maternal iliac fossa as a large, long vessel running parallel to the uterus. The uterine artery is seen branching around the external iliac artery and is located medial to the iliac artery but lateral to the uterus. The operator should try to identify the vessel first on real-time, to save actual Doppler time. If it is technically impossible to get good duplex images, the sonographer must search up and down the medial aspect of the external iliac artery until the proper signal is obtained (Fig. 19-8C, D).

FETAL DESCENDING AORTA

Most studies of fetal blood flow have evaluated volume flow and velocity in the aorta. In 1979 Gill used a modified 8-transducer water-path transducer to perform the first flow studies. He estimates that he achieved errors of less than 10%.[19]

Various investigators have used a linear-array transducer with a pulsed Doppler probe at a fixed angle of 45 degrees. The fixed angle helps ensure that the angle of insonation of the Doppler beam

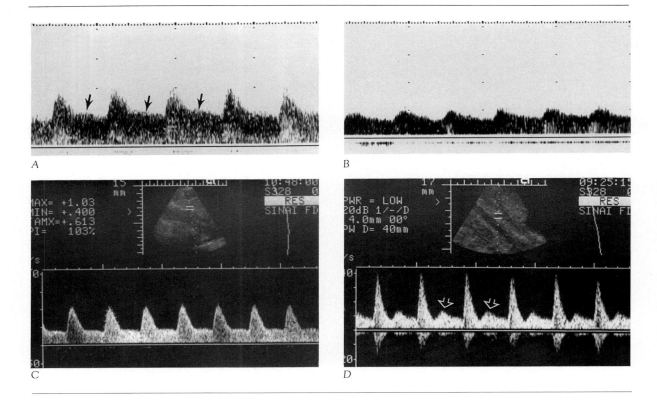

FIGURE 19-8. (A) Normal uterine artery waveform demonstrates a normal S/D ratio. Note the high diastolic flow (arrows). (B) Normal arcuate artery waveform on the same patient. (C) Duplex image of normal uterine artery. (D) An abnormal uterine artery at 32 weeks' gestation. Note the high S/D ratio and the arrow demonstrating the persistence of the "notch."

is less than 60 degrees from the direction of flow of the red blood cells.[46] The fetal descending aorta and umbilical vein are the vessels most often studied with flow velocity. The descending aorta should be examined just above the level of the diaphragm. The transducer should be parallel to the aorta. The sample gate should be opened beyond the lumen walls, to ensure even insonation of the vessel.

Gill[18] has shown that for low beam-flow angles increasing the gate to exceed the lumen diameter will compensate in part for the inadequate beam width.

The aortic flow velocity waveform shows rapid acceleration during systole. From peak systole to end-diastole there is rapid deceleration. There is no reversal of flow during diastole in normal fetuses.

The S/D, RI, and PI show little change in the third trimester, except for a slight increase in end-diastolic flow.

CEREBRAL BLOOD FLOW

In a normal pregnancy there is continuous forward flow in the fetal internal carotid artery throughout the cardiac cycle. With fetal growth retardation there is a marked increase in internal carotid flow and a decrease in cerebral resistance.[50] Intrauterine asphyxia alters blood flow to the fetal organs and brain, which may ultimately cause brain damage.

To sample the internal carotid artery a biparietal diameter is first obtained with duplex sonography. The internal carotid artery appears anterior to the thalamus on either side of the midline. This is the

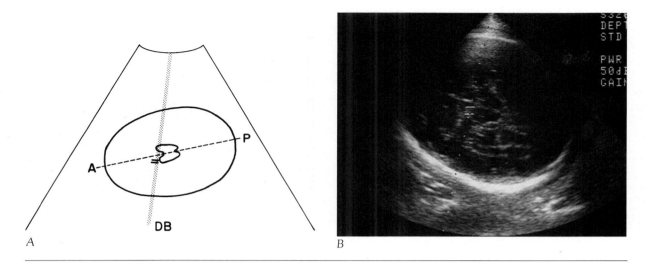

FIGURE 19-9. (A) Diagrammatic representation and (B) sonogram representing Doppler sample gate in internal carotid artery.

level of bifurcation into the middle and anterior cerebral arteries (Figs. 19-9A,B). In normal pregnancy the internal carotid S/D ratio and PI decrease with advancing gestational age, signifying decreasing resistance. In the face of IUGR and hypoxic stress, a drop in cerebral S/D ratio and PI signify a marked decrease in resistance, and perhaps increased blood flow to the brain. This is believed to be a brain-sparing effect.

FACTORS THAT AFFECT WAVEFORMS

Most investigators perform fetal Doppler studies with the patient supine or semirecumbent. According to Marsal[33] the patient should be semirecumbent to avoid supine hypotension. When fetal breathing occurs, flow patterns in the umbilical vein are modulated (Fig. 19-10). This is because the increase in tracheal or intrapleural pressure increases venous return to the heart. Fetal breathing may be associated with an irregular heart rate, owing to respiratory sinus arrhythmia. Doppler sampling should not be performed during episodes of fetal breathing movements.

As fetal blood flow is affected by irregularities in the fetal heart rate pattern, Doppler examination should not be performed during episodes of fetal bradycardia or tachycardia. Normal waveforms are

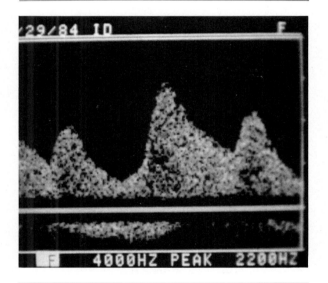

FIGURE 19-10. Alterations in umbilical artery waveforms caused by fetal breathing.

altered by changes in heart rate or rhythm. With extrasystolic beats there is a lower peak and mean velocity. The first post-extrasystolic beat shows an increase in blood velocity that does not fully com-

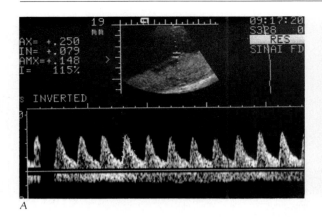
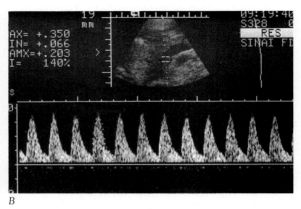

FIGURE 19-11. Duplex sonogram demonstrates differences in umbilical Doppler waveform depending on sampling location. (A) Umbilical placental insertion (mean S/D ratio, 3.1) and (B) fetal umbilical insertion (mean S/D ratio, 5.3).

pensate for the extrasystolic beat. Compensation does occur, however, over the next three or four beats.[32,33]

The influence of pharmacologic agents on uterine and fetal blood flow is variable and controversial. Joupilla and others have observed no major change in umbilical vein flow associated with the mother's smoking or being administered oxygen, caffeine, labetolol, alcohol, or anesthesia.[25-28] Medications that alter heart rate, such as beta-mimetics (ritodrine, terbutaline) used for tocolysis, may lower Doppler S/D ratios in the fetal aorta and uterine artery, thus confusing interpretation of the waveforms.[37]

IDENTIFYING PLACENTAL AND FETAL INSERTION

Investigators have noted the clinical significance of the effect of waveform sampling site on Doppler ratios. This is more pronounced in the fetal umbilical circulation than in the maternal uterine circulation. The uterine circulation is composed of multiple vessels that branch and that are fed by collateral vessels. The umbilical circulation consists of the umbilical cord itself. Because resistance to blood flow is greater at the fetal umbilical cord insertion than at the placental cord insertion (Fig. 19-11),[35] it is very important to obtain a fetal umbilical waveform sample as close to the placental cord insertion as possible.

Several theories might possibly explain the lower ratio at the placental cord insertion than at the fetal cord site. One is that the changes in arterial diameter or wall elasticity may alter the waveform. Another is that pressure changes across the fetal abdominal wall lead to changes in resistance. The third explanation is that the decrease in the ratio may be the result of dampening and attenuation of the propagated wave. If sampling location is not known and ratios are high, the sonographer should take multiple samples at different locations along the cord to see whether the results are consistent. The accuracy of Doppler measurements depends on consistent and uniform measurement techniques.

INTRAUTERINE GROWTH RETARDATION

A question that has been pondered for years is "Is the baby simply small or is the baby's growth retarded?" This question is not easily answered; small-for-dates studies require accurate dating since every small baby is not growth retarded. Doppler ultrasound is the newest parameter to be used to determine the presence of stress in the fetal environment, therefore determining fetal well-being.

There are two types of intrauterine growth retardation (IUGR): symmetric and asymmetric. The first type may be manifest before 28 weeks and usually results in a symmetrically small fetus. This type

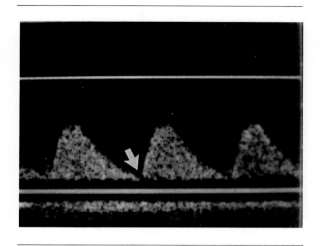

FIGURE 19-12. CW Doppler waveform demonstrating absent end-diastolic flow (*arrow*) in a fetus compromised by IUGR.

is due to infection, a chromosomal anomaly, or environmental factors such as drug ingestion or radiation exposure. Asymmetric IUGR is usually manifest after 28 weeks and results in asymmetric fetal growth with a small abdomen and appropriate biparietal diameter (BPD). This type of IUGR is secondary to maternal lupus, hypertension, or toxemia of pregnancy. Placental infarcts and circumvallate placenta may also hinder fetal growth.

Doppler ultrasound has shown that in fetuses with asymmetric IUGR vascular resistance increases in the aorta and umbilical artery and decreases in the internal carotid artery. This phenomenon ensures blood flow to the brain at the expense of the extremities, reinforcing the head-sparing theory. Increased vascular resistance is reflected by diminished or absent diastolic flow, leading to an increased SD ratio or PI. Extreme cases of elevated resistance causing absent or reverse end-diastolic flow velocity waveforms are associated with high rates of morbidity and mortality.[42] Trudinger and colleagues[47,48] demonstrated that a small-for–gestational-age fetus with an increased umbilical artery S/D ratio is at a much higher risk for a poor outcome than a small fetus with normal S/D ratio. Recent data[5] suggest that umbilical artery velocimetry

may be predictive of IUGR at an earlier age than sonographic estimation of fetal weight.

In a series by Berkowitz and colleagues[6] a growth-retarded fetus with an abnormal S/D ratio was found to be at risk for early delivery, reduced birth weight, decreased amniotic fluid at birth, admission to the neonatal intensive care unit, neonatal complications associated with IUGR, and a prolonged hospital stay. Trudinger[47] and Rochelson and colleagues[43] have reported similar results. Absent or reversed end-diastolic flow velocity waveform in the umbilical artery or the fetal aorta is associated with increased perinatal morbidity and mortality (Fig. 19-12). It has also been shown that elevated uterine artery S/D ratios and a persistent notch are associated with stillbirth, premature birth, and IUGR in patients with hypertensive disorders.[15]

Maternal Disease

Adequacy of fetal nutrition and oxygenation depend on an adequate blood supply from the maternal circulation. Maternal diseases that can compromise proper oxygenation and nutrition include hypertension, collagen vascular disease, renal disease, diabetes, and malnutrition. It is believed that the failure of the trophoblastic invasion of the spiral arteries at the deciduomyometrial junction produces a constriction in the spiral arteries and may lead to preeclamptic pregnancies. This results in increased resistance in the maternal uterine and arcuate artery circulations. Notching may also persist in the waveform (Fig. 19-13).

In early pregnancy and in nonpregnant women, the uterine artery waveform has a notch at the beginning of the diastolic phase of the cardiac cycle. A true notch represents a deceleration of at least 50 Hz below the maximum diastolic velocities and rarely occurs after the 20th week of gestation. In nonpregnant women and in early pregnancy, the uterine artery waveform has a high pulsatility with reduced diastolic velocity. In the second trimester there is a decrease in impedance that continues until 24 weeks' gestation.[9] One reason for this is the invasion in the myometrial portion of the spiral arteries, which occurs around 16 weeks' gestation.[9] The presence of a notch or persistently elevated ratios implies that the pregnancy suffers from inadequate nutrition and oxygenation (Fig. 19-13).

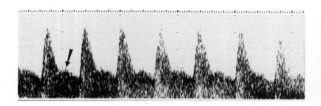

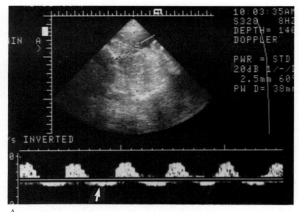

FIGURE 19-13. PW Doppler waveform representing the persistence of a notch (*arrow*) in the maternal uterine circulation.

Cohen-Overbeek[11] reported that the maternal arcuate artery Doppler waveform shows increased ratios in patients with high blood pressure or proteinuria and in mothers of growth-retarded fetuses, owing to increased resistance.

Multiple Gestations

Multiple gestations are associated with increased morbidity and mortality. This is due mainly to problems associated with premature delivery and growth discrepancies. Up to 30 to 32 weeks, twins grow at the same rate as singletons; thereafter they grow more slowly. Sonography and Doppler can be used to screen multiple gestations for abnormal and discordant growth. Pathologic conditions that induce discordancy include twin-to-twin transfusion syndrome, an anomalous fetus with a normal co-twin, or growth retardation in one twin because of uteroplacental insufficiency.[23]

In the twin-to-twin transfusion syndrome the fetuses' venous and arterial circulations communicate causing both twins to be adversely affected. One twin is a "donor," who becomes anemic and growth retarded (Fig. 19-14A). The "recipient" twin becomes polycythemic and can suffer congestive heart failure due to volume overload (Fig. 19-14B). The perinatal mortality associated with twin-to-twin transfusion syndrome may be as high as 70%.[4] Abnormal umbilical artery Doppler waveforms may identify the fetus at risk and may help to study the pathophysiology of abnormal circulation.

Growth disturbance may be seen in only one

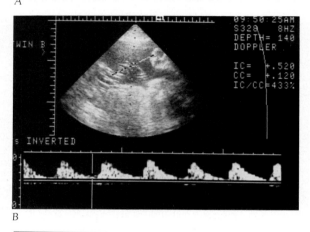

FIGURE 19-14. Duplex sonograms from growth-retarded twins of a patient with a renal transplant. (*A*) Twin A was severely growth retarded and died in the neonatal period. Umbilical artery waveforms showed reverse end-diastolic flow (*arrow*). (*B*) Twin B had elevated umbilical artery S/D ratio but was appropriate for gestational age at delivery and was discharged home alive and well.

twin in the face of congenital anomalies or localized uteroplacental insufficiency. In most cases of congenital anomalies the growth of the normal co-twin lags significantly.[23] Partial abruption, infarction of the placenta, or differences in local blood supply can produce one twin with IUGR and a normal co-twin. Doppler studies may aid in deter-

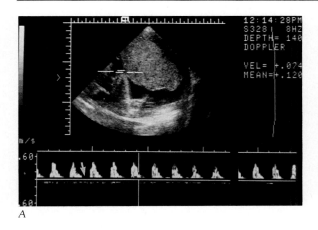

A

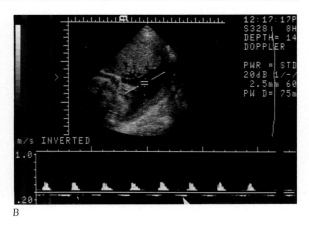

B

FIGURE 19-15. Doppler umbilical waveform from a 29-week fetus after intravascular intrauterine blood transfusion for Rh isoimmunization. Pretransfusion umbilical artery S/D Doppler ratio was 2.8. Immediately after transfusion the ratio increased to 5. (A) Doppler tracing 3 minutes after transfusion. There is no end-diastolic flow in the waveform (*arrow*). (B) Doppler tracing 6 minutes after transfusion: reversal of flow (*arrow*) occurred, followed by cardiac asystole. Emergency cesarean section was performed. The baby's Apgar score was 5, 7, and it suffered from mild respiratory distress syndrome.

mining the cause of growth discrepancy and assessing well-being.[16]

In severe oligohydramnios, when it is difficult to differentiate between cords, the Doppler sampling should be taken from a loop of cord close to the fetal abdomen. The ratios will be slightly higher than at the placental insertion site, but this will ensure true sampling of each twin.

Diabetes

Diabetes in pregnancy can lead to altered fetal growth, ranging from macrosomia (classes A and B) to IUGR (classes D, R, or F). Mothers with class C diabetes are not immune to vascular compromise.

Gill[17] studied fetal umbilical venous blood flow in diabetic patients and found flow rates to be consistently higher than control values. When "low flow" was noted in a diabetic mother there was a significantly higher incidence of hypoxia and neonatal morbidity. Abnormal umbilical artery Dopp-

ler waveform has also been associated with poor outcome in diabetic pregnancies.[7]

Fetal Anemia

Since the introduction of Rh(D) immunoglobulin in 1968, the incidence of Rh factor sensitization has been dramatically reduced. Unfortunately it is not eliminated, and an increasing proportion of sensitized pregnancies are due to atypical antibodies such as Kell. Recent investigations have linked the severity of the disease with increased umbilical vein blood flow.[20,29]

Doppler investigation of the fetal cardiac, arterial, and venous circulation may aid in identifying the anemic fetus, thereby providing a noninvasive means of determining optimal timing of intrauterine blood transfusion. It has been our experience that absence of end-diastolic flow or reversal of flow following intrauterine blood transfusion is associated with fetal morbidity. These patients should be followed extremely closely (Fig. 19-15).

Future Directions

Doppler ultrasound is gaining acceptance in the surveillance and management of the fetus at risk for poor perinatal or neonatal outcome. Both very high umbilical S/D ratios and absent end-diastolic flow have been associated with fetal and neonatal death. Complete reversal of umbilical artery blood flow is associated with impending fetal demise; therefore, delivery should be expedited.

It is just as important to evaluate the maternal vessels as it is to evaluate the fetal side of the circulation. Abnormal waveform readings can be early signs of a predisposing condition and should not be ignored. The finding of an abnormal fetal or uterine waveform necessitates careful monitoring, which should include repeated Doppler examinations, growth scans, and tests of fetal well-being. These can be suggested to the attending obstetrician.

With the advent of duplex Doppler sonography one can be very specific as to which vessels to study. Vessels from the umbilical cord to the intricate circle of Willis have been studied. Recently, color flow mapping has been added to help us further understand the complicated fetal circulatory pathways—not only of the vessels but also of the organs they supply. It is anticipated that Doppler studies will help us take better care of the fetus in addition to providing a noninvasive means of studying the pathophysiology of disease states.

References

1. Baker DW: Pulsed ultrasonic Doppler blood flow sensing. IEEE Transsonics-Ultrasonics. 1970; 17:170.
2. Baker DW, Watkins D. Aphase-coherent pulsed Doppler system for cardiovascular measurement. Proc. 20th Alliance for Engineering in Medicine and Biology, Stockholm; 1967; 27:2.
3. Barcroft J, Flexner LB, McClurkin T. The output of the fetal heart in the goat. J Physiol. 1934; 82:498–508.
4. Benirschke K, Kim CK. Multiple pregnancies. N Engl J Med. 1973; 288:1276.
5. Berkowitz GS, Chitkara U, Rosenberg J, et al. Sonographic estimation of fetal weight and Doppler analysis of umbilical artery velocimetry in the prediction of intrauterine growth retardation: A prospective study. Am J Obstet Gynecol. 1988; 5:1149–1153.
6. Berkowitz GS, Mehalek K, Chitkara U, et al. Doppler umbilical velocimetry in the prediction of adverse outcome in pregnancies at risk for intrauterine growth retardation. Am J Obstet Gynecol. 1988; 5:742–746.
7. Bracero L, Schulman H, Fleischer A, et al. Umbilical artery velocity waveform in diabetic pregnancy. Obstet Gynecol. 1986; 68:654–658.
8. Burns P. Doppler flow estimations in the fetal and maternal circulations: Principles, techniques, and some limitations. In: Maulick D, McNellis D, eds. Doppler Ultrasound Measurement of Maternal-Fetal Hemodynamics. 1st ed. New York: Perinatology Press; 1987.
9. Campbell S, Cohen-Overbeek TE. Doppler investigation of the uteroplacental circulation during pregnancy. In: Maulick D, McNellis D, eds. Doppler Ultrasound Measurement of Maternal-Fetal Hemodynamics. 1st ed. New York: Perinatology Press; 1987.
10. Campbell S, Diaz-Recasens J, Griffin DR, et al. New Doppler technique for assessing uteroplacental blood flow. Lancet. 1983; 1:675–677.
11. Cohen-Overbeek T, Pearce J, Campbell S. The antenatal assessment of uteroplacental and fetoplacental blood flow using Doppler ultrasound. Ultrasound Med Biol. 1985; 2:329.
12. DeSa DJ. Pathology of the placenta. In: Perrin E, ed. Pathology of the Placenta. 2nd ed. New York: Churchhill Livingstone; 1984.
13. Doppler CJ. Uber das farbige Licht der Dopplersterne. Abhand Lungen der Koniglishen Bohmischen Gesellschaften der Wissenchaften. 1842; 2:465.
14. Farmikides G, Schulman H, Saldana L, et al. Surveillance of twin pregnancy with umbilical artery velocimetry. Am J Obstet Gynecol. 1985; 153:789–792.
15. Fleisher A, Schulman H, Farmikides G, et al. Uterine artery velocimetry in pregnant women with hypertension. Am J Obstet Gynecol. 1986; 154:806–813.
16. Giles WB, Trudinger BJ, Cook CM. Fetal umbilical artery velocity time waveforms in twin pregnancies. Br J Obstet and Gynaecol. 1985; 92:490.
17. Gill RW. Performance of the mean frequency Doppler demodulator. Ultrasound Med Biol. 1979; 5:237–247.
18. Gill RW. Accuracy calculations for ultrasonic pulsed Doppler blood flow measurements. Austral Phys Eng Sci Med. 1982; 5:51–57.
19. Gill RW. Measurement of blood flow by ultrasound accuracy and sources of error. Ultrasound Med Biol. 1985; 11:4,625–641.
20. Gill RW, Kosoff G, Warren PS, et al. Umbilical venous flow in normal and complicated pregnancy. Ultrasound Med Biol. 1984; 10:349.
21. Gosling RG, King DH. Ultrasound angiography. In: Marcus AW, Adamson L, eds. Arteries and Veins. Edinburgh: Churchhill Livingstone; 1975.
22. Hill M, Lande I, Grossman J. Duplex evaluation of

fetoplacental and uteroplacental circulation. In: Grant EG, White EM, eds. Duplex Sonography. 1st ed. New York: Springer-Verlag; 1988.

23. Hobbins JC, Winsberg F, Berkowitz RL. Third-trimester complications. In: Hobbins JC, Winsberg F, Berkowitz RL, eds. Ultrasonography in Obstetrics and Gynecology. 2nd ed. Baltimore: Williams & Wilkins; 1983.

24. Itzkovitz J. Maternal-fetal hemodynamics. In: Maulik D, McNellis D, eds. Ultrasound Measurements of Maternal-Fetal Hemodynamics. 1st ed. New York: Perinatology Press; 1987.

25. Joupilla P, Kirkinen P, Eik-Nes S. Acute effect of maternal smoking on the human fetal blood flow. Br J Obstet Gynaecol. 1983; 90:7.

26. Joupilla P, Kirkinen P, Koivula A, et al. The influence of maternal oxygen inhalation on placental and umbilical venous blood flow. Eur J Obstet Gynecol Reprod Biol. 1983; 16:151.

27. Joupilla P, Kirkinen P, Koivula A, et al. Ritodrine infusion during late pregnancy: Effects on fetal and placental blood flow, prostacyclin and thromboxane. Am J Obstet Gynecol. 1985; 151:1028.

28. Joupilla P, Kirkinen P, Koivula A, et al. Labetol does not alter the placental and fetal blood flow or maternal prostanoids in preeclampsia. Br J Obstet Gynaecol. 1986; 93:543.

29. Kirkinen P, Joupilla P, Eik-Nes SH. Umbilical vein blood flow in Rhesus isoimmunization. Br J Obstet Gynaecol. 1983; 90:640.

30. Kirkinen P, Joupilla P, Koivula A, et al. The effect of caffeine on placental and fetal blood flow in human pregnancy. Am J Obstet Gynecol. 1983; 147:939.

31. Lind J, Wegelius C. Human fetal circulation changes in the cardiovascular system at birth and disturbances in the postnatal closure of the foramen ovale and ductus venosus. Cold Spring Harbor Symposium on Quantitative Biology. 1954; 19:109–125.

32. Lingman G, Dahlstrom JA, Eik-Nes SH, et al. Haemodynamic evaluation of fetal heart arrhythmias. Br J Obstet Gynaecol. 1984; 91:647.

33. Marsal K, Lindblad A, Lingman G, et al. Blood flow in the fetal descending aorta: Intrinsic factors affecting movements and cardiac arrhythmias. Ultrasound Med Biol. 1984; 10:339–348.

34. Mehalek K, Berkowitz G, Chitkara U, et al. Comparison of continuous-wave and pulsed-wave S/D ratios of umbilical and uterine arteries. Am J Obstet Gynecol. 1988; 72:603.

35. Mehalek K, Rosenberg J, Berkowitz GS, et al. Umbilical and uterine artery flow velocity waveforms: Effect of the sampling site on Doppler ratios. J Ultrasound Med. 1989; 4:171–176.

36. Miller M, Church C, Barnett S. Bioeffects of Doppler ultrasound in the maternal-fetal context. In: Maulik D, McNellis D, eds. Doppler Ultrasound Measurements of Maternal-Fetal Hemodynamics. 1st ed. New York: Perinatology Press; 1987.

37. Nimrod C, Davies D, Harder J, et al. Doppler evaluation of the impact of betamimetic therapy on human fetal aortic and umbilical blood flow. Proceedings of the Society of Perinatal Obstetricians. Sixth Annual Meeting, San Antonio, Feb 1986.

38. Nyquist H. Certain topics in telegraph transmission theory. Trans Am Inst Electrical Eng 1928; 47:617–644.

39. Peronneau P, Deloche A, Bui-Mong-Hung, et al. Debitmetrie ultrasonore. Developpements et applications experimentales. Eur Surg Res. 1969; 1:147.

40. Peronneau P, Hinglais H, Pellet M, et al. Velocimetre sanguin par effet Doppler a l'emission ultrasonore pulsée. L'onde Electrique. 1970; 59:369.

41. Pourcelot L. Application clinques de l'examen Doppler transcutanie. In: Peronneau P, ed. Velometric Ultrasonor Doppler. Paris:10 Inserm; 1974; 34:625.

42. Rochelson BL, Schulman H, Farmakides G, et al. The significance of absent end-diastolic velocity in umbilical artery velocity waveforms. Am J Obstet Gynecol. 1987; 156:1213–1218.

43. Rochelson BL, Schulman H, Fleischer A, et al.: The clinical significance of Doppler umbilical artery velocimetry in the small-for–gestational-age fetus. Am J Obstet Gynecol. 1987; 156:1223.

44. Satomura S. A study on examining the heart with ultrasonics. I. Principles. II. Instruments. Jpn Circ J. 1956; 20:227.

45. Stuart B, Drumm J, Fitzgerald DE, et al. Fetal blood velocity waveforms in normal and complicated pregnancies. Br J Obstet Gynaecol. 1980; 87:780.

46. Tonge HM, Wladimiroff JW, Noordam MJ, et al. Blood flow velocity waveforms in the descending fetal aorta: Comparison between normal and growth-retarded pregnancies. Obstet Gynecol. 1986; 67:851–855.

47. Trudinger BJ, Giles WB, Cook CM. Flow velocity waveforms in the maternal uteroplacental and fetal umbilical placental circulation. Am J Obstet Gynecol. 1985; 152:155–163.

48. Trudinger BJ, Giles WB, Cook CM, et al. Fetal umbilical artery flow velocity waveforms and placental resistance. J Obstet Gynaecol. 1985; 92:23.

49. Wallenburg HCS. Physiology and pathophysiology of the uteroplacental circulation. J Drug Ther Res. 1986; 11:381–383.

50. Wladimiroff JW, Tonge HM, Stewart PA. Doppler ultrasound assessment of cerebral blood flow in the human fetus. Br J Obstet Gynaecol. 1986; 93:471–475.

CHAPTER **20**

Abnormal First-Trimester Gestations

PAULA S. WOLETZ, STEVEN R. GOLDSTEIN

In the second and third trimesters of pregnancy, diagnostic ultrasound is used primarily to determine gestational age, identify multiple gestations, evaluate fetal anatomic structures, and assess fetal well-being. Until very recently, ultrasound examination was indicated in the first trimester only to establish the presence of an intrauterine pregnancy (or verify an ectopic pregnancy) and predict its viability. Its role is now being expanded.

While debate continues over the routine use of ultrasound during pregnancy, few, if any, researchers advocate routine scanning in the first trimester. In 1984, a National Institutes of Health task force addressed the issue of routine obstetric ultrasound and found it offered no demonstrable improvement in perinatal outcome[16]; however, a recent large-scale study in Sweden concluded that significant benefit is obtained from a single routine obstetric sonogram. The results of this study suggest that scanning take place at about the 15th week of pregnancy.[17] Routine first-trimester ultrasound is sometimes seen in private obstetric practice, but it is not the accepted standard of care in the United States at this time. More information is available about fetal anatomy early in the second trimester than in the first, and correlation can be made with maternal serum α-fetoprotein levels. A secondary concern is that the first trimester, with its rapid cell growth and differentiation, is the period of greatest susceptibility to physical and chemical insults. Re-

sultant abnormalities may not be manifested immediately. Finally, caution must be exercised when introducing any unnecessary influences to the intrauterine environment, particularly at this stage. Although no significant bioeffects have been documented at the current diagnostic levels of ultrasound, prudence demands a conservative approach to the use of a modality that is still under investigation.

When a patient reports a problem during the first trimester of pregnancy, or when the clinician perceives an unusual finding or discrepancy, ultrasound is often the method of choice to confirm or rule out the clinician's suspicions. Therefore, this discussion of abnormal first-trimester pregnancies is organized according to the most commonly presenting clinical symptoms (Table 20-1). They include vaginal bleeding, size-dates discrepancy, and other abnormalities detectable in the first trimester. Ectopic pregnancy, hydatidiform mole, and co-existing masses are discussed in depth in other chapters.

Vaginal Bleeding

Clinically, pregnancy is confirmed after a woman has missed a menstrual period and has had a positive urine or serum pregnancy test. A surprisingly large number of undetected pregnancies are aborted spontaneously before a woman has missed

347

Table 20-1. Clinical indications for first-trimester ultrasound examination

Clinical Findings	Sonographic Findings	Diagnosis
First-trimester bleeding, closed cervical os	Embryo with clearly identifiable heartbeat	Viable pregnancy
	Embryo with absence of cardiac activity as observed by two experienced observers for at least 3 minutes each	Spontaneous abortion (embryo demise or missed abortion)
	No identifiable embryo in a gestational sac (GS) of 25 mm or larger, or no yolk sac in a GS 20 mm or larger	Blighted ovum (anembryonic pregnancy)
	No intrauterine GS identified; GS <20 mm without yolk sac; GS <25 mm without identifiable embryo	Equivocal findings
	Normal GS partly surrounded by crescent-shaped sonolucent area	Subchorionic hemorrhage
Profuse bleeding, dilated cervix (imminent abortion)	Empty uterus	Complete abortion
	GS located in cervix or vagina	Inevitable abortion
	No GS; complex collection in the uterus	Incomplete abortion
Unsure of dates	Measure mean-sac diameter (MSD) or crown-rump length (CRL)	Sonographic age
Size-dates discrepancy (large for dates)	Early gestation in a normal uterus, MSD or CRL corresponds with LMP	Sonographic gestational age corresponds with menstrual age
	CRL or BPD, etc. more advanced than LMP indicates	Incorrect dates
	Early gestation within an enlarged or irregularly shaped uterus	R/O fibroid uterus or uterine anomalies
	More than one GS or more than one embryo within a single sac	Multiple pregnancy
Size-dates discrepancy (small for dates)	Early gestation in a normal uterus, MSD or CRL corresponds with LMP	Sonographic gestational age corresponds with menstrual age
	Normal gestation less advanced than LMP indicates	Incorrect dates
	Empty uterus	R/O ectopic vs complete abortion vs nongravid uterus
	Embryo with absence of cardiac activity	Embryo demise
	No identifiable embryo within a GS 25 mm or larger, or no yolk sac in a GS 20 mm or larger	Blighted ovum

her menstrual period, and thus neither she nor her obstetrician are ever aware of the pregnancy and its loss. Of those pregnancies that progress to the point of detection, approximately one-quarter are complicated by some degree of first-trimester bleeding.[4] When vaginal bleeding occurs with a closed cervical os in a pregnancy of less than 20 weeks, the diagnosis is threatened abortion. While other factors not related to the pregnancy (such as cervical polyps) may be responsible for the bleeding, first consideration goes to establishing the viability of the pregnancy.

Traditionally it has been said that half of all women with threatened abortion eventually abort and half proceed to a normal outcome. Though various attempts to influence these results have been investigated, none holds much promise for increasing the proportion of successful pregnancies. Most likely this is because many spontaneous abortions are thought to be due to chromosomal abnormalities that are not compatible with life. The value of ultrasound in threatened abortion lies not in any endeavor to alter the outcome of the pregnancy but in the ability to predict which pregnancies will continue successfully to term. At the same time, we can rule out the possibility of ectopic pregnancy, as discussed in Chapter 21.

Examination of the intrauterine gestational sac

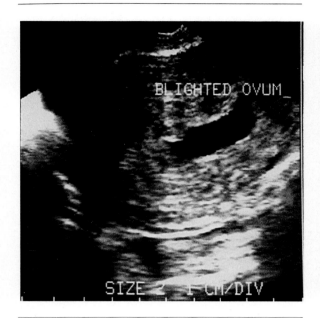

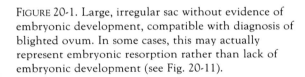

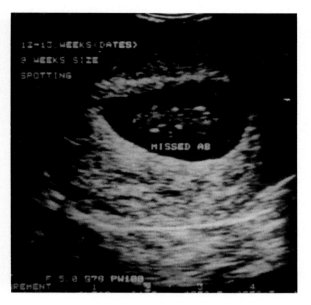

FIGURE 20-1. Large, irregular sac without evidence of embryonic development, compatible with diagnosis of blighted ovum. In some cases, this may actually represent embryonic resorption rather than lack of embryonic development (see Fig. 20-11).

FIGURE 20-2. Missed abortion in a patient with a history of vaginal spotting. Ultrasound examination is performed 12 to 13 weeks after LMP when, upon clinical examination, the fetus was only 9 weeks' size. The sonogram reveals an embryo with a CRL of 2.3 cm and no cardiac activity.

and its contents enables the sonographer to determine whether the patient's condition is an early viable pregnancy or an abnormal development. A mean sac diameter (MSD) can be obtained by measuring the height, width, and depth of the gestational sac and calculating their average. These measurements are taken at the fluid-chorionic tissue interface. Using transabdominal scanning technique an embryo should be apparent in all gestational sacs with an MSD of 25 mm or larger. A vaginal probe enables earlier visualization of the embryo, but definitive thresholds have not yet been established for this modality. Using 25 mm as a cutoff point, the absence of an embryo at this time is indication of an abnormal gestation with a poor prognosis.[11] This is commonly referred to as a blighted ovum, or anembryonic pregnancy. Blighted ova may occur when the embryo has died and been resorbed or development ceases prior to the formation of a discrete embryo (Fig. 20-1).[6]

In examining gestational sacs with an MSD under 25 mm, the sonographer should attempt to locate a yolk sac. The yolk sac can be identified before the embryo can be visualized; it should be evident in all gestational sacs that have attained an MSD of 20 mm or more.[12] Its absence in a sac of this size is sonographic proof of a nonviable pregnancy.

As mentioned in Chapter 12, the heartbeat is often identified before the embryo is visualized, and it serves as a marker to locate the embryonic pole. In clearly definable embryos, the absence of cardiac activity is diagnostic of embryo demise (Fig. 20-2). It is advisable for the sonographer to scan the embryo for a full three minutes before assuming embryo demise, and the findings should be confirmed by another observer (usually the radiologist or obstetrician). A dead embryo that is not expelled from the uterus is termed a missed abortion.[14]

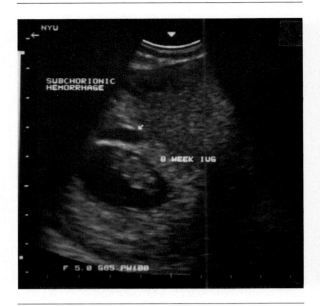

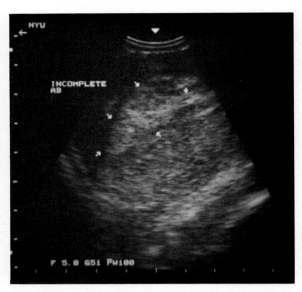

FIGURE 20-3. Patient at 8 weeks after LMP with normal embryo; cardiac activity is demonstrated on real-time examination. Patient was scanned because of vaginal bleeding. Crescent-shaped area outside gestational sac (*small white arrow*) represents subchorionic hemorrhage.

FIGURE 20-4. Irregular heterogeneous, dense endometrial echo (outlined by *white arrows*) compatible with a diagnosis of incomplete abortion.

An important caveat for the sonographer: diagnosis depends on adequate visualization and cannot be made when studies are technically limited, whether by the equipment's resolution capacities, fibroids, or patient habitus. Transvaginal scanning greatly reduces the limitations these factors impose. If there is any doubt, follow-up scans are indicated after an appropriate interval.

The presence of a sonographically identifiable intrauterine embryo with an obviously pulsating heart is the best predictor of a favorable outcome. Among patients with threatened abortion who demonstrate a living embryo, 84 to 98% successfully carry to term.[2,15,18] The range in estimates is due largely to the patient populations from which the data were collected. As might be expected, the highest success rates were obtained from exclusively private patients (presumably more affluent, better nourished, and more likely to receive prenatal care), whereas the lower rates reflected a large clinic population from a lower socioeconomic stratum.[15] Nonetheless, visualization of embryonic heart activity is a very reassuring sign.

Occasionally, a normal-looking gestational sac may be partially surrounded by a crescent-shaped sonolucent collection (Fig. 20-3). This is evidence of a subchorionic hemorrhage (bleeding between the endometrium and the gestational sac). Coexistence of a subchorionic hemorrhage with embryonic heart activity leads to a slightly reduced continuation rate. Approximately 70% of these pregnancies continue to term.[7]

When the patient is noted to have profuse bleeding and the cervical os has begun to dilate, abortion is said to be inevitable and imminent. A sonogram may be requested to inform the obstetrician of the progress or completion of the evacuation of the uterine contents. Sonographically, a gestational sac may be seen in the cervix or vagina as it is expelled. If the uterus appears empty and has moderate to bright endometrial echoes, the patient has had a complete abortion. A complex collection of echoes within the endometrial cavity indicates incomplete abortion (Fig. 20-4). These ultrasound

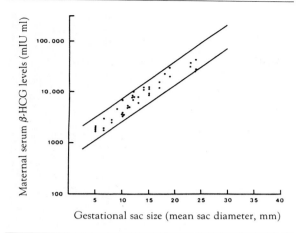

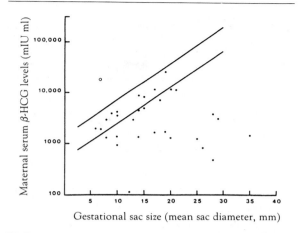

FIGURE 20-5. Correlation of mean sac diameter with simultaneous serum HCG level for 39 normal gestations. Solid lines represent 95% confidence limits. (From Nyberg D, et al. Threatened abortion: sonographic distinction of normal and abnormal gestational sacs. Radiology. 1986;158:395.)

FIGURE 20-6. Mean sac diameter compared with serum HCG levels for 31 abnormal gestations. In 20 cases (65%), the HCG level was disproportionately low. Only one woman (with a molar pregnancy) had an elevated HCG determination (O). (From Nyberg D, et al. Threatened abortion: sonographic distinction of normal and abnormal gestational sacs. Radiology. 1986;158:395.)

findings may determine whether the patient requires dilation and curettage.

Size-Dates Discrepancy

When a patient is unsure of her last normal menstrual period (LMP), her clinician may request a sonogram to date the pregnancy. Although this is usually requested early in the second trimester, several factors, such as the presence of uterine fibroids, maternal obesity, surgical scars, or multiple gestation, may make it difficult for the obstetrician to estimate the size of the uterus, from which the gestational age is estimated. Because other aspects of pregnancy management (e.g., methods of termination, interpretation of α-fetoprotein levels, timing of chorionic villi sampling or amniocentesis) hinge on the correct assessment of the duration of pregnancy, the patient may be sent for ultrasound evaluation in the first trimester.

A mean sac diameter of 5 mm can be obtained by the 5th week after LMP using transvaginal transducer, but other fluid collections in the endometrial cavity can have a similar appearance. It is therefore important to correlate the MSD to the level of human chorionic gonadotropin (HCG).[10] A 5-mm MSD should correspond to an HCG level of 1800 mIU/ml (2nd International Standard). The MSD and serum levels should continue to rise proportionally in normal pregnancies (Figs. 20-5, 20-6). By the 8th week LMP, HCG levels start to plateau, but by this time the embryo should be seen clearly on ultrasound and crown-rump length (CRL) can be measured. Normal embryos are consistently identified by the time their CRL reaches 5 mm or more.

When the obstetrician reports that the patient is large for dates, the gestational age should be estimated from either MSD or CRL. The pregnancy may simply be more advanced than was anticipated. The uterus should be surveyed carefully to rule out the presence of leiomyomas (Fig. 20-7). If fibroids are found, the sonographer should be able to demonstrate their number, size, and location for future follow-up; however, care must be taken not to mistake a focal myometrial contraction for a fibroid. These contractions are transient thickenings of a portion of the myometrium (Fig. 20-8). They

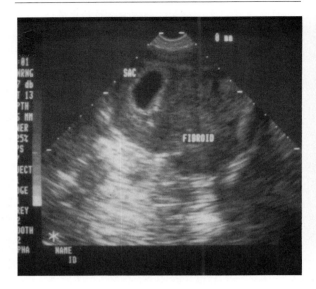

FIGURE 20-7. Sonogram of patient who presented at 7 weeks dates with a 14-week–sized uterus reveals a 7-week intrauterine gestation within a large myomatous uterus.

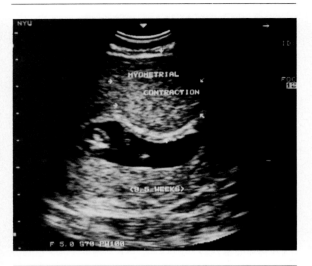

FIGURE 20-8. Sonographic appearance of a focal myometrial contraction (*arrows*). Note how the gestational sac is indented. This should not be confused with a fibroid uterus. This is extremely important when performing chorionic villus sampling. The patient with a focal myometrial contraction may be allowed to walk about for 15 to 20 minutes before the scan is repeated.

tend to indent the gestational sac or endometrial cavity, whereas fibroids more often distort the outer contours of the uterus.[19]

A large-for-dates uterus accompanied by hyperemesis and elevated serum HCG levels may be an indication of hydatidiform mole (see Chapter 22). Another cause of an enlarged uterus is a multiple gestation (Fig. 20-9). The uterus must be scanned carefully in several planes to establish the number of conceptuses and to rule out uterine anomalies such as septate uterus that may distort a gestational sac and in some planes make a singleton appear to be twins (Fig. 20-10). It is also important to keep in mind the large number of early pregnancies that fail to develop. While some are shed and the woman experiences vaginal bleeding, others are simply resorbed. As with a single pregnancy, this process can occur with one or more of a multiple gestation and is known as the "vanishing twin" (Fig. 20-11). In as many as 70% of cases, when twins are identified at or before 10 weeks' gestational age, only a singleton survives to be born.[5]

When the uterus is smaller than expected, careful measurements are again taken to establish the

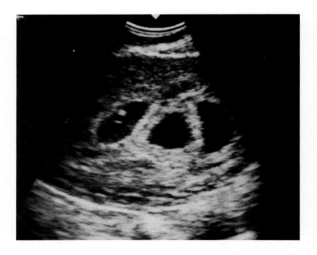

FIGURE 20-9. Sonogram performed transvaginally revealed three distinct gestational sacs at 6 weeks after LMP. Note that the sac on the left contains a yolk sac and small embryonic disc which are seen in this projection. Multiple gestation is a common source of size-dates discrepancy.

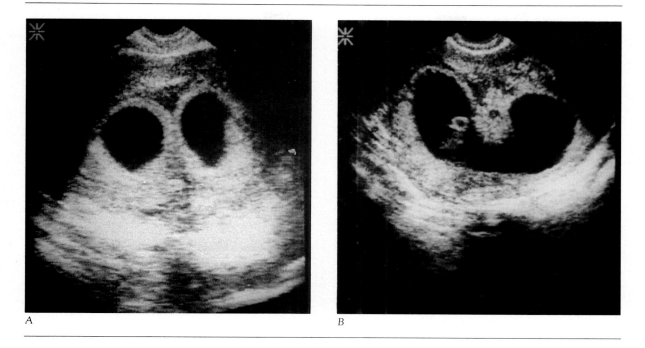

A B

FIGURE 20-10. (A) Sonogram reveals an apparent twin gestation. (B) Sonogram of the same patient taken at slightly different scan angle reveals a septate uterus containing a single intrauterine pregnancy. Careful scanning will help avoid misdiagnosing a twin gestation.

FIGURE 20-11. Sonogram reveals 2 yolk sacs contained within the same gestational sac 6 weeks after LMP. The patient subsequently experienced vaginal bleeding. Follow-up scan at that time (2 weeks after initial study) revealed a single viable intrauterine gestation with cardiac activity. This represents an example of the vanishing twin. The mechanism of such embryonic resorption may be the same one by which singletons transform into "empty sacs."

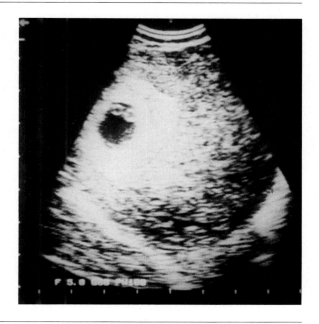

gestational age. If the development of the gestational sac and its contents are indeed less advanced than the patient's dates would indicate, again, correlation with the HCG levels is in order. Once spontaneous abortion and blighted ovum have been ruled out, sequential sonograms should be performed to establish a normal rate of growth. While most cases of intrauterine growth retardation (IUGR) are due to uteroplacental insufficiency, and therefore occur in the third trimester (or, in severe cases, in the second), congenital anomalies, particularly those associated with chromosomal abnormalities and certain congenital viral infections, cause disturbed growth patterns as well.[14] IUGR associated with triploidy (admittedly a rare occurrence) has been identified in the first trimester.[1]

Abnormalities Identified in the First Trimester

Great care must be taken when scanning a first-trimester patient to avoid both misinterpreting normal appearances and processes and offering premature reassurances. Perhaps the most obvious example in the first category is mistaking normal extraabdominal bowel migration and rotation for an omphalocele. As discussed in Chapter 12, in the normal embryo, bowel begins migrating into the proximal portion of the umbilical cord at about 6 weeks' gestational age. It is often seen sonographically at 8 to 10 weeks, and by 11 weeks it begins to return to the abdominal cavity. In most cases, the extraabdominal mass of bowel never exceeds 10 mm in greatest diameter and the fetal anterior abdominal wall appears normal by 14 weeks' gestational age. Embryonic omphalocele has been diagnosed when the diameter of the herniated mass was larger than the abdominal diameter and had the homogeneous appearance of liver rather than the heterogeneous echo pattern of bowel. Follow-up studies revealed the persistence of the mass beyond the 14th week of gestation.[3]

Nuchal blebs, seen as sonolucent neck masses, are a common developmental anomaly that occurs in about 40% of all embryos at about the 9th week after LMP. The majority of these blebs regress; the remainder can progress and result in defects of the skull, meninges, or lymphatic system. When there is lymphatic involvement, cystic hygroma or the more extensive jugular lymphatic obstructive sequence occurs. Any cystic neck mass visualized in a gestation of less than 10 weeks must be followed before a diagnosis is made.[8] Successful diagnosis of cystic hygroma has been made transvaginally at 10 weeks' gestation and confirmed by demonstrating an increase in the size of the mass at 11 weeks.[13]

Early multiple gestations should be surveyed carefully in the first trimester. A bifid appearance of the embryonic pole may indicate conjoined twins. When the sonographer is unable to demonstrate separation of the embryos, and their heads are repeatedly seen at the same level, suspicion of this anomaly is strong. At least one case of conjoined twins has been diagnosed sonographically in the first trimester, seen again on repeat scans, and confirmed at autopsy following spontaneous abortion.[9]

Normal appearance in the first trimester does not necessarily assure a normal fetus by the second trimester. In one example, visualizing a normal amount of cortical tissue at 10 weeks' gestation could not preclude abnormal structure and vascularization and resultant degeneration that gave rise to anencephaly as seen at 16 weeks.[8] It is therefore unwise to either confirm or exclude a diagnosis prematurely.

Conclusion

First-trimester ultrasound examination, especially when coupled with quantitative serum HCG levels, provides the most accurate evaluation of early problem pregnancies. Its greatest strengths at this time are in predicting viability and gestational age. A growing area, though one fraught with pitfalls, is the early identification of congenital anomalies. Great care and detailed knowledge of normal embryonic processes can reduce the rates of false-negative and false-positive diagnoses, but the sonographer must remain aware of the possibility of anomalies that will not be manifest until the second trimester. As the field of first-trimester ultrasound examination expands, competent ultrasound practitioners will continue to play an important role in the management of early pregnancy.

References

1. Benacerraf BR. Intrauterine growth retardation in the first trimester associated with triploidy. J Ultrasound Med. 1988; 17:153–154.

2. Cashner KA, Christopher CR, Dysert GA. Spontaneous fetal loss after demonstration of a live fetus in the first trimester. Obstet Gynecol. 1987; 70:827–830.

3. Curtis JA, Watson L. Sonographic diagnosis of omphalocele in the first trimester of fetal gestation. J Ultrasound Med. 1988; 7:97–100.

4. Fantel AG, Shepard TH. Basic aspects of early (first-trimester) abortion. In: Iffy L, Kaminetzky HA, eds. Principles and Practices of Obstetrics and Perinatology. New York: Wiley; 1981; 1.

5. Finberg HJ, Birnholz JC. Ultrasound observation in multiple gestation with first-trimester bleeding: The blighted twin. Radiology. 1979; 132:137–142.

6. Goldstein SR. Endovaginal Ultrasound. New York: Alan R. Liss; 1988.

7. Goldstein SR, et al. Subchorionic bleeding in threatened abortion: Sonographic findings and significance. Am J Roentgenol. 1983; 141:975–978.

8. Hill LM, Thomas ML, Kislak S, et al. Sonographic assessment of the first-trimester fetus: A cautionary note. Am J Perinatol. 1988; 5:13–15.

9. Maggio M, Callen NA, Hamod KA, et al. The first-trimester ultrasonographic diagnosis of conjoined twins. Am J Obstet Gynecol. 1985; 152:833–835.

10. Nyberg DA, Filly RA, Filho DL, et al. Abnormal pregnancy: Early diagnosis by US and serum chorionic gonadotropin. Radiology. 1986; 158:393–396.

11. Nyberg DA, Laing FC, Filly RA. Threatened abortion: Sonographic distinction of normal and abnormal gestation sacs. Radiology. 1986; 158:397–400.

12. Nyberg DA, Mack LA, Harvey A, et al. Value of the yolk sac in evaluating early pregnancies. J Ultrasound Med. 1988; 7:129–135.

13. Reuss A, Pipers L, van Swaaij E, et al. First-trimester diagnosis of recurrence of cystic hygroma using a vaginal ultrasound transducer. Eur J Obstet Gynecol Reprod Biol. 1987; 26:271–273.

14. Sanders RC, James AE. The principles and practice of ultrasonography in obstetrics and gynecology. 3rd ed. Norwalk, CT: Appleton-Century-Crofts; 1985.

15. Siddiqi TA, Caligaris JT, Miodovnik M, et al. Rate of spontaneous abortion after first-trimester sonographic demonstration of fetal cardiac activity. Am J Perinatol. 1988; 5:1–4.

16. U.S. Department of Health and Human Services, Public Health Service, National Institutes of Health. Diagnostic Ultrasound Imaging in Pregnancy. NIH Publication No. 84-667. Washington, DC: US Government Printing Office; 1984.

17. Waldenström U, Exelsson O, Nilsson S, et al. Effects of routine one-stage ultrasound screening in pregnancy: A randomized controlled trial. Lancet. 1988; II:585–588.

18. Wilson RD, Kendrick V, Wittman BK, et al. Spontaneous abortion and pregnancy outcome after normal first-trimester ultrasound examination. Obstet Gynecol. 1986; 67:352.

19. Wilson RL, Worthen NJ. Ultrasonic demonstration of myometrial contractions in intrauterine pregnancy. AJR. 1979; 132:243–247.

CHAPTER 21

Sonographic Assessment of Ectopic Pregnancy

FRANK CERVANTES

An ectopic pregnancy is one in which the fertilized ovum implants in any area outside the endometrial cavity. Before the advent of modern diagnostic techniques, patients died from hemorrhage secondary to rupture because the diagnosis was not made in time for surgical intervention. The maternal mortality rate from ectopic pregnancy declined markedly starting in 1970, from 3.5 deaths per thousand, and more gradually in recent years with an overall sevenfold decrease to 0.5 deaths per thousand in 1983. Currently, 40 to 50 women die each year in the United States as a result of ectopic pregnancy. The incidence of extrauterine pregnancy has been reported to be 1.4 ectopic pregnancies for every 100 reported pregnancies.[5]

Ultrasound used in conjunction with clinical presentation and radioimmunoassay provides anatomic images that contribute to making the diagnosis. A thorough understanding of sonographic features, implantation sites, scanning technique, and differential diagnoses is necessary for the sonographer to perform a sonographic evaluation of a patient at risk for ectopic pregnancy. A knowledge of the physiology of conception and gestation, along with an awareness of the meaning of pertinent laboratory values, clinical symptoms, and predisposition to ectopic pregnancy, supplements the information provided by diagnostic images.

Tubal Ectopic Pregnancy

Normal implantation occurs in the upper corpus or fundal region of the uterine cavity.[2] Most ectopic gestations occur in the fallopian tubes (Fig. 21-1). Nontubal ectopic implantation sites such as the ovaries (2 to 3% of ectopic pregnancies) abdomen (1.4%), cervix, interligamentous and rudimentary horn occur rarely. The narrow tubular structure of the fallopian tubes and their unique location in the true pelvis with an opening into the peritoneal cavity account for the occurrence of abdominal pregnancies.

ETIOLOGY

The fallopian tube is derived bilaterally from the Müllerian duct system and is the only connection between the peritoneal cavity and the endometrial cavity.[22] As the ovum is expelled from the dominant follicle and is swept up by the fimbriae into the oviduct, certain conditions may impede its normal course and cause it to implant in the fallopian tube.

Mechanical obstruction and abnormalities in the movement of the embryo through the tube may result in ectopic implantation. Alteration of the tubal transport mechanism and intrinsic embryonic abnormalities cause most ectopic pregnancies to be located in the fallopian tube.[26] Causes of ectopic pregnancy include scar tissue from previous ectopic pregnancy, reduced tubal motility secondary to pelvic inflammatory disease, follicle-stimulating hormone (FSH) therapy, in vitro fertilization procedures, and the use of an intrauterine contraceptive device (IUD). An IUD is far more effective in preventing implantation in the uterus than it is at preventing implantation in an ectopic location.[7] Processes responsible to a lesser extent for ectopic pregnancy are induced abortion, tubal surgery for infertility or sterilization, conservative management of ectopic pregnancy, delayed childbearing, and douching.[5]

A history of previous ectopic pregnancy increases the likelihood of an extrauterine pregnancy. Among women who have had an ectopic pregnancy, the subsequent overall conception rate is approximately 60%. Of these, 50% are intrauterine and 10% are repeat ectopic gestations. Tubal scarring from the first ectopic pregnancy probably accounts for the second ectopic pregnancy or contributes to infertility.

One of the most prevalent contributors to mechanical obstruction is pelvic inflammatory disease (PID) and associated salpingitis. Antibiotic therapy is used to treat the patient. Treatment of salpingitis and PID results in the scarring of epithelial tissue which reduces motility in the tube.[22] Congenital abnormalities of the fallopian tube and tubal ligations are also responsible for causing implantation in the oviduct. Transmigration of the fertilized ovum is another process that can culminate in a tubal pregnancy. Internal transmigration occurs when the ovum is fertilized in one tube and migrates across the uterus to enter the opposite tube and implant there. External transmigration occurs when fertilization occurs in the cul-de-sac, progresses to the blastocyst disc stage, and is then picked up by the fimbriae and implants in the contralateral tube. Demonstration of a contralateral corpus luteum cyst supports this transmigration theory.

A malformed embryo may be predisposed to ectopic implantation if the propulsive mechanism of the tube is inhibited or rendered ineffective by an abnormality. Grossly abnormal chromosome patterns have been noted in a number of ectopic pregnancies.[26]

Uterine and adnexal masses can interfere with the normal function of the tube. Myomas, endo-

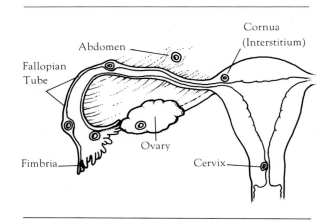

FIGURE 21-1. Sites of implantation of the fertilized ovum in an ectopic pregnancy.

metriomas, adnexal masses, and pelvic adhesions can result in kinking of the tube or narrowing of the lumen.

Where an ectopic gestation is implanted depends on various mechanisms and sequences of events. Pavinstein and colleagues found that the majority of tubal pregnancies occur in the ampullary portion; other locations include the isthmus, the fimbria, and the interstitium. The interstitial (cornual) pregnancy, which is the least common, is the one that may go undetected, as it is surrounded by myometrium, which allows for greater growth than the less vascular wall of the oviduct. Because the maternal veins lie adjacent, massive hemoperitoneum may result from late rupture of this form of ectopic pregnancy.

Upon implantation within the tubal mucosa, there is invasion by the villous trophoblast into the endosalpinx and subsequent layers of the oviduct. Bleeding may occur and may be seen in the cul-de-sac and other dependent areas where free fluid collects.

Other Implantation Sites
Cervical Implantation
Cervical pregnancy—when a fertilized ovum implants below the level of the internal os—is rare

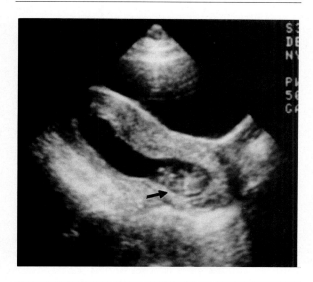

FIGURE 21-2. A longitudinal scan of a cervical ectopic prenancy shows the fetus in the cervical region (*arrow*).

(Fig. 21-2). It is postulated that any factor that alters the entire endometrium or a portion of it, making it unsuitable for uterine implantation, may increase the risk of cervical pregnancy. Endometritis, Ascherman's syndrome, an IUD, previous cesarean section, and leiomyomas are such factors.[2] The clinician must first consider an impending abortion in progress, because of the similar location. An abortion in progress would demonstrate a more complex sonographic appearance than implantation of the blastocyst below the internal os. Ectopic implantation is diagnosed histologically if cervical glands are found opposite the placental attachment site, and fetal elements must not be present in the corpus of the uterus.[15]

ABDOMINAL IMPLANTATION

An abdominal pregnancy is defined as primary or secondary. In the primary sort, (1) both tubes and ovaries are normal, with no evidence of recent or remote injury; (2) there is no evidence of uteroperitoneal fistulas; and (3) the pregnancy is adherent to the peritoneal surface without evidence of secondary implantation after primary implantation in the tube. Most secondary abdominal pregnancies result from tubal abortion or rupture with extension and implantation of a viable placenta on the peritoneal surfaces.[24] Early diagnosis of abdominal pregnancy is of the utmost importance in light of the possibility of massive hemorrhage secondary to separation of the placenta from its attachment to bowel or other peritoneal viscera.[2]

OVARIAN IMPLANTATION

Ovarian pregnancy is a rare type of ectopic pregnancy with certain established identifying features. The tube and the fimbriae on the affected side must be intact. The gestational sac must occupy the normal position of the ovary. The gestational sac must be connected to the uterus by the uteroovarian ligament, and ovarian tissue must be identified histologically in the wall of the sac. An ovarian pregnancy is classified as primary or secondary. The primary, or interfollicular, type presumably results from failure of the ovum to be extruded from the follicle; fertilization subsequently occurs within the early corpus luteum. The secondary type probably results from an early tubal abortion that implants on the ovarian surface.[2]

Clinical Information

Symptoms of acute ectopic pregnancy include vaginal spotting or bleeding, abdominal pain, amenorrhea, adnexal tenderness or palpable adnexal mass, and a positive pregnancy test. Tubal rupture results in intraperitoneal hemorrhage, which may cause pain referred to the shoulder as the abdomen fills with blood.[6] Severe abdominal pain is due to peritoneal reaction to the blood.[7] Less acute pelvic discomfort suggests a chronic ectopic pregnancy. Symptoms are recurrent, intermittent, low-grade fever associated with a palpable solid mass.[11] Patients with chronic ectopic pregnancies have higher lactic dehydrogenase (LDH) levels than patients with acute ectopic symptoms.[3] Certain signs and symptoms suggest abdominal pregnancy: abdominal pain, nausea or vomiting late in pregnancy, pain on fetal movements, sudden cessation of fetal movement, and fetal movement high in the mother's abdomen.[2]

Laboratory tests are based on the production of human chorionic gonadotropin (HCG) by the embryo. The urine pregnancy test is moderately reliable, but it might react to luteinizing hormone (LH) in the urine. The result may be false positive for patients with PID and false negative for those with early abnormal pregnancy. The development of a radioimmunoassay (RIA) that specifically measures serum HCG (as opposed to LH) has revolutionized the diagnosis of early pregnancy-related disorders. The estimation of serum levels of HCG is clinically superior to the measurement of any other pregnancy protein or biochemical parameter.[23] With intrauterine pregnancy, HCG normally becomes detectable in the bloodstream 7 to 10 days after ovulation, and serum concentration increases exponentially, paralleling the early proliferation of the trophoblast. An abnormally rapid increase may indicate the presence of hydatidiform mole; decreasing concentrations indicate a nonviable pregnancy, such as a spontaneous abortion or ectopic implantation.[19]

Kadar and colleagues report that in women with HCG levels exceeding 6500 mIU/ml sonography should demonstrate a gestational sac; its absence is evidence for an ectopic pregnancy. More recently, detection of a gestational sac at HCG levels exceeding 1800 mIU/ml has been presented as a threshold for visualization of the sac on transvaginal scans, and its absence is evidence of an ectopic pregnancy, as ectopic pregnancies are associated with lower HCG levels than normal pregnancies.

Nyberg and coworkers have conducted studies in which absence of an intrauterine gestational sac combined with HCG levels greater than 1800 mIU/ml correctly identified 47% of ectopic pregnancies. They report that an HCG level of 1800 mIU/ml corresponds to a gestation sac that is approximately 5 to 6 mm in diameter; an HCG level of 3250 mIU/ml corresponds to a sac of approximately 8 mm in average diameter.[16]

Increased serum amylase has been reported in association with ruptured tubal pregnancy, owing to release of tubal amylase when rupture occurs. When an ectopic gestation ruptures, tubal amylase may be released into the peritoneal cavity.[13]

Alternate Diagnostic Modalities

Other diagnostic modalities for evaluating ectopic pregnancy may be used when sonographic findings are equivocal. Although criteria for differentiating between the echogenic decidual reaction and a true intrauterine gestation have been established, when a gestational sac cannot be conclusively identified sonographically, other diagnostic procedures must be used. A uterine curettage may be diagnostic since recovery of chorionic villi confirms intrauterine pregnancy, whereas recovery of decidual tissue alone suggests extrauterine pregnancy.[16] It must be remembered that the incidence of simultaneous intrauterine and extrauterine implantation of twins is increasing.

Culdocentesis is used widely to diagnose hemoperitoneum in patients with suspected ectopic pregnancy.[20] This procedure has value only for diagnosing *ruptured* tubal pregnancy. There is also the possibility of a false positive result, because culdocentesis cannot predict the site of hemorrhage. Clinical findings with ruptured, but not actively bleeding, corpus luteum cyst may closely resemble those of ectopic pregnancy and can yield a positive result on culdocentesis.[27]

Laparoscopy has replaced laparotomy for diagnosis of ectopic pregnancy. Early unruptured ectopic pregnancy without hemoperitoneum can be diagnosed only by laparoscopy or laparotomy.[12] Laparoscopy may be used when sonographic findings are inconclusive (Fig. 21-3).

Sonographic Technical Protocol

Optimal visualization of the uterus and adnexa is crucial in the sonographic evaluation of a suspected ectopic pregnancy. The sonographer must be familiar with the patient's medical and surgical history and clinical presentation in order to better correlate the sonographic findings and formulate the differential diagnosis. The single most important function of ultrasound in the evaluation of ectopic pregnancy is to establish the presence of a viable intrauterine pregnancy. A sac is usually noted 4 to 5 weeks after the last menstrual period (LMP) with transabdominal scanning and 3 to 4 weeks after LMP with transvaginal technique; sonographic appearance may suggest an intrauterine pregnancy, but this does not exclude the possibility of an ectopic pregnancy. The decidual reaction, which takes place with both extrauterine and intrauterine pregnancy, may resemble a sac. Demon-

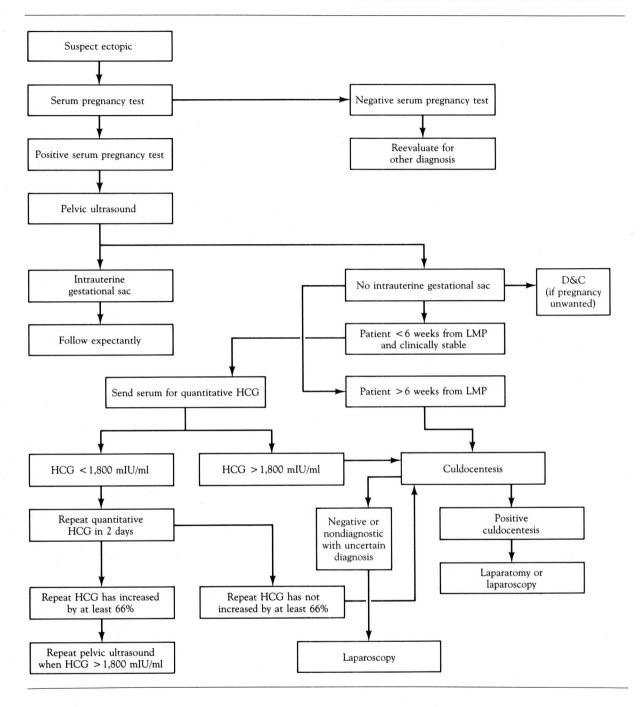

FIGURE 21-3. Management of stable patients with suspected ectopic pregnancy.

stration of a fetal pole with cardiac activity definitively locates the gestation.

Transvaginal scanning has been shown to be almost essential in examinations for possible ectopic pregnancy[17]; however, transabdominal scans usually are performed first, to obtain more complete views of the adnexa, fundal region, flanks, and abdomen.[8] In order to optimize visualization, appropriate bladder filling and transducer selection are important technical aspects. The urinary bladder should be filled enough to cover the uterine fundus. Certain conditions, such as an enlarged leiomyomatous uterus, may prohibit tolerable bladder distension, and the sonographer should use other means, such as patient positioning. Placing the patient in an oblique position will shift the bladder to better visualize the right- and left-side lower quadrants. Placing the patient in the Trendelenburg position may afford a better view of the uterine fundus facilitated by bladder displacement. An overly distended bladder and submucosal fibroids may both contribute to the eccentric location of an early gestational sac. To differentiate, the patient should be scanned again after voiding partially.

The sonographer must now systematically evaluate all potential sites of implantation and must look for other sonographic diagnostic criteria. Evaluation of the endometrial cavity begins by noting the degree of prominence of the endometrial echo and its contents. Decidual reaction, saclike structures, fluid and other echoes are some of the endometrial criteria. All other areas of the uterus must be evaluated for potential implantation sites. Both adnexa and adnexal regions should be scrutinized. Special attention needs to be given to any suspicious masses. They should be demonstrated from a variety of scanning planes, and every technique available, such as looking for peristalsis, should be used to make sure the mass is not a segment of normal bowel. Any complex adnexal mass that has a pole with cardiac activity outside the endometrial cavity is definitely an ectopic pregnancy. A complex mass can represent an ectopic gestation at one of its stages of growth or rupture. When there is clinical suspicion of an ectopic pregnancy, all adnexal findings should be noted, characterized, and treated as potential ectopic pregnancy until proven otherwise.

Sonographic evaluation also includes the hepa-

TABLE 21-1. Scanning protocol for ectopic pregnancy employing transabdominal and/or transvaginal transducers

1. Be acquainted with clinical history, pregnancy test results, and last menstrual period.
2. Use bladder distention (transabdominal scanning) and appropriate transducer (3.5 MHz).
3. Examine endometrial cavity in sagittal and transverse planes for signs of ectopia:
   Decidual cast versus double sac sign
   Absence of gestational sac
   Gestational sac located in cervical area
   Gestational sac located in cornual region
   Gestational sac in asymmetric location
   Fluid in endometrial cavity
4. Examine adnexa in sagittal and transverse planes for signs of ectopia:
   No rupture: look for fetal cardiac motion in adnexal mass
   Acute rupture: variable complex adnexal mass with free fluid
   Chronic ruptured: echogenic complex mass that may gravitate to cul-de-sac region
5. Examine cul-de-sac for the presence of fluid, blood, or embryonic tissue from ruptured sac or tube.
6. Examine hepatorenal space for free fluid.
7. Describe sonographic findings and establish a preliminary impression.

torenal space (Morison's pouch) and paracolic gutters (flank areas) to check for the extent of free fluid, such as blood from ruptured ectopic implantation or peritoneal fluid from a ruptured ovarian cyst. Certain cul-de-sac masses may also be bowel related and can be differentiated by administering a fluid enema and observing for peristalsis with real-time ultrasonography. The sonographer may be faced with a patient who exhibits severe abdominal discomfort, which is a further complication to an already difficult and sensitive examination. This stressful environment should not be allowed to compromise a comprehensive evaluation (Table 21-1).

Sonographic Characteristics

UTERINE

The demonstration of a viable intrauterine pregnancy occupying a high fundal position within the endometrium is the usually conclusive sonographic information that rules out an ectopic pregnancy.

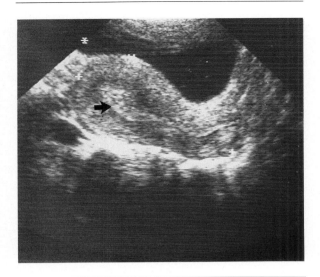

FIGURE 21-4. A longitudinal scan demonstrates prominent endometrial echoes (*arrow*) that normally occur during the secretory phase of the menstrual cycle. This appearance is similar to the decidual reaction of pregnancy.

The coexistence of intrauterine and extrauterine gestations (heterotopic pregnancy) occurs 1 in 6000 cases and is considered a rare phenomenon.[9] A viable intrauterine gestation may be visualized transabdominally from 5 to 6 weeks after LMP, depending on the mother's body habitus. Vaginal transducers detect gestational sacs and cardiac activity about 10 days earlier than transabdominal ones. Suggestive transvaginal sonographic findings of an intrauterine pregnancy, such as visualization of a double sac sign, a yolk sac, or a gestational sac, eliminate the likelihood of an ectopic implantation.

The normal prominence of the endometrial echo during the secretory phase of the endometrial cycle may appear similar to the decidual reaction of the endometrial lining as it prepares for implantation in response to both intrauterine and extrauterine pregnancies (Figs. 21-4, 21-8A). Therefore, this finding in itself is not a diagnostic criterion. The appearance of a saclike structure with a perimeter of high-amplitude echoes, which is due to tro-phoblastic reaction, can be somewhat suggestive of an early intrauterine pregnancy.

Demonstration of the double sac sign is a stronger and more reliable indicator of an early intrauterine pregnancy. The double sac, which consists of two concentric rings surrounding a portion of the gestational sac, is thought to represent the decidua parietalis (decidua vera) adjacent to the decidua capsularis. In contradistinction, the pseudogestational sac of an ectopic pregnancy is composed of a single decidual layer surrounding an intraendometrial fluid collection and thus demonstrates a single echogenic ring.[7] Intrauterine gestations are clearly distinguished by their asymmetric sonographic pattern, as opposed to the circular decidual sac that is associated with an ectopic pregnancy and postovulation.[14]

An interstitial pregnancy demonstrates a gestational sac adjacent to the uterine cornua and not completely surrounded by myometrium (Fig. 21-5). A cervical ectopic pregnancy demonstrates a gestational sac below the level of the internal os; however, owing to the rarity of this type of cervical ectopic pregnancy, it more frequently represents an inevitable abortion. The sonographer should keep in mind that a bicornuate uterus may demonstrate a decidual reaction in the nongravid horn and the

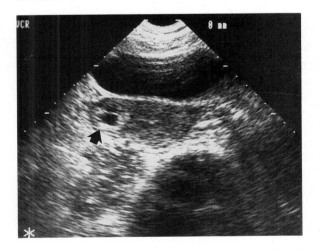

FIGURE 21-5. A transverse scan demonstrates an unruptured right cornual gestational sac (*arrow*).

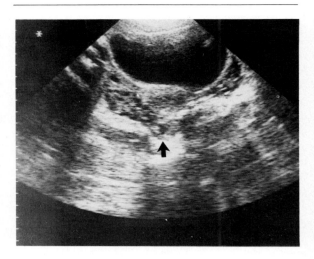

FIGURE 21-6. A transverse scan demonstrates a gestational sac (*arrow*) in contact with the medial aspect of the right adnexa extending posterior to the uterus.

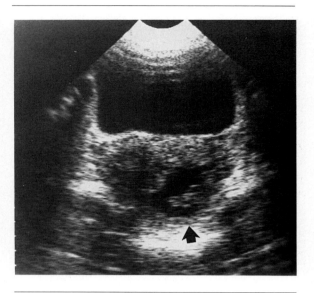

FIGURE 21-7. A transverse view demonstrates a complex mass in the left adnexa. This proved to be an unruptured left-sided ectopic pregnancy extending into the cul-de-sac region (*arrow*).

gestational sac in the other, resembling an extrauterine gestational sac.

It is important to be aware of intrauterine findings that can simulate pertinent sonographic diagnostic criteria. Fluid collections in the uterus may appear similar to an early pregnancy. A decidual cast may sometimes develop a hematoma, which can simulate an early saclike structure. Depending on the degree of organization, blood clots simulate a fetal pole. Bladder overdistention may compress the gestational sac, compromising evaluation. It may also displace the gestational sac, giving the false impression of an impending abortion, a cervical pregnancy, or a cornual pregnancy. Other structures that may represent an abnormal first-trimester intrauterine pregnancy, such as a blighted ovum or a missed abortion, can seem to meet ectopic pregnancy criteria.

ADNEXAL

Unruptured Tubal Pregnancy. An adnexal mass is palpated in a significant number of patients with an ectopic pregnancy. Adnexal sonographic findings are, predictably, more common in patients with an unruptured ectopic pregnancy than in patients with an intrauterine pregnancy.[21] The sono-

graphic appearance of these masses is highly variable, and a number of other lesions mimic them sonographically. Ultrasound may provide definitive diagnosis of an ectopic pregnancy only if an ectopic gestational sac is visible outside the uterus and fetal heart movements are demonstrable within it. Certain sonographic findings may suggest an unruptured ectopic pregnancy. An echogenic ring is usually noted (due to trophoblastic reaction) with a sonolucent central portion (Fig. 21-6). This saclike structure may be located adjacent to or distant from either ovary. Because location may be influenced by bladder filling or bowel arrangement, all areas of the pelvis should be evaluated for suspicious extrauterine masses (Fig. 21-7). A corpus luteum cyst may be found on the contralateral side of an ectopic gestation, as a result of its migrating through the uterus, or on the ipsilateral side.

An extrauterine sac may also appear as a complex mass with both solid and cystic areas, which prior to rupture can mimic other pelvic masses. A pelvic hematocele, corpus luteum cysts with inter-

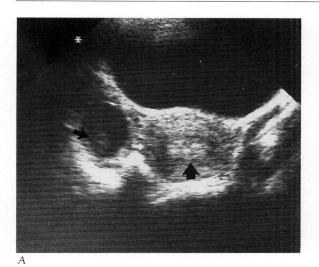
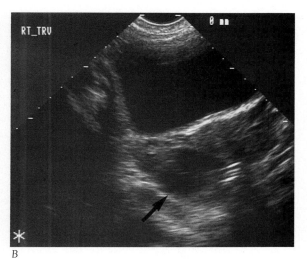

A   B

FIGURE 21-8. (A) A transverse scan demonstrates a complex, primarily cystic, right-sided mass. Observation of a fetal pole with cardiac motion (*small arrow*) proved it to be an ectopic pregnancy. A prominent decidual reaction was also noted (*large arrow*). (B) A transverse scan demonstrates a complex, primarily cystic, right-sided mass representing a hemorrhagic cyst (*arrow*) The low-level echoes are caused by the hemorrhagic debris.

nal bleeding, tuboovarian abscess, or pelvic inflammatory disease collections are some of the more common conditions that can sonographically simulate ectopic pregnancy (Fig. 21-8). Other masses that can give the appearance of ectopic pregnancy are small serous and mucinous cystadenomas, cystic teratomas, and single endometriomas. Echoes may be seen within these neoplasms, making them difficult to differentiate from ectopic implantation. It is important to remember that any of these masses can coexist with an ectopic pregnancy. Fluid-filled bowel loops should be differentiated from an ectopic pregnancy by looking for peristalsis.

Because they look similar on sonographic examination ovarian ectopic pregnancies are often indistinguishable from more common tubal ectopic pregnancies. This makes a true ovarian pregnancy difficult to identify.[10]

Ruptured Tubal Pregnancy. Acute rupture of a tubal pregnancy initiates formation of a complex mass, which shows further changes as it proceeds to the chronic stage. When there is a partial or complete rupture of the tubal pregnancy a variety of sonographic appearances occur initially that enlarge the differential diagnosis. When rupture occurs, blood and gestational contents add to the complex nature of the adnexal mass (Fig. 21-9). The presence of hemoperitoneum that becomes more complex in appearance as the mass develops may simulate a tuboovarian abscess and pelvic adhesions. This debris may gravitate to the cul-de-sac area or surround the adnexa and develop into a ruptured chronic ectopic gestation.

The presence of free fluid in the cul-de-sac, around the uterus and adnexa, subphrenic spaces, and paracolic gutters is part of the sonographic evaluation of the patient with acute rupture of an ectopic pregnancy (Fig. 21-10). The volume and sonographic appearance of free intraperitoneal fluid is a valuable sign in the diagnosis of ectopic pregnancy. Fluid in the cul-de-sac may be exudate, in the presence of pelvic inflammatory disease, or blood, in patients with an ectopic pregnancy or rupture of other abdominal viscera.[4] Acquaintance with a patient's menstrual history may also suggest that cul-de-sac fluid is the result of her ovulatory phase. Aside from identifying cardiac activity in the extragestational sac, adnexal findings tend to be nonspecific, and a differential diagnosis is proposed in conjunction with the clinical and laboratory findings. One must also consider the concurrent presence of other neoplasms or lesions that further complicate the sonographic presentation.

Chronic ectopic pregnancy is a form of tubal pregnancy in which growth of trophoblastic tissue early in gestation causes gradual disintegration of the tubal wall and slow or repeated episodes of hemorrhage. The presence of blood, trophoblastic tissue, and disrupted tubal tissue in the peritoneal cavity incites an inflammatory response, which seals off the area, creating a pelvic hematocele.[3] The echogenicity of the mass may be similar to that of the uterus, obscuring its borders and creating the "indefinite uterus" sign. Sonographically, one may see a complex extrauterine mass in the region of the adnexa and cul-de-sac that conforms to the spaces that it occupies. Echogenic foci and sonolucent areas may contribute to a highly complex and variable appearance, depending on the degree of clot and mass organization. The sonographic appearances of endometriosis and chronic PID are similar to those of chronic ectopic pregnancy.

Abdominal Pregnancy. Most abdominal pregnancies are diagnosed sonographically at a later gestational age than tubal pregnancy. A first-trimester abdominal pregnancy may be difficult to distinguish by sonographic criteria from an unruptured tubal pregnancy. Rupture of a tubal ectopic gestation generally occurs between 6 and 12 weeks, so the finding of an extrauterine gestation of 12 or more weeks' duration should suggest the diagnosis of an abdominal pregnancy (Fig. 21-11). Certain clinical signs and symptoms suggest the presence of an abdominal pregnancy.[1] Sonographically, a number of specific findings are associated with an abdominal pregnancy. The most frequent and reliable one is an empty uterus separate from the fetus.[25] Extragestational findings in abdominal pregnancy are listed in Table 21-2.

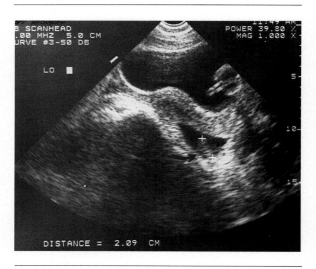

FIGURE 21-9. A longitudinal scan of a ruptured ectopic pregnancy in the cul-de-sac (*curved arrow*). A fetal pole was seen within the blood and disrupted tubal contents.

The sonographer must also be aware of the variability in the appearance of a dead fetus. Signs of intrauterine and extrauterine fetal demise are similar; however, documentation becomes more difficult in abdominal pregnancies, owing to the lack of amniotic fluid and to maceration of fetal parts. This further complicates interpretation, as the fetus may simulate other conditions such as calcific changes in the leiomyomatous uterus. Additional

TABLE 21-2. Sonographic findings in abdominal pregnancy

Oligohydramnios
No placenta-myometrium interface
Poor definition of placenta
    May be seen attached to maternal intestine
    Lack of chorionic plate
Close location of fetal parts to maternal abdominal wall
Unusual fetal presentation
Maternal bowel gas anterior or intermingled with fetal parts
Pseudoprevia created by empty uterus superior to maternal bladder and free fluid

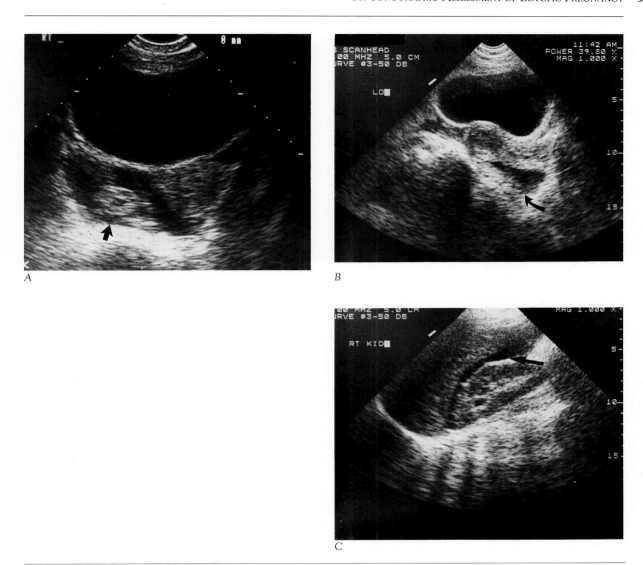

FIGURE 21-10. (A) A complex right adnexal mass (*arrow*) represents a gestational sac surrounded by fluid and blood resulting from the tubal rupture. (B) In this sagittal scan of the same patient free fluid is seen in the cul-de-sac (*curved arrow*). (C) Fluid in the hepatorenal space of the same patient (*arrow*).

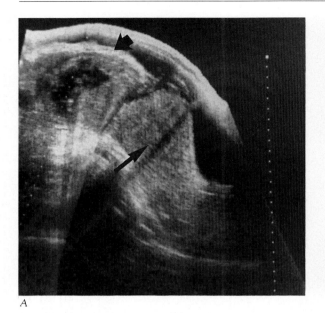
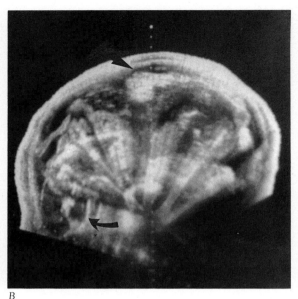

A

B

FIGURE 21-11. (A) A longitudinal scan of an empty uterus (*long arrow*). The abdominal pregnancy is visible superior to the fundus (*short arrow*). (B) A transverse scan superior to the fundus shows the abdominal pregnancy, bowel (*straight arrow*), and right kidney (*curved arrow*). (Courtesy of Charles Odwin, Bronx, NY.)

diagnostic imaging modalities such as radiography and hysterosalpingography can be used to confirm sonographic findings. Unfortunately, the diagnosis of abdominal pregnancy is missed in a significant percentage of patients. One must carefully document criteria that firmly establish an intrauterine pregnancy (placental-myometrial interface), especially when other abnormal features are seen on the sonogram.

Transvaginal Scanning

Transvaginal sonography has become an integral part of evaluating women who are suspected of having an ectopic pregnancy when conventional transabdominal sonography fails to show a living intrauterine or extrauterine embryo.[17] Transvaginal sonography uses a higher-frequency transducer (5.0 to 7.5 MHz) and is also placed closer to the cul-de-sac and adnexal regions, allowing better evaluation of uterine content and extrauterine

structures (Fig. 21-12). Since transvaginal scanning does not require a full urinary bladder, it expedites evaluation in emergency situations.

Owing to the variable locations of the adnexa, transabdominal scanning may still be necessary for a complete evaluation. Although transvaginal scanning is sufficient in early pregnancy, occasionally structures that are superior to the uterus and are outside the field of view of the transvaginal probe may be difficult to delineate.[8] The presence of free fluid can be detected transvaginally only in the pouch of Douglas; other collection sites can be out of the field of view of the transducer, making it difficult to quantitate the amount of fluid.

Treatment of Ectopic Pregnancy

The treatment of ectopic pregnancy is surgical. Laparotomy is indicated as soon as the diagnosis of tubal pregnancy is made. One operation is total salpingectomy; however, when the tube has not rup-

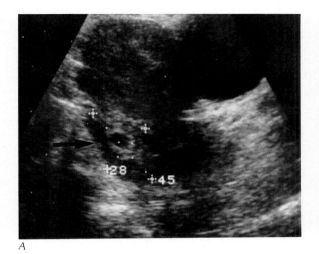

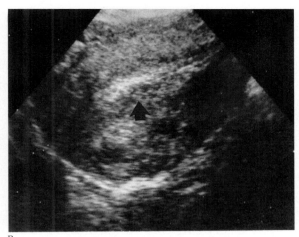

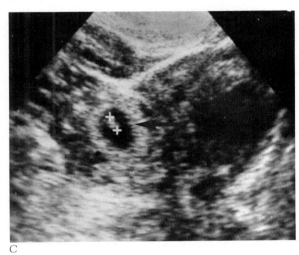

A

B

C

FIGURE 21-12. (A) A sagittal transabdominal scan displays a complex mass containing a saclike structure (*arrow*) posterior to the uterus. (B) A transvaginal scan of the same patient demonstrates a decidual reaction but no evidence of an intrauterine gestational sac (*arrow*). (C) An adnexal transvaginal scan of the same patient reveals a viable extrauterine gestation (*arrow*).

tured—and sometimes when it has—salpingostomy with removal of the pregnancy and conservation of the tube is feasible. Ruptured contents, such as old blood, clots, and conceptus debris (chronic pregnancy), are removed from the peritoneal cavity during surgery. A hysterectomy may be necessary in cases of ruptured interstitial pregnancy, as the cornua may be so damaged that repair is time consuming, unsatisfactory, and accompanied by considerable blood loss.[6] Methotrexate has shown promise as a nontraumatic way of resolving early tubal ectopic pregnancy. Preliminary data suggest that methotrexate may be effective in inducing tubal abortion and reabsorption of ectopic pregnancy. Preliminary experience suggests that it is a safe and relatively effective alternative to surgery for patients with early ectopic pregnancy.[18]

Regardless of gestational age or fetal condition, the clinical management of abdominal pregnancy is surgical. The maternal mortality rate for abdominal pregnancy is in the range of 4 to 18%. The fetal mortality rate is 90%, and the prevalence of fetal deformity ranges from 1 to 100%. Three different ways for dealing with the placenta are described: It can be removed; it can be left in situ and allowed to be reabsorbed; methotrexate can be given to hasten reabsorption.[24]

Conclusion

Unfortunately, despite new techniques such as transvaginal scanning, ultrasound cannot always produce a definitive diagnosis. The combination of clinical findings, HCG values, patient history, and other diagnostic tests increases the degree of certainty when ectopic pregnancy is suspected. A methodical evaluation of pelvic organs, adnexal regions, and dependent body areas for free fluid provides a routine for the sonographer that can contribute diagnostic information. When sonographic results are equivocal and the patient is stable, serial β-HCG assays and repeat scans give the questionable intrauterine sac time to develop.

The sonographer plays a critical role in the diagnostic component of the patient's evaluation; with all its potential, technology requires a skillful and conscientious operator to maximize its effectiveness.

References

1. Athey PA. Ectopic pregnancy. Ultrasound in Obstetrics and Gynecology. In: Athey PA, Hadlock FP, eds. 2nd ed. Moody, 1985.
2. Bayless RB. Nontubal ectopic pregnancy. Clin Obstet Gynecol. 1987; 30:191–199.
3. Bedi D, Fagan C, Nocera R. Chronic ectopic pregnancy. J Ultrasound Med. 1981; 3:347–352.
4. deCrespigny LC. The value of ultrasound in ectopic pregnancy. Clin Obstet Gynecol. 1987; 30:136–147.
5. Dorfman SF. Epidemiology of ectopic pregnancy. Clin Obstet Gynecol. 1987; 30:176.
6. Droegemueller W. Ectopic pregnancy. In: Danforth D, ed. Obstetrics and Gynecology. 4th ed. New York: Harper & Row; 1982.
7. Filly RA. Ectopic pregnancy: The role of sonography. Radiology. 1987; 162:661–668.
8. Fleischer A. Sonography in early intrauterine pregnancy emphasizing transvaginal scanning. Presented at 12th Annual Spring Weekend Symposium in Diagnostic Ultrasound. SUNY Health Science Center at Brooklyn, 1988.
9. Fleischer A, Jeanty P. Obstetrical sonography. In: Fleischer J, ed. Diagnostic Sonography Principles and Clinical Application. Philadelphia: WB Saunders; 1989.
10. Fleischer A, Boehr F, James A. Sonographic evaluation of ectopic pregnancy. In: Sanders RC, James AE Jr, eds. The Principles and Practice of Ultrasonography in Obstetrics and Gynecology. 2nd ed. Norwalk, CT: Appleton-Century-Crofts; 1980.
11. Fleischer A, Cartwright P, DiPietro D, et al. Evaluation of ectopic pregnancy. In: Sanders RC, James AE Jr, eds. The Principles and Practice of Ultrasonography in Obstetrics and Gynecology. 3rd ed. Norwalk, CT: Appleton-Century-Crofts; 1985.
12. Hallat J. Tubal conservation in ectopic pregnancy: A study of 200 cases. Am J Obstet Gynecol. 1986; 154:1216–1221.
13. Hannon Z, Guzick D. Tubal pregnancy: The significance of serum and peritoneal fluid amylase. Obstet Gynecol. 1985; 66:396.
14. Hansmann M, Hackeloer B, Staudach A. Ultrasound Obstet Gynecol: Berlin: Springer-Verlag; 1985; 60.
15. Laughlin CL, Lee TG, Richards RC. Ultrasonographic diagnosis of cervical ectopic pregnancy. J Ultrasound Med. 1983; 2:137–138.
16. Nyberg D, Filly R, Laing F, et al. Ectopic pregnancy diagnosis by sonography correlated with quantitative HCG levels. J Ultrasound Med. 1987; 6:145–150.
17. Nyberg D, Mack LA, Jeffrey RB Jr, et al. Endovaginal sonographic evaluation of ectopic pregnancy: A prospective study. AJR. 1987; 149:1181–1186.
18. Ory SJ, Villanueva AL, Sand PK, et al. Conservative treatment of ectopic pregnancy with methotrexate. Am J Obstet Gynecol. 1986; 154:1299–1306.
19. Pittway D. BHCG dynamics in ectopic pregnancy. Clin Obstet Gynecol. 1987; 30:130–132.
20. Romero R, Copel J, Kadar N, et al. Value of culdocentesis in the diagnosis of ectopic pregnancy. Obstet Gynecol. 1985; 65:519.
21. Romero R, Kadar N, Castro D, et al. The value of adnexal sonographic findings in the diagnosis of ectopic pregnancy. Am J Obstet Gynecol. 1988; 158:52–54.
22. Russell JB. The etiology of ectopic pregnancy. Clin Obstet Gynecol. 1987; 30:183–184.
23. Seppala M, Purhonen M. The use of HCG and other pregnancy proteins in the diagnosis of ectopic pregnancy. Clin Obstet Gynecol. 1987; 30:148–152.
24. Spanta R, Roffman L, Grissan T, et al. Abdominal pregnancy: Magnetic resonance identification with ultrasonographic follow-up of placental involution. Am J Obstet Gynecol. 1987; 157:887–889.
25. Stanley JH, Horger EO III, Fagan CJ, et al. Sonographic findings in abdominal pregnancy. AJR. 1986; 147:1043–1046.
26. Weckstein LN. Current perspective on ectopic pregnancy. Obstet Gynecol Surv 1985; 40:259–272.
27. Weckstein LN, Boucher AR, Tucker H, et al. Accurate diagnosis of early ectopic pregnancy. Obstet Gynecol. 1985; 65:393–397.

CHAPTER **22**

Gestational Trophoblastic Disease

Marie DeLange, Phil-Ann Tan-Sinn, Gerald L. Grube

Gestational trophoblastic diseases are rare but important conditions that constitute a range of benign and malignant processes, including hydatidiform mole, invasive mole, and choriocarcinoma. Sonography plays a crucial role in diagnosing hydatidiform mole, in evaluating its progression to invasive mole or choriocarcinoma, and in monitoring the efficacy of treatment. By correlating the sonographic findings with clinical and laboratory findings, obstetric and gynecologic conditions with similar sonographic appearances can be distinguished from gestational trophoblastic disease.

Gestational trophoblastic diseases are related to abnormalities of the trophoblast. The trophoblast, from which the chorion and amnion are derived, provides the attachment to the uterine wall, invading the wall and its vessels to supply nutrition to the embryo.[7] Gestational trophoblastic disease results from a combination of male and female gametes. Nongestational trophoblastic disease does not involve a gestational event and includes testicular and ovarian choriocarcinoma.[6]

Hydatidiform Mole

Hydatidiform mole is the most common neoplasm that arises from the trophoblast. Complete hydatidiform moles arise from fertilization of a defective ovum by a single sperm that duplicates, yielding a homozygous mole of 46,XX karyotype, or from fer-

tilization of one ovum by two sperm, resulting in a heterozygous mole with 46,XX or 46,XY karyotype.[9] A defective ovum fertilized by a single sperm with a Y sex chromosome would not be viable without some X-linked genetic material.[7]

Histologically, complete hydatidiform moles are characterized by hydropic degeneration and swelling of the chorionic villus stroma, absence of blood vessels in the swollen villi, proliferation of the trophoblastic epithelium to varying degrees, and absence of fetus and amnion (Fig. 22-1).[12]

A partial (incomplete) hydatidiform mole results from a normal egg with a 23,X haploid chromosome set being fertilized by two sperm carrying either sex chromosome, giving a karyotype of 69,XXY, 69,XXX, or 69,XYY. A triploid karyotype of XXY can also result from fertilization of a normal egg by a sperm with a 46,XY diploid set.[9] A partial mole has focal and less advanced hydatidiform changes with slowly progressing swelling of some avascular villi while vascular villi are spared. The hyperplasia of the trophoblast is focal rather than generalized.[12] There may be a fetus, fetal parts, or just an amniotic sac. Approximately 5% of hydatidiform moles are incomplete or partial.

Both complete and partial hydatidiform moles are regarded clinically as benign trophoblastic disease, although the complete moles, especially the rare heterozygous type, have a definite malignant potential. Partial moles have very little malignant

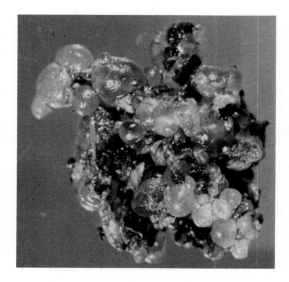

FIGURE 22-1. Grapelike clusters of hydropic villi in a specimen from a complete hydatidiform mole.

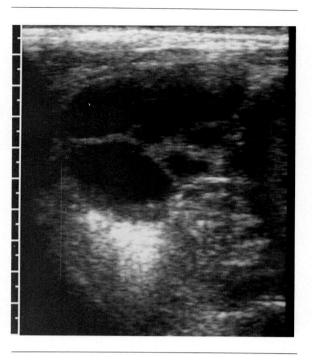

FIGURE 22-2. Transverse view of an enlarged ovary with theca lutein cysts.

potential.[7] Complete heterozygous moles are 1000 times more likely to precede choriocarcinoma than a complete homozygous mole.[4]

Ovarian theca lutein cysts are found in 20 to 35% of patients with hydatidiform mole and are caused by overstimulation of lutein elements by large amounts of chorionic gonadotropin (HCG) secreted by the proliferating trophoblast.[12] They are bilateral, contain multiple cysts and septa, and are largest when HCG production is greatest (at 12 to 24 weeks' gestation; Fig. 22-2). Theca lutein cysts may twist and hemorrhage, causing areas of solid echogenicity that correspond with areas of thrombus.

Sonography's role is to assess and determine whether there has been regression of the cysts following uterine evacuation of the molar pregnancy. Theca lutein cysts may persist 2 to 4 months after evacuation, which may cause confusion when performing serial follow-up studies for recurrence of the molar pregnancy.

INCIDENCE
Hydatidiform moles occur in one out of every 1,000 to 2,000 pregnancies in the United States and Eu-

rope.[1,12] The highest national incidence occurs in the far eastern countries, especially Taiwan, Japan, and Indonesia, and is 10 times greater than that in the U.S.; however, an epidemiologic study of oriental women in the U.S. did not find them to be at significantly greater risk of molar pregnancy than women of other races in the U.S.[1] The prevalence in Mexico is twice that in the U.S.[7,12]

Women 46 years or older and 14 years or younger are at higher risk for a molar pregnancy.[1,9] Women between 20 and 29 years of age are at lowest risk. Although ovarian hydatidiform moles are rare, they have been reported; the estimated incidence is 1 in 25,000 to 40,000 gestations.[13] Risk of recurrence of hydatidiform mole increases by 2 to 3% with each subsequent pregnancy.[1,7]

SYMPTOMS AND COMPLICATIONS
A woman who is considered to be pregnant may experience vaginal bleeding, which may follow a missed period. Spotting or bleeding of a brownish discharge has been described in 97% of women

with a molar pregnancy. Some pass grapelike clusters of maternal blood and molar tissue.[7] Other common clinical symptoms are discrepant uterine height, hyperemesis, and preeclampsia.

On physical examination the uterus in the majority of cases is noted to be large for gestational age, which may be due to rapid proliferation of the trophoblastic tissue; however, the uterine size also may be consistent with or small for the gestational age.[7]

Hyperemesis and preeclampsia occur in approximately 25% of cases and are thought to be caused by the increased levels of β-HCG in the bloodstream. Projectile vomiting and nausea are some of the clinical findings with hyperemesis gravidarum. With eclampsia or preeclampsia, varying degrees of proteinuria and hypertension are present. Preeclampsia occurs more frequently in cases of complete than partial molar pregnancies.[9]

With a nonmolar gestation, pregnancy-induced hypertension usually occurs after the 24th week of pregnancy. A molar pregnancy must, therefore, be considered when hypertension and elevated β-HCG are present before the 24th gestational week.

The following complications may develop as a result of a molar pregnancy:

1. Hemorrhage from an existing mole or local invasion.
2. Anemia due to maternal blood loss.
3. Rupture or hemorrhage of theca lutein cysts.
4. Pulmonary embolization or pulmonary edema due to the migration of trophoblastic tissue through the uterine veins.
5. Hyperthyroidism associated with 2 to 10% of cases due to elevated β-HCG levels, which stimulate thyroxine production.
6. Progression to invasive mole or choriocarcinoma.

LABORATORY FINDINGS
Hydatidiform moles usually show elevated serum β-HCG levels (>100,000 mIU/ml). This is especially significant if the levels are persistently high or continue to rise beyond 100 days after the last menstrual period, when normally there is a decline in HCG level.[12]

Ultrasound-guided chorionic villus sampling has been performed with coexistent molar and normal gestations in separate sacs to determine the karyotype of the molar pregnancy (because a triploid karyotype would have a low malignant potential and the pregnancy might be allowed to continue).[8]

SONOGRAPHIC APPEARANCE
Reported cases of first-trimester molar pregnancy document that a variable appearance is possible. Some first-trimester moles may have an appearance that simulates a blighted ovum, missed abortion, degenerating leiomyoma, or hydropic placenta (Fig. 22-3, Table 22-1). Others may demonstrate a small echogenic mass filling the entire uterine cavity.[6] In any of these situations, careful clinical correlation is important in differentiating these possible causes (Table 22-2).

The more advanced hydatidiform mole, which contains numerous hydropic villi, can be well-visualized by sonography. Owing to the hydropic villi, uterine enlargement greater than is appropriate for dates may be present. The hydatidiform mole appears as a large soft tissue mass containing cystic spaces of varying sizes (Fig. 22-4). This appearance has previously been referred to as a snowflake or lacy pattern. No fetal parts are seen. When the tumor volume is small, the myometrium may be perceived as less echogenic soft tissue surround-

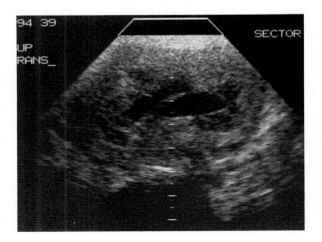

FIGURE 22-3. Missed abortion with an irregular gestational sac and placental degeneration.

Table 22-1. Sonographic appearance of gestational trophoblastic disease

Trophoblastic Process	Sonographic Appearance
Hydatidiform mole (first trimester)	May have appearance of a blighted ovum, threatened abortion, or variable echogenicity filling the entire uterus without the characteristic vesicular appearance[1]
Hydatidiform mole (after first trimester)	Large soft tissue mass of low- to moderate-amplitude echoes filling the uterine cavity and containing fluid-filled spaces
Incomplete or partial mole	May present as a gestational sac which is relatively large and intact surrounded by a thick rim of placentalike echoes with well-defined sonolucent spaces within. It may be empty or contain a disproportionally small viable or nonviable fetus. Echogenic fetal parts may be visualized with or without normal placenta.
Coexisting mole and fetus	Concurrent presence of normal-appearing placenta and fetus and a separate area of cystic vesicular appearance
Invasive mole	Enlarged uterus with foci of increased echogenicity and cystic spaces in the myometrium
Choriocarcinoma	Cystic to solid areas of necrosis, coagulated blood, or tumor tissue invading and extending as a mass outside the uterine wall with metastatic lesions located in the liver

Table 22-2. Differential diagnoses of hydatidiform mole

Missed abortion
Hydropic placenta
Degenerating leiomyoma
Endometrial carcinoma
Adenomyosis

Invasive Mole (Chorioadenoma Destruens)

The invasive mole (chorioadenoma destruens) is classified clinically as malignant, nonmetastatic trophoblastic disease. These all result from malignant progression of hydatidiform moles; approximately 15 to 18% manifest these changes. Histologically the invasive mole is distinguished by excessive trophoblastic overgrowth and penetration by the trophoblastic elements, including whole villi, into the depths of the myometrium, sometimes penetrating through the uterine wall and involving the peritoneum, adjacent parametrium, or vaginal vault. Such moles show local invasion but not widespread metastasis.[12] The diagnosis of invasive mole is made primarily from the myometrial tissue if hysterectomy is performed.

Invasive trophoblastic disease is recognizable sonographically by the presence of hemorrhagic necrosis within the myometrium, which appears as irregular anechoic and echogenic areas in the homogeneously hypoechoic myometrium (Fig. 22-6). Sonography should not be considered a screening procedure for invasive trophoblastic disease because in some cases no recognizable textural abnormalities of the uterus can be demonstrated.[6]

Choriocarcinoma

Choriocarcinoma is classified clinically as malignant, metastatic gestational trophoblastic disease. Microscopically, choriocarcinoma is characterized by sheets of highly malignant trophoblast of both cytotrophoblast and syncytiotrophoblast elements with no villous structures. Choriocarcinoma, the most malignant form of gestational trophoblastic disease, has an incidence of approximately 1 in 40,000 pregnancies in the U.S.[3] Two to five percent of hydatidiform moles progress to choriocarcinoma. Approximately 50% of choriocarcinomas

ing the echogenic mass that fills the uterus. These classic sonographic findings are specific only for a second-trimester hydatidiform mole.[11] The identification of fetal parts within or adjacent to the molar tissue helps to classify an incomplete mole (Fig. 22-5). With a significant rise in the β-HCG level, bilateral, multicystic, multiseptate ovarian theca lutein cysts may be identified in the adnexa.

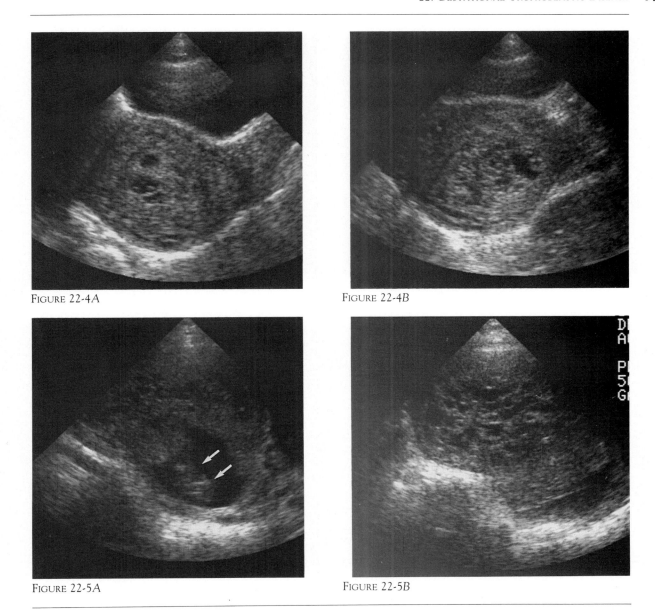

FIGURE 22-4A

FIGURE 22-4B

FIGURE 22-5A

FIGURE 22-5B

FIGURE 22-4. Longitudinal (A) and transverse (B) views of a complete mole filling the uterine cavity at 10 weeks after LMP.

FIGURE 22-5. Longitudinal (A) and transverse (B) views of a partial molar pregnancy demonstrating a fetal pole (arrows) surrounded by a large multicystic mass.

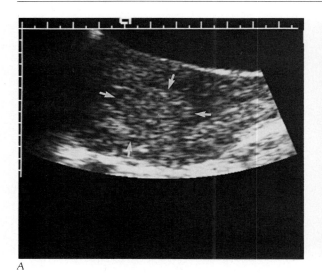
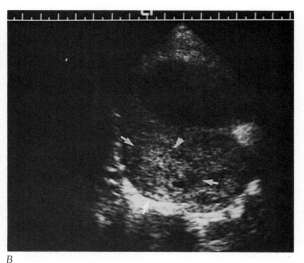

A   B

FIGURE 22-6. Longitudinal (A) and transverse (B) views of an invasive mole with an echogenic lesion surrounded by a hypoechoic rim, invading peripherally into the uterine wall (arrows).

develop from a hydatidiform mole, and 50% evolve from a normal-term pregnancy, ectopic pregnancy, or spontaneous abortion.

Generally this condition is first suspected clinically in a patient with a history of gestational trophoblastic disease who has undergone evacuation of the uterine contents but presents with continued vaginal bleeding, persistently elevated β-HCG levels, and/or persistent theca lutein cysts. Sonographically, choriocarcinoma may present with marked hemorrhagic necrosis in the myometrium. The factors involved in malignant transformation of the trophoblast are unknown. The tumor spreads rapidly through the uterus and disseminates either locally in the pelvis or by hematogenous spread to the lungs, lower gastrointestinal tract, central nervous system, liver, and urinary tract. The lungs and vagina are the most common sites of metastases.[12]

Fetus and Coexisting Mole
Several reports in the literature have noted a molar pregnancy associated with a living fetus. Unfortu-nately their statistics included patients whose placenta had undergone hydropic degeneration as well as those with a proliferating trophoblast in a classic hydatidiform mole.[2,5,13]

A coexisting complete mole and a normal fetus in a normal gestational sac arise from transformation of the trophoblast of one of two dizygotic twin placentas.[16] Ultrasound examination may suggest the diagnosis by demonstrating fetal echoes adjacent to a trophoblastic process (Fig. 22-7). However, the findings should ultimately be confirmed histologically, as these lesions are considered to have the same malignant potential as the more classic hydatidiform mole.

Sonographic Differentiation
Sonographers should be alert for a possible hydatidiform mole when sonographic findings include an enlarged uterus containing complex echoes without evidence of a viable fetus. The sonographic appearance of a leiomyoma is most often homogeneous to complex, rounded, and well-circumscribed. It does not transmit sound well and

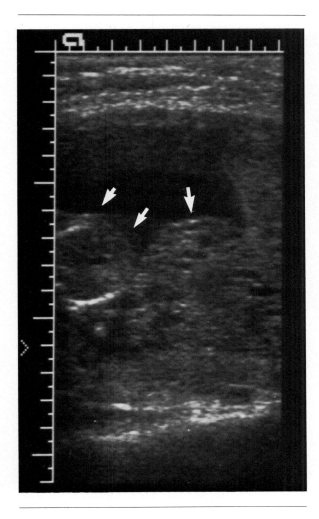

FIGURE 22-7. Transverse view of a fetal abdomen adjacent to apparently multicystic molar tissue in a coexisting mole (*arrows*).

occupies only a portion of the uterus. A mole, on the other hand, occupies the entire uterus and has the appearance of placental tissue with anechoic areas. Detection of fetal parts or a viable fetus is very important in evaluating for coexisting or partial mole. When scanning the uterus for coexisting fetal parts, various gain settings and postprocessing techniques should be utilized to better resolve subtle echogenic areas that may represent fetal parts. Scans should also be performed of the liver to look for metastases. Patients who have undergone evac-

uation of a molar pregnancy can be followed sonographically to assess the uterine contents and the resolution of theca lutein cysts.

Doppler Examination

Duplex Doppler ultrasound can be used to evaluate for gestational trophoblastic neoplasia and to differentiate from other similar-looking conditions in the first trimester. Doppler waveform analysis of the uterine artery flow in the first trimester of normal pregnancy, as well as in patients with hydropic degeneration of the placenta, incomplete abortion, and degenerating fibroids, will demonstrate a high impedance pattern characterized by little diastolic flow. The patient with gestational trophoblastic neoplasia shows considerably increased peak systolic flow and markedly increased overall uterine artery flow with increased peak systolic frequency and end-diastolic frequency (Fig. 22-8). This difference is thought to be due to the large, thin-walled vascular spaces in the areas of trophoblastic neoplasia, with consequent low impedance and high-velocity flow with increased signal amplitude. In a normal pregnancy, increased blood flow and decreased impedance do not occur until the late second and third trimester, when there is invasion of the spiral arteries. Color flow duplex Doppler ultrasound may also prove useful by graphically demonstrating the flow within the tumor vessels in the area of persistent trophoblastic neoplasia.

Treatment

Following confirmation of the molar pregnancy by sonographic evaluation of the pelvis, most women undergo cervical dilation and suction and curettage of the trophoblastic contents from the uterine cavity.

The patient is placed on oral contraception for 1 year to prevent pregnancy-induced elevation of β-HCG. A quantitative β-HCG test is performed every 1 to 2 weeks following primary treatment until results of three consecutive tests are normal, then monthly for 6 months, and then every other month for 6 months. Regression should occur within 2 to 3 months. Recurrence is suspected if the β-HCG level reaches a plateau and remains there for 3 consecutive weeks or increases over 2 weeks.

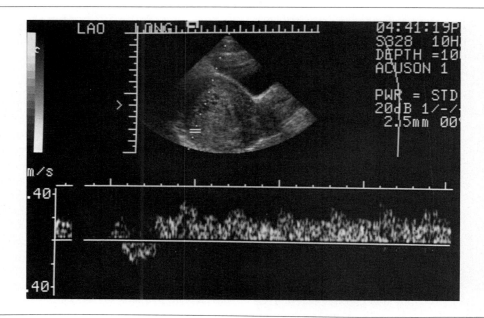

Figure 22-8. Doppler velocity tracing demonstrates increased diastolic flow in a patient with recurrent gestational trophoblastic disease.

Recurrent molar pregnancy confined to the pelvic region is treated with single-agent chemotherapy such as methotrexate or actinomycin D. The risk of toxicity from these agents is high, but their use has been found to decrease the incidence of persistent gestational trophoblastic disease by 90%.[7,10] Multiple chemotherapeutic agents are used for widespread or persistent disease.

Surgical intervention, such as hysterectomy or hysterotomy, is performed only for control of local tumor symptoms and if fertility is not a concern. Older women in the high-risk category and women with invasive trophoblastic disease are the most likely candidates for surgery.

The course of treatment for choriocarcinoma depends on whether the woman is in the low- or high-risk group for malignancy.[6,12] Women in the high-risk group will have a urine level of β-HCG greater than 100,000 mIU/24 hours or serum levels of β-HCG greater than 40,000 mIU/ml. Liver or brain metastasis is present in the high-risk group. Single-agent chemotherapy will have failed and the duration of the disease will be greater than 4 months. Radiation therapy may be used in conjunction with chemotherapy for brain or liver metastases. If choriocarcinoma is associated with a term pregnancy, the woman is also considered to be at high risk.

Conclusion

Ultrasound is a sensitive modality for detecting gestational trophoblastic disease. When correlated with the patient's clinical history and β-HCG values, ultrasound findings can further assist in follow-up of recurrent or invasive trophoblastic disease.

References

1. Atrash HK, Hogne JR, Grimes DA. Epidemiology of hydatidiform mole during early gestation. Am J Obstet Gynecol. 1986; 154:906–909.
2. Bree RL, Silver TM, Wicks JD, et al. Trophoblastic disease with coexistent fetus: A sonographic and clinical spectrum. J Clin Ultrasound. 1978; 6:310–314.

3. Callen PW. Ultrasonography in evaluation of gestational trophoblastic disease. In: Callen PW, ed. Ultrasonography in Obstetrics and Gynecology. 2nd ed. Philadelphia: WB Saunders; 1988; 20.

4. Fisher RA, Sheppard DM, Lawler SD. Two patients with complete hydatidiform mole with 46,XY karyotype. Br J Obstet Gynecol. 1984; 91:690–693.

5. Fleischer AC, James AE, Krause DA, et al. Sonographic patterns in trophoblastic diseases. Radiology. 1978; 126:215–220.

6. Fleischer AC, Jones HW III, James AE. Sonography of trophoblastic disease. In: Sanders RC, James AE, eds. The Principles and Practice of Ultrasonography in Obstetrics and Gynecology. 3rd ed. Norwalk, CT: Appleton-Century-Crofts; 1985.

7. Heath JM, Bu TH, Brereton WF. Hydatidiform moles. Am Family Phy. 1985; 31:123–131.

8. Hertzberg BS, Kurtz AB, Wagner AB, et al. Gestational trophoblastic disease with coexistent normal fetus: Evaluation by ultrasound-guided chorionic villus sampling. J Ultrasound Med. 1986; 5:467–469.

9. Hiscock K. Ultrasound diagnosis of partial hydatidiform mole: A case report and review. J Diagn Med Sonogr. 1987; 3:91–94.

10. Kim DS, Moon H, Kim KT. Effects of prophylactic chemotherapy for persistent trophoblastic disease in patients with complete hydatidiform mole. Obstet Gynecol. 1986; 67:690–694.

11. Munyer TP, Callen PW, Filly RA, et al. Further observations on the sonographic spectrum of gestational trophoblastic disease. J Clin Ultrasound. 1981; 9:349–358.

12. Pritchard JA, Mac Donald PC, Gant NG. Abnormalities of the placenta and fetal membranes. In: Williams' Obstetrics. 17th ed. Norwalk, CT: Appleton-Century-Crofts; 1985.

13. Sauerbrie EE, Salem S, Fayle B. Coexistent hydatidiform mole and live fetus in the second trimester. Radiology. 1980; 135:45.

14. Switzer JM, Weckstein ML, Campbell LF, et al. Ovarian hydatidiform mole. J Ultrasound Med. 1984; 3:471–473.

15. Szulman AE, Surti U. The syndromes of hydatidiform mole I. Cytogenic and morphologic conditions. Am J Obstet Gynecol. 1978; 131:20–27.

16. Szulman AE, Surti U. The syndromes of hydatidiform mole. II. Morphologic evaluation of the complete and partial mole. Am J Obstet Gynecol. 1978; 132:20–27.

17. Taylor JW, Schwartz PE, Koharn EI. Gestational trophoblastic neoplasia: Diagnosis with Doppler ultrasound. Radiology. 1987; 165:445–448.

CHAPTER 23

Sonography of the Abnormal Fetal Head, Neck, and Spine

JANE STRELTZOFF, GLENN ISAACSON, FRANK A. CHERVENAK

Anomalies of the head, neck, and spine are among the most commonly diagnosed fetal malformations. The impact of any defect in this vital part of the body may be profound. The normal sonographic anatomy of these areas is described in Chapter 14; the most common anomalies are described in this chapter.

Anencephaly

Anencephaly is a congenital anomaly in which the cerebral hemispheres and overlying skull and scalp are absent. The incidence of anencephaly, one of the most common congenital disorders in the world, varies with geography, race, and sex. Anencephaly occurs most frequently in areas where spina bifida is also very common. In 1984 its incidence in Northern Ireland was as high as 4.7 in 10,000 deliveries, whereas in the United States it was 2.6. Anencephaly was the first malformation diagnosed with sufficient certainty that physicians were willing to perform elective abortion on the basis of sonographic findings.[3,29,33,45]

The diagnosis of anencephaly is made when the upper portion of the cranial vault cannot be visualized (Fig. 23-1A). This bony structure normally can be seen after 14 weeks if the head is not hidden in the mother's pelvis. The area of the cerebrovasculosa, a vascular malformation seen in this disorder, may appear as an ill-defined mass of heterogeneous density above the level of the orbits (Fig.

23-1B). Hydramnios due to poor fetal swallowing may complicate these pregnancies.

The diagnosis of anencephaly can be made with extraordinary accuracy. In the combined experiences of six centers, over 130 cases have been detected with no false positive diagnoses.[9,36] Anencephaly is a lethal anomaly. The recurrence rate increases with the number of previous affected fetuses, as do all neural tube defects.

Ventriculomegaly and Hydrocephalus

Ventriculomegaly, an abnormal increase in the volume of the cerebral ventricles, has many different causes. Ventriculomegaly may be due to intraventricular or extraventricular obstruction, increase in cerebrospinal fluid (CSF) production, or a relative decrease in the amount of brain substance. The term hydrocephalus is often reserved for ventriculomegaly resulting from increased CSF pressure.

Although an abnormally increased head circumference or biparietal diameter may suggest the diagnosis of ventriculomegaly, examination of the intracranial contents is necessary for accurate diagnosis. This is particularly true because enlargement of the ventricles and lateral displacement of the choroid plexus precedes cranial enlargement (Fig. 23-2).

For evaluating the volume of the cerebral ventricles, measurements of the bodies of the lateral ventricles are useful.[32] The lateral ventricle–to–

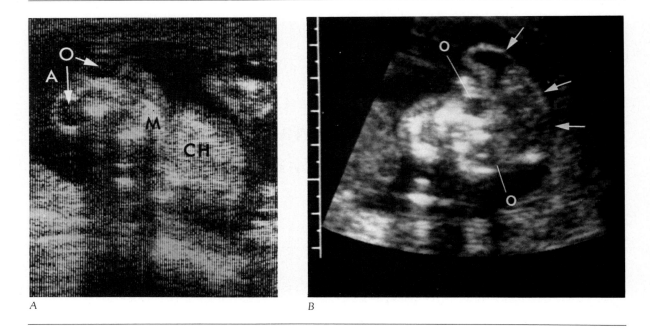

A   *B*

FIGURE 23-1. (*A*) Sonogram demonstrates absence of cranium in a fetus with anencephaly (A, absent cranium; O, orbits; M, mandible; CH, chest). (*B*) Coronal sonogram demonstrates fetal anencephaly with protruding cerebrovasculosa (*arrows*) and orbits (O). (A from Chervenak FA, Farley MA, Walters L, et al. When is the termination of pregnancy during the third trimester morally justifiable? N Engl J Med. 310:501, 1984.)

hemispheric ratio, as described by Jeanty and colleagues[30] and Johnson and associates[31] is a valuable tool in the diagnosis of ventriculomegaly. Correlation of the lateral ventricle–to–hemispheric width ratio with the Jeanty nomogram has proved to be an accurate predictor of fetal ventriculomegaly over a wide range of gestational ages,[4] including those less than 24 weeks.[5] It should be noted, however, that the absence of ventriculomegaly at one point in gestation does not preclude its developing later. Serial examinations are indicated for a pregnancy at risk. With ventriculomegaly other parts of the ventricular system, such as frontal horns, occipital horns, and third ventricle, can be seen to be dilated (Fig. 23-3).

Certain pitfalls in the early detection of fetal ventriculomegaly have been described.[5] These include an artifactual hyperechoic area of sonographic "dropout" in the distal hemisphere and re-verberation artifacts in the proximal hemisphere (Fig. 23-4).[40]

As the natural history of ventricular enlargement early in gestation is uncertain,[10] the diagnosis of ventriculomegaly is most secure if progressive ventricular enlargement is documented with serial sonography. Once fetal ventriculomegaly is diagnosed, it is essential to search for associated anomalies, which have been reported to occur in 83% of cases.[6] Although spina bifida is the most common one, associated structural anomalies may affect any organ system. In addition to meticulous real-time sonographic evaluation, amniocentesis should be performed to determine the fetal karyotype.

The prognosis for hydrocephaly does not depend on the severity of the hydrocephalus. Associated anomalies may portend a poor prognosis (e.g., holoprosencephaly, thanatophoric dysplasia with cloverleaf skull). The outcome for isolated hy-

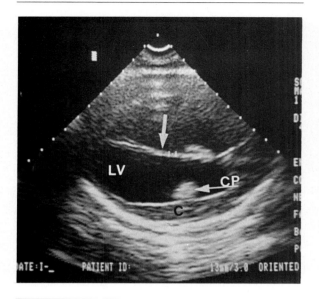

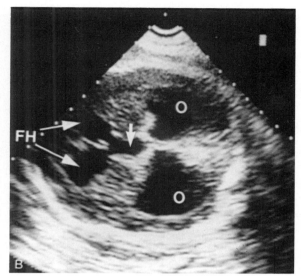

FIGURE 23-2. Transverse cranial sonogram demonstrates hydrocephalus with dilated lateral ventricle (LV), choroid plexus (CP), compressed cerebral cortex (C), and arrow pointing to midline echo.

FIGURE 23-3. Transverse cranial sonogram demonstrates hydrocephalus with dilated frontal horns (FH), occipital horns (O), and third ventricle (*arrow*).

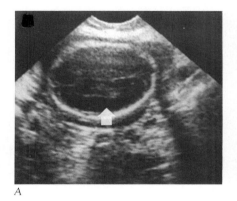

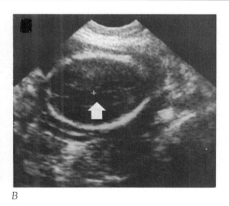

FIGURE 23-4. (A) On transverse cranial sonogram arrow points to hypoechoic area of "dropout" in normal fetus. (B) In transverse cranial sonogram of same fetus arrow points to the lateral ventricle. (From Chervenak FA, Berkowitz RL, Tortora M, et al. Diagnosis of ventriculomegaly before fetal viability. Obstet Gynecol. 1984; 64:652.)

drocephalus ranges from normal to severely deficient. A range of anomalies may be associated with hydrocephalus (Table 23-1).

Microcephaly

Microcephaly means *small head*. Its diagnosis, therefore, is based on biometry rather than on morphology. In general, a small head is the product of an underdeveloped brain, whether as a primary defect or as a part of a more extensive malformation syndrome. Although different biometric standards have been described to define microcephaly, a head perimeter 3 standard deviations or more below the mean for age seems workable, and the correlation with mental retardation is very high.[44]

The biparietal diameter (the biometric parameter most commonly measured by sonography) is unreliable in the prediction of microcephaly (a 44% false positive rate in one study).[16] Compression of the fetal head in normal pregnancies with resultant dolichocephaly accounts for many of these errors. A nomogram of head circumference as a function of gestational age, which corrects for such compressive changes, has proved to have greater predictive value. Further aids to diagnosis include nomograms of ratios of head circumference to abdominal perimeter and of femur length to head circumference. At the present time, it appears that multiple fetal measurements should be utilized for greater accuracy.[16,18]

The prognosis for microcephaly varies, but most affected children are mentally retarded. In general, the smaller the head the worse is the prognosis. As with other malformations, the association with other anomalies increases the likelihood of a poor outcome. Risk of recurrence depends on underlying causes.

Holoprosencephaly

Holoprosencephaly describes a variety of abnormalities of the brain and face that result from incomplete cleavage of the primitive prosencephalon (forebrain; Fig. 23-5). Holoprosencephaly is divided into alobar, semilobar, and lobar categories, defined by the degree of separation of the cerebral hemispheres. The alobar variety shows no evidence of division of cerebral cortex. Thus, the falx cerebri

TABLE 23-1. Anomalies associated with 27 documented cases of fetal hydrocephalus

ANOMALY	NO. OF CASES
Intracranial anomalies	10
Microcephaly	3
Hypoplasia of corpus callosum	3
Encephalocele	2
Arteriovenous malformation	2
Arachnoid cyst	2
Cebocephaly	1
Extracranial anomalies	17
Meningomyelocele	7
Lumbosacral	6
Thoracolumbar	1
Renal	5
Dysplastic kidneys	2
Unilateral renal agenesis	2
Bilateral renal agenesis	1
Cardiac	4
Ventricular septal defect	2
Tetralogy of Fallot	1
Tricuspid hypoplasia	1
Gastrointestinal	2
Colon and anal agenesis	1
Malrotation of bowel	1
Cleft lip/palate	3
Meckel's syndrome	2
Gonadal dysgenesis	1
Sirenomelia	1
Arthrogryposis	1
Dysplastic phalanges	1
Chromosomal anomaly	
Trisomy 21	3
Mosaic (46,XY/48,XY, +7, +8)	1
Balanced translocation (long arm chromosome 12 and short arm chromosome 5)	1
No anomaly	5

(Modified from Chervenak FA, Berkowitz RL, et al. The diagnosis of fetal hydrocephalus. Am J Obstet Gynecol. 1983;147:703.)

and interhemispheric fissures are absent and there is a single common ventricle (Fig. 23-6). The semilobar and lobar varieties represent higher degrees of brain development. The semilobar type demonstrates partially separated brain while the lobar type shows complete separation of the hemisphere. Microcephaly is usually present because of decreased cortical mass, but macrocephaly may be seen if hydrocephalus develops.

The prechordal mesoderm, an embryonic con-

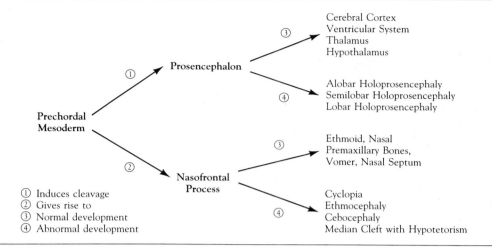

FIGURE 23-5. Embryology of holoprosencephaly and midline facial defects. (From Chervenak FA, Isaacson G, Mahoney MJ, et al. The obstetric significance of holoprosencephaly. Obstet Gynecol. 1984; 63:115.)

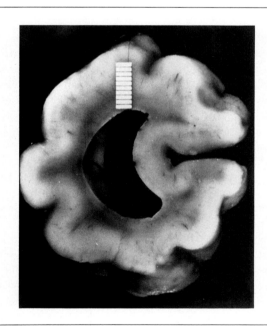

FIGURE 23-6. An example of alobar holoprosencephaly with absent interhemispheric fissure and common ventricle. (From Chervenak FA, Isaacson G, Hobbins JC, et al. The diagnosis and management of fetal holoprosencephaly. Obstet Gynecol. 1985; 66:322.)

nective mass between the oral cavity and the undersurface of the neural tube, is thought to be responsible for both the production of the nasofrontal process and the division of the prosencephalon. The nasofrontal process gives rise to the ethmoid, nasal, and premaxillary bones and to the vomer and the nasal septum. Failure of these structures to develop normally can result in the varying degrees of hypotelorism, cleft lip and palate, and nasal malformation that are seen in this disorder. The prosencephalon develops from the most rostrad part of the neural tube and gives rise to the cerebral hemispheres, thalamus, and hypothalamus. Failure of its sagittal division can result in a common ventricle, a fused thalamus, and a cortex with neither lobes nor an interhemispheric fissure (Fig. 23-7).[23]

In holoprosencephaly, a spectrum of midline facial anomalies may be seen. Indeed, certain facies predict the presence of the alobar type. Cyclopia, the presence of a single median bony orbit with a fleshy proboscis above it, is the most severe malformation. In cebocephaly, hypotelorism is associated with a normally placed nose and a single nostril (Fig. 23-8). Hypotelorism with a midline facial cleft also predicts the presence of alobar holoprosencephaly. Holoprosencephaly may also be associated

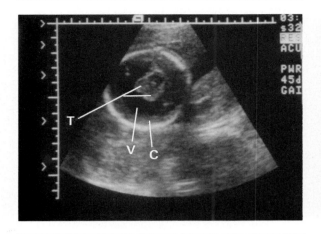

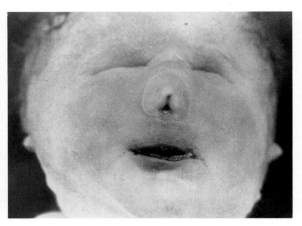

Figure 23-7. Transverse sonogram of fetus with alobar holoprosencephaly demonstrates single common ventricle (V), compressed cerebral cortex (C), and prominent thalamus (T).

Figure 23-8. Cebocephaly with hypotelorism and normally placed nose with a single nostril. (From Chervenak FA, Isaacson G, Mahoney MJ, et al. The obstetric significance of holoprosencephaly. Obstet Gynecol 1984; 63:115.)

with milder forms of midline facial dysplasia or normal facies.[23]

Just as there is incomplete sagittal division of the brain in holoprosencephaly, a series of midline facial anomalies of varying severity are seen. Orbital abnormalities ranging from mild hypotelorism to cyclopia (a single orbit) may be present. The nose may have two nostrils, a single midline nostril, or it may be replaced by a fleshy proboscis, and a variety of midline facial clefts may be present.

Alobar holoprosencephaly may be diagnosed before birth if two criteria are met. The midline echo generated by the interhemispheric fissure should be absent (Fig. 23-9). Hypotelorism can be detected by measuring inner and outer orbital distances, which are then compared to a standard nomogram (Fig. 23-10). Even when these strict criteria are used, some cases of alobar holoprosencephaly may be missed. Further, the pathologic changes in lobar and semilobar holoprosencephaly may be too subtle to be detected by antenatal ultrasound.[12]

The alobar forms of holoprosencephaly carry a poor prognosis. More subtle forms may be associated with minimal neurologic deficits. Recurrence rates increase with associated chromosomal abnormalities (e.g., autosomal recessive and, rarely, autosomal dominant).

Cephalocele

Cephaloceles are protrusions of the meninges and frequently of brain substance through a defect in the cranium. The term includes encephaloceles, which contain brain tissue, and cranial meningoceles, which do not. In the western world, 75% of these lesions are occipital, but cephaloceles may be parietal, frontal, or nasopharyngeal.

Although cephaloceles usually result from a defect in neural tube closure, they may be seen in the amnion rupture sequence or amniotic band syndrome or in association with a variety of malformation syndromes (e.g., Meckel's syndrome).[22]

Sonographically, cephaloceles appear as saclike protrusions about the head not covered with bone. The diagnosis can be made with certainty only if a defect in the skull is detected (Fig. 23-11); however, such a defect may be small and difficult to visualize. When a defect is present, its position may be determined using the bony structures of the face and spine and the midline echo for orientation. Ultrasound has not been a reliable technique for differentiating between meningoceles and encephaloceles with a small amount of brain tissue. When brain tissue has herniated, it gives the sac a complex appearance. Furthermore, extrusion of a large

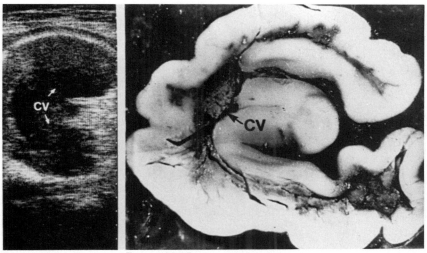

FIGURE 23-9A   FIGURE 23-9B

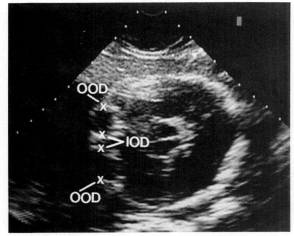

FIGURE 23-10

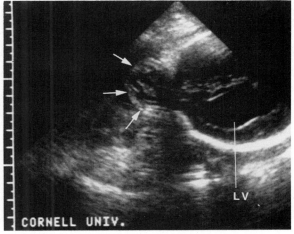

FIGURE 23-11

FIGURE 23-9. (A) Sonogram through fetal head demonstrates common ventricle (CV) and absence of midline structures. (B) Transverse section of fetal brain at autopsy demonstrating a collapsed common ventricle (CV), failure of separation of cerebral hemispheres, and absence of corpus callosum. (From Chervenak FA, Isaacson G, Mahoney MJ, et al. The obstetrical significance of holoprosencephaly. Obstet Gynecol. 1984; 63:115.)

FIGURE 23-10. Transverse sonogram through the orbits demonstrates an inner orbital distance (IOD) of 14 mm and an outer orbital distance (OOD) of 43 mm, both decreased for gestational age of 28 weeks. (From Chervenak FA, Isaacson G, Mahoney MJ, et al. The obstetrical significance of holoprosencephaly. Obstet Gynecol. 1984; 63:115.)

FIGURE 23-11. Sonogram demonstrates occipital encephalocele with protruding brain (*arrows*) and hydrocephalus with enlarged lateral ventricle (LV).

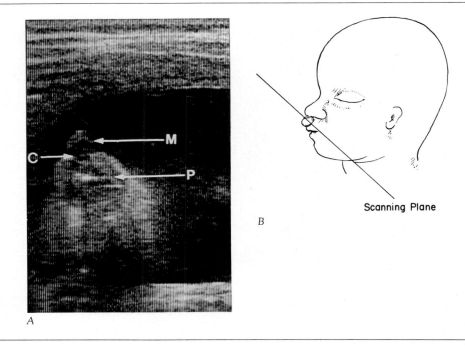

FIGURE 23-12. (A) Sonogram along an oblique plane through lower part of fetal face shows intact palate, cleft lip, and a mass protruding from lip (C, cleft; M, mass; P, palate). (B) Demonstration of oblique scanning plane for sonogram. (From Chervenak FA, Tortora M, Mayden K, et al. Am J Obstet Gynecol. 1984; 149:95.)

amount of brain substance may result in microcephaly. Hydrocephalus is commonly associated with cephaloceles.[13] Encephaloceles, in general, carry a poor prognosis. Pure meningoceles may have a favorable prognosis.

Facial Clefts

Failure of lip fusion, normally complete by 35 days of intrauterine life, may impair subsequent closure of the palatal shelves, leading to cleft lip and cleft palates.[42] In order to demonstrate a facial cleft before birth, the lower portion of the face must be anterior and clearly visualized. Both sagittal and oblique coronal planes of study may be useful. Undulating tongue movements,[20] hypertrophied tissue at the edge of the cleft,[19] and hypertelorism[19] have all been described as useful adjuncts in the diagnosis of a facial cleft. Nevertheless, clefts are subtle changes in the face, and their diagnosis is difficult and inconsistent (Figs. 23-12, 23-13).

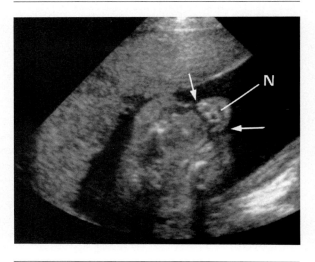

FIGURE 23-13. Sonogram along an oblique plane through lower part of fetal face demonstrates bilateral cleft lip (*arrows;* N, nose).

Cystic Hygroma

Cystic hygromas are congenital malformations of the lymphatic system that appear as either single or multiloculated cavities filled with fluid. They arise most often about the neck. In fetal life, a more generalized lymphatic disorder exists characterized by cystic hygromas of the posterior triangle of the neck with various degrees of lymphedema. Fetal lymphatic vessels drain into two large sacs lateral to the jugular veins. If these jugular lymph sacs fail to communicate with the venous system, they may enlarge as they fill with lymph and form cystic hygromas. This failure in lymphatic drainage may also result in the generalized edema of hydrops fetalis (Fig. 23-14).[11,43]

Several sonographic features aid in the diagnosis of fetal cystic hygromas. Hygromas are generally located on the posterolateral neck, are cystic in appearance, and are frequently divided by random, incomplete septa. As they arise from paired jugular lymph sacs, which may enlarge to meet at the posterior midline, a septum representing the nuchal ligament may be visualized (Fig. 23-15). Associated hydrops is manifest sonographically as ascites, pleural effusion, pericardial effusion, and skin edema.[14] Other craniocervical masses that must be

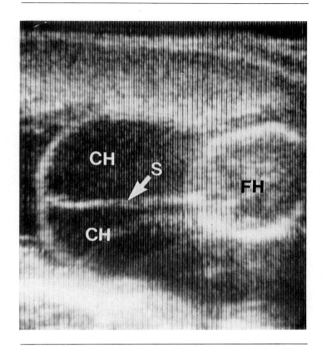

FIGURE 23-15. Transverse sonogram shows a cystic hygroma with a midline septum. The hygroma is slightly larger than the fetal head (CH, cystic hygroma; S, septum; FH, fetal head). (Chervenak FA, Isaacson G, Blakemore KJ, et al. Fetal cystichygroma cause and natural history. N Engl J Med. 1983; 309:822.)

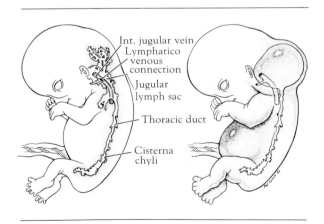

FIGURE 23-14. Lymphatic system in a normal fetus (*left*) with a patent connection between the jugular lymph sac and the internal jugular vein and a cystic hygroma and hydrops from a failed lymphaticovenous connection (*right*). (Chervenak FA, Isaacson G, Blakemore KJ, et al. Fetal cystichygroma cause and natural history. N Engl J Med. 1983; 309:822.

differentiated from cystic hygromas include cystic teratomas, cephalocele, branchial cleft cyst, and nuchal edema.[41]

Prognosis for cystic hygroma varies. If the hygroma is detected along with fetal hydrops, the condition is fatal. An isolated hygroma may have a good outcome.

Spina Bifida and Meningomyelocele

Spina bifida refers to a defect in the spine resulting from a failure of the two halves of the vertebral arch to fuse. These lesions usually occur in the lumbosacral and cervical regions. If the meninges protrude through the defect, the lesion is designated a meningocele; if neural tissue is included, it is a meningomyelocele.

Sonographically, spina bifida is seen as a splaying

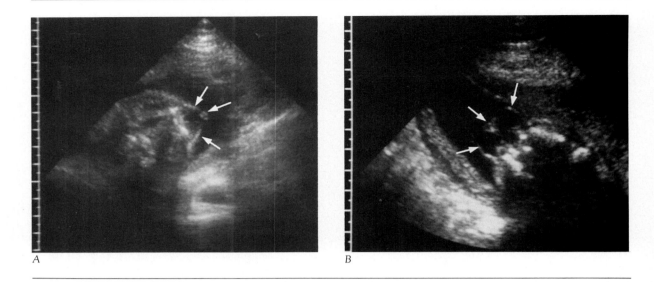

A *B*

FIGURE 23-16. (*A* and *B*) Transverse sonograms with arrows pointing to meningomyelocele.

of the posterior ossification centers of the spine giving the vertebral segment a **U**-shape (Fig. 23-16). The posterior ossification centers should be more widely spaced than those in vertebral segments above and below the defect. It should be noted that there is normally progressive widening of the spinal canal in the cervical region. Although the defect may be visualized on longitudinal scanning, meticulous transverse examinations of the entire vertebral column are necessary to detect smaller defects. When a meningocele or a meningomyelocele is present and intact, a protruding sac may be detected (Fig. 23-17). While detection of small spina bifida defects, especially in the sacral area, remains a challenge,[27,39] sonographic signs of Arnold-Chiari malformation are of adjunctive value.[2,28]

Although spina bifida may be detected during routine ultrasound examination, many are found as a result of careful ultrasound examinations in pregnancies in which elevation of maternal serum α-fetoprotein had been detected. Amniotic fluid α-fetoprotein determination may have an adjunctive role in the diagnosis of smaller lesions.[35]

The prognosis for spina bifida is dependent on the level of the lesion. Bowel and bladder dysfunction, inability to walk, and complications due to associated hydrocephalus may occur.

Arnold-Chiari Malformation

The Arnold-Chiari malformation is an anomaly of the hindbrain that has two components. The first is a variable displacement of a tongue of tissue derived from the inferior cerebellar vermis into the upper cervical spinal canal. The second is a similar caudal dislocation of the medulla and fourth ventricle. It has been stated that most, if not all, cases of spina bifida are complicated by the Arnold-Chiari malformation and that 90 to 95% of these patients show hydrocephalus.[2,28]

▶

FIGURE 23-18. (*A*) Diagram of "banana" and "lemon" signs in fetus with spina bifida. (*B*) Transverse sonogram of normal fetal head in an 18-week fetus at level of cavum septi pellucidi (*left*). Transverse section of fetal head at level of cavum septi pellucidi in an 18-week fetus with open spina bifida showing "lemon" sign (*right*). (*C*) Suboccipital bregmatic view of fetal head in an 18-week fetus with a normal cerebellum and cisterna magna (*left*). Suboccipital bregmatic view of fetal head in an 18-week fetus with open spina bifida, demonstrating "banana" sign (+) (*right*). (Nicolaides KM, Campbell S, Gabbe SG, et al. Ultrasound screening for spina bifida: Cranial and cerebellar signs. Lancet, 1986; 2:72.)

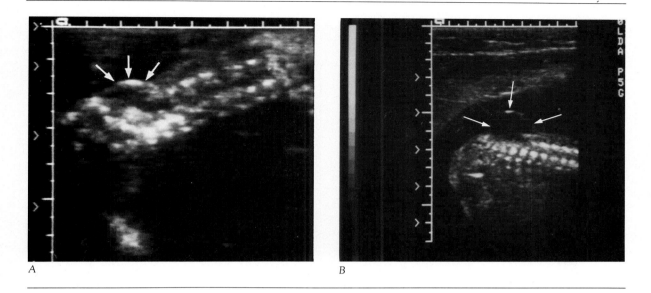

FIGURE 23-17. (A and B) Longitudinal sonograms with arrows pointing to meningomyelocele.

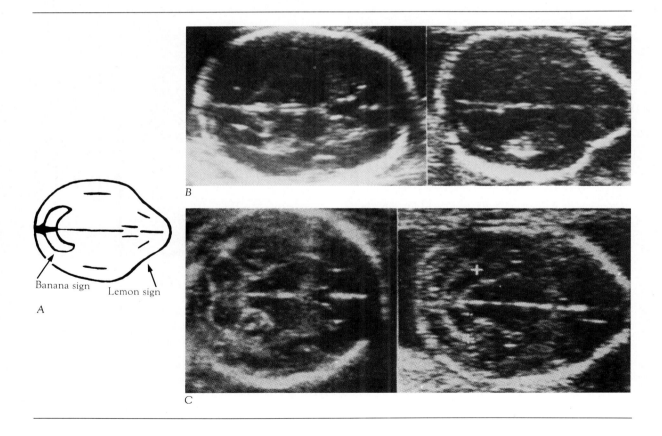

The Arnold-Chiari malformation can serve, therefore, as an important marker for spina bifida. Two characteristic sonographic signs (the lemon and the banana) of the Arnold-Chiari malformation have been described. A scalloping of the frontal bones can give a lemonlike configuration to the skull of an affected fetus in axial section during the second trimester. The caudal displacement of the cranial contents within a pliable skull is thought to produce this scalloping effect. Similarly, as the cerebellar hemispheres are displaced into the cervical canal, they are flattened anteroposteriorly and the cisterna magna is obliterated, thereby producing a flattened, centrally curved, bananalike sonographic appearance. In extreme cases, the cerebellar hemispheres may be absent from view during fetal head scanning. This characteristic cranial appearance should alert the sonographer to search for spina bifida and has led to its diagnosis in a fetus not previously suspected of having the disorder (Fig. 23-18).[37]

Teratomas

Teratomas are neoplasms composed of a wide variety of tissues foreign to the anatomic site in which they arise. They are the most common tumor in neonates, occur in a variety of locations, and are usually histologically benign.

Sacrococcygeal teratomas comprise over 50% of these lesions at birth; others include intracranial, palatal, cervical, mediastinal, retroperitoneal, and

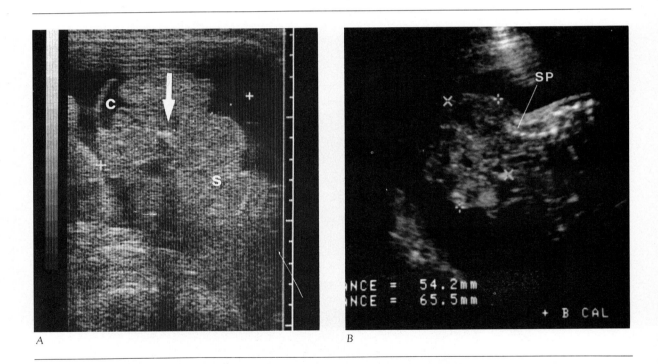

A   *B*

FIGURE 23-19. (A) Sonogram through a teratoma of fetus with midline facial teratoma demonstrates a complex mass with solid (S) and cystic (C) components. The arrow points to areas of calcification with acoustic shadowing (H, head; T, thorax). (Chervenak FA, Tortora M, Moya FR, et al. Antenatal sonographic diagnosis of epignathus. J Ultrasound Med. 1984; 3:235.) (B) Longitudinal sonogram demonstrates a sacrococcygeal teratoma outlined by crosses protruding beneath the sacral spine (SP).

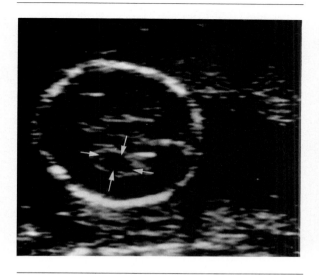

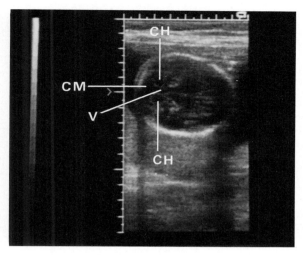

FIGURE 23-20. Transverse sonogram of fetal head at 20 weeks' gestation with choroid plexus cyst (*arrows*) in distal hemisphere.

FIGURE 23-21. Transverse sonogram of fetal head at 22 weeks of gestation demonstrates absence of cerebellar vermis, with contiguity of cisterna magna (CM), fourth ventricle (V), and cerebellar hemisphere (CH). Dandy-Walker malformation is demonstrated.

gonadal teratomas.[25] The diagnosis of these lesions is particularly important as they may be resected after birth and the infant cured.

It is not possible to make diagnoses by ultrasound, yet several morphologic features may help to distinguish teratomas from other lesions in similar locations. By ultrasound, teratomas appear both cystic and solid (Fig. 23-19). The solid components may not be homogeneous in density and may contain calcifications. The cysts frequently have irregular and angulated borders. A variety of anomalies have been reported in association with fetal teratomas, including gastrointestinal fistulas. Hydramnios is commonly present.[15] Fetal outcome is generally good with teratomas that are benign and isolated. Isolated sacrococcygeal teratomas have a better prognosis than those that arise from vital organs, are found intracranially, or occur along the facial midline.

Choroid Plexus Cysts

Small areas of cystic dilatation may be noted in the choroid plexus of the lateral ventricles of the normal, developing fetus (Fig. 23-20). Generally they resolve before the end of the second trimester without sequelae.[21] An association with trisomy 18 and bilateral choroid plexus cysts has been described.[38] These lesions are usually transient and without clinical significance.

Rare Anomalies

As experience with ultrasound increases and the resolution of the equipment improves, the list of rare anomalies of the fetal neural axis detected before birth continues to grow. Several "cystic" lesions have been detected. Hydranencephaly, appearing as a large, echo-spared area within the head, is distinguished from hydrocephalus by the absence of frontal, temporal, and parietal cerebral cortex.[32] Dandy-Walker cyst,[24] porencephalic cyst,[32] arachnoid cyst,[32] and cerebral atrophy all display echo-spared areas as well.[10] Craniofacial duplication,[17] vein of Galen malformation,[26] intracranial hemorrhage,[34] fetal goiter,[1] and cloverleaf skull[7] add to the list of rare anomalies detected by antenatal ultrasound (Fig. 23-21).

References

1. Barone CM, van Natta FC, Kourides IA, et al. Sonographic detection of fetal goiter, an unusual case of hydramnios. J Ultrasound Med. 1985; 4:625.

2. Bell JE, Gordon A, Maloney AFJ. The association of hydrocephalus and Arnodl-Chiari malformation with spina bifida in the fetus. Neuropathol Appl Neurobiol. 1980; 6:29.

3. Campbell S, Johnstone FD, Hold EM, et al. Anencephaly: Early ultrasonic diagnosis and active management. Lancet. 1972; 2:1226.

4. Chervenak FA, Berkowitz RL, Romero R, et al. The diagnosis of fetal hydrocephalus. Am J Obstet Gynecol. 1983; 147:703.

5. Chervenak FA, Berkowitz RL, Tortora M, et al. Diagnosis of ventriculomegaly before fetal viability. Obstet Gynecol. 1984; 64:652.

6. Chervenak FA, Berkowitz RL, Tortora M, et al. The management of fetal hydrocephalus. Am J Obstet Gynecol. 1985; 151:933.

7. Chervenak FA, Blakemore KJ, Isaacson G, et al. Antenatal sonographic findings of thanotophoric dysplasia with cloverleaf skull. Am J Obstet Gynecol. 1983; 146:984.

8. Chervenak FA, Duncan C, Ment LR, et al. The perinatal management of meningomyelocele. Obstet Gynecol. 1984; 63:376.

9. Chervenak FA, Farley MA, Walter L, et al. When is termination of pregnancy during the third trimester morally justifiable? N Engl J Med. 1984; 310:501.

10. Chervenak FA, Hobbins JC, Wertheimer I, et al. The natural history of ventriculomegaly in a fetus without obstructive hydrocephalus. Am J Obstet Gynecol. 1985; 152:574.

11. Chervenak FA, Isaacson G, Blakemore KJ, et al. Fetal cystic hygroma. Cause and natural history. N Engl J Med. 1983; 309:822.

12. Chervenak FA, Isaacson G, Hobbins JC, et al. The diagnosis and management of fetal holoprosencephaly. Obstet Gynecol. 1985; 66:322.

13. Chervenak FA, Isaacson G, Mahoney MJ, et al. Diagnosis and management of fetal cephalocele. Obstet Gynecol. 1984; 64:86.

14. Chervenak FA, Isaacson G, Tortora M. A sonographic study of fetal cystic hygroma. J Clin Ultrasound. 1985; 5:311.

15. Chervenak FA, Isaacson G, Touloukian R, et al. The diagnosis and management of fetal teratomas. Obstet Gynecol. 1985; 66:666.

16. Chervenak FA, Jeanty P, Cantraine F, et al. The diagnosis of fetal microcephaly. Am J Obstet Gynecol. 1984; 149:512.

17. Chervenak FA, Pinto MM, Meller CI, et al. The obstetric significance of fetal craniofacial duplication. J Reprod Med. 1985; 30:74.

18. Chervenak FA, Rosenberg J, Brightman R, et al. A prospective study of the accuracy of ultrasound in predicting fetal microcephaly. Obstet Gynecol. 1984; 69:908.

19. Chervenak FA, Tortora M, Mayden K, et al. Antenatal diagnosis of median cleft face syndrome: Sonographic demonstration of cleft lip and hypertelorism. Am J Obstet Gynecol. 1984; 149:94.

20. Christ JE, Meininger MG. Ultrasound diagnosis of cleft lip and cleft palate before birth. Plast Reconstr Surg. 1981; 6:854.

21. Chudleigh P, Pearce JM, Campbell S. The prenatal diagnosis of transient cysts of the fetal choroid plexus. Prenatal Diag. 1984; 4:135.

22. Cohen MM, Lemire RJ. Syndromes with cephaloceles. Teratology. 1982; 25:161.

23. DeMeyer W, Zeman W. Alobar holoprosencephaly (arhinencephaly) with median cleft lip and palate. Confin Neurol. 1963; 23:1.

24. Depp R, Sabbagha RE, Brown TJ. Fetal surgery for hydrocephalus: Successful in utero ventriculoamniotic shunt for Dandy-Walker syndrome. Obstet Gynecol. 1983; 61:710.

25. Gonzalez-Crussi F. Extragonadal Teratomas. Atlas of Tumor Pathology. 2nd ser, fascicle 18. Bethesda, MD: Armed Forces Institute of Pathology; 1982:1–198.

26. Hirsch JH, Cyr D, Eberhardt H, et al. Ultrasonic diagnosis of an aneurysm of the vein of Galen in utero by duplex scanning. J Ultrasound Med. 1983; 2:231.

27. Hobbins JC, Grannum PAT, Berkowitz RL, et al. Ultrasound in the diagnosis of congenital anomalies. Am J Obstet Gynecol. 1979; 134:331.

28. Hobbins JC, Venus I, Tortora M, et al. Stage II ultrasound examination for the diagnosis of fetal abnormalities with an elevated amniotic fluid alpha-fetoprotein concentration. Am J Obstet Gynecol. 1982; 142:1026.

29. International Clearinghouse for Birth Defects Monitoring Systems. Annual Report. 1983.

30. Jeanty R, Dramaix-Wilmet M, Delbeke D, et al. Ultrasonic evaluation of fetal ventricular growth. Neuroradiology. 1981; 21:127.

31. Johnson ML, Dunne, MG, Mack LA, et al. Evaluation of fetal intracranial anatomy by static and real-time ultrasound. J Clin Ultrasound. 1980; 8:311.

32. Last RJ, Tompsett DH. Casts of the cerebral ventricles. Br J Surg. 1953; 40:525.

33. Lorber J, Ward AM. Spina bifida—A vanishing nightmare? Arch Dis Child. 1985; 60:1086.

34. Lustig-Gilman I, Young BK, Silverman F, et al. Fetal intraventricular hemorrhage: Sonographic diagnosis

and clinical implications. J Clin Ultrasound. 1983; 11:277.

35. McIntosh R. The incidence of congenital malformations: A study of 5964 pregnancies. Pediatrics. 1954; 14:505.

36. Murken JD, Stengel-Rutkowski S, Schwinger E. Prenatal Diagnosis of Genetic Disorders. Stuttgart: Ferdinand Enke; 1979:94–192.

37. Nicolaides KM, Campbell S, Gabbe SG, et al. Ultrasound screening for spina bifida: Cranial and cerebellar signs. Lancet. 1986; 2:72.

38. Nicolaides KM, Rodeck CH, Gosden CM. Rapid karyotyping in nonlethal malformations. Lancet 1986; 1:283.

39. Pearce JM, Little D, Campbell S. The diagnosis of abnormalities of the fetal central nervous system. In: Saunders RC, James AE, eds. The Principles and Practice of Ultrasonography in Obstetrics and Gynecology. 3rd ed. Norwalk, CT: Appleton-Century-Crofts; 1985: 246–248.

40. Reuter KL, D'Orsi CJ, Raptopoulos VD, et al. Sonographic pseudosymmetry of the prenatal cerebral hemispheres. J Ultrasound Med. 1982; 1:91.

41. Sabbagha RE, Tamura RK, Dal Campo S, et al. Fetal cranial and craniocervical masses: Ultrasound characteristics and differential diagnosis. Am J Obstet Gynecol. 1980; 138:511.

42. Smith DW. Recognizable Patterns of Human Malformation: Genetic, Embryologic and Clinical Aspects. 3rd ed. Philadelphia: WB Saunders; 1982: 174–175.

43. Smith DW. Recognizable Patterns of Human Malformation: Genetic, Embryologic and Clinical Aspects. 3rd ed. Philadelphia: WB Saunders; 1982: 472–473.

44. Warkany J. Microcephaly: Congenital Malformations. Chicago: Year Book Medical Publishers; 1971:237–244.

45. Warkany J. Congenital Malformations. Notes and Comments. Chicago: Year Book Medical Publishers; 1971:189–200.

CHAPTER 24

Abnormalities of the Fetal Chest, Abdomen, and Pelvis

Harris L. Cohen, Martha Newelt, Raymond Atwood

Knowledge of normal anatomy and biometry of the fetal thorax, abdomen, and pelvis, and their contents, combined with the excellent resolution of today's ultrasound equipment and meticulous sonographic technique, have allowed continued improvement in the evaluation of normal and abnormal fetuses.

Thorax

The thorax should be evaluated for overall size and symmetry of its bony and soft tissue elements. Masses extending from the thorax should be excluded. Normal intrathoracic contents should consist of homogenous, relatively symmetric lung parenchyma surrounding the central heart and mediastinum. Evaluation of the sonographic image for assymetry, mass, or mediastinal shift is helpful in detecting possible intrathoracic pathology.

The Bony Thorax and Its Soft Tissues

A few abnormalities long enough or large enough to appear to involve the thorax may actually extend from the head and neck. Encephaloceles and myelomeningoceles have associated calvarial and spinal abnormalities, respectively. The key differential diagnosis for a cystic mass in the region of the neck or upper thorax, when there is no abnormality of the spine or calvarium, includes fetal edema and cystic hygroma.[76]

Fetal edema may be focal at the neck but is more often associated with fetal hydrops and an increase in soft tissue thickness, forming a halo pattern around the neck, thorax, or abdomen (Fig. 24-1). Nuchal area edema has been associated with nonimmune fetal hydrops, fetal demise, and some skeletal dysplasias.[76,127] The antenatal presence of abnormal and excessive skin or soft tissue in the nuchal area of a fetus has also been associated with trisomy 21 (Down's syndrome).[7] Amniocentesis can be performed to karyotype a fetus with a thick nuchal area.[25]

Cystic hygromas, benign abnormalities of lymphatic origin occurring in one of every 6000 pregnancies, are thought to occur from a failure in the development of normal lymphatic venous communication. The lymphatic sacs dilate, and sonographically they appear as unilocular or multilocular cystic masses. Most (80%) originate from the posterolateral neck (Fig. 24-2). Approximately half of cystic hygromas are evident in antenatal life and 10% are bilateral.[125] They may be seen extending to or originating from the thorax (Fig. 24-3) or the mediastinum as well as the axilla or groin.[143] Internal solid elements seen on the sonographic image probably represent surrounding connective tissue or hemangiomatous elements.[25]

The differentiation of cystic hygroma from the

statistically less likely thoracic wall hemangioma is difficult. Large hemangiomas may be associated with cardiac dilatation owing to the presence of arteriovenous shunting and increased blood return to the heart.[143] Cystic hygromas may spontaneously resolve before birth, possibly owing to further development of lymphatic channel communication with the venous system. This is thought by some to be the cause of the webbed neck of patients with Turner's syndrome, a condition with an abnormal fetal karyotype (XO) and a frequent association with cystic hygroma.[126] Cystic hygromas may also cause venous obstruction; affected fetuses develop ascites, pleural effusions, generalized edema, an enlarged edematous placenta, or cystic cutaneous lymphangiectasia, and their prognosis is poor.[112] Generally, fetuses with cystic hygroma and hydrops succumb in utero or shortly after birth.[17,25]

Other soft tissue masses involving the thorax are uncommon. The soft tissues of the thorax are normally thin, but they may be generally increased in fetuses of diabetic mothers, owing to subcutaneous fat deposition or, as noted, in patients with fetal anasarca or edema, owing to subcutaneous fluid.[37,47] Teratomas with combined cystic and solid components have been described. They may increase in size during pregnancy, growing more solid (echogenic) in appearance.[25] Hamartomas, benign nonneoplastic overgrowths of the normal cellular elements of an affected area, often arise within a rib. They may have disproportionately large intrathoracic components capable of displacing the fetal heart and causing respiratory insufficiency. Early diagnosis with complete resection is curative.[12]

The clavicles may be absent or hypoplastic in several syndromes, including cleidocranial dysplasia, Holt-Oram syndrome, and pyknodysostosis. Thick ribs may be noted in mucopolysaccaridoses as well as several skeletal syndromes; diagnoses on prenatal ultrasound is often difficult.

Pulmonary Hypoplasia. Biometry allows evaluation of the thorax for pulmonary hypoplasia and syndromes involving the size of the chest wall. Pulmonary hypoplasia is associated with a poor prognosis. It is rarely of primary origin; usually it is secondary to lung compression in utero. Causes are numerous (Table 24-1) and are related to lung compression from intrathoracic masses or abdomi-

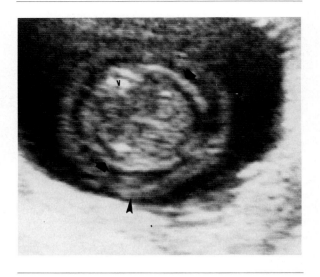

Figure 24-1. Fetal hydrops of upper abdomen is imaged in the transverse oblique plane. A halo of soft tissue (*arrowheads*) surrounds the fetal body (*arrows*; v, vertebral body).

nal masses that prevent the downward movement of the diaphragms or have an intrathoracic component. The small thorax of several skeletal dysplasias is associated with lung hypoplasia. In oligohydramnios of any cause, the lack of transmitted fluid pulsations on the chest wall, said to be necessary for tracheobronchial tree development, is thought to be the cause of the associated pulmonary hypoplasia. Prognosis, is related to the degree of hypoplasia.[15,21,124,125,138,147]

Lung hypoplasia may be diagnosed by gestalt, noting a small chest cavity in relation to a larger abdominal cavity. Thoracic circumference-to-abdominal circumference ratios average 0.89. Measurements that are under 0.77 (>2 SDs) are considered abnormal.[77,125,138] A prominent heart in the thorax of a fetus without cardiac disease is suggestive of pulmonary hypoplasia (Fig. 24-4).[21]

THE MEDIASTINUM

Mediastinal masses are rare in the fetus and few have been imaged antenatally. These include me-

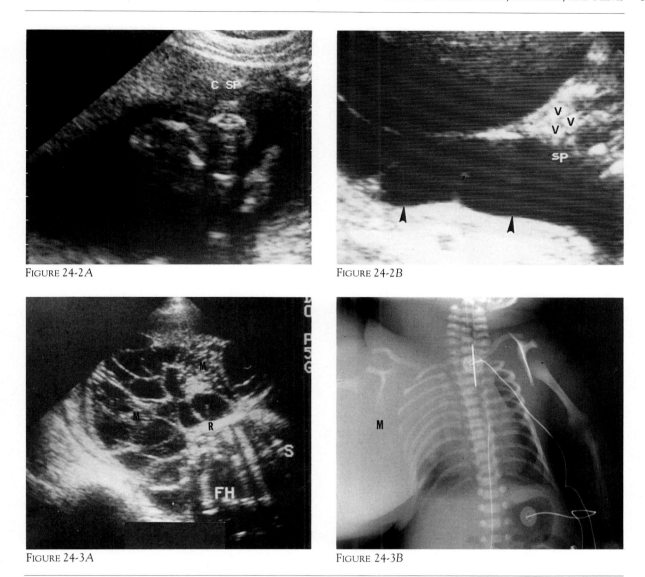

Figure 24-2A

Figure 24-2B

Figure 24-3A

Figure 24-3B

Figure 24-2. (A) Transverse view of a normal cervical spine shows converging posterior elements of a normal cervical vertebral body (*arrows*). No masses are seen to extend from the neck. (B) This transverse plane view shows a multilocular cystic mass (hygroma, *arrowheads*) posterior to the neck of the fetus. The hygroma is posterior and lateral to the three ossification centers (v) of the normal vertebral body seen at this level.

Figure 24-3. Cystic hygroma of the thoracic wall. (A) An ultrasound image in the coronal oblique plane shows a multilocular, predominantly cystic, mass (M) extending from the echogenic ribs (R) of the right thoracic wall (S, spine; FH, area of fetal heart). (B) Anteroposterior neonatal chest film reveals a soft tissue mass (M) off the right thorax.

Table 24-1. Causes of pulmonary hypoplasia

Intrathoracic masses that compress developing lung
    Pleural effusion
    Pulmonary cyst
    Teratoma
    Meningocele
    Hemangiomas

Abdominal mass effects that prevent downward
    displacement of the diaphragm or compress
    developing lung tissue
    Ascites
    Renal mass
    Diaphragmatic hernia

Oligohydramnios with a lack of transmitted fluid
    pulsation on the chest wall said to be necessary for
    tracheobronchial tree development
    Bilateral renal agenesis or obstruction
    Bilateral ureteral obstruction
    Bladder outlet obstruction, usually urethral atresia
    Prolonged rupture of membranes

Small thorax as part of a skeletal dysplasia
    Thanatophoric dwarfism
    Jeune's syndrome
    Ellis-Van Creveld syndrome
    Hypophosphatasia
    Cleidocranial dysostosis
    Metatrophic dwarfism
    Campomelic dwarfism

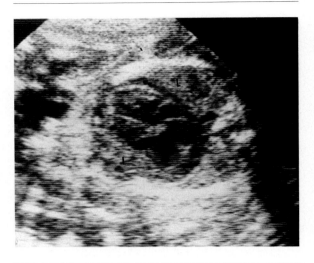

Figure 24-4. Hypoplastic lungs. A transverse oblique plane view through the thorax demonstrates that the heart takes up more than its usual one-third of the intrathoracic space. Although the cause was initially thought to be cardiomegaly, autopsy revealed a normal-sized heart in a fetus with hypoplastic lungs related to oligohydramnios of renal origin (L, lung parenchyma).

diastinal (including intrapericardial) teratoma,[26] enteric cyst,[101] lymphangioma, and mediastinal meningocele.[4] All may be associated with pleural effusion. Mass impression on the esophagus may lead to polyhydramnios because of an obstructed upper gastrointestinal tract, and mass impression on the vena cava may compromise blood return and lead to the development of fetal hydrops.

The Lungs

Normal fetal lungs should be symmetrically echogenic. Half of all intrathoracic abnormalities noted on fetal examination are pleural effusions.[4] The other abnormalities noted consist primarily of cystic masses within the lung parenchyma and masses that cause cardiac or mediastinal shift.[143] The most predominant cystic masses of the lung include the typically unilocular bronchogenic cyst and the multicystic image of cystic adenomatoid malformation, types II and III.

Bronchogenic Cyst. Four cases of bronchogenic cyst have been diagnosed antenatally.[3,4,143] Bronchogenic cysts may be unilocular (Fig. 24-5) or multilocular. They may displace mediastinal structures, although this is an uncommon finding in neonatal life. Bronchogenic cysts result from abnormal budding of the ventral diverticulum of the primitive foregut and are lined by epithelium similar to that of a normal bronchus. They may contain cartilage, muscle, or mucus glands.[25] They may be found within the lung parenchyma or mediastinum, often communicating with the trachea or mainstem bronchi.[3]

Cystic Adenomatoid Malformation. Excluding diaphragmatic hernias, cystic adenomatoid malformation (CAM) is the most frequently identified mass in the fetal chest.[25] Accounting for 25% of congenital lung malformations,[119] it is typically a unilateral disorder involving a lung lobe or part of one, although bilateral involvement may occur. Rarely, CAM may involve an entire lung.[35] It is characterized histologically as an adenomatoid in-

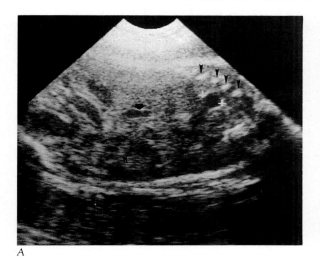

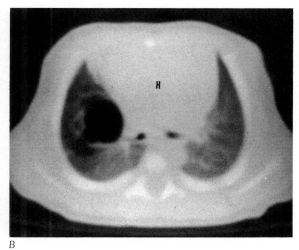

A   B

FIGURE 24-5. Bronchogenic cyst. (A) On a left parasagittal plane view of chest and abdomen crosses mark off an echo-free mass within the normally echogenic lung. Ribs can be seen anteriorly (*small arrowheads*). The right kidney (K) as well as a small portion of the abdominal aorta (*large arrowhead*) may be noted in the abdomen. (B) Axial CT view of neonate's thorax demonstrates a low-density area in the left thorax consistent with air filling the bronchogenic cyst (H, heart).

crease of terminal respiratory elements leading to the development of a pathologic mass consisting of multiple cysts of different sizes (Table 24-2).[25,111,119]

Three forms of CAM have been described. Type I consists of a single large cyst (usually 3 to 7 cm, but at least 2 cm) with a trabeculated wall and, often, smaller cystic outpouchings. Broad fibrous septa and mucigenic cells may be responsible for areas of echogenicity within the mass. Type II CAM is a mass made up of multiple uniform-sized cysts of about 1.5 cm diameter. Types I and II appear cystic on ultrasound examination (Fig. 24-6). Type III consists of multiple very small cysts (0.5 to 5.0 mm), that, like the multiple small cysts of infantile polycystic kidney disease, present numerous reflecting surfaces to the ultrasound beam. Because they cannot be resolved individually, the mass appears as a single, solid, homogenously echogenic structure.[94,111,140] There are associated renal, cardiac, and gastrointestinal malformations; as with all space-occupying lung masses, there may be associated fetal hydrops, ascites, and polyhydramnios. The mass may expand and cause a greater than

normal increase in thoracic diameter as well as inversion of the diaphragm or, as in one case report, decrease in relative size during the pregnancy.[35,119]

Stillbirth and premature labor are common. Many neonates present with respiratory distress at birth. Of 19 reported cases of CAM diagnosed antenatally, however, nine infants have survived. The association with fetal hydrops appears more indicative of a poor fetal outcome than the exact histologic type of CAM.[25]

The differential diagnosis of the type III, solid-appearing, CAM includes pulmonary sequestration, rhabdomyoma, mediastinal teratoma, and herniated liver, spleen, or, rarely, kidney.[25,119] The differential diagnosis of type I and II lesions includes cystic lung and mediastinal masses as well as pleural and pericardial effusions. Key considerations in the differential diagnosis are the fluid-filled stomach and bowel in diaphragmatic hernias.[119]

Pulmonary Sequestration. A pulmonary sequestration is a solid nonfunctioning mass of lung tissue that

Table 24-2. Cystic adenomatoid malformations

Type	Histologic Findings	Sonographic Appearance[94,111,140]	Differential Diagnoses[25,119]
I	Single large cyst, usually 3–7 cm but at least 2 cm; trabeculated wall with smaller cystic outpouchings	Usually unilateral May involve a lung lobe or part of a lung lobe Rarely involves entire lung Can be bilateral Single large cyst with smaller cystic outpouchings visualized superior to the diaphragm in the fetal lung Can have echogenic areas within the cyst	Bronchogenic cyst Mediastinal mass Pleural and pericardial effusions Fluid-filled stomach and bowel in diaphragmatic hernia
II	Mass made up of multiple similar-sized cysts, 1.5 cm in diameter	Usually unilateral May involve a lung lobe or part of a lobe Rarely involves entire lung Can be bilateral Multiple similar sized cysts seen in the fetal lung replacing normal lung parenchyma	Same as Type I
III	Multiple small cysts (0.5–5 mm)	Cysts too small to be resolved sonographically appear as a single solid echogenic mass in the fetal lung	Pulmonary sequestration Rhabdomyoma Mediastinal teratoma Herniated liver, spleen, or rarely kidney

lacks communication with the tracheobronchial tree and has a systemic arterial blood supply (and, in the extralobar type, a systemic venous drainage). These masses are spherical, highly echogenic, and often at the lung base. There is a bronchiectatic form that may simulate the ultrasound image of type I and II CAM.[25,91]

Pleural Effusion and Fetal Hydrops. More than 50% of ultrasound-diagnosed intrathoracic pathology is pleural effusion.[143] Any fluid in the pleural space of a fetus is abnormal,[44] and there is a reported 15% mortality associated with this fetal ultrasound finding.

Pleural fluid may be an isolated finding, but more typically it is part of other fetal pathology, which may or may not be imaged. It is most often seen in association with fetal hydrops,[44,88,110] a condition associated with excessive fluid accumulations within the fetal soft tissues and body cavities. The two types of hydrops are immune and nonimmune.

Immune hydrops (or erythroblastosis fetalis)

usually occurs in a fetus whose mother has been sensitized, usually in previous pregnancies, by a blood factor histoincompatibility, usually Rhesus (Rh) factor, and an immune reaction between maternal immunoglobulin G (IgG) and the fetal blood factor (acting as an antigen) results. This reaction leads to significant fetal morbidity and mortality with a small amount of ascites, usually an early sign of impending decompensation into full-blown immune hydrops with sonographic findings of profound skin thickening (>5 mm), placental thickening (>4 cm), significant pleural and pericardial effusions, ascites, hepatomegaly and splenomegaly, and polyhydramnios. At one time Rh incompatibility was the cause of 98% of all immune hydrops. The development of Rhogam to protect the Rh-negative mother from histoincompatibility reactions with a future Rh-positive fetus reduced this to about 90%.[18]

Nonimmune hydrops has a high incidence of fetal mortality, ranging between 50 and 98%.[18] The sonographic findings are similar to those of immune hydrops. Causes include fetal cardiac ar-

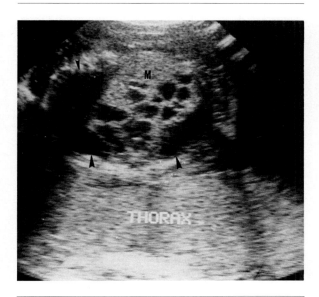

FIGURE 24-6. Transverse oblique plane. Multiple cysts are noted in the lung parenchyma of this patient with cystic adenomatoid malformation (M) and surrounding pleural effusion (*arrowheads*).

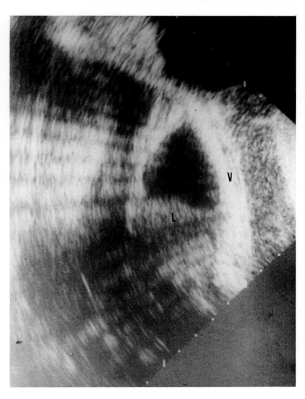

FIGURE 24-7. Pleural effusion. Right parasagittal plane view shows a triangular echo-free area above the liver (L) and anterior to the vertebral column (V).

rhythmias or anomalies (e.g., hypoplastic left heart and supraventricular tachycardia, said to be the probable cause of many of the cases labeled idiopathic), intrauterine infection (any of the TORCH—*t*oxoplasmosis, *r*ubella, *c*ytomegalovirus, *h*erpes—infections), chromosomal abnormalities (Turner's syndrome, trisomy 18 or 21), abdominal or pulmonary masses leading to venous obstruction (CAM or neuroblastoma), congenital hematologic disorders (α-thalassemia, an extremely common cause in Asia), renal abnormalities (congenital nephrosis), and maternal causes (diabetes, toxemia)[26,44,118] Hydrothorax unrelated to hydrops usually has an extrathoracic cause, but intrathoracic pathology such as CAM has been noted to be responsible for its development.[107]

On ultrasound examination, sonolucent fluid is seen within one or both hemithoraxes, conforming to the shape of the chest cavity and its diaphragmatic contour (Fig. 24-7). If large, the pleural effusion may flatten or even evert the diaphragm.[44,68,86]

Mortality from pleural effusion is affected by the underlying cause as well as by the development of pulmonary hypoplasia, which may occur if there is significant mass effect early in lung development. In an attempt to decrease this possibility, midtrimester thoracocentesis under ultrasound guidance was performed on a fetus who at birth showed no thoracic abnormality.[6]

Pleural effusions may be chylous, appearing as anechoic as serous pleural effusions owing to the absence of chylomicrons in the fetus.[44] Chylothorax is caused by overaccumulation of lymph. It is most often unilateral and right-sided. It occurs twice as often in male infants and is observed in association with congenital pulmonary lymphangiectasia, tracheoesophageal fistula, trisomy 21, and extralobar pulmonary sequestration.[120]

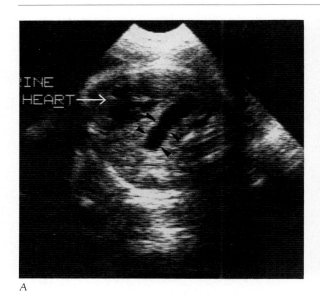
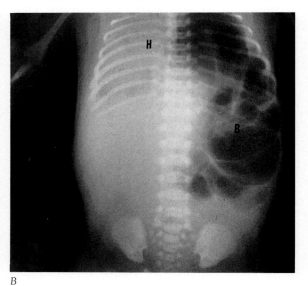

A

B

Figure 24-8. Diaphragmatic hernia. (A) On this transverse oblique view of a fetal chest, the heart has been shifted to the right chest *(arrow)*. A tubular lucency *(arrowheads)* within the chest is a loop of bowel. (B) On AP film of the chest and abdomen a radiolucency from air-filled bowel (B) is noted below the left hemidiaphragm and within the left chest of this neonate. The heart (H) has been shifted into the right chest, accounting for some of the "white out" of the right lung field.

DIAPHRAGMATIC HERNIA

Congenital diaphragmatic hernia (CDH; incidence one in every 5000 to 10,000 pregnancies) results from defective diaphragm formation or fusion.[96] These defects may result in the most common diaphragmatic hernia, the posterolateral Bochdalek, and in other types, including retrosternal and anteromedial (Morgagni) hernias and diaphragmatic eventration.[59,121] Left-sided involvement is five times more common than right-sided,[84] which may be due to the presence of the liver, whose mass is known to prevent craniad progression of bowel and thereby moderate symptoms and improve prognosis. Involvement is usually unilateral and the disorder is somewhat more common in male infants.[121]

There are familial forms of CDH, but these are bilateral in 20% of cases rather than the 3% bilaterality noted in sporadic cases, with a 2 to 1 male predominance and fewer associated anomalies.[44,59] One Finnish study showed a 2% recurrence risk among subsequent siblings.[102]

Abdominal contents acting as an intrathoracic mass can lead to pulmonary hypoplasia, which may be bilateral despite a unilateral diaphragmatic lesion.[59] Overall mortality is 50 to 80%,[2] which figure includes 35% stillbirths. CDH is associated with major congenital anomalies of other body systems. Associated cardiovascular and central nervous system anomalies are the most lethal.[14]

On fetal ultrasound examination (Fig. 24-8) the stomach, bowel, or other organs may be seen in the chest, often posteriorly. Fluid-filled structures are readily differentiated from echogenic lung parenchyma. Occasionally peristalsis may be noted in herniated small bowel. To rule out cystic abnormalities of the lung simulating CDH the sonographer must search the abdomen to prove it contains

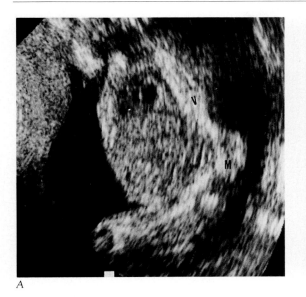
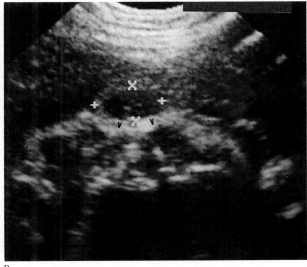

A   B

FIGURE 24-9. Myelomeningocele. (A) On a sagittal plane view a mass (M) consisting of a myelomeningocele is seen to extend posteriorly from the fetal vertebral column (V). (B) On the transverse plane view, crosses surround the mass, which lies posterior to divergent posterior elements of a vertebral body (v). No normal skin line was seen.

no stomach; the condition is often accompanied by a smaller abdominal circumference measurement. Often the heart and mediastinum shift away from the side of herniation. With fetal breathing, the abdominal organs may descend on the normal side and, paradoxically, ascend on the affected side. Polyhydramnios and pleural effusions may be noted. One series reported a 55% survival rate among patients with CDH without associated polyhydramnios (as opposed to 11% when polyhydramnios was associated).[53] Smaller defects and herniation later in gestation are also associated with improved prognosis. A careful sonographic search should be made for other congenital anomalies.[17,25,44,120]

Management of these cases should include karyotyping, fetal echocardiography, and delivery at a tertiary center. Experimental work with surgery in utero in fetal lambs[139] has paved the way for similar work in humans. There is no indication that early delivery improves the prognosis.[120]

Abdomen

SCANNING TECHNIQUES

A general fetal abdominal survey should evaluate the anterior abdominal wall to see that it is intact. This is most important at the site of umbilical cord entry.

No masses should extend from the vertebral column or posteriorly (Fig. 24-9). Posterior elements of the vertebral bodies should converge or appear parallel. Any divergence of the posterior elements, particularly in the presence of defects in the overlying skin or posterior masses, suggests the presence of a meningocele or myelomeningocele. Protrusions from the abdominal side walls should also be sought, although they are unusual. The soft tissues of the abdominal wall should not be thickened, a finding noted in hydrops fetalis but also in the offspring of diabetic (type C) mothers.[124]

Abdominal situs is determined by noting the liver's position on the opposite side of the cardiac apex. This is best accomplished by caudad and craniad angulation of the transducer in the transverse plane. Complete situs inversus (cardiac apex on right and liver on left) can be diagnosed only by meticulous attention to fetal position and visualized anatomy.[131] In cases of correct abdominal situs, transverse images of the abdomen show the spine, stomach, and umbilical vein in clockwise relation when the fetus is in cephalic presentation and counterclockwise when the fetus is breech.

Abdominal circumference (AC) should be measured to assess conformity with accepted measurements for gestational age. Biometric evaluation of abdominal circumference allows assessment of the nutritional status of the fetus. Assymetric intrauterine growth retardation (IUGR) will show a smaller AC, owing to loss of glycogen stores in the liver and the resultant decrease in liver size; there will be no associated decrease in head circumference (HC) or femur length (FL) measurements. HC/AC and FL/AC ratios are, therefore, used to determine IUGR.[77,124]

The remainder of the routine fetal abdominal survey includes evaluation of the transverse AC view for the presence of a fluid-filled stomach and assessment of the liver. A transverse view at the level of the kidneys may reveal renal obstruction. Coronal and longitudinal views may supplement the transverse views in further evaluating any area of concern.

PERITONEUM AND ASCITES

Ascites (Fig. 24-10) represents fluid in the peritoneum. True fetal ascites is always abnormal. Depending on the amount, the fluid may be seen only in dependent portions of the fetus (e.g., the pelvis in a fetus in breech position) or, in large amounts, surrounding and shifting intraperitoneal structures superiorly, inferiorly, or laterally. Intraperitoneal fluid is seen best in the subhepatic space, flanks, and lower abdominal cavity or pelvis. The retroperitoneal structures such as the kidneys lie posterior to the free fluid. With patency of the processus vaginalis, ascitic fluid may extend into the scrotum as apparent hydroceles. In studies of intrauterine transfusions, the presence of at least 10 ml of intraperitoneal fluid at 22 weeks and 15 ml at 26 weeks is required before fetal ascites can be detected sonographically.[55]

Commonly noted in association with the multi-

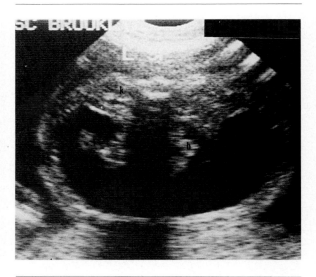

FIGURE 24-10. Ascites. On transverse plane view fluid is seen within the peritoneal cavity of this fetus with hydrops. Echogenic masses in the fluid are normal bowel loops (b). The retroperitoneal right kidney (k) is posterior to the ascites.

ple findings of fetal hydrops, fetal ascites may develop as an isolated finding in bowel perforation or as urinary ascites from bladder outlet obstruction or renal forniceal rupture.[87] Heart failure, infections, tumors, and twin-twin transfusions are other causes. Sonography typically demonstrates only 25 to 50% of the causes.[12]

If fetal ascites is detected, the sonographer and sonologist should investigate further, seeking bowel dilatation (indicating bowel obstruction), dilatation of the pyelocalyceal system or bladder (genitourinary problem), or intraabdominal cysts or peritoneal calcification indicative of bowel perforation and resultant meconium peritonitis or pseudocyst formation.[44] Because normal peristalsis is necessary to extrude meconium, this phenomenon usually is not seen until the 5th month of fetal life.[29]

If sterile meconium, associated with bowel perforation, is extruded into the peritoneal cavity, an intense foreign body reaction occurs. Punctate echogenicities develop over time, owing to the resultant irritative peritonitis caused by meconium and

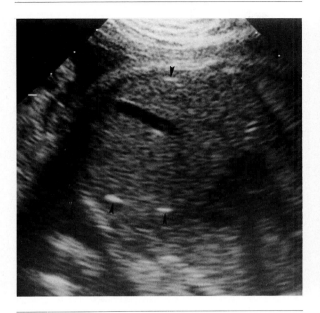

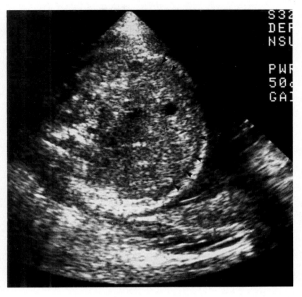

FIGURE 24-11. Peritoneal calcification. Transverse oblique plane view shows highly echogenic linear densities (*arrowheads*) at the liver periphery. This fetus probably had a bowel perforation.

FIGURE 24-12. A hypoechoic band (*arrowheads*) at the inner aspect of the echogenic abdominal wall echoes represents the abdominal wall musculature, creating the image of pseudoascites.

its subsequent calcification. This calcification is most easily detected around the liver (Fig. 24-11). Localized fibrotic reactions may cause walls to form about the areas of greatest meconium concentration within the peritoneum, forming meconium pseudocysts. These complex calcified masses may simulate retroperitoneal teratomas or calcified neuroblastomas. Other causes of peritoneal recess calcification include infections from TORCH organisms.[29,36,40,59,79]

PSEUDOASCITES

A hypoechoic band positioned along the inner aspect of the echo produced by the anterior abdominal wall and its subcutaneous tissue may simulate a small amount of ascites. This image of pseudoascites (Fig. 24-12) is created by the hypoechoic quality of the abdominal wall musculature sandwiched between the highly echogenic subcutaneous and preperitoneal fat. Unlike true ascites, it does not outline parts of the falciform ligament or umbilical vein, nor does it surround other abdominal organs.[11,54,124]

Liver and Spleen

The normal fetal liver has a homogenous appearance. Although congenital anomalies are rare, atypical echogenicities can be seen in association with extramedullary hematopoiesis.[59] The fetal liver enlarges in association with immune or non-immune causes of hydrops. If the longest liver length to the right of the aorta on coronal image increases more than 5 mm in a week, isoimmunization must be ruled out.[77] The umbilical vein is enlarged in hydrops, and in association with placental chorioangioma. It is notable that macrosomic fetuses have large livers whereas growth-retarded infants have small livers.[59]

Solitary liver cysts may develop because of interruption of the development of the intrahepatic biliary tree. A 10.5-cm cyst has been reported.[19] There are several types of choledochal cysts. The most common is cystic dilatation of the common bile duct, which may be seen in an intrahepatic or subhepatic location, but other types include multiple intrahepatic and extrahepatic cysts or a common bile duct diverticulum. Antenatal detection and early surgery may prevent the development of some severe consequences, especially the development of biliary cirrhosis and portal hypertension.[28,32,57]

Diffuse liver calcification may be noted in intrauterine infections such as toxoplasmosis and herpes simplex. Calcified portal thromboemboli have been reported on autopsy and plain films of newborn and stillborn infants.[10,44]

Antenatal detection of a case of late third-trimester gallstones has been reported. Like gallstones reported in neonates, they disappeared, possibly due to postnatal hydration or because they are not gallstones but tumefactive sludge.[8,70]

Liver masses are unusual but have been reported. The most common vascular tumor of the neonatal liver is the infantile hemangioendothelioma, which may be associated with hepatomegaly, anemia, or high-output congestive heart failure. Sonography has shown these masses to be of variable mixed echogenicity in neonates. Reports have been made of the antenatal detection of hemangiomas in fetuses of 31 and 32 weeks, respectively.[59,99,113]

The fetal spleen is enlarged in cases of Rh and other isoimmunization (owing to extramedullary hematopoiesis or hydrops) and in chronic infections such as toxoplasmosis, cytomegalovirus, rubella, and syphilis.[78,133] It may be enlarged in such inborn metabolic errors as Gaucher's, Niemann-Pick, or Wolman's disease. The antenatal diagnosis of a congenital splenic cyst can be made if a cyst is noted in the left upper quadrant and is separable on sonography from the imaged kidney and adrenal gland. Asplenia and polysplenia may be associated with congenital heart disease. Antenatal diagnosis is difficult.[31,59,81,133]

Kidney, Ureters, and Bladder

Fetal malformations are noted once in every 200 births. Urinary tract abnormalities represent between 35 and 50% of these.[21,58]

By 12 weeks' gestational age, the kidneys should have attained their normal position and the blood supply should be established. By 15 weeks' gestational age the kidneys may be visualized sonographically as symmetric paraspinal masses. If assymetry is noted, a search of the fetal abdomen may reveal an ectopic kidney, which occurs in 1 in 2000 pregnancies. An unusual kidney shape may be due to a single horseshoe kidney, a duplicated system, a tumor, or fused or nonfused crossed ectopia.[21,42,60,66]

A renal pelvis greater than 1.0 cm in anteroposterior diameter or a dilated urethra is considered abnormal. The normal ureters are not visualized unless they are obstructed. The bladder, which may appear quite large in normal fetuses, should be seen either on initial or Lasix-enhanced examinations of fetuses older than 15 weeks, to rule out bilateral dysfunction or obstruction. The bladder size should change to demonstrate fetal voiding and rule out outlet obstruction; wall thickening, another sign of outlet obstruction, should also be excluded.[21,48,57]

Amniotic Fluid

Amniotic fluid is a dialysate of maternal serum, essential for the maintenance of an even fetal temperature and biochemical homeostasis. Its presence allows fetal movement and growth and is thought to be essential for the development of the tracheobronchial tree.[21]

Amniotic fluid volume should average 60 ml at 12 weeks' gestation, increasing 20 to 25 ml per week until 16 weeks and then increasing 50 to 100 ml per week until 20 weeks. The mean fluid volume at 20 weeks is 500 ml. The fetus may contribute to amniotic fluid volume by fluid transfer across the fetal skin surfaces, including skin, cord, chorion, and amnion. Fetal urine production begins at 12 weeks, but the amount is insignificant until the 18th to 20th weeks of gestation. By the late third trimester the fetus is producing approximately 450 ml of urine per day. Beyond 20 weeks, transudation of fluid across fetal surfaces is inadequate to maintain normal amniotic volume, and the fetus essentially modifies fluid volume and composition only by swallowing and urination.[21,46,135]

Normal amniotic fluid volume may be maintained by one functioning kidney and a nonob-

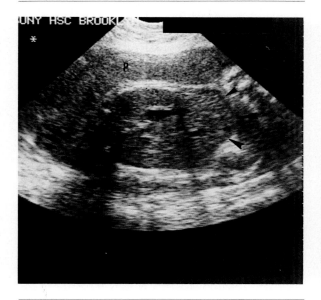

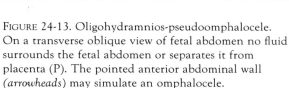

FIGURE 24-13. Oligohydramnios-pseudoomphalocele. On a transverse oblique view of fetal abdomen no fluid surrounds the fetal abdomen or separates it from placenta (P). The pointed anterior abdominal wall (*arrowheads*) may simulate an omphalocele.

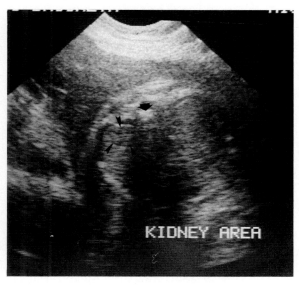

FIGURE 24-14. Renal agenesis. Kidney is simulated by normal adrenal gland. The image was made in the transverse plane at the level of the kidneys. Oval masses on either side of the vertebral body (*arrow*) look like kidneys. At autopsy there were no kidneys but prominent, normal adrenals (*arrowheads*, right adrenal).

structed genitourinary (GU) tract. Oligohydramnios of fetal origin is due to abnormality of the GU tract, usually bilateral renal agenesis, urethral atresia, or bilateral nonfunctional renal dysplasia. The diagnosis of oligohydramnios is somewhat subjective and is related to fetal gestational age. Sonographically, less fluid surrounds the fetus, crowding fetal parts and tending also to obscure imaging of fetal anatomy. Compression of the fetal abdomen may cause a pseudoomphalocele image (Fig. 24-13), a finding that may also be simulated by uterine contractions.[21,46,97,128]

RENAL AGENESIS

Bilateral renal agenesis is the most severe anomaly of the GU system. It occurs at the rate of 1 to 3 cases per 10,000 live births, predominantly in males. It has been noted to recur in a 5% rate within affected families.[21,30]

Severe oligohydramnios will be noted between the 16th and 28th weeks of gestation. The adrenal gland may simulate the kidney, and, in association with renal agenesis may take on a more globular shape (Fig. 24-14). The most helpful sonographic finding of agenesis is the failure to detect the fetal bladder despite repeated examinations and furosemide challenge.[21,30,83,145]

Early neonatal death associated with renal agenesis is due to pulmonary hypoplasia. Affected infants are often in breech presentation, deliver prematurely, and have Potter's-type facies and features (flattened nose, epicanthic folds, low-set ears, receding chin, hypertelorism, brachycephaly, and talipes equinovarus) owing to the lack of cushioning typically provided in utero by the surrounding amniotic fluid.[21,30,97,114] Evaluating a fetus for unilateral renal agenesis is difficult because the secondary signs—absent bladder filling and oligohydramnios—are not observable because the fetus has one functioning kidney.

FETAL HYDRONEPHROSIS

Sonography allows ready detection of fetal hydronephrosis. Small amounts of anechoic fluid may be seen in the renal pelvis, in sharp contrast with the normal echogenicity of the renal parenchyma.

After 24 weeks' gestation it is quite common to see at least some dilatation of the central renal pelvis. One study showed anteroposterior measurements of the renal pelvis to be as wide as 1 to 2 mm in 41% and 3 to 11 mm in 18% of a group of normal fetuses. Theories as to the cause include the influence of maternal hormones and maternal fluid volume expansion, although experimental work with sheep has shown no change in fetal urine production with maternal volume expansion.[21,62,85,135]

A grading system (Table 24-3) has been developed to assess fetal hydronephrosis in relation to neonatal clinical outcome. Grade I dilatation (Fig. 24-15) is considered physiologic. Grade II (Fig. 24-16) and grade III are considered intermediate hydronephrosis. Fifty percent of this group required postnatal surgical intervention. All patients with grade IV (Fig. 24-17) and grade V required surgical intervention.[48]

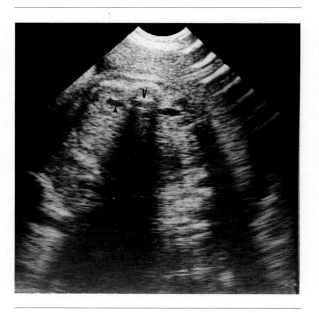

FIGURE 24-15. Transverse plane view of bilateral physiologic dilatation of fetal renal pelvis. Echo-free urine is seen in each renal pelvis. Anteroposterior dimension of this dilatation is less than 5 mm. No postnatal abnormality was noted (V, vertebral body; *arrowhead*, right renal pelvis).

TABLE 24-3. Grading system for fetal hydronephrosis

Grade I, Physiologic dilatation
    Renal pelvis: <1 cm in AP diameter
    Calyces: Not visualized
    Cortex: Unremarkable
Grade II
    Renal pelvis: 1.0–1.5 cm
    Calyces: Not visualized (normal)
    Cortex: Unremarkable
Grade III
    Renal pelvis: >1.5 cm
    Calyces: Slight dilatation
    Cortex: Unremarkable
Grade IV
    Renal pelvis: >1.5 cm
    Calyces: Moderately dilated
    Cortex: No significant abnormality
Grade V
    Renal pelvis: >1.5 cm
    Calyces: Severe dilatation
    Cortex: Atrophic
Percentage of patients that required surgery based on
    grade: Gr. I, 0%; Gr. II, 39%; Gr. III, 62%; Gr. IV,
    100%; Gr. V, 100%

(Data from Grignon A, Filion R, Filiatrault D, et al. Urinary tract dilatation in utero. Radiology. 1986;160:645–647.)

We tend to follow patients with fetal dilatations of 8 mm or greater. Postnatal confirmation of hydronephrosis should not be made within the first two days of life because relative neonatal dehydration and relatively low glomerular filtration rate may contribute to a falsely normal appearance to the newborn renal pelvis.[21,78]

A dilated renal pelvis can be caused by obstruction at any level of the urinary tract. It may be the result of vesicoureteral reflux or be related to prune belly syndrome. The majority of these suspicious fetal kidneys prove to be normal at birth. Cases of prenatally imaged fetal GU tract dilatation that proved in neonatal life to be unrelated to obstruction and without evidence of vesicoureteral reflux have engendered a decidedly conservative approach to intrauterine intervention, particularly for unilateral GU system dilatation.[21,48,58]

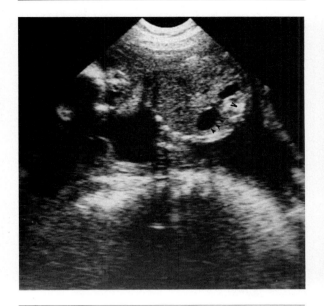

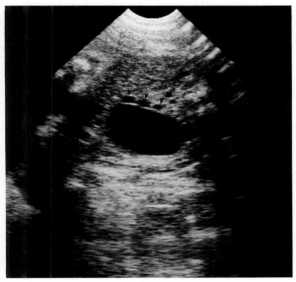

FIGURE 24-16. Grade II dilatation. On transverse plane view arrowheads point to 1.3-cm dilatation of left renal pelvis. Dilatation on the right was physiologic. At birth, the baby had a UPJ obstruction on the left and a normal right kidney (V, vertebral body).

FIGURE 24-17. Grade IV dilatation. Longitudinal oblique plane view demonstrates a 3-cm dilatation of the renal pelvis with mild to moderate dilatation of calyces (*arrowheads*). There was renal cortex, although it is difficult to see on this view.

GENITOURINARY TRACT OBSTRUCTION

Early diagnosis of renal obstruction and subsequent early pediatric surgery for correction is necessary to ensure future renal function. A long-term follow-up study of patients with severe obstructive uropathy noted improvement or normalization of renal function when surgery was performed within the first year of life. If surgery was not performed until after age 2 years, patients experienced progressive deterioration of renal function.[21,48,92]

The most common cause of congenital obstructive hydronephrosis is ureteropelvic junction (UPJ) obstruction, which occurs in 1 of every 1258 newborns and is bilateral in almost one-third of cases. Bilateral involvement is usually asymmetric; severe bilateral involvement is unusual. Progressive dilatation during antenatal life is common, particularly with the higher grades of obstruction.[49,135]

Ureterovesical junction obstruction (UVJ) is rare and is typically due to a renal duplication anomaly consisting, unilaterally or bilaterally, of two renal collecting systems and ureters and their associated obstruction, usually of the upper moiety alone, by an ectopic ureterocele. Prenatal diagnosis is often limited by the small size of the upper moiety and the changing size of the ureterocele owing to intravesical pressures. Ureteroceles found outside the bladder may simulate any pelvic cystic mass, including ovarian cyst, anterior meningocele, and hydrocolpos. Primary megaureter can cause obstruction by lack of peristalsis in a focal portion of distal ureter, but severe hydronephrosis is unusual.[21,49,103,134]

Bladder outlet obstructions are seen with posterior urethral valves (PUV), urethral atresia, and the caudal regression syndrome. In each case there may be retrograde filling and dilatation of bladder, ureters, and renal pelvis. The bladder wall may be thickened.

In PUV (Fig. 24-18), predominantly a male abnormality, redundant membranous folds in the posterior urethra lead to varying degrees of GU system obstruction. Typically, there is a thick-walled dilated bladder, and often an apparent di-

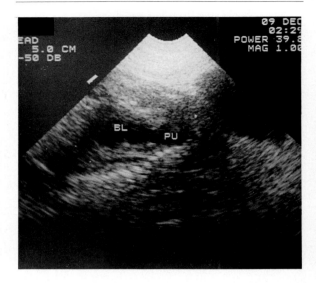

FIGURE 24-18. Posterior urethral valves. Transverse oblique view at level of bladder and posterior urethra shows urine in the bladder (BL) and the posterior urethra (PU), which normally is not imaged. There is some increased thickness to the bladder wall. The valve itself was not imaged antenatally but was noted on a neonatal voiding cystourethrogram.

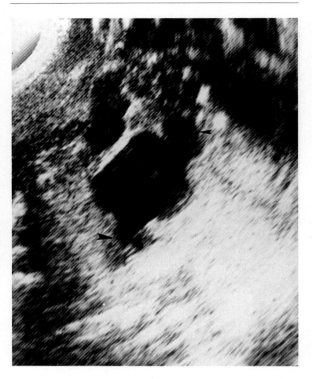

FIGURE 24-19. Urethral atresia. Coronal plane view shows dilated ureters (*small arrowheads*) leading to a dilated bladder with a conical outlet at the histopathologically proven point of urethral atresia (*large arrowhead*). This fetus died as a newborn of complications related to pulmonary hypoplasia.

lated posterior urethra. If the obstructed urine refluxes with pressure into the renal pelvis, there may be forniceal rupture and the development of a perirenal urinoma or urinary ascites. Severe hydronephrosis is seen in about 15% of cases. Severe hydronephrosis may lead to Potter's syndrome. Late, incomplete, or transient obstruction may lead to little, if any, renal damage. Females with dilated bladders may have caudal regression syndrome, in which anal atresia and a persistent cloaca may obstruct bladder and bowel.[43,57,61,86]

Complete urethral atresia (Fig. 24-19) is similar to severe PUV. Sonographic evidence of an enlarged bladder, dilated urethra, bilateral hydronephrosis, oligohydramnios, and cystic renal dysplasia (Potter's type IV) may be seen.[21,43,61]

PRUNE BELLY SYNDROME

Fetal ascites, when not due to hydrops, is due to GU system abnormality. It can distend the fetal abdomen and has been implicated in the development of the lax abdominal musculature of prune belly syndrome. Of 14 infants with posterior urethral obstruction reviewed by Hayden and colleagues, 77% had the prune belly triad of deficient abdominal musculature, cryptorchidism, and GU anomaly. Whether this is truly prune belly syndrome, a sporadic mesodermal defect occurring in 1 in 40,000 births and usually associated with dilated, tortuous ureters and ineffective peristalsis, or pseudo-prune belly syndrome is unknown. Both disorders may show undulation of the anterior abdominal wall of the fetus when the transducer is used to tap on the mother's abdominal wall.[57,61,144]

TABLE 24-4. Fetal renal dysplasia

TYPE	INVOLVEMENT	SONOGRAPHIC APPEARANCE	ASSOCIATED FINDINGS
TYPE I, Autosomal recessive polycystic kidney disease (RPK) or infantile polycystic kidney disease	Bilateral	1- to 2-mm cysts too small to be seen sonographically; massively enlarged homogeneous echogenic kidneys taking up most of the abdomen's space	Oligohydramnios, bladder not visualized, neonatal death due to pulmonary hypoplasia
TYPE II, Multicystic dysplastic kidney (MDK) (*most common*)	Usually unilateral	Multiple large anechoic cysts of varying size, the largest not being central; kidney size varies from small to normal to large; reniform shape is often lost; echogenicity between cysts is due to proliferation of connective tissue	Amniotic fluid level and lung development unaffected in unilateral dysplasia
TYPE III, Autosomal dominant polycystic kidney disease (DPK) or adult polycystic disease	Uncommon in neonatal life; bilateral disease usually presents in adult life		
TYPE IV, Cystic renal dysplasia	Occurs secondary to an early GU tract obstruction; can be seen in severe cases of posterior urethral valves; commonly seen in urethral atresia	Moderately enlarged echogenic kidneys with scattered small cysts	Significant oligohydramnios

RENAL DYSPLASIA

Renal dysplasia occurs at the rate of two to four cases for every 1000 births. Cystic dysplasias have been classified into four types: type I, autosomal recessive polycystic kidney disease (RPK), also known as infantile polycystic kidney disease; type II, multicystic dysplastic kidney or MDK; type III, autosomal dominant polycystic kidney disease (DPK), also known as adult polycystic kidney disease; and type IV, cystic renal dysplasia. There is controversy regarding concepts involving RPK and DPK as well as their pathologic diagnosis (Table 24-4).[21,38,106]

RPK affects both kidneys and its reported incidence is two cases in 110,000 births,[120] with a 25% recurrence rate in affected families. Saccular dilatations of the collecting tubules create multiple small cysts, typically, 1 to 2 mm and therefore too small to be resolved as cysts on sonography. The classic image is that of massively enlarged, homogenously echogenic kidneys (Fig. 24-20) taking up most of the abdomen's space. Unlike other dysplasias, there is no increase in connective tissue within these kidneys. Affected fetuses tend to have severe oligohydramnios because of bilateral renal dysfunction, and the bladder is not imaged. Neonatal death is usually due to pulmonary hypoplasia. Cases have been reported of normal-looking kidney images evolving during fetal life into those typical of infantile polycystic kidney.[21,51,52,89]

The MDK is the most common of the cystic renal dysplasias. Usually unilateral, the amniotic

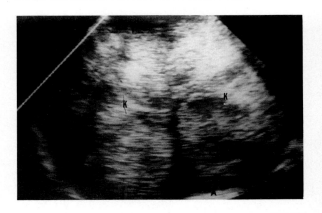

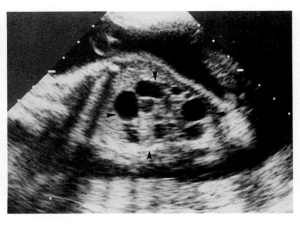

FIGURE 24-20. Infantile polycystic kidney disease. Transverse oblique view of abdomen shows echogenic enlarged kidneys (K, *arrowheads*) taking up most of this newborn's abdomen. A high near-field gain setting is responsible for the apparent increase in the echogenicity of the anterior third of the kidneys.

FIGURE 24-21. Multicystic dysplastic kidney. Longitudinal view shows multiple cysts of varying sizes in this right renal mass (*arrowheads*) that retains a relatively reniform shape. The left kidney was normal.

fluid level—and therefore fetal lung development—is unaffected. An abnormality in the contralateral kidney is not uncommon, and contralateral ureteropelvic junction obstructions are often seen. Bilateral MDK (19% incidence in one study of contralateral MDK disease) or MDK with contralateral renal agenesis (11%) is incompatible with life. There is a question of at least partial genetic influence in this disorder, which has a 3 to 5% familial recurrence rate. The sonographic image (Fig. 24-21) consists of multiple large anechoic cysts of variable size the largest of which is not central (more typical of hydronephrosis). The kidney may vary in size from small to normal to large, but the reniform shape is often absent. Increased echogenicity between the cysts is usually due to connective tissue proliferation. The renal pelvis and proximal ureter are absent or atretic. Histologically, these kidneys typically consist of thick-walled cysts, small groups of tubules, and poorly formed glomeruli. Nephrons, although few in number, can produce urine, which is why these dysplastic kidneys have been reported occasionally to increase in size. Many reports of disappearing MDKs may, in part, be related to eventual cessation of any urine production.[21,56,74,108,132]

Autosomal dominant (or adult) polycystic kidney disease is rarely seen in antenatal life. Case reports note cysts interspersed in the cortex and medulla of bilaterally enlarged kidneys. Small cysts may not be resolved and the kidneys may appear only echogenic. Although adult PKD is a bilateral disease, there may be asymmetry of involvement. Amniotic fluid levels may be normal or decreased.[38,90,116,122]

Type IV dysplasia occurs secondary to an early obstruction of the GU tract. Usually seen in severe cases of posterior urethral valves, it is commonly seen in association with the more severe obstruction of urethral atresia (Fig. 24-22). It has been reported in the caudal regression syndrome with persistent cloaca and other obstructions. There is significant oligohydramnios and moderately enlarged kidneys with small to medium capsular or parenchymal (usually peripheral) cysts. Depending on the site of obstruction distal obstructions of long standing may also show bladder wall thickening and enlargement as well as ureteral dilatation and a tortuous ureteral course.[6,21,89]

RENAL TUMORS

Fetal renal hamartomas (congenital mesoblastic nephromas) are the most common renal neoplasms of the first few months of life. They have been noted

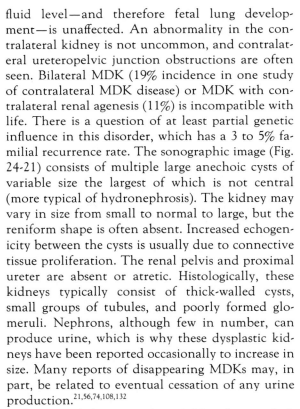

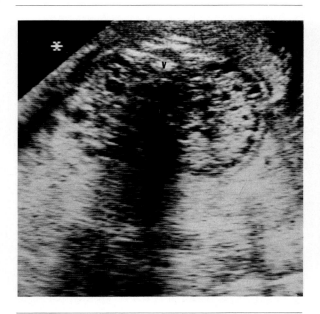

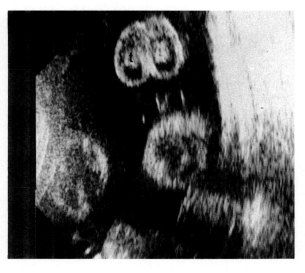

FIGURE 24-23. Hydrocele. In a coronal view, fluid surrounds each testicle (t, right testis) in this scrotum surrounded by amniotic fluid.

FIGURE 24-22. Cystic renal dysplasia, type IV. Transverse plane image shows scattered cysts, mostly peripheral, in these enlarged kidneys of a fetus with GU tract obstruction due to urethral atresia (v, vertebral body).

antenatally as unilateral echogenic masses. Bilateral fetal renal tumors may be simulated by the enlarged but functioning kidneys associated with tyrosinosis, glycogen storage diseases, and other congenital metabolic disorders.

RENAL VEIN THROMBOSIS

Renal vein thrombosis (RVT) is a well-known entity in neonates that often presents with palpably enlarged kidney(s) and associated hematuria or varying degrees of renal failure. Theoretical etiologies include septicemia, maternal diabetes, prenatal steroid administration, and congenital renal defects. Linear echoes or densities within the kidneys suggest the pathognomonic intrarenal calcification within thrombosed renal vessels.[13,65,107]

Scrotum

Fetal hydroceles (Fig. 24-23) are very common. A variable amount of fluid remaining from normal testicular descent into the scrotum can be seen sur-

rounding the testes. These hydroceles do not increase in size and tend to be resorbed within the first 9 months of life. Enlarging hydroceles indicate continued patency of the processus vaginalis and continued communication with the peritoneum and are readily noted in fetal ascites. Increasing scrotal volume may indicate an inguinal hernia. Intrascrotal extension of meconium peritonitis may produce echogenic or calcified intrascrotal masses.[21,71,93]

Adrenal

In the presence of renal agenesis, the adrenal gland may assume a more circular shape and simulate a kidney, particularly as viewed on transverse section.

Anencephalic fetuses have small adrenal glands, allegedly because no ACTH is produced.[15] The adrenal gland also weighs less in the offspring of preeclamptics and patients with antepartum hemorrhage.[34]

The diagnosis of congenital malignant neoplasms is very rare. Most of those discovered antenatally have been neuroblastomas, the most common extracranial solid malignancy of children. At least four instances of antenatal detection of adrenal neuroblastomas have been reported. The sonographic pattern is nonspecific: mixed cystic and solid, solid, and hyperechoic masses are reported. The asymmetry of these masses may help differentiate them from fetal adrenal hemorrhage.[34,41]

The Intraluminal Gastrointestinal Tract
Esophagus

Rapid proliferation of the esophageal epithelium during the fetal embryonic period creates almost complete closure of the esophageal lumen. One infant in every 2500 live births, predominantly males, may have a complication thought to be due to this esophageal maldevelopment or to unequal partitioning of the foregut into the esophagus and trachea resulting in esophageal atresia.[59] Several types are described. The most common consists of a proximal esophageal pouch with communication with the more distal gastrointestinal (GI) tract through a fistula between the tracheobronchial tree of the respiratory tract, usually at or near the tracheal bifurcation, and the more distal esophagus. Communication with the more distal GI tract significantly reduces the number of fetuses that present with polyhydramnios due to impaired swallowing. Polyhydramnios (Fig. 24-24) has been reported in 76% of affected fetuses but in only 8% of those with an associated fistula. Another helpful sign for the antenatal diagnosis of this entity is the absence of a fluid-filled stomach. Even fetuses with a fistula may have only partly filled stomachs. Cases have been reported of actual antenatal visualization of the area of esophageal atresia. This finding requires the fortuitous presence of fluid in the proximal esophagus at the time of imaging.[33,59,115]

Esophageal atresia is associated with Down's syndrome and other chromosomal abnormalities and is part of the VATER or VACTERL association (*v*ertebral abnormalities, *a*nal atresia, *c*ardiac abnormalities, *t*racheo*e*sophageal, *r*enal, and *l*imb {or *r*adius} abnormalities). Fetuses should be viewed for each of these abnormalities if any one of them is present.[124,144]

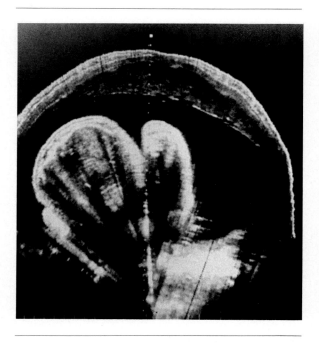

FIGURE 24-24. Polyhydramnios and esophageal atresia. Transverse plane view through gravid uterus demonstrates polyhydramnios. This fetus proved at birth to have esophageal atresia without distal GI tract communication. The atresia itself was not imaged antenatally.

Stomach

A fluid-filled stomach noted in the left upper quadrant may allow the sonographer or sonologist to image adjacent normal structures, such as the spleen, and to rule out other abnormalities besides esophageal atresia without fistula—abdominal situs inversus, diaphragmatic hernia, upper GI tract obstruction. The absence of stomach fluid can be seen on a physiologic basis in oligohydramnios or in the purported stress of nonimmune hydrops, despite polyhydramnios.[10,44]

Duplications of Stomach and Bowel. Duplications can exist throughout the bowel. They are probably due to errors of GI lumen recanalization, and in the stomach in particular, to errors in the development of normal inpouching of the longitudinal folds. Stomach duplication is the least common, although 109 cases have been reported in the literature through 1984.[10]

Antenatal diagnoses of duplications have been made in all parts of the GI tract. They are typically echoless cystic structures, occasionally filled with echogenic hemorrhagic or inspissated material. Echogenic inner walls may be seen, owing to the mucosal lining.[9,69,96,141]

SMALL BOWEL AND GASTROINTESTINAL TRACT OBSTRUCTIONS

Causes of small bowel obstruction include the aforementioned intestinal duplications as well as bowel atresia or stenosis, midgut volvulus and congenital peritoneal bands, internal hernias, and Hirschsprung's disease when it involves the entire colon.[105]

Duodenal atresia occurs in one in 10,000 births. As a result of failure of recanalization during the embryonic period, there is usually a membrane or diaphragm in the duodenum in its descending (second) or horizontal (third) portion. Less often, the duodenal atresia is due to transverse diaphragms, blind-ending loops connected by a linear fibrous attachment or unconnected blind loops. Fluid filling the stomach and the duodenum at the site of obstruction creates the classic double bubble image (Fig. 24-25), which according to some can be imaged at about 24 weeks, when swallowed fluid amounts exceed the resorptive capacity of the gut. Cases diagnosed before 24 weeks have been reported. The double bubble image is nonspecific and can be seen in other entities, including duodenal stenosis (typically involving the third or fourth portion of the duodenum), annular pancreas (a ring of anomalously rotated pancreas encircling the descending portion of the duodenum), and in association with anomalous peritoneal bands associated with abnormal bowel rotation, and often midgut volvulus.[44,59,123]

Almost half of duodenal atresia cases are associated with other anomalies (Table 24-5). One-fifth are cardiovascular, 22 to 40% are bowel malrotations, and as many as one-third are associated with trisomy 21. About 50% of affected fetuses show symmetric growth retardation, and, as with any high GI tract obstruction, many (45%) have polyhydramnios. Seven percent have associated esophageal atresia and tracheoesophageal fistula. Early

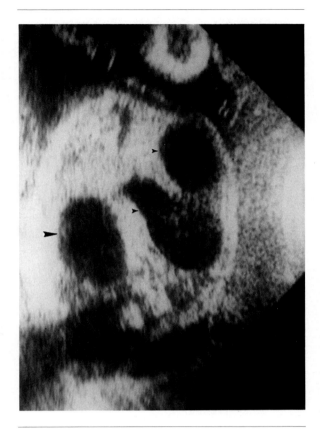

FIGURE 24-25. Double bubble sign. Transverse oblique plane view shows fluid-filled stomach (*small arrowhead*), in this case visualized with a little more anatomic detail than the classic single bubble of stomach and second bubble of proximal duodenum (*large arrowhead*). Although typically it is due to duodenal atresia, the double bubble sign is nonspecific. In this case it was due to a more distal jejunal atresia.

TABLE 24-5. Prevalence of anomalies associated with duodenal atresia[39,44,59,100]

ANOMALY	PREVALENCE (%)
Cardiovascular	20
Bowel malrotation	22–40
Trisomy 21	33
Symmetric growth retardation	50
Polyhydramnios	45
Esophageal atresia or tracheoesophageal fistula	7

neonatal surgery is associated with a good GI tract result.[39,44,59,100]

Duodenal atresia may be part of an apple-peel or Christmas tree form of intestinal atresia, extensive atresia involving most of the small bowel to the proximal ileum. This is thought to be due to prenatal obstruction of either the right colic or marginal branch of the superior mesenteric artery. Impaired blood supply to the jejunum and ileum are thought to be responsible for jejunoileal atresia (Fig. 24-26), which occurs with a frequency of once in every 12,500 to 20,000 births. Twenty to thirty percent of these cases are associated with polyhydramnios. Although there may be one long atresia or multiple small areas of atresia, antenatal ultrasound examination shows only dilated loops of bowel.[59,82,123]

The findings of polyhydramnios, a disproportionately dilated proximal small bowel, the failure to detect normal colon until late pregnancy, fetal ascites or peritoneal calcifications, decreased or absent peristalsis in dilated bowel loops noted over a period of time, and a large abdominal circumference for gestational age should make the examiner suspicious of a small bowel obstruction. Lack of bowel contents entering the large bowel can produce microcolon.[44] Perforations are the cause of ascites and meconium peritonitis. Proximal lesions are associated with higher incidences of polyhydramnios. Peristalsis is not always easy to determine in the small bowel and it is not seen in large bowel. Functional causes of bowel dilatation may simulate obstruction, for example, the rare congenital chloridorrhea, with its profuse chloride diarrhea, dilated small bowel, and microcolon.[44,50]

Midgut Volvulus

The bowel attains its normal position and configuration after a 270-degree rotation, of which the first 180 degrees occurs in the extraembryonic coelom at the base of the umbilical cord (in weeks 6 through 10). The remaining 90 degrees occurs within the fetal abdomen. If the small bowel fails to enter the abdominal cavity and rotate properly or if the long mesenteric attachments that fix the bowel to the posterior abdominal wall fail to develop the bowel will be malrotated and may twist about the axis of the superior mesenteric artery, resulting in poor vascular flow to the small bowel dis-

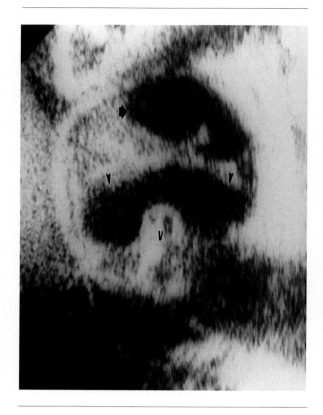

Figure 24-26. Jejunal atresia. Fluid fills a dilated transverse duodenum (*arrowheads*) noted crossing the midline vertebral body (v). This suggests normal bowel rotation. More distal bowel dilatation was noted, suggesting jejunal atresia, although the specific site of obstruction could not be determined antenatally (*arrow*, stomach).

tal to the point of obstruction or volvulus. If it is not untwisted surgically, infarction will result.[20,23,59]

Midgut volvulus is usually diagnosed in the first days of life, as the infant presents with distention, obstruction, or bilious vomiting. Antenatal diagnosis has been made by noting mild polyhydramnios, an echogenic mass under the fetal liver, and slightly dilated bowel loops. It is logical that one may note, antenatally, the typical neonatal sonographic image of a fluid-filled proximal duodenum with an arrowhead twist at the point of descending or transverse duodenal obstruction.[20,24,129]

COLON

Obstruction is more difficult to diagnose in the large bowel than in the small bowel. There is no increase in amniotic fluid level. Normal colon tends to be seen only later in pregnancy (third trimester), and peristalsis is not seen. The major causes of large bowel obstruction are imperforate anus, or anal atresia, and Hirschsprung's disease (an aganglionosis of part or the entire colon). Focal bowel dilatation has been reported as an antenatal clue. Total colonic Hirschsprung's disease is a particularly difficult diagnoses to make because of the lack of a normal segment of bowel for comparison.[59,105,142]

Dilated bowel is also an antenatal sonographic sign of cystic fibrosis (CF), an inherited (autosomal recessive) dysfunction of the exocrine and mucus-producing glands, most particularly of the pancreas, biliary tract, intestines, and bronchi, with associated disturbances of mucus and electrolyte secretion. It is the most common lethal genetic condition among Caucasians, occurring at a frequency of once in 2000 live births.[45,105,137]

A colon diameter greater than 18 mm in a preterm fetus is considered abnormal. Fetuses have been treated antenatally by the addition of urografin (a hyperosmolar agent) to the amniotic cavity. Within the bowel it can draw fluid into the meconium and loosen it.[105,130]

Obstruction of the small bowel (meconium ileus) may lead to perforation and the previously noted complications and findings of meconium peritonitis. Noteworthy, however, is the fact that few cases of meconium peritonitis described antenatally are due to CF, even though 30 to 40% of infantile meconium peritonitis and nearly 100% of infantile meconium ileus cases are associated with CF.[45]

Abdominal Wall Defects

Abdominal wall defects occur at a rate of one in 2500 births and vary in type and complexity. The two most common types, omphalocele and gastroschisis, have been well evaluated by sonography. Other abdominal wall defects range from the mundane umbilical hernia, with its linea alba defect and protruding bowel covered by skin and subcutaneous tissue, to the complex defects of cloaca or bladder extrophy, ectopia cordis, amniotic band syndrome, and the limb–body wall complex. The development of the anterior abdominal wall is based on fusion of four ectomesodermal folds, a cephalic, a caudal, and a pair of lateral folds. Knowledge of the particular defect and its associated abnormalities is necessary for proper decision making with regard to continuation of pregnancy, method of delivery, and surgical treatment (Table 24-6).[59,104,121]

OMPHALOCELE

Omphalocele (Fig. 24-27) is a midline defect that occurs in one in 5800 births. It may be due to failure of fusion of the lateral ectomesodermal folds or to persistence of the body stalk in an area normally occupied by abdominal wall.[104,121]

Abdominal viscera, covered by an amnion/peritoneal sac, protrudes through a midline defect (2 to 10 cm) into the base of the umbilical cord. The omphalocele typically contains liver, but it may contain other viscera, usually large or small bowel, and no liver.[59,104]

Omphaloceles are often (29 to 66%) associated with other anomalies whose presence affects prognosis for the worse. Gastrointestinal anomalies are found in 30 to 50% of cases—usually bowel malrotation, but sometimes atresia or stenosis of small bowel, bowel duplication, biliary atresia, or omphalomesenteric fistula. Cardiovascular anomalies (20%) usually consist of ventricular septal defects, as well as tetralogy of Fallot, and atrioventricular valve abnormalities. Fifteen to twenty percent of patients have a chromosomal abnormality, including trisomies 13, 18, and 21.[59,72,104]

The smaller the abdominal wall defect and the fewer the associated anomalies, the better the prognosis. Defects greater than 5 cm tend to have an adverse outcome. The presence of spleen or heart in the sac leads to a poor outcome.[67,98,121]

Omphaloceles are part of several significant fetal malformation syndromes. One-seventh of omphalocele cases are associated with the Beckwith-Wiedemann syndrome (organomegaly, macroglossia, hypoglycemia, hemihypertrophy, and increased risk for Wilm's tumor).[59,121] Cloacal extrophy involves a low omphalocele with cloacal or bladder extrophy and variable caudal abnormalities (e.g., anal atresia and lower limb defects).[104]

TABLE 24-6. Anomalies involving the body wall

TYPE OF ANOMALY	DESCRIPTION	SONOGRAPHIC APPEARANCE	DIAGNOSTIC CONSIDERATIONS
Omphalocele	Herniation of abdominal viscera into the base of the umbilical cord; liver involvement common	Complex membrane-enclosed sac; midline anterior wall defect continuous with umbilical cord. Size varies with amount of involved viscera.	29–66% association with other anomalies
Gastroschisis	Herniation of abdominal viscera through an off-midline defect in the abdominal wall, usually located just to the right of the umbilicus; liver involvement very unusual	Free-floating bowel loops not bound by a sac. Insertion of the umbilical cord is normal.	Associated GI anomalies are common; anomalies of other systems are rarely seen
Umbilical cord hernia	Protrusion of a small amount of intestine at the umbilicus	Similar to omphalocele; covered by skin and subcutaneous tissue, usually less than 2–4 cm	Limited clinical significance; associated anomalies are unusual
Bladder extrophy	Congenital failure of abdominal wall to develop over bladder; urinary bladder may be everted (inside may protrude through abdominal wall)	Variable: May see a fluid-filled intrapelvic portion of bladder with a contiguous extraabdominal mass with echogenicity similar to that of soft tissue. More commonly, no fluid-filled intrapelvic bladder is seen.	Most common in males; may be associated w/ GI, GU, and musculoskeletal anomalies; must be differentiated from urachal cyst
Ectopic cordis	Defect of the lower sternum and anterior abdominal wall; heart protrudes into extrathoracic sac covered by skin or a thin membrane	Beating heart protrudes through anterior abdominal wall into amniotic fluid	Often associated w/ amniotic band syndrome; other associated anomalies include craniofacial and limb deformities and omphalocele; very poor prognosis
Limb-body wall complex (LBWC)[104]	Complex of anomalies including lateral body wall defects of thorax and abdomen with herniation of viscera; cranial, craniofacial, spinal, and limb anomalies common	Herniated viscera within a complex membrane-involved mass, severe scoliosis, cranial defects, spinal defects	A severe form of amniotic band syndrome is thought to play a major role in pathogenesis; no genetic predisposition has been identified; not compatible with life

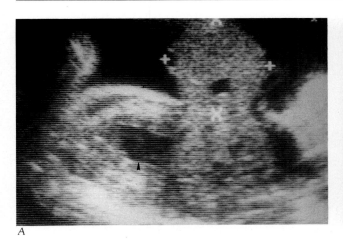
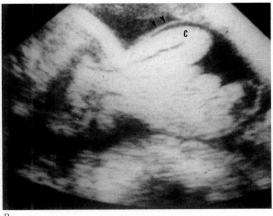

A

B

FIGURE 24-27. Omphalocele. (A) Coronal view. A large mass, marked off by crosses, is seen extending anterior to the abdomen. The abdominal cavity appears small owing to a decrease in its contents (*arrowhead*, heart). (B) Transverse oblique view of anterior abdominal wall shows that the omphalocele sac (*arrowheads*) contains colon (c). On another view the sac was seen to enter the umbilical cord. Matching images of anterior abdominal wall, omphalocele, and cord helps to confirm the diagnosis, although this is sometimes difficult with large omphaloceles.

Sonographically there is a variable number of organs within a sac extending from the abdomen into the base of the cord. Occasionally antenatal evidence of a sac membrane enables omphalocele to be differentiated from gastroschisis on postnatal examination when the sac ruptures during delivery.

GASTROSCHISIS

Gastroschisis (Fig. 24-28) is a smaller defect (2 to 4 cm) that is off midline, typically just to the right of it, and unrelated to the umbilical cord. Theoretical causes include abnormal involution of the right umbilical vein and disruption of the omphalomesenteric artery.[27] Gastroschisis occurs once in every 10,000 to 20,000 pregnancies. Except for bowel malrotation and jejunal or ileal atresia, associated anomalies are probably related to vascular compromise of the malrotated bowel and are far less common than with omphalocele. Bowel abnormalities related to vascular compromise are noted more often with the smaller abdominal wall defects.[59,104,124]

The herniated viscera, usually small or large bowel (rarely liver), are not covered by a sac. This fact leads to the development of a fibrinous coating on the bowel, probably the result of chemical peritonitis produced by its contact with fetal urine in the amniotic fluid.[75,104,121] Although there is active debate over the method of delivery, most clinicians favor cesarean section to avoid further contamination of the uncovered eviscerated bowel. Surgical closure is done primarily or in stages; a Silastic covering is placed over the bowel and abdominal wall defect between operations.[73,80]

Sonographically, this abnormality has been noted as early as 14 to 16 weeks. The diagnosis can typically be made by visualizing free-floating small bowel loops in the amniotic fluid. Sometimes the image may simulate omphalocele, and the sonographer or sonologist must attempt to rule out involvement with the midline umbilical cord.

PATENT URACHUS AND BLADDER EXTROPHY

The urachus connects the allantoic stalk to the anterior cloaca. Normally, around week 12, patency is obliterated and the urachus becomes the median

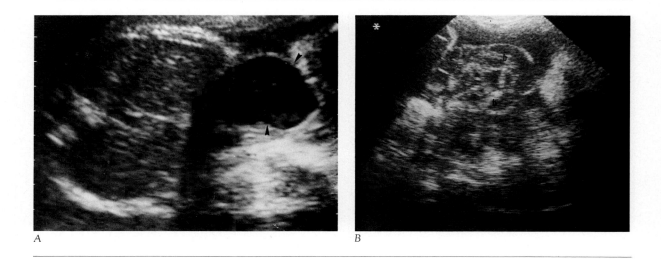

FIGURE 24-28. Gastroschisis. (A) In this transverse oblique view the stomach (*arrowheads*) is seen extending through an off-midline anterior wall defect. (B) In the transverse view several loops of small bowel (b), without a covering sac, are seen in the amniotic fluid surrounding the fetus.

vesicular ligament. Partial obliteration can lead to cystic masses between the bladder and umbilicus along the anterior abdominal wall—urachal cysts (cystic masses along the duct's course) and urachal sinuses (cystic masses that communicate with the anterior abdominal wall but not with the bladder. Rarely, patent urachus (complete communication between bladder and anterior abdominal wall at the umbilicus) may occur (1 to 2.5 per 100,000 deliveries, twice as often in boys as in girls). It has been noted antenatally as a cystic mass extending from bladder apex to anterior abdominal wall at the umbilicus. The abnormality is limited and is not associated with other significant congenital abnormalities. The mass may be noted extraabdominally and therefore may require differentiation from the more serious problem of bladder extrophy.[109]

Bladder extrophy is a more common (one in 25,000 to 40,000 births, three times more common in boys) and serious anomaly, associated with other GU, GI, and musculoskeletal abnormalities. Failure of development of a primitive streak of mesoderm in the allantoic extension of the cloacal membrane leads to variable presentations of bladder extrophy, including split bony symphysis, divergent rectus muscles, and exteriorization of the bladder. The extraabdominal mass, in variants that have an intrapelvic portion of fluid-filled bladder, are said to be echogenic, simulating omphalocele more than patent urachus.[95,109]

Pelvis

The normal fetal pelvis is small. Masses within it typically extend into the abdomen. The only routinely visualized normal organ is the fluid-filled bladder. In the third trimester, the meconium-filled echopenic and tubular rectosigmoid may be noted. Normal muscle groups are often seen to be separated by echogenic fascial lines. The two major groups of abnormality in this area are those of the female genital system, seen as masses within and extending beyond the pelvis, and sacrococcygeal teratomas, noted as predominantly external masses with variable internal pelvic extension. The posterior soft tissues, made up predominantly of the gluteal muscles, should be symmetric.

teric duplications, or mesenteric cysts. They may simulate hydrometrocolpos. Pedunculation can cause a gynecologic mass to present in a high abdominal location where its area of origin is obscured. Bilateral multiseptate cystic pelvic masses in a female fetus suggest an ovarian origin.[25,85,117]

Ovarian cysts, unlike hydrometrocolpos, are said not to compress the GU system, although they can compress bowel. This may be responsible for the one case in ten associated with polyhydramnios, when very large, ovarian cysts may cause dystocia. Ovarian cysts may be noted in association with hypothyroidism.[25,64,85]

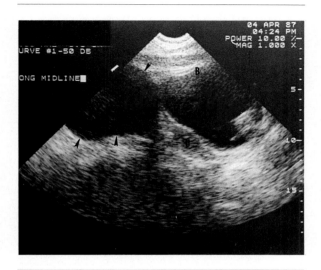

FIGURE 24-29. Ovarian cyst. Longitudinal view of pelvis shows a large cystic mass (*arrowheads*) superior to this newborn's uterus (U) and bladder (B). The mass extends into the abdomen, simulating an abdominal mass.

Female Genital System

Despite maternal hormone stimulation, antenatal visualization of vagina, uterus, or ovary is possible only if there is abnormal enlargement or a pelvic mass.[85]

Hydrometrocolpos, a cystic dilatation of the vagina and uterus due to mucus accumulation proximal to a point of obstruction, is noted as a hypoechoic mass posterior to the bladder that may occasionally compress the lower ureters, leading to hydronephrosis. When the obstruction is due to vaginal atresia or a vaginal membrane there may be associated genitourinary tract abnormalities.[1,22,25,85]

Fetal ovarian cysts are noted infrequently on ultrasound examination and are nearly always benign. They probably develop in response to maternal hormonal stimulation. Small follicular cysts not visualized on fetal examination are found in as many as one-third of autopsy specimens. Ovarian cysts may be unilocular (Fig. 24-29) or multiseptate masses that typically rise into the abdomen when enlarged. Internal echogenicity may be noted as the result of complications of torsion or hemorrhage. They may be simulated by urachal cysts, en-

Sacrococcygeal Teratoma

The sacrococcygeal teratoma (SCT) is the most common tumor noted in neonatal life. Associated morbidity and mortality related to prematurity, dystocia, traumatic delivery, and intratumor hemorrhage make antenatal diagnosis very important. The increased incidence (2 to 4% in newborns, 60% in 4-month-old infants) of malignant components discovered in SCTs, as time goes on, suggests the need for early diagnosis and excision to prevent malignant degeneration.[25,63]

Typically noted as a large mass off the fetal rump, SCT occurs in one in every 40,000 births, more often in twin gestations. Affected females outnumber males by a ratio of four to one. SCT develops during fetal life, and its growth tends to parallel that of the fetus. The pregnancy is often large for gestational age. These masses may have significant intrapelvic extensions and have been classified according to the degree of exterior component or intrapelvic extension (Table 24-7). There are no associated sacral vertebral anomalies,

TABLE 24-7. Classification of sacrococcygeal teratoma

Type I	Predominantly *external* component, minimal presacral or intrapelvic extension
Type II	Predominantly *external* component, significant *intrapelvic* extension
Type III	Small external component, significant *intrapelvic/intraabdominal* component
Type IV	No apparent external component, predominantly *presacral* or *intrapelvic* tumor

(Data from Hogge W, Thiagarajah S, Barber V, et al. Cystic sacrococcygeal teratoma. J Ultrasound Med. 1987;6:707.)

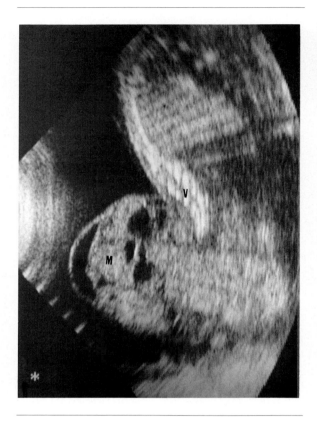

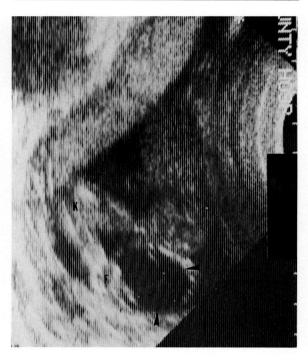

FIGURE 24-31. Cystic sacrococcygeal teratoma. On the sagittal view a cystic mass (*arrowheads*) extends from this fetus' rump as if the fetus were sitting on it (K, knee; F, foot).

FIGURE 24-30. Sacrococcygeal teratoma. Sagittal view shows a predominantly solid mass (M) extending from the patient's sacral area. No vertebral column (v) abnormality was noted.

References

1. Abraham D, Koenigsberg M, Hoffman-Tretin J. The prenatal ultrasound appearance of hydrometrocolpos. J Diagn Med Sonogr. 1985; 1:115–116.
2. Adzick N, Harrison M, Glick P, et al. Diaphragmatic hernia in the fetus: Prenatal diagnosis and outcome in 94 cases. J Pediatr Surg. 1985; 20:357–361.
3. Albright E, Crane J, Schakelford G. Prenatal diagnosis of bronchogenic cyst. J Ultrasound Med. 1988; 7:91–95.
4. Avni E, Vanderelst A, Van Gansbeke D, et al. Antenatal diagnosis of pulmonary tumours: Report of two cases. Pediatr Radiol. 1986; 16:190–192.
5. Beck A. The effect of intrauterine urinary obstruction upon the development of the fetal kidney. J Urol. 1971; 105:784–789.
6. Benacerraf B, Frigoletto F Jr. Mid-trimester fetal thoracentesis. J Clin Ultrasound. 1985; 13:202–204.
7. Benacerraf B, Brass V, Laboda L, et al. A sono-

although the incidence of associated vertebral anomalies in other locations is increased.[63,134]

On antenatal examination, those with external masses are easiest to diagnose. The tumors may be solid or of mixed (Fig. 24-30) echogenicity with interspersed or peripheral cystic components. About 15% of SCTs are cystic (Fig. 24-31). There is little correlation between size and consistency and ultimate prognosis. The imaging of increased echogenicity or echogenicity and shadowing due to contained calcification is variable. The intrapelvic mass may be noted when mass effect causes bowel or ureteral dilatation or by anterior compression of the bladder. Cystic intrapelvic SCTs may simulate anterior meningocele, ovarian cyst, or bladder.[25,63,136]

graphic sign for detection of Down syndrome. Am J Obstet Gynecol. 1985; 151:1078–1079.

8. Beretsky I, Lankin D. Diagnosis of fetal cholelithiasis using real-time high resolution imaging employing digital detection. J Ultrasound Med. 1983; 2:381–383.

9. Bidwell J, Nelson A. Prenatal ultrasonic diagnosis of congenital duplication of the stomach. J Ultrasound Med. 1986; 5:589–591.

10. Blanc W, Berdon W, Baker D, et al. Calcified portal vein thromboemboli in newborn and stillborn infants. Radiology. 1967; 88:287–292.

11. Bowie J. Sonography of fetal abdominal abnormalities. In: Sanders R, James A, eds. The Principles and Practice of Ultrasonography in Obstetrics and Gynecology. 3rd ed. Norwalk, CT: Appleton-Century-Crofts; 1985.

12. Brar M, Cubberley D, Baty B, et al. Chest wall hamartoma in a fetus. J Ultrasound Med. 1988; 7:217–220.

13. Brill P, Mitty H, Strauss L. Renal vein thrombosis: A cause of intrarenal calcification in the newborn. Pediatr Radiol. 1977; 6:172–175.

14. Butler N, Claireaux A. Congenital diaphragmatic hernia as a cause of perinatal mortality. Lancet. 1962; 1:659–663.

15. Callan N, Colmorgen H, Weiner S. Lung hypoplasia and prolonged preterm ruptured membranes: A case report with implication for possible prenatal ultrasonic diagnosis. Am J Obstet Gynecol. 1985; 151:756–757.

16. Carter R, Waterston D, Aberdeen E. Hernia and eventration of the diaphragm in childhood. Lancet. 1962; 1:656–659.

17. Chervenak F, Isaacson G, Blakemore KJ, et al. Fetal cystic hygroma: Cause and natural history. N Engl J Med. 1983; 309:822–825.

18. Chinn D. Ultrasound evaluation of hydrops fetalis. In: Callen P, ed. Ultrasonography in Obstetrics and Gynecology. 2nd ed. Philadelphia: WB Saunders; 1988.

19. Chung W. Antenatal detection of hepatic cyst. J Clin Ultrasound. 1986; 14:217–219.

20. Cloumer M, Fried A, Selke A. Antenatal observation of midgut volvulus by ultrasound. J Clin Ultrasound. 1983; 11:286–288.

21. Cohen H, Haller J. Diagnostic sonography of the fetal genitourinary tract. Urol Radiol. 1987; 9:88–98.

22. Cohen H, Haller J. Pediatric and adolescent genital tract abnormalities. In: Babcock D, ed. Neonatal and Pediatric Ultrasonography. New York: Churchill Livingstone; 1989.

23. Cohen H, Haller J. Fluid aided US of the pediatric upper gastrointestinal tract. Appl Radiol. 1988; 17:28–35.

24. Cohen H, Haller J, Mestel A, et al. Neonatal duodenum: fluid-aided US examination. Radiology. 1987; 164:805–809.

25. Comstock C. Fetal masses: Ultrasound diagnosis and evaluation. Ultrasound Quart. 1988; 6:229–256.

26. Cyr D, Guntheroth W, Nyberg D, et al. Prenatal diagnosis of an intrapericardial teratoma. A cause for nonimmune hydrops. J Ultrasound Med. 1988; 7:87–90.

27. DeVries P. The pathogenesis of gastroschisis and omphalocele. J Pediatr Surg. 1980; 15:244–251.

28. Dewbury K, Aluwihare M, Birch S, et al. Prenatal ultrasound demonstration of a choledochal cyst. Br J Radiol. 1980; 53:906–907.

29. Dillard J, Edwards D, Leopold G. Meconium peritonitis masquerading as fetal hydrops. J Ultrasound Med. 1987; 6:49–51.

30. Dubbins P, Kurt A, Wapner R, et al. Renal agenesis: spectrum of in utero findings. J Clin Ultrasound. 1981; 9:189–193.

31. Elieser S, Ester F, Ehud W, et al. Fetal splenomegaly, ultrasound diagnosis of cytomegalovirus infection: A case report. J Clin Ultrasound. 1984; 12:520–521.

32. Elrad H, Mayden K, Ahart S, et al. Prenatal ultrasound diagnosis of choledochal cyst. J Ultrasound Med. 1985; 4:553–555.

33. Eyheremendy E, Fister M. Antenatal real-time diagnosis of esophageal atresia. J Clin Ultrasound. 1983; 11:395–397.

34. Ferraro E, Fakhry J, Aruny J, et al. Prenatal adrenal neuroblastoma. Case report with review of the literature. J Ultrasound Med. 1988; 7:275–278.

35. Fine C, Adzick N, Doubilet P. Decreasing size of a congenital cystic adenomatoid malformation in utero. J Ultrasound Med. 1988; 7:405–408.

36. Fleischer A, Davis R, Campbell L. Sonographic detection of a meconium-containing mass in a fetus. A case report. J Clin Ultrasound. 1983; 11:103–105.

37. Fleischer A, Killam A, Boehm F, et al. Hydrops fetalis: Sonographic evaluation and clinical implications. Radiology. 1981; 141:163–168.

38. Fong K, Rahmani M, Rose T, et al. Fetal renal cystic disease: Sonographic-pathologic correlation. AJR. 1986; 146:767–773.

39. Fonkalsrud E, DeLorimer A, Hays M. Congenital atresia and stenosis of duodenum. A review compiled from members of the surgical section of the American Academy of Pediatrics. Pediatrics. 1969; 43:79–83.

40. Foster M, Nyberg D, Mahony B, et al. Meconium peritonitis: Prenatal sonographic findings and their clinical significance. Radiology. 1986; 165:661–665.

41. Gadwood K, Reynes C. Prenatal sonography of metastatic neuroblastoma of the neck. J Clin Ultrasound. 1983; 11:512–515.

42. Giulian B. Prenatal ultrasonographic diagnosis of fetal renal tumors. Radiology. 1984; 152:69–70.

43. Glazer G, Filly R, Callen P. The varied sonographic appearance of the urinary tract in the fetus and the newborn with urethral obstruction. Radiology. 1982; 144:563–568.

44. Goldstein R, Callen P. Ultrasound evaluation of the fetal thorax and abdomen. In: Callen P, ed. Ultrasonography in Obstetrics and Gynecology. 2nd ed. Philadelphia: WB Saunders; 1988.

45. Goldstein R, Filly R, Callen P. Sonographic diagnosis of meconium ileus in utero. J Ultrasound Med. 1987; 6:663–666.

46. Graham D, Sanders R. Amniotic fluid. Semin Roentgenol. 1982; 17:210–218.

47. Graham D, Sanders R. Sonographic evaluation of the fetal chest. In: Sanders R, James A Jr, eds. The Principles and Practice of Ultrasonography in Obstetrics and Gynecology. 3rd ed. Norwalk, CT: Appleton-Century-Crofts; 1985.

48. Grignon A, Filion R, Filiatrault D, et al. Urinary tract dilatation in utero. Classification and clinical applications. Radiology. 1986; 160:645–647.

49. Grignon A, Filiatrault D, Homsy Y, et al. Ureteropelvic junction stenosis: Antenatal ultrasonographic diagnosis, postnatal investigation and follow-up. Radiology. 1986; 160:649–651.

50. Groli C, Zucca S, Cesaretti A. Congenital chloridorrhea: antenatal ultrasonographic appearance. J Clin Ultrasound. 1986; 14:293–295.

51. Gruenewald S, Crocker E, Walker A, et al. Antenatal diagnosis of urinary tract abnormalities: Correlation of ultrasound appearance with postnatal diagnosis. Am J Obstet Gynecol. 1984; 148:278–283.

52. Habif D, Berdon W, Yeh M. Infantile polycystic disease: In utero sonographic diagnosis. Radiology. 1984; 152:143–146.

53. Harrison M, Adzick N, Nakayama D, et al. Fetal diaphragmatic hernia: Fatal but fixable. Semin Perinatol. 1985; 9:103–112.

54. Hashimoto B, Filly R, Callen P. Fetal pseudoascites: Further anatomic considerations. J Ultrasound Med. 1986; 5:151–152.

55. Hashimoto B, Filly R, Callen P. Sonographic detection of fetal intraperitoneal fluid. J Ultrasound Med. 1986; 5:203–204.

56. Hashimoto B, Filly R, Callen P. Multicystic dysplastic kidney in utero: Changing appearance on US. Radiology. 1986; 159:107–109.

57. Hayden S, Russ P, Pretorius D, et al. Posterior urethral obstruction: Prenatal sonographic findings and clinical outcome in fourteen cases. J Ultrasound Med. 1988; 7:371–375.

58. Helin I, Persson P. Prenatal diagnosis of urinary tract abnormalities by ultrasound. Pediatrics. 1986; 78:879–883.

59. Hill L. Sonographic detection of fetal gastrointestinal anomalies. Ultrasound Quart. 1988; 6:35–68.

60. Hill L, Peterson C. Antenatal sonographic diagnosis of fetal pelvic kidneys. 1987; 6:393–396.

61. Hill L, Breckle R, Gehrking W. The prenatal detection of congenital malformations by ultrasonography. Mayo Clin Proc. 1983; 5:805–826.

62. Hoddick W, Filly R, Mahony B, et al. Minimal renal pyelectasis. J Ultrasound Med. 1985; 4:85–89.

63. Hogge W, Thiagarajah S, Barber V, et al. Cystic sacrococcygeal teratoma. Ultrasound diagnosis and management. J Ultrasound Med. 1987; 6:707–710.

64. Jafri S, Bree R, Silver T. Fetal ovarian cysts: sonographic detection and association with hypothyroidism. Radiology. 1984; 150:809–812.

65. Jayogopal S, Cohen H, Brill P, et al. Neonatal renal vein thrombosis. Demonstration by CT and US. Pediatr Radiol. 1990; 20:2.160–162.

66. Jeffrey R Jr, Laing F, Wing V, et al. Sonography of the fetal duplex kidney. Radiology. 1984; 153:123–124.

67. Jones P. Exomphalos. A review of 45 cases. Arch Dis Child. 1963; 38:180–187.

68. Jouppila P, Kirkinen P, Herva R, et al. Prenatal diagnosis of pleural effusions by ultrasound. J Clin Ultrasound. 1983; 11:516–519.

69. Kangerloo H, Sample W, Harven G, et al. Ultrasonic evaluation of abdominal gastrointestinal duplication in children. Radiology. 1979; 131:191–194.

70. Keller M, Markle B, Laffey P, et al. Spontaneous resolution of cholelithiasis in infants. Radiology. 1985; 157:345–348.

71. Kenney P, Spirt B, Ellis D, et al. Scrotal masses caused by meconium peritonitis: Prenatal sonographic diagnosis. Radiology. 1985; 154:362.

72. Kim S. Omphalocele. Surg Clin North Am. 1976; 56:361–371.

73. Kirk E, Wah R. Obstetric management of the fetus with omphalocele or gastroschisis. A review and report of one hundred and twelve cases. Am J Obstet Gynecol. 1983; 146:512–518.

74. Kleiner B, Filly R, Mack L, et al. Multicystic dysplastic kidney: Observations of contralateral disease in the fetal population. Radiology. 1986; 161:27–29.

75. Kluck P, Tibboel D, van der Kamp A, et al. The effect of fetal urine on the development of the bowel in gastroschisis. J Pediatr Surg. 1983; 18:47–50.

76. Knochel J, Lee T, Melendez M, et al. Fetal anomalies involving the thorax and abdomen. Radiol Clin North Am. 1982; 20:297–310.

77. Kurtz A, Goldberg B. Fetal body measurements. In:

Obstetrical Measurements in Ultrasound. A Reference Manual. Chicago: Year Book Medical Publishers; 1988.

78. Laing F, Burke V, Wing V, et al. Postpartum evaluation of fetal hydronephrosis: Optimal timing for follow-up sonography. Radiology. 1984; 152:423–424.

79. Lauer J, Craddock T. Meconium pseudocyst: prenatal sonographic and antenatal radiologic correlation. J Ultrasound Med. 1982; 1:333–335.

80. Lenke R, Hatch E Jr. Fetal gastroschisis: A preliminary report advocating the use of cesarean section. Obstet Gynecol. 1986; 67:395–398.

81. Lichman J, Miller E. Prenatal ultrasonic diagnosis of splenic cyst. J Ultrasound Med. 1988; 7:637–638.

82. Lyrenis S, Cnattingius S, Lingberg B. Fetal jejunal atresia and intrauterine volvulua—A case report. J Perinatol Med. 1982; 10:247–248.

83. McGahan J, Myracle M. Adrenal hypertrophy: Possible pitfall in the sonographic diagnosis of renal agenesis. J Ultrasound Med. 1986; 5:265–268.

84. McNamara J, Eraklis A, Gross R. Congenital posterolateral diaphragmatic hernia in the newborn. J Thorac Cardiovasc Surg. 1968; 55:55–59.

85. Mahony B. The genitourinary system. In: Callen P, ed. Ultrasonography in Obstetrics and Gynecology. 2nd ed. Philadelphia: WB Saunders; 1988.

86. Mahony B, Filly R. The genitourinary system in utero. Clin Diagn Ultrasound. 1986; 18:1–21.

87. Mahony B, Callen P, Filly R. Fetal urethral obstruction: US evaluation. Radiology. 1985; 157:221–224.

88. Mahony B, Filly R, Callen P, et al. Severe non-immune hydrops fetalis: Sonographic evaluation. Radiology. 1984; 151:757–761.

89. Mahony B, Filly R, Callen P, et al. Fetal renal dysplasia: Sonographic evaluation. Radiology. 1984; 152:143–146.

90. Main D, Mennuti M, Cornfeld D, et al. Prenatal diagnosis of adult polycystic kidney disease. Lancet. 1983; 2:337.

91. Mariona F, McAlpin G, Zador I, et al. Sonographic detection of fetal extrathoracic pulmonary sequestration. J Ultrasound Med. 1986; 5:283–285.

92. Mayor G, Genton N, Torado A, et al. Renal function in obstructive nephropathy: Long-term effects of reconstructive surgery. Pediatrics. 1975; 56:740–743.

93. Meizner I, Katz M, Zamora E, et al. In utero diagnosis of congenital hydrocele. J Clin Ultrasound. 1983; 11:449–451.

94. Miller R, Sieber W, Unis E. Congenital cystic adenomatoid malformation of the lung. Pathol Ann. 1980; 15:387–407.

95. Mirk P, Calisti A, Fileni A. Prenatal sonographic diagnosis of bladder extrophy. J Ultrasound Med. 1986; 5:291–293.

96. Moore K. Body cavities, primitive mesenteries, and diaphragm. In: The Developing Human: Clinically Oriented Embryology. 3rd ed. Philadelphia: WB Saunders; 1982.

97. Moore P, Mencini R, Spitz H. Sonographic diagnosis of hydramnios and oligohydramnios. Semin Ultrasound CT MR. 1984; 5:157–169.

98. Moore T. Gastroschisis and omphalocele: Clinical differences. Surgery. 1977; 82:561–568.

99. Nakamoto S, Dreilinger A, Dattel B, et al. The sonographic appearance of hepatic hemangioma in utero. J Ultrasound Med. 1983; 2:239–241.

100. Nelson L, Clark C, Fishburne J, et al. Value of serial sonography in the in utero detection of duodenal atresia. Obstet Gynecol. 1982; 59:657–660.

101. Newnham J, Crues J, Vinstein A, et al. Sonographic diagnosis of thoracic gastroenteric cyst in utero. Prenatal Diagn. 1984; 4:467–471.

102. Norio R, Kaarininen H, Rapola J, et al. Familial congenital diaphragmatic defects. Aspects of etiology, prenatal diagnosis and treatment. Am J Med Genet. 1984; 17:471–483.

103. Nussbaum A, Dorst J, Jeffs R, et al. Ectopic ureterocele: Their varied sonographic manifestations. Radiology. 1986; 159:227–235.

104. Nyberg D, Mack L. Abdominal wall defects. In: Callen P, ed. Ultrasonography in Obstetrics and Gynecology. 2nd ed. Philadelphia: WB Saunders; 1988.

105. Nyberg D, Hastrup W, Watts H, et al. Dilated fetal bowel. A sonographic sign of cystic fibrosis. J Ultrasound Med. 1987; 6:257–260.

106. Osthanondh V, Potter E. Pathogenesis of polycystic kidneys. Arch Pathol. 1964; 77:459–512.

107. Patel R, Connors J. In utero sonographic findings in fetal renal vein thrombosis with calcifications. J Ultrasound Med. 1988; 7:349–352.

108. Pedicelli G, Jequier S, Bowen A, et al. Multicystic dysplastic kidneys: Spontaneous regression demonstrated with US. Radiology. 1986; 161:23–26.

109. Persutte W, Lenke R, Kropp K, et al. Antenatal diagnosis of fetal patent urachus. J Ultrasound Med. 1988; 7:399–403.

110. Petres R, Redwine F, Cruikshank D. Congenital bilateral chylothorax: Antepartum diagnosis and successful intrauterine surgical management. JAMA. 1982; 248:1360–1361.

111. Pezzuti R, Isler R. Antenatal ultrasound detection of cystic adenomatoid malformation of lung: Report of case and review of the recent literature. J Clin Ultrasound. 1983; 11:342–346.

112. Phillips H, McGahan J. Intrauterine fetal cystic hy-

gromas. Sonographic detection. AJR. 1981; 136:799–802.

113. Platt L, Devore G, Benner P, et al. Antenatal diagnosis of a fetal liver mass. J Ultrasound Med. 1983; 2:521–522.

114. Potter E. Bilateral absence of ureters and kidneys. Obstet Gynecol. 1965; 25:3–12.

115. Pretorius D, Meier P, Johnson M. Diagnosis of esophageal atresia in utero. J Ultrasound Med. 1983; 2:475–476.

116. Pretorius D, Lee M, Manco-Johnson M, et al. Diagnosis of autosomal dominant polycystic kidney disease in utero and in the young infant. J Ultrasound Med. 1987; 6:249–255.

117. Preziosi P, Fariello G, Moiorana A, et al. Antenatal sonographic diagnosis of complicated ovarian cysts. J Clin Ultrasound. 1986; 14:196–198.

118. Queenan J, O'Brien G. Diagnostic ultrasound in erythroblastosis fetalis. In: Sanders R, James EA Jr. The Principles and Practice of Ultrasonography in Obstetrics and Gynecology. 3rd ed. Norwalk, CT: Appleton-Century-Crofts; 1985.

119. Rempen A, Feige A, Wunsch P. Prenatal diagnosis of bilateral cystic adenomatoid malformation of the lung. J Clin Ultrasound. 1987; 15:3–8.

120. Romero R, Pilu G, Jeanty P, et al. The lungs. In: Prenatal Diagnosis of Congenital Anomalies. East Norwalk, CT: Appleton & Lange; 1988.

121. Romero R, Pilu G, Jeanty P, et al. The abdominal wall. In: Prenatal Diagnosis of Congenital Anomalies. East Norwalk, CT: Appleton & Lange; 1988.

122. Romero R, Pilu G, Jeanty P, et al. The urinary tract and adrenal glands. In: Prenatal Diagnosis of Congenital Anomalies. East Norwalk, CT: Appleton & Lange; 1988.

123. Romero R, Pilu G, Jeanty P, et al. The gastrointestinal tract and intraabdominal organs. In: Prenatal Diagnosis of Congenital Anomalies. East Norwalk, CT: Appleton & Lange; 1988.

124. Sabbagha R, Comstock C. Abnormalities of the chest and gastrointestinal tract. In: Sabbagha R, ed. Diagnostic Ultrasound Applied to Obstetrics and Gynecology. 3rd ed. Philadelphia: JB Lippincott; 1987.

125. Sabbagha R, Sheik Z. Skeletal abnormalities. In: Diagnostic Ultrasound Applied to Obstetrics and Gynecology. 3rd ed. Philadelphia: JB Lippincott; 1987.

126. Sabbagha R, Chervenak F, Isaacson G. External body defects. In: Sabbagha R, ed. Diagnostic Ultrasound Applied to Obstetrics and Gynecology. 3rd ed. Philadelphia: JB Lippincott; 1987.

127. Sabbagha R, Dalcampo S, Shkolnick A. Correlative anatomy. In: Sabbagha R, ed. Diagnostic Ultrasound Applied to Obstetrics and Gynecology. 3rd ed. Philadelphia: JB Lippincott; 1987.

128. Salzman L, Kuligowska E, Semine A. Pseudoomphalocele: pitfall in fetal sonography. AJR. 1986; 146:1283–1285.

129. Samuel N, Dicker D, Feldberg D. Ultrasound diagnosis and management of fetal intestinal obstruction and volvulus in utero. J Perinatal Med. 1984; 12:333–337.

130. Samuel N, Dicker D, Landman J, et al. Early diagnosis and intrauterine therapy of meconium plug syndrome in the fetus: Risks and benefits. J Ultrasound Med. 1986; 5:425–428.

131. Sarti D. Ultrasound evaluation of normal and abnormal fetal anatomy. In: Sarti D, ed. Diagnostic Ultrasound. Text and Cases. 2nd ed. Chicago: Year Book Medical Publishers; 1987.

132. Schifer T, Heller R. Bilateral multicystic dysplastic kidneys. Pediatr Radiol. 1988; 18:242–244.

133. Schmidt W, Yarkoni S, Jeanty P, et al. Sonographic measurements of the fetal spleen: Clinical implications. J Ultrasound Med. 1985; 4:667–672.

134. Schoenecker S, Cyr D, Mack L. Sonographic diagnosis of bilateral fetal renal duplication with ectopic ureteroceles. J Ultrasound Med. 1985; 4:617–618.

135. Seeds J. Antenatal sonographic assessment of the genitourinary tract. In: Sanders R, Hill M, eds. Ultrasound Annual 1986. New York: Raven Press; 1986.

136. Sheth S, Nussbaum A, Sanders R, et al. Prenatal diagnosis of sacrococcygeal teratoma: Sonographic-pathologic correlation. Radiology. 1988; 169:131–136.

137. Simpson J, Elias S. Genetic amniocentesis. In: Sabbagha R, ed. Diagnostic Ultrasound. Applied to Obstetrics and Gynecology. Philadelphia: JB Lippincott; 1987.

138. Skiptunas S, Weiner S. Early prenatal diagnosis of asphyxiating thoracic dysplasia (Jeune's syndrome). Value of fetal thoracic measurement. J Ultrasound Med. 1987; 6:41–43.

139. Soper T, Pringle K, Schofield J. Creation and repair of diaphragmatic hernia in the fetal lamb: Techniques and survival. J Pediatr Surg. 1984; 19:33–40.

140. Stocker T, Madewell J, Drake RT. Congenital cystic adenomatoid malformation of the lung: Classification and morphologic spectrum. Hum Pathol. 1977; 8:155–171.

141. van Dam L, deGroot C, Hazeborek F, et al. Intrauterine demonstration of bowel duplication by ultrasound. Eur J Obstet Gynecol Reprod Biol. 1984; 18:229–232.

142. Vermesh M, Mayden K, Confino E, et al. Prenatal sonographic diagnosis of Hirschsprung's disease. J Ultrasound Med. 1986; 5:37–39.

143. Weiss J, Cohen H, Haller J, et al. Cystic abnormalities of the fetal thorax. Sonographic evaluation. J

Diag Med Sonogr. 1987; 3:172–176.

144. Witt D, Hall J. Multiple congenital anomaly syndromes. In: Rudolph A, Hoffman J, Axelrod S, eds. Pediatrics. 18th ed. East Norwalk, CT: Appleton & Lange; 1987.

145. Wladimiroff J. Effect of furosemide on fetal urine production. Br J Obstet Gynaecol. 1975; 82:221–224.

146. Woodard J. Prune belly syndrome. In: Kelalis P, King R, Belman A, eds. Clinical Pediatric Urology. 2nd ed. Philadelphia: WB Saunders; 1985.

147. Zimmer E, Weintraub Z. Antenatal diagnosis of a fetus with an extremely narrow thorax and short limb dwarfism. J Clin Ultrasound. 1984; 12:112–114.

CHAPTER 25

Normal and Abnormal Fetal Limbs

BIRGIT BADER-ARMSTRONG

The fetal long bones routinely measured during an ultrasound examination to determine gestational age (GA) are the femur and the humerus. The femur is considered more accessible to ultrasound than the humerus because it is not overshadowed by the head or chest and because the legs tend to move less than the arms. When it is impossible to obtain good measurements of the femur and humerus, other long bones can be assessed. GA estimation nomograms are available for most bones from the 12th week to term (Appendixes J–L).

In addition to dating the pregnancy, measurement and evaluation of the limbs documents their existence, whether they are properly mineralized and formed, and how they are positioned. A skeletal abnormality is often a characteristic of a syndrome involving other organs. Such a finding should alert the sonographer to proceed with a thorough fetal anatomic examination and to obtain a family history for any genetically transmitted skeletal abnormalities.

In this chapter, we explain how to scan long bones and how to determine whether a limb is normal or abnormal, and we discuss the most prevalent fetal limb malformations with their associated anomalies (Table 25-1).

Normal Fetal Limbs

ANATOMY

It is the calcium content of the bones that generates the high-amplitude reflection on ultrasound and permits imaging of the appendicular and axial skeleton. The diaphysis (shaft) of the long bone is the primary ossification center and may be especially well-visualized in the first trimester via a transvaginal approach (Fig. 25-1). The epiphysis is separated from the shaft by a layer of cartilage and is the secondary ossification center (Fig. 25-2). The two epiphyseal plates seen on ultrasound are the distal femoral epiphysis (visible at 32 to 35 weeks) and the proximal tibial epiphysis (visible by 34 or 35 weeks). The proximal humeral epiphysis does not form until term.

The metacarpals and phalanges of the fetal hand are visible in the second trimester (Fig. 25-3); the carpal bones ossify after birth. The talus, calcaneus, metatarsals, and phalanges of the foot begin to calcify during the second trimester.

SONOGRAPHIC TECHNIQUE

To image the femur, the examiner should scan in a transverse plane through the fetal trunk toward the bladder. The bright echoes on either side of the bladder are the iliac bones. The femur is found lat-

TABLE 25-1. Skeletal dysplasias and their associated anomalies

Dysplasia	Curved or Bowed Long Bones	Hypo-mineralization	Bone Fractures	Radial Aplasia	Polydactyly	Macrocephaly	Heart Disease	Narrow Thorax
Achondrogenesis		x	x					x
Achondroplasia						x		x
Asphyxiating thoracic dysplasia					x		x	x
Camptomelia	x	x				x		x
Ellis-van Creveld syndrome					x		x	
Holt-Oram syndrome				x			x	
Hypophosphatasia	x	x	x					
Osteogenesis imperfecta	x	x	x					
Roberts' syndrome		x		x			x	
Short rib-polydactyly syndrome					x			x
TAR				x			x	
Thanatophoric dwarfism	x	x				x		x
VACTERL associations				x	x		x	

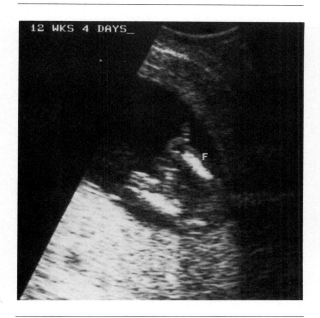

FIGURE 25-1. Femur (F) was imaged at 12.5 weeks using a transvaginal probe.

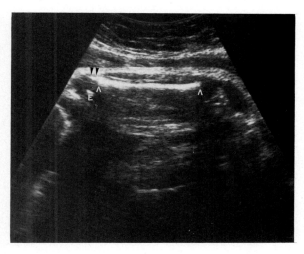

FIGURE 25-2. Femur at 37 weeks demonstrates the end points of the ossified shaft (*white arrows*), reflections from the lateral aspect of the distal femoral epiphyseal cartilage (*black arrows*), and the distal femoral epiphysis (E).

eral and caudad to the ilium. Rotating the transducer until the longest axis of the shaft is obtained is a hand-eye coordination task that requires practice. A normal shaft is fairly straight, symmetric, and evenly ossified. In the lower leg, the tibia (the medial shaft) is thicker than the fibula.

Care must be taken to ensure that the longest dimension of the ossified shaft is visualized and that the ends of the image are sharply defined. The ends may be blunted or slightly curved. In a normal pregnancy, mild bowing of either femoral shaft produced by the curved medial border of the femur may be seen after 18 weeks' GA. The posterior lying femur often has a more pronounced bowing, mimicking skeletal dysplasia (Fig. 25-4). Mild artifactual bowing should not cause an inaccurate measurement, but if the transducer is not perpendicular to the shaft, an oblique view is obtained and the measurement is artificially shortened. Acoustic shadowing should fall perpendicular to and behind the long bone, to verify the correctness of the scanning plane. The femur length can be overestimated by several millimeters

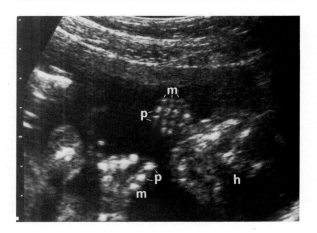

FIGURE 25-3. Fetal hands at 18 weeks' gestation show the phalanges (p) and metacarpals (m) (fetal head, h).

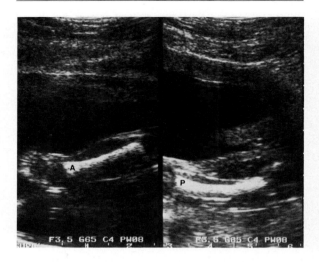

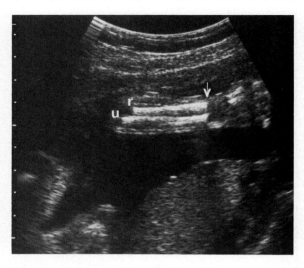

FIGURE 25-4. Femurs at 21 weeks' gestation. The shaft of the anterior femur (A) has slight normal curvature. The posterior femur (P) exhibits a more pronounced artifactual bowing.

FIGURE 25-5. Radius (r) and ulna (u) at 25 weeks' gestation. Note that the distal radius and ulna end at the same point (*arrow*).

by including the "distal femur point," which is believed to be a reflection from the smooth surface of the lateral aspect of the distal femoral epiphyseal cartilage, and therefore not part of the ossified femoral shaft (Fig. 25-2).[10] Normal growth patterns of the long bones have been established to determine GA.[11,12,25] Be sure the tables used in your laboratory are appropriate for your patient population and type of equipment used (linear or sector scanner). Serial measurements of fetal long bones are useful in the diagnosis of skeletal dysplasias; in the presence of such conditions long bone growth may be appropriate in early pregnancy then may drop below the 10th percentile for GA in the second trimester.

To measure the humerus, the operator scans in transverse sections toward the fetal shoulders and rotates the transducer on the scapula. The transducer is gently rocked back and forth, to be certain only one bone (the humerus) is seen and not two (the radius and ulna). Obtaining a good image of the shaft of the humerus in late pregnancy requires more patience than imaging the femur, as the upper arm is often wedged between the trunk and the uterine wall. When evaluating the lower arm, the sonographer should document that the distal radius and ulna end at the same point (Fig. 25-5). This is a helpful landmark for assessing lower arm reductions. The ulna is the longer of the two bones.

Several technical factors may limit the sonographer's ability to visualize limbs. Limbs located in the near field are often difficult to delineate. An acoustic standoff pad shifts the focal zone of the transducer to the region of interest. Oligohydramnios results in poor overall resolution of the crowded fetus. Limbs may be tucked under the trunk or lie in a bizarre position. A transvaginal approach may be helpful when scanning a pregnancy complicated by severe oligohydramnios (Fig. 25-6). With polyhydramnios, the fetus is often very active or may lie beyond the focal range of the transducer. The patient can be positioned on her elbows and knees, so that the operator can scan the abdomen from beneath.

Patience is the key to obtaining a good diagnostic scan. A fetus that remains in an unfavorable position may be encouraged to move by having the

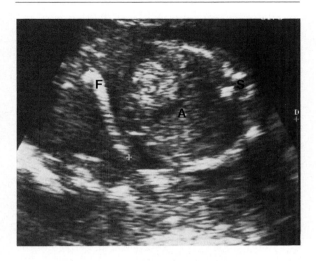

FIGURE 25-6. A 17-week pregnancy was complicated by severe oligohydramnios. An initial transabdominal scan was unable to identify or measure any fetal limbs. A transvaginal approach demonstrated a femur length (F) consistent with 16 weeks' gestation. Fetal abdomen (A) and spine (S) are seen in cross section.

TABLE 25-2. Lethal dysplasias

Achondrogenesis
Asphyxiating thoracic dysplasia*
Camptomelic dysplasia*
Ellis-van Creveld syndrome*
Homozygous achondroplasia
Hypophosphatasia*
Osteogenesis imperfecta type II
Roberts' syndrome
Short rib–polydactyly syndrome
TAR syndrome*
Thanatophoric dysplasia
VACTERL associations*

*Mildly affected persons may survive.

patient get off the table and empty her bladder or take a short walk. A last resort is to have the patient return the next day.

Abnormal Fetal Limbs

Skeletal dysplasia is abnormal development of the cartilaginous and osseous tissues resulting in bones that appear shortened, deformed, or thin or that fail to form at all. Some syndromes are uniformly lethal, and others are lethal in their more severe forms (Table 25-2).

Most forms of short-limbed dwarfism are inherited. In autosomal dominant forms of dwarfism, such as achondroplasia, there is a 50% chance that an affected parent will pass the trait to the offspring. When both parents are affected, the fetus has a 25% chance of not inheriting the gene from either parent and, so, of being normal; a 50% chance of receiving the gene from one parent and being affected; and a 25% chance of inheriting the gene from both parents. The latter genotype is homozygous and is associated with the most severe form of dysplasia. When both parents are carriers of the gene for an autosomal recessive trait there is a 25% chance that the fetus will receive two genes for that trait and, therefore, inherit the dysplasia. When unaffected parents have a child with a skeletal dysplasia as the result of spontaneous mutation the risk of recurrence in subsequent pregnancies is minimal.

As a group, skeletal dysplasias are rare and are not always detectable prenatally by ultrasound. For example, osteogenesis imperfecta type IV is not severe enough to be demonstrated in utero. Fetuses affected with heterozygous achondroplasia may exhibit normal femur length growth patterns until 21 to 26 weeks' gestation.[14] A sporadic occurrence of this form of dwarfism may be missed if the patient is scanned only during the first trimester or early second trimester.

Short-limb dysplasia is classified into four descriptive categories. *Rhizomelia* is shortening of a proximal extremity such as the humerus or femur. *Mesomelia* is middle-segment limb shortening that affects the radius, ulna, tibia, and fibula. *Acromelia* is a distal extremity shortening involving the hands and feet. *Micromelia* is shortening of an entire extremity.

SONOGRAPHIC TECHNIQUE

Skill, patience, and an accurate patient history are the major components of a good ultrasound examination when there is a suspicion of skeletal dysplasia. Although a detailed examination, including

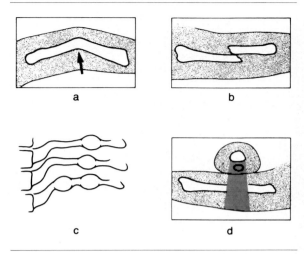

FIGURE 25-7. Appearance of fractures. (A) Highly angled shaft, (B) overlapping segments of bone, (C) beading of the ribs caused by the callus formation at the fracture site, (D) sonographic pitfall. "Gap" caused by shadowing from fetal limb is not a fracture. (Donnenfeld AE, Mennuti MT. Second trimester diagnosis of fetal skeletal dysplasias. Obstet Gynecol Sur. 1987;4d:204.)

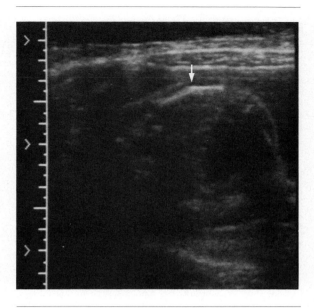

FIGURE 25-8. Sonogram of fracture site (arrow) in a femur. (Filly RA, Golbus MS. Ultrasonography of the normal and pathologic fetal skeleton. Rad Clin North Am. 1982;20:321.)

a finger and toe count, is beyond the time restrictions of a routine ultrasound examination, a closer look is certainly indicated when a patient presents with a history of genetically transmitted skeletal abnormalities or whenever a bone abnormality is noted on routine examination.

Protocol for Scanning a Fetus at Risk.
Document and measure each limb.
Look for:

1. True bowing of the femurs, which may result in a short-for–GA measurement, versus the curved medial border of the normal femur.
2. A sharply angulated midshaft, indicating a fracture (Figs. 25-7, 25-8).
3. Shadowing from other fetal limbs may artificially shorten a long bone or even create a gap that mimics a fracture (Fig. 25-9).
4. Abnormal skeletal mineralization, which makes bones appear thin, unevenly mineralized, or, in the cranium, difficult to visualize (Fig. 25-10).

Determine dominant category of limb shortening (Table 25-3).

Note whether the the distal radius and ulna end at the same point to rule out radial hypoplasia (Fig. 25-5).

Measure thoracic circumference–to–abdominal circumference ratio (normal ratio .89)[3] to rule out an abnormally narrow thorax, which may cause respiratory distress at birth.

Check for any other associated abnormalities such as polyhydramnios, polydactyly, prominent skin folds, cleft lip or palate, and three-vessel umbilical cord.

Perform a fetal cardiac examination to evaluate a fetus with skeletal malformations associated with congenital heart disease.

Table 25-4 lists skeletal dysplasias by their ultrasound findings. When a genetically transmitted skeletal dysplasia is suspected, a genetic amniocentesis for chromosomal analysis may be indicated to confirm the diagnosis. Fetoscopy may be consid-

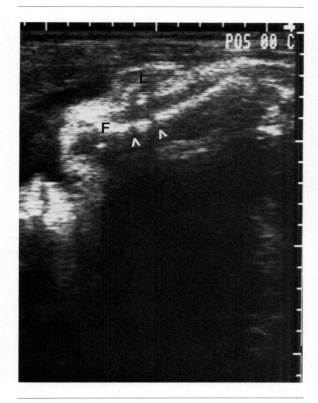

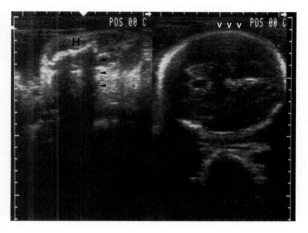

FIGURE 25-10. Osteogenesis imperfecta type II. The humerus (H) is short, misshapen, and shows uneven acoustic shadowing due to faulty mineralization (*black arrowheads*). The cranium is poorly mineralized.

FIGURE 25-9. Sonographic pitfall. Shadowing from fetal limb (L) may artificially shorten a femur (F) or may create gaps mimicking fractures (*arrowheads*).

TABLE 25-3. Dominant category of limb shortening in skeletal dysplasias

SKELETAL DYSPLASIA	DOMINANT CATEGORY
Achondrogenesis	Micromelia*
Achondroplasia	Rhizomelia†
Asphyxiating thoracic dysplasia	Mesomelia‡
Camptomelic dysplasia	Mesomelia, rhizomelia
Congenital hypophosphatasia	Micromelia
Ellis-van Creveld syndrome	Rhizomelia
Hypophosphatasia	Micromelia
Osteogenesis imperfecta	Micromelia
Radial aplasia, hypoplasia	Mesomelia
Short rib–polydactyly syndrome	Micromelia
Thanatophoric dysplasia	Micromelia

*Shortening of entire extremity
†Shortening of proximal extremity
‡Middle segment limb shortening (radius, tibia)

ered to visualize limbs of suspected fetuses in early pregnancy. A plain film of the abdomen may also be helpful. Often, the prognosis for the fetus is the determining factor in the patient's decision to terminate the pregnancy. Should the pregnancy continue, an accurate diagnosis is helpful for planning subsequent obstetric care.

SKELETAL DYSPLASIAS

Thanatophoric Dysplasia. Thanatophoric (death-producing) dysplasia is one of the more common forms of lethal congenital short-limbed dwarfism. Its etiology is unknown. It presents sonographically as extreme micromelia, bowed long bones, narrow thorax, protruding abdomen (champagne cork appearance), general hypomineralization of all bones, and short ribs (Fig. 25-11).[4,13,16] Associated abnor-

malities of the head are macrocephaly due to hydrocephalus and frontal bossing (protruding forehead). Thanatophoric dwarfism with cloverleaf skull occurs when premature closure of the coronal and lambdoid sutures causes the temporal bones to bulge. This gives the head a trilobular, or clover-

Table 25-4. Sonographic findings in skeletal dysplasias

Curved or bowed long bones
Camptomelic dysplasia
Hypophosphatasia
Osteogenesis imperfecta
Thanatophoric dysplasia

Hypomineralization
Achondrogenesis
Camptomelic dysplasia
Hypophosphatasia
Osteogenesis imperfecta
Short rib–polydactyly syndrome
Thanatophoric dysplasia

Narrow thorax
Achondrogenesis type I
Achondroplasia
Asphyxiating thoracic dysplasia
Camptomelic dysplasia
Short rib–polydactyly syndrome
Thanatophoric dysplasia

Polydactyly
Asphyxiating thoracic dysplasia*
Ellis-van Creveld syndrome
Short rib–polydactyly syndrome
VACTERL association*

Radial aplasia or hypoplasia
Holt-Oram syndrome
Roberts' syndrome
TAR
VACTERL associations

Bone fractures
Achondrogenesis
Hypophosphatasia
Osteogenesis imperfecta

Heart disease
Asphyxiating thoracic dysplasia
Ellis-van Creveld syndrome
Holt-Oram syndrome
Roberts' syndrome
Short rib–polydactyly syndrome*
VACTERL association*

Macrocephaly
Achondroplasia
Camptomelic dysplasia*
Thanatophoric dysplasia

*Does not occur in all cases

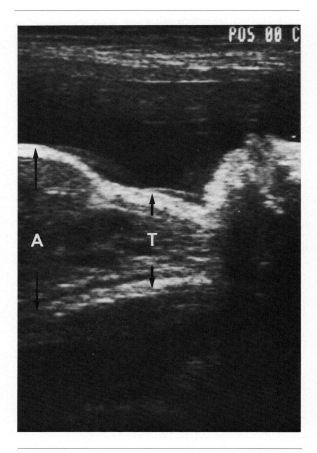

Figure 25-11. Longitudinal view of a thanatophoric dwarf. The thorax (T) is narrow and the abdomen (A) protrudes, giving a champagne cork appearance.

leaf, appearance (Fig. 25-12).[29,32] Massive polyhydramnios is a prominent feature and may lead to premature labor.[30] The infant dies shortly after birth from cardiorespiratory failure.

Achondroplasia. Achondroplasia is inherited in an autosomal dominant manner, but it frequently appears as a spontaneous disorder. It falls within the rhizomelia category of skeletal dysplasia with associated limb bowing.[14] The hands have short fingers in a trident configuration. Occasional associated findings are macrocephaly, frontal bossing, and hydrocephalus.[25] Serial femur length measurements may fall within the normal range up to 26 weeks' gestation. A normal life expectancy is possible, although the person may suffer from spinal problems, pulmonary compromise, and difficulties during pregnancy due to a small pelvis. Adult height

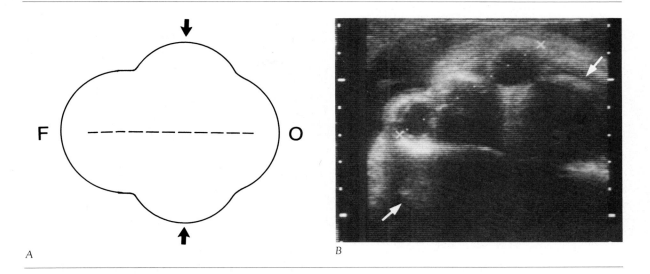

A   *B*

FIGURE 25-12. (A) Schematic diagram. Bulging of the temporal bones (*arrows*); occiput (O); frontal bone (F). (Weiner CP, Williamson RA, Bonsib SM. Sonographic diagnosis of cloverleaf skull and thanatophoric dysplasia in the second trimester. J Clin Ultrasound 1986;14:463-465.) (B) Only the bulging of the temporal bones (*arrows*) can be seen on this transverse view of the cloverleaf skull of a thanatophoric dwarf. Markers are measuring outer orbital distance.

averages 49 inches for women and 52 inches for men. The homozygous form, inherited from two parents who are heterozygous achondroplastic dwarfs, is a lethal condition.

Achondrogenesis. Achondrogenesis types I and II may be autosomal recessive conditions or may occur spontaneously. Type I is characterized by micromelia, a narrow thorax with extremely short ribs, and polydactyly. Type II is more severe and presents with extreme micromelia, a short thorax, and protruding abdomen. Although the entire skeleton shows varying degrees of hypomineralization, the spinal column is especially affected.[17] The short, thin fetal ribs may show evidence of multiple fractures. This condition may be associated with polyhydramnios and hydrops (Fig. 25-13)[2]; however, excess skin folds over a shortened frame may also give the appearance of hydrops.[19] Achondrogenesis results in stillbirth or neonatal death due to pulmonary hypoplasia.

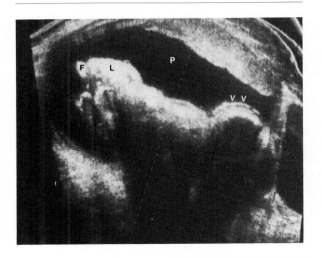

FIGURE 25-13. Fetus affected by achondrogenesis. The lower limbs (L) are short, and the foot (F) is seen. There is scalp edema (*arrowheads*) and marked polyhydramnios (P).

Short Rib–Polydactyly Syndrome. This syndrome may have a similar appearance to achondrogenesis. It is differentiated by additional findings of polydactyly, cardiac and genitourinary anomalies, and cleft lip.[5,9,23] Transmission is autosomal recessive. Manifestations of the dysplasia vary, and four types of short rib–polydactyly syndrome have been identified. Each has a fatal prognosis.

Asphyxiating Thoracic Dysplasia. This rare, autosomal recessive disease is also known as Jeune's syndrome. Major findings on ultrasound examination are shortening of the extremities, funnel-shaped chest with short, horizontal ribs, and renal dysplasia.[6,15] Occasionally, polydactyly occurs. Severity of the disease varies. The majority of affected infants die within the first year from respiratory failure and infections. A few survive through early adulthood.

Ellis-van Creveld Syndrome. Features of this rare chondroectodermal dysplasia vary widely. There is an autosomal recessive mode of inheritance. Most often, only the femurs are shortened, rather than both the humeri and femurs. An atrial septal defect occurs in over 50% of those affected with this syndrome. A partial or pseudo-cleft lip and postaxial polydactyly (an extra digit on the medial side) may also be seen if it contains a bony structure. With proper postnatal care, half of those affected can survive into adulthood.[20,25]

Osteogenesis Imperfecta. This dysplasia is an inherited collagen disorder characterized by varying degrees of hypomineralization of the entire skeleton. Bones are fragile and may become deformed or easily fractured.[33] Sillence and coworkers[27] classified osteogenesis imperfecta (OI) into four groups.

Type I occurs most frequently and is autosomal dominant. Diagnosis in utero is difficult because fractures usually occur after birth.

Type II, the most severe form, has an autosomal recessive transmission pattern. Its major sonographic landmarks include long bones and ribs which are shortened, bowed, or fractured, and decreased acoustic shadowing behind hypomineralized long bones.[1,7,22] The outline of the skull may be irregular and intracranial structures unusually well-visualized owing to a thin cranium (Figs. 25-8,

25-10). Amniocentesis should be considered to evaluate the pryophosphate level. A high value may indicate OI.[28] Most fetuses are stillborn or die early in the neonatal period of cardiorespiratory complications and infections.

Type III may be either autosomal recessive or autosomal dominant. Long bone fractures may be present at birth or may not appear until the child begins to walk. Although the child may survive into adulthood, long bones and spine become progressively deformed.

Type IV is an autosomal dominant condition and the mildest manifestation of the disease. The life span may be normal, but the person may be short of stature.

Camptomelic Dysplasia. The term camptomelic, coined from the Greek word for "bent limb," describes the characteristic findings of bowed long bones (Fig. 25-7). The tibia and fibula are most severely affected. It must be noted that some fetuses affected with camptomelic dysplasia do not have bowed limbs. Associated abnormalities include shortened and poorly ossified long bones, and a narrow, barrel-shaped thoracic cage.[5,8,31] Occasional findings include hydrocephalus, macrocephaly, cleft palate, and polyhydramnios. This is a rare form of short-limbed dwarfism. Many cases are sporadic; however, autosomal recessive transmission is suggested. The majority of affected children die in early infancy from respiratory failure.

Congenital Hypophosphatasia. Hypophosphatasia is an autosomal recessive metabolic disorder. The principal sonographic finding is severe hypomineralization of the entire skeleton. The calvarium is especially difficult to demonstrate and is easily compressed by its environment. Ribs are short and have a beaded appearance. Limbs are bowed, fractured, and shortened. Polyhydramnios may be present.[5,17,34] There is a wide variation in the severity of this syndrome. Those who are severely affected die early in infancy from respiratory failure. The osseous anomalies of mildly affected infants tend to improve in time.

LIMB ABNORMALITIES
Some limb abnormalities, such as polydactyly and most limb reductions, are features of more complex

genetic disorders. Other limb abnormalities result from maternal conditions and embryonic malformations. Limb abnormalities are not life-threatening in themselves. The prognosis for the fetus depends on whether other disorders are involved.

Polydactyly. Polydactyly is the presence of extra fingers or toes either on the medial aspect (postaxial) or lateral aspect (preaxial). It is a frequent finding in several genetic syndromes such as trisomy 13 and short rib–polydactyly syndrome. The extra digit may be visualized on ultrasound if it contains a bony structure.

Limb Reduction Abnormality. Limb reduction is the congenital absence of one or more limbs or segments of limbs. The following terms are often used:

Amelia:	absence of one or more limbs
Hemimelia:	absence of one or more extremities below elbow or knee
Acheiria:	absence of one or more hands
Apodia:	absence of one or more feet
Adactyly:	absence of one or more digits from hands or feet
Phocomelia:	absence of proximal portion of extremity with hand or foot attached to trunk

Radial Aplasia, Hypoplasia. Approximately 25 syndromes are characterized by radial aplasia or hypoplasia. Some, such as trisomy 13, 18, and 22, have genetic origins (Fig. 25-14). Other causes are exogenous agents such as thalidomide and some cases are idiopathic. To determine whether the radius is hypoplastic, the examiner should note whether the distal end of the radius lines up with the distal end of the ulna (see Fig. 25-5). Also, the hand on the affected limb is radially deviated (club hand).

Holt-Oram syndrome. Transmission is autosomal dominant. Other findings include congenital heart disease, absence of thumbs, and phocomelia.

Thrombocytopenia–absent radius (TAR) syndrome. This is an autosomal recessive blood disorder. Absence of the radius usually is bilateral. The sonographic feature in this syndrome that differentiates it from other absent radius syndromes is the presence of five fully formed digits. In other syn-

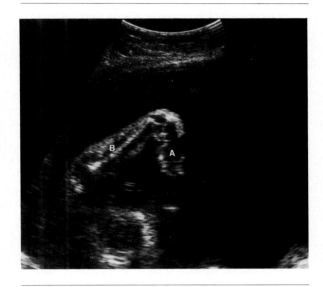

FIGURE 25-14. Radial aplasia in a fetus affected by trisomy 18. The hand (A) is seen attached to the end of the humerus (B).

dromes, the thumb may not be formed. Unilateral or bilateral absence of the ulna and humerus may also be noted. Occasional findings include heart defects or renal anomalies. Infant mortality is approximately 40%, owing to hemorrhage early in infancy.

Roberts' syndrome. This is a symmetric dysmorphism syndrome involving upper and lower limbs with an autosomal recessive transmission pattern. Additional findings include cleft lip or palate, phocomelia, and growth deficiency. Occasional findings are frontal encephalocele, renal and cardiac abnormalities, and polyhydramnios.

VACTERL association (vertebral anomalies, anal atresia, cardiac anomalies, tracheoesophageal fistula, renal anomalies, limb dysplasia). At least three features of this association must be demonstrated to make a diagnosis. A single umbilical artery may be seen.

Club Foot. Club foot is characterized by medial deviation and inversion of the sole of the foot. Although club foot is part of many genetic syndromes, an individual may have only a genetic

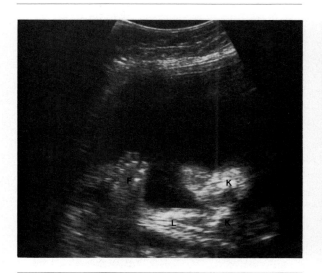

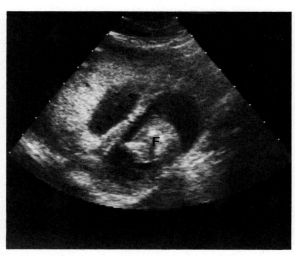

FIGURE 25-15. Medial deviation of a club foot (F). The lower leg (L) and both knees (K) are seen on the same plane.

FIGURE 25-16. Amniotic band (*arrowheads*) is attached from uterine wall to uterine wall. Fetal parts (F) are seen on one side of the band.

predisposition to laxity of joint ligaments. It is also associated with spina bifida and nongenetic conditions such as caudal regression syndrome, muscular dystrophy, lead poisoning, oligohydramnios, and positional constraint. On ultrasound, the club foot can be imaged on the same frontal plane as the lower leg and is almost at a right angle with the ankle (Fig. 25-15). A normal foot is seen in transverse section and perpendicular to the lower leg.

Amniotic Band Syndrome. The exact explanation for the formation of amniotic bands is unknown. It is thought that they probably occur after rupture of the amnion in early pregnancy. On ultrasound, bands appear as strings or cords attached from one uterine wall to another, or from the uterine wall to a fetal part (Fig. 25-16). These strands are known to entangle and amputate fetal limbs and digits. Those that attach themselves to the fetus cause mutilating deformities.[18,21] Amniotic bands detected by ultrasound have been reported to disappear as the pregnancy continued, leaving little or no evidence of their formation at delivery.[24]

Sirenomelia Sequence. Sirenomelia is an embryonic defect in the primitive streak stage that results in the fusion of the lower extremities (Fig. 25-17). It is associated with pregnancies that are complicated by poorly controlled diabetes and by monozygotic twinning. Other anomalies include absence of bladder, genital defects, renal agenesis, and oligohydramnios.

Multiple Gestation. Skeletal abnormalities occurring in multiple gestations include conjoined twins, sirenomelia, and acardiac twin. An acardiac fetus (having no heart) will present with a partial or absent upper trunk, amelia, or rudimentary limbs.

Maternal Conditions and Associated Limb Abnormalities. Maternal disease processes, medications, substance abuse, and exposure to radiation or industrial chemicals affect the environment of the fetus and may cause skeletal growth abnormalities. Obtaining a detailed and accurate medical and social history from the mother is very important.

Limb measurements below the 10th percentile

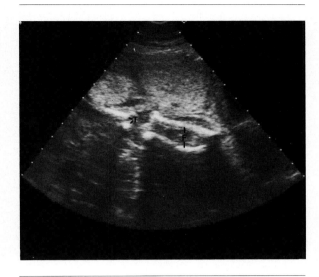

FIGURE 25-17. Sirenomelia detected at 23 weeks' gestation in the fetus of a diabetic mother. The proximity of the two femurs (F) and the proximal ends of both tibias (T) indicate fusion of the lower extremities.

are consistent with severe intrauterine retardation, fetal alcohol syndrome, drug abuse, and other conditions that are conducive to small-for-dates babies. Environmental compression due to oligohydramnios or uterine tumors can deform limbs. As a historical note, pregnant women in Europe used thalidomide in the 1960s as a remedy for nausea. During clinical trials in the United States, phocomelia was observed and therefore the FDA never approved its sale for pregnant women.

References

1. Bader B, Warner RW. Osteogenesis imperfecta type II: A review for sonographers. J Diagn Med Sonogr. 1987; 3:275–280.
2. Benacerraf B, Osathanondh R, Bieber FR. Achondrogenesis type I: Ultrasound diagnosis in utero. J Clin Ultrasound. 1984; 12:357.
3. Chitkara U, Rosenberg J, Chervenak FA, et al. Prenatal sonographic assessment of the fetal thorax: Normal values. Am J Obstet Gynecol. 1987; 156:1069–1074.
4. Cremin BJ, Ross JL. Case report 386. Skeletal Radiol. 1986; 15:495–498.
5. Donnenfeld AE, Mennuti MT. Second-trimester diagnosis of fetal skeletal dysplasias. Obstet Gynecol Surv. 1987; 42:199–217.
6. Elejalde BR, deElejalde MM, Pansch D. Prenatal diagnosis of Jeune's syndrome. Am J Med Genet. 1985; 21:433.
7. Filly RA, Golbus MS. Ultrasonography of the normal and pathologic fetal skeleton. Rad Clin North Am. 1982; 20:311–323.
8. Fryns JP, van den Berghe K, van Assche A, et al. Prenatal diagnosis of camptomelic dwarfism. Clin Genet. 1981; 19:199.
9. Gembruch U, Hansmann M, Fodisch HJ. Early prenatal diagnosis of short rib-polydactyly (SRP) syndrome type I (Majewski) by ultrasound in a case at risk. Prenatal Diagn. 1985; 5:357–362.
10. Goldstein RB, Filly RA, Simpson G. Pitfalls in femur length measurements. J Ultrasound Med. 1987; 6:203–207.
11. Hadlock FP, Harrist RB, Deter RL, et al. Ultrasonically measured fetal femur length as a predictor of menstrual age. AJR. 1982; 138:875–878.
12. Jeanty P, Rodesch F, Delbeke D, et al. Estimation of gestational age from measurements of fetal long bones. J Ultrasound Med. 1984; 3:75–79.
13. Kaufman RL, Rimoin DL, McAlister WH, et al. Thanatophoric dwarfism. Am J Dis Child. 1970; 120:53–57.
14. Kurtz AB, Filly RA, Wapner RJ, et al. In utero analysis of heterozygous achondroplasia: Variable time of onset as detected by femur length measurements. J Ultrasound Med. 1986; 5:137–140.
15. Lipson M, Waskey J, Rice J, et al. Prenatal diagnosis of asphyxiating thoracic dysplasia. Am J Med Genet. 1984; 18:273.
16. Loong EPL. The importance of early prenatal diagnosis of thanatophoric dysplasia with respect to obstetric management. Eur J Obstet Gynecol Reprod Biol. 1987; 25:145–152.
17. McGuire J, Manning F, Lange I, et al. Antenatal diagnosis of skeletal dysplasia using ultrasound. Birth defects: Orig Art Ser. 1987; 23:367–384.
18. Mahony BS, Filly RA, Callen PW, et al. The amniotic band syndrome: Antenatal sonographic diagnosis and potential pitfalls. Am J Obstet Gynecol. 1985; 152:63–68.
19. Mahony BS, Filly RA, Copperberg PL. Antenatal sonographic diagnosis of achondrogenesis. J Ultrasound Med. 1984; 3:333.
20. Mahoney MJ, Hobbins JC. Prenatal diagnosis of chondroectodermal dysplasia (Ellis-van Creveld syn-

drome) with fetoscopy and ultrasound. N Eng J Med. 1977; 297:258.

21. Malinger G, Rosen N, Achiron R, et al. Short communications: Pierre Robin sequence associated with amniotic band syndrome. Ultrasonographic diagnosis and pathogenesis. Prenatal Diagn. 1987; 7:455–459.

22. Metz E, Goldhofer W. Sonographic diagnosis of lethal osteogenesis imperfecta in the second trimester: Case report and review. J Clin Ultrasound. 1986; 14:380–383.

23. Naumoff P, Young LW, Mazler J, et al. Short rib-polydactyly syndrome type III. Radiology. 1977; 122:443–447.

24. Papp Z, Toth Z, Csecsei K, et al. Letter to the editor. Are there "innocent" amniotic bands? Am J Med Genet. 1986; 24:207–209.

25. Scott CI. Dwarfism. Summit, NJ: Ciba-Geigy; 1988; 40:3–30.

26. Seeds JW, Cefalo RC. Relationship of fetal limb lengths to both biparietal diameter and gestational age. Obstet Gynecol. 1982; 60:680–685.

27. Sillence DO, Rimoin DL, Danks DM. Clinical variability in osteogenesis imperfecta—Variable expressivity or genetic heterogeneity. Birth Defects: Orig Art Ser. 1979; 15:113–129.

28. Solomons CC, Gottesfeld K. Prenatal biochemistry of osteogenesis imperfecta. Birth Defects. 1979; 15:69.

29. Stamm ER, Pretorius DH, Rumack CM, et al. Kleeblattschadel anomaly: In utero sonographic appearance. J Ultrasound Med. 1987; 6:319–324.

30. Thompson BH, Parmley TH. Obstetric features of thanatophoric dwarfism. Am J Obstet Gynecol. 1971; 109:396.

31. Thurmon TF, DeFraites EB, Anderson EE. Familial camptomelic dwarfism. J Pediatr. 1973; 83:841.

32. Weiner CP, Williamson RA, Bonsib SM. Sonographic diagnosis of cloverleaf skull and thanatophoric dysplasia in the second trimester. J Clin Ultrasound. 1986; 14:463–465.

33. White RD, Lewis PE, Sanders RC. Prenatal sonographic diagnosis of osteogenesis imperfecta: Case reports. Virginia Med. 1984; 3:218–220.

34. Wladimiroff JW, Niermeijer MF, van der Harten JJ, et al. Early prenatal diagnosis of congenital hypophosphatasia: Case report. Prenatal Diagn. 1985; 5:47.

CHAPTER 26

Observing Fetal Maturation Through Fetal Movement and Fetal Breathing

CATHERINE A. WALLA, LAWRENCE D. PLATT

Interest in the nature of fetal activity has led to the scientific study of fetal movements and breathing over the last 100 years. Noninvasive observations in utero of the qualitative and quantitative aspects of fetal motor behavior throughout the course of pregnancy have been achieved only recently, with linear-array real-time ultrasonography. The visualization of fetal activity in terms of the current status of that activity and of its development has proven vital to the assessment of fetal condition. Recent basic and clinical investigations have indicated that not only the presence of fetal movement and breathing but also their development is a direct reflection of the status of the fetal central nervous system (CNS). The ultimate goal of clinical investigations of fetal motor behavior has been antenatal identification of fetuses with a compromised CNS in order to allow a more informed diagnosis concerning either the therapy or the timely delivery of that fetus. In this chapter we address the clinical applications of fetal movements and breathing in the determination of fetal health.

Fetal Body Movements

As early as 1885, Preyer[44] studied fetal movements directly, in aborted living fetuses with intact gestational sacs, and by palpation of the mother's abdomen. He was convinced that spontaneous fetal limb movement occurred prior to 16—and probably even 12 weeks'—gestation. More detailed studies of fetal movements have been carried out on exteriorized fetuses, but the impact of determination of the physiologic state of the fetus was not known. Other methods that have been used to detect and analyze fetal movements have included maternal perception,[7,18,46,51,56] piezoelectric crystals,[52,55] surface electrodes,[19] tocodynamometers,[16] and unprocessed Doppler signals.[63] While these methods have afforded quantification of prenatal motor behavior, they do not define the quality of fetal movements or the correlation of one type of movement to another. The introduction of ultrasound techniques has opened a new vista of analysis of fetal motor behavior.

FETAL MOVEMENT IN EARLY GESTATION

A detailed classification of individual movement patterns of the fetus was developed by three independent research groups led by Birnholz,[3] Ianniruberto and Tanjani,[21] and DeVries.[12] A comparison of these studies of early fetal motor activity demonstrates that although there are some discrepancies in the observed time of onset of the various types of movements, there is successive development from simple movements involving the whole fetal body to more complex movements (Table 26-1). DeVries group's[12] examination of the qualitative aspects of the development of fetal movement determined a specific sequence of emergence of the movements that was evident in all fetuses studied.

Table 26-1. Classification and week of onset of fetal movements

Week of Onset	de Vries et al. (1982)	Week of Onset	Birnholz et al. (1978)	Week of Onset	Ianniruberto and Tajani (1981)
7	Just discernible movements			6–7	Vermicular movements
8	Startle	7–16	Twitch	8–18	Jerky global flexion and extension
8	General movements	12–16	Combined/repetitive simultaneous or serial movements of head, trunk, and limbs	11–18	Jumps, with change of lying position
9	Hiccoughs	24	Vigorous diaphragmatic excursions	22	Sudden rhythmic diaphragm movements
10	Breathing movements	24	Respiratory	13–14	Breathing movements
9	Isolated arm or leg movement	10–12	Independent limb movements	12–13	Isolated and/or independent movement of limbs
9	Isolated retroflexion of head	14	Isolated extension of head		
9–10	Isolated rotation of head	14	Isolated rotation of head	12–13	Head rotation
10	Isolated anteflexion of head	14	Isolated flexion of head		
10–11	Jaw movements			13–14	Opening of mouth
12	Sucking and swallowing	24	Probable thumb sucking	13–14	Swallowing
10	Hand-face contact	16	Hand-face contact	12–13	Hands in contact w/ hand, face, or mouth
10	Stretch			16	Global extension
11	Yawn			12–13	Rotation, with change in lying position
10	Rotation of fetus				

(From deVries JIP, Visser GH, Prechtl HFR. Fetal motility in the first half of pregnancy. Clin Develop Med. 1984;94:46.)

It was discovered that all movements that could be identified in the term fetus were present by age 15 weeks. It should be noted that the morphologic appearance (Table 26-2) of movement patterns varies little throughout pregnancy once the patterns emerge.

The earliest movement of the fetus can be appreciated as early as 6 to 7 weeks. By 8 weeks, general movements of the limbs, trunk, and head can be identified. A "startle" motion was also seen in this period. Hiccoughs were observed as early as 9 weeks. Fetal breathing movements, both regular and irregular, have been identified as early as 10 weeks—as solitary movements or in combination with jaw opening or swallowing. Identification was made at 10 weeks of the rotation of the fetus (Fig. 26-1) and of active locomotion resulting in position change.

Quantitatively, very young fetuses have been found to gradually increase the amount of time they spend moving. By 11 weeks, a plateau of the incidence of total activity was observed: the fetus moves approximately 21 to 30% of the time (Table 26-3). A wide range of activity was demonstrated between individual fetuses (25 to 91%).[14]

Fetal Movement in Late Gestation
Analysis of fetal movement patterns during the second half of pregnancy is characterized by the development of (1) periodicity of individual move-

Table 26-2. Classification of fetal movement patterns

Movement	Description of Movement
Just discernible movements	Slow and small shifting of the fetal contour, lasting from 0.5 to 2 seconds
Startle	Quick generalized movement always initiated in limbs and sometimes spreading to neck and trunk. Flexion or extension of limbs usually of large amplitude but can be small or just discernible. Movements last about 1 second.
General movements	Applicable if the whole body is moved but no distinctive pattern or sequence of body parts can be recognized
Hiccoughs	Jerky contraction of diaphragm, abrupt displacement of diaphragm, thorax, and abdomen
Breathing movements	"Inspiration" consists of fluent, simultaneous movement of diaphragm (caudad direction), leading to movements of thorax (inward) and abdomen (outward)
Isolated arm or leg movements	May be rapid or slow and may involve extension, flexion, external and internal rotation, or abduction and adduction of an extremity without movement in other body parts
Isolated retroflexion of the head	Displacement of the head can be small or large. Large movements may cause overextension of the spine.
Isolated rotation of the head	Head may turn from a midline position to one side and back. This movement is often associated with hand-face contact.
Isolated anteflexion of the head	Carried out slowly; may occur alone or together with hand-face contact, when sucking can be observed.
Sucking and swallowing	Rhythmic bursts of regular jaw opening and closing at rate about one per second may be followed by swallowing. Swallowing consists of displacements of tongue and/or larynx.
Hand-face contact	Hand slowly touches face and fingers frequently extend and flex
Stretch	Carried out slowly; consists of forceful extension of back, retroflexion of head, and external rotation and elevation of arms
Yawn	Prolonged wide opening of jaws followed by quick closure, often with retroflexion of head and sometimes elevation of arms
Rotation of fetus	Rotation occurs around sagittal or transverse axis. Complete change around transverse axis is achieved by complex general movement, including alternating leg movements. Rotation around longitudinal axis can result from leg movements with hip rotation or from rotation of head followed by trunk rotation.

(From deVries JIP, Visser GHA, Prechtl HFR. The emergence of fetal behaviour. I. Qualitative aspects. Early Human Develop. 1982;7:301.)

ments, (2) a fixed combination of individual movements, and (3) the association of fetal heart rate patterns and fetal movement. These facets of movement can be related to CNS maturation.

An inverse relationship exists between gestational age and both the incidence and the mean number of fetal movements (Table 26-3). As gestational age increases the number and incidence of movements decrease.[16,32,33,36,37] Thus, as the fetus matures during the second half of pregnancy, the incidence of motor activity decreases from a maximum of 21% in the 20- to 22-week fetus[11] to 10% in the 30- to 40-week fetus.[37] A similar decrease in the average number of movements observed in an hour can also be demonstrated with increasing ges-

tational age. Fetuses at 24 to 26 weeks move an average of 53 times per hour; 26- to 28-week fetuses, 46 times[32]; and 30- to 40-week fetuses 31 times.[37]

It should be noted that although younger fetuses move more often the movements are of shorter duration than those observed at a later gestational age.[32] This aspect of fetal motor behavior can be related to the gradual maturation of the CNS. Dobbing and Sands[18] reported that by the beginning of the third trimester the number of neurons in the CNS has reached the adult level. These neurons continue to exhibit hypertrophy—an increase in dendritic arborization and synaptic connections. This second phase of brain growth is associated with glial cell hyperplasia and neuron myelination.

Based on the above evidence, Nasello-Paterson and coworkers[32] have suggested that the fetus at 24 to 28 weeks might experience a "short circuit" effect in transmission of nerve impulses to the neuromuscular junction. Alternatively, relatively few of these fetuses' motor units may be innervated. Transmission of nerve impulses to muscle would result in sporadic, uncontrolled movements.[32] These fetuses do not, therefore, have well-defined periods of rest or activity.

The second half of pregnancy is also characterized by the establishment of a circadian pattern of motion (see Table 26-3). Twenty-four–hour observations of fetal movements have demonstrated that 24- to 28-week fetuses move more often during the late night–early morning hours (11:00 PM to 8:00 AM).[32] In 30- to 40-week fetuses the active period is briefer, and movements increase only from 9:00 PM to 1:00 AM.[37]

Correlations of fetal movements with fetal heart rate have been found as early as 20 to 22 weeks.[11] The interaction between movements and heart rate accelerations becomes more evident by 32 weeks' gestation. The number and amplitude of fetal heart rate accelerations associated with movements increase as the fetus approaches 32 weeks,[37] so it appears that at that point the probability that a nonstress test will be reactive increases.

There was no significant evidence that change in movements could be associated with maternal meals.[32,37] Feeding a patient prior to an ultrasound examination will not increase the chance of observing fetal movements.

Fetal Breathing Movements

Fetal breathing movements were first described by Ahlfeld in 1888.[1] This early investigation involved the observation of periodic rhythmic intrauterine fetal movements in the periumbilical area of pregnant women. The belief that breathing movements were part of the fetus' repertoire of motor behavior was in doubt until direct evidence was provided by Dawes,[8,9] who performed in utero studies on fetal lambs. This basic research performed on fetal lambs aroused clinical interest in the utilization of fetal breathing movements as a measure of the fetus' condition. Both A-mode ultrasound[4] and tocodynamometers[54] have been used to detect human fetal respiratory movements, but real-time

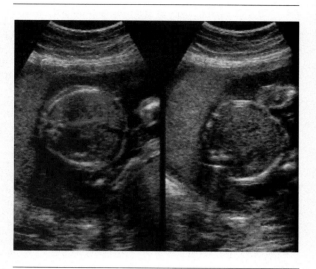

FIGURE 26-1. A cross-sectional scan of a 15-week fetus demonstrates rotation of its body.

ultrasound has proven to be the method of choice for qualitative and quantitative investigations of fetal breathing, as it has for fetal movements.

Several clinical studies have been performed utilizing real-time ultrasonography. In humans Connors and associates[6] studied the effects of maternal inhalation of various concentrations of carbon dioxide mixtures. It was discovered that the incidence of fetal breathing movements correlated significantly with maternal end-tidal carbon dioxide pressure (PCO_2). Fetal breathing movements increased during periods of hypercapnia and decreased with maternal hyperventilation.

Human fetal breathing movements have been observed during maternal hypoxemia and its resolution. Manning and Platt[25] reported cessation of fetal respirations in the presence of a maternal PO_2 no greater than 40 mm Hg. Conversely, when the maternal PO_2 was 60 mm Hg or more, fetal breathing movements were present 23 to 80% of the time.

A reduction of human fetal breathing movements can be attributed to other causes. For example, operative manipulation of the human fetus can significantly decrease the incidence of fetal breathing movements. Fetal breathing movements have been observed to be partially inhibited up to 2 days after amniocentesis.[27] Human fetal breathing movements have also been found to be decreased

Table 26-3. Characteristics of fetal movement according to gestational age

Investigators	Period of Observation (Hours)	Gestational Age (Weeks)	Prevalence of Movement (%)	Movements per Hour	Hours of Most Movement
de Vries et al., 1988	1	11	21–30	—	—
de Vries et al., 1987	6	20–22	5–21	—	2200–2400
Nasello-Paterson et al., 1988	24	24–26	13	53	2300–0800
Nasello-Paterson et al., 1988	24	26–28	12	46	2300–0800
Patrick et al., 1982	24	30–40	10	31	2100–0100

or abolished by maternal ingestion of sedatives[4,25] and of alcohol.[24]

Fetal Breathing Early in Gestation

In general, movement patterns have an obvious effect on the development of the fetus. Fetal breathing movements have been considered as a preparatory exercise for extrauterine breathing.[41] These particular movements are considered essential to fetal lung growth. Fetal respiratory activity enhances both neuromuscular and skeletal develop-

ment of the respiratory system and makes possible the appropriate respiratory epithelial development of the gas-exchanging surfaces of the lung.[23]

Breathing can easily be observed in the fetus by obtaining a longitudinal sectional view with a real-time scanner. The diaphragm moves caudad, simultaneously drawing the anterior chest wall inward and the anterior abdominal wall outward (Fig. 26-2). The earliest such movements have been observed is at 10 weeks' gestation. They tend to be regular. Fetal breathing at this gestational age may

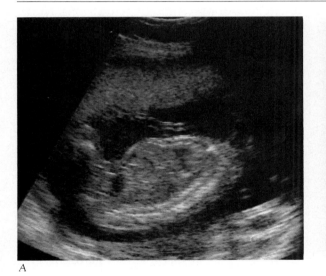

A

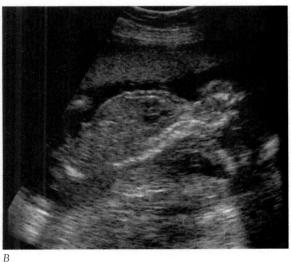

B

Figure 26-2. Fetal breathing movements of an 18-week fetus. Compare the inward location of the chest wall (A; inspiration) to its outward location during expiration (B; expiration).

be observed alone or in combination with jaw opening, swallowing, or general body movement.[11] Fetal hiccoughs, jerky contractions of the diaphragm that can be viewed as a particular kind of breathing, have been recognized as early as 9 weeks. On scan, hiccoughs are seen as an abrupt displacement of the diaphragm, thorax, and abdomen. They may occur singly, but most often follow each other in regular succession.[11] Other researchers have not observed these movements until 22 to 24 weeks (Table 26-1).[3,21]

DeVries and coworkers[14] have observed that the incidence of hiccoughs is high during early gestation (9 to 13 weeks) and that it decreases as gestational age increases. In contrast, the frequency breathing movements have is directly related to gestational age. No daily patterns were found in fetal breathing movements in early gestation.[11]

Fetal Breathing Late in Gestation

Manning and Platt[27] described five patterns of fetal breathing that can be recognized in the second half of pregnancy (Table 26-4)—regular, irregular, irregular slow, and periodic accelerated breathing and hiccoughs. Before 26 weeks' gestation the breathing pattern was especially irregular and slow.

Overall, the incidence of fetal breathing has been found to increase with increasing maturity of the fetus (Table 26-5). Twenty-four–hour observations of respiratory movement have demonstrated a 13.7% incidence in 24- to 26-week fetuses[35] and a 31% incidence in fetuses at 30 to 40 weeks' gesta-

Table 26-4. Patterns of fetal breathing movements

Pattern of FBM	Characteristics of Patterns	Rate (breaths/min)
Regular	Regular in rate and amplitude	40–60
Irregular	Observed in the fetus <26 weeks gestational age; highly irregular in rate and amplitude	20–100
Irregular slow	Slow, large-amplitude	6–20
Periodic accelerated	Rising and falling changes in rate and amplitude	30–90
Hiccoughs	Irregular, intermittent, large-amplitude breaths of short duration	6–20

(From Manning FM, Platt LD. Fetal breathing movements. Antepartum monitoring of fetal conditions. Clin Obstet Gynecol. 1979;6:335–349.)

tion.[36,38,48,49] This incidence of breathing decreases dramatically beginning as early as 3 days prior to the initiation of labor and persists until delivery (Table 26-6).[5,48]

As the fetus matures, the duration of apneic intervals increases (see Table 26-5). The longest apneic interval observed in the 24- to 26-week fetuses was relatively brief (12 minutes[35]), as opposed to the 122-minute interval of the 38- to 39-week fetus.[36]

Table 26-5. Characteristics of fetal breathing movements according to gestational age

Investigators (Hours' Observation)	Gestational Age (weeks)	Prevalence of FBM (%)	Mean Hourly Respiratory Rate	Longest Apneic Interval (min)	Hours of Most Movement
de Vries et al., 1987 (6)	20–22	1–40	—	—	1300–1500 2200–2400
Natale et al., 1988 (24)	24–26	13.7	42.8	12	2300–0200
Natale et al., 1988 (24)	26–28	14.2	43.9	14	0200–0500
Patrick et al., 1980 (24)	30–31	31	58.3	68	0400–0700
Patrick et al., 1978 (8)	34–35	31.8	49.1	—	—
Patrick et al., 1980 (24)	38–39	31	47	122	0400–0700

TABLE 26-6. Incidence of fetal breathing movements observed prior to and during labor at term

INVESTIGATORS	OBSERVATION PERIOD	PREVALENCE OF FETAL BREATHING MOVEMENTS (%)
Carmichael et al., 1984	3 days prior to onset of labor	22.2
Carmichael et al., 1984	12 hours prior to onset of labor	11.4
Richardson et al., 1979	Latent phase of labor	8.3
Richardson et al., 1979	Active phase of labor	0.8

The fetus' respiratory rate per hour gradually increased from 24 to 31 weeks' gestation, but as term approached it decreased again (Table 26-5).

A circadian pattern of fetal breathing appears early in the second half of pregnancy. At 24 to 26 weeks, the frequency of fetal breathing movements increases between 11:00 PM and 2:00 AM.[35] It is interesting to note that, as the fetus matures it gradually alters the timing of this pattern so as to demonstrate that by 30 to 39 weeks, the greatest number of fetal respiratory movements are observed between 4:00 AM and 7:00 AM.[36]

In opposition to fetal movement observations, a significant increase in breathing was observed in 30- to 32-week fetuses after the mother had a meal.[34]

Clinical Significance of Fetal Movements and Breathing

Motor behavior of the fetus, including both movement and breathing, have been demonstrated to be a normal fetal function throughout gestation. It has been suggested that a decrease, cessation, or change in fetal motor behavior may be an indication of a change in the fetus' condition. Prior to the utilization of real-time ultrasonography maternal perception of fetal movements was the principal mode of assessing fetal movements.

Clinical applications of the results of investigational studies of fetal movements and respiratory activity have revolved around attempts to find more accurate methods for the assessment of fetal health. Quantification of fetal movements has been used to assess fetal well-being in pregnancies complicated by factors such as diabetes[15] and congenital malformations.[45] In fetuses of diabetic mothers, for example, it was discovered that the length of active periods does not increase with gestational age as it does in normal pregnancies, indicating maturational delay in the development of active-quiet cycles. The anomalous fetus gave evidence of being less active than those with no defects.

Fetal breathing has been considered an indicator of fetal condition because it is part of the normal motor repertoire. Platt and colleagues[41] demonstrated a significant relationship between the presence or absence of fetal breathing movements in the last observation before delivery and the resulting Apgar score. In the presence of respiratory activity, the fetus was found to be more likely to have an Apgar score of at least 7. Manning and associates[31] correlated the presence or absence of breathing movements and reactivity of the nonstress test with the Apgar score. Taken separately, the absence of fetal breathing or nonreactivity each was equally accurate in predicting neonatal outcome. When the tests were used in combination and when both results were abnormal, the findings were significantly better at predicting which fetuses were likely to have an abnormality.

Fetal Biophysical Profile

Manning and Platt's findings culminated in development of the fetal biophysical profile.[28] Five variables were used to develop an assessment tool for the fetus in utero: fetal breathing movement, fetal movements, fetal tone, the nonstress test (indicating fetal heart rate reactivity), and amniotic fluid volume. These variables were chosen because they are initiated and regulated by the fetus' CNS, and it is thought that the presence of any given variable is indirect evidence of a functioning and intact neurologic system. The absence of one of these variables does not necessarily imply that something is amiss; absence of any one of these variables (excluding amniotic fluid volume) may reflect a sleep-rest state rather than a depressed CNS. Fetal biophysical activities are initiated by nerve impulses that arise from different anatomic sites in the brain.

It has been hypothesized that fetal tone is regulated by the cortex, fetal movement by the cortex nuclei, breathing by the ventral surface of the fourth ventricle, and the NST by the posterior hypothalamus and medulla.[58] Alterations in any one of these four components of the profile are considered to be acute indicators of fetal asphyxia. Decreased amniotic fluid volume, on the other hand, is thought to be an indicator of chronic asphyxial insults to the fetus. With sustained or frequent asphyxia, cardiac output is distributed away from the fetal lungs, kidneys, and intestinal tract and toward the heart, brain, and placenta. This results in decreased urine production and lung fluid, leading to oligohydramnios. The sensitivity of the central nervous system to any given depressant factor is unknown, but Manning and colleagues[28] have suggested that it varies. To support this hypothesis, when several variables were combined, the false negative and false positive rates dropped significantly; at the same time the incidence of abnormal outcomes increased with the number of abnormal variables in a fetus' profile. Manning and Platt thought this instrument (the biophysical profile) particularly important as it would indicate gradations of fetal well-being or compromise (rather than an all-or-none diagnosis) and create a circumstance by which the direction and degree of change in fetal condition could be determined.

The biophysical profile was used to measure the five fetal parameters during a single observation period. Except for the nonstress test, all variables were recorded by real-time ultrasound. During the observation period each variable was coded as normal or abnormal, according to specific criteria. The criteria as originally[28] reported were as follows:

Nonstress Test. Reactive (normal) if two or more heart rate accelerations of at least 15 beats per minute in amplitude and at least 15 seconds' duration associated with fetal movement(s) in a 10-minute period

Fetal Breathing Movements. Present (normal), the presence of at least one episode of fetal breathing of at least 60 seconds' duration within a 30-minute observation period

Fetal Movements. Present (normal), the presence of at least three discrete episodes of fetal movements within a 30-minute observation period

Fetal Tone. Normal upper and lower extremities in position of full flexion and head flexed on chest; at least one episode of extension of extremities with return to position of flexion and/or extension of spine with return to position of flexion

Amniotic Fluid Volume. Normal, fluid evident throughout the uterine cavity; largest pocket of fluid greater than 1 cm in vertical diameter.

For scoring purposes, each variable was arbitrarily assigned a score of 2 when normal and of 0 when abnormal. Thus, the highest possible score was 10. The lowest score, indicating all variables were abnormal, was 0. A combined score of either 10 or 8 was regarded as normal. A score of 6 was equivocal and indicated that the profile should be repeated within 12 hours. A score of 4, 2, or 0 was considered to indicate fetal compromise.

Current use of the biophysical profile (Table 26-7) at Los Angeles County/University of Southern California Medical Center demonstrates the reassessment of the value of decreased amniotic fluid in evaluating fetal condition. The amniotic fluid index (AFI), described in Chapter 27, has replaced the parameter of one pocket of amniotic fluid. In analyzing this method, Phelan and associates[39] suggested that an AFI of 5.0 cm or less indicates oligohydramnios. An additional advantage of utilizing the AFI is that ultrasonographers have the ability to follow quantitative changes of the amniotic fluid with advancing gestational age. Serial measurements of AFI may be an effective means of assessing fetal status throughout pregnancy.[40]

A second alteration in the original criteria of the biophysical profile is the duration of fetal breathing. Currently, observation of a 30-second period of regular breathing within a 30-minute test period is considered normal. (Originally the observation period was 60 seconds.) This modification was instituted subsequent to assessing Manning and coworkers'[29] utilization of a 30-second observation of fetal breathing.

RELATIONSHIP OF THE BIOPHYSICAL PROFILE SCORE TO FETAL WELL-BEING

Several studies examining the benefits of the fetal biophysical profile have been published since the initial observations were made. Manning and coworkers[30] have now reported that the biophysical

Table 26-7. Scoring the fetal biophysical profile

Parameter	Normal Finding (Score 2)	Abnormal Finding (Score 0)
Nonstress test	Reactive: Two or more fetal heart rate accelerations of at least 15 bpm in amplitude and at least 15 sec duration in 10 min within a 40-min test period	Nonreactive: One or fewer fetal heart rate accelerations of at least 15 bpm and 15 sec duration in 10 min within 40-min test period
Fetal breathing movements	The presence of at least one episode of sustained fetal breathing of at least 30 sec duration within a 30-min observation period	The absence of fetal breathing or the absence of an episode of breathing of at least 30 sec duration during a 30-min observation period
Fetal body movements	The presence of at least three discrete episodes of fetal movements in a 30-min period; simultaneous limb and trunk movement count as a single movement	Two or fewer discrete fetal movements in a 30-min observation period
Fetal tone	Upper and lower extremities in position of full flexion and head flexed on chest; at least one episode of extension of extremities with return to position of flexion and/or extension of spine with return to position of flexion	Extremities in position of extension or partial flexion; spine in position of extension; fetal movement not followed by return to flexion
Amniotic fluid volume	AFI more than 5.0 cm	AFI 5.0 cm or less

Score interpretation: 10, 8: Normal; repeat in 4 to 7 days (depending on indication).
　　　　　　　　　　　6: Equivocal; repeat within 12 hours.
　　　　　　　　4, 2, 0: Abnormal; consider delivery.

profile was performed in 19,221 high-risk pregnancies and that the corrected perinatal mortality rate decreased significantly. Further investigations of fetal biophysical profile have shown similar promising results.[10,53,58]

Recent studies by Vintzileos and colleagues[57–59] have suggested the use of a modified fetal biophysical profile as an early predictor of fetal infection in patients with premature rupture of the membranes. It was discovered that a biophysical profile score of 7 or less (of a possible 12) was a good predictor of impending fetal infection in this group. The absence of fetal breathing and a nonreactive NST were the first signs of impending infection; decreased tone and fetal movement were late manifestations.

The biophysical profile has also been found to have a significant relationship to fetal acid-base status at the time of testing. In a prospective study of 124 patients undergoing cesarean section prior to the onset of labor, it was discovered that a low profile score indicated fetal acidosis (pH <7.20). Further, the first signs of fetal acidosis were the loss of fetal breathing and nonreactivity of the NST.[61,62]

A recent prospective study compared the bio-physical profile to the nonstress test to determine which was more predictive of fetal well-being.[42] No significant difference was found in the negative predictive value, the sensitivity, or the specificity of the two tests in attempting to identify overall abnormal outcome as measured by the presence of perinatal mortality, fetal distress in labor, low 5-minute Apgar score, or small for gestational age infants. A statistical difference was found between the profile and the nonstress test for a positive predictive value in determining a composite of the above abnormal outcome. In this instance, the positive predictive value of the profile was significantly greater than that of the NST.

Fetal maturation may be a significant variable in the assessment of the profile's parameters. Baskett[2] observed that the incidence of abnormal nonstress tests and of abnormal fetal breathing movements are inversely related to gestational age. The fetus at 26 to 33 weeks was more likely to have an equivocal profile because of nonreactivity or abnormal fetal breathing as compared to fetuses of 34 to 41 weeks' gestational age. It is suggested, therefore, that the biophysical profile be interpreted in relation to the fetus' gestational age, although these

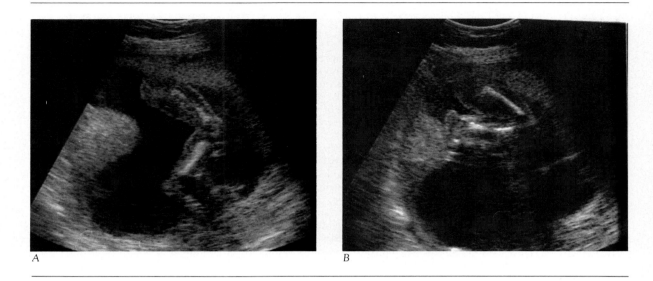

A   B

FIGURE 26-3. (A) Extension and (B) flexion of the leg of an 18-week fetus.

findings have not been investigated by others. Currently, the biophysical profile is being utilized to assess high-risk pregnancies ranging from 25 weeks' gestational age to 44 weeks.[30,42,57]

FUTURE DEVELOPMENTS OF THE FETAL BIOPHYSICAL PROFILE: ACOUSTIC STIMULATION

Like other antepartum fetal assessment techniques (such as the NST or the contraction stress test [CST]), in general, the fetal biophysical profile is highly specific but relatively insensitive. In order to improve the sensitivity of the biophysical profile, Divon and colleagues[17] suggested that response to acoustic stimulation be used as a measure of fetal tone. After 25 weeks' gestation, the normal fetus demonstrates auditory startle behavior[21] similar to the neonatal Moro reflex. Upon stimulation with sound, it was found that the fetuses respond with a significant increase in movements and a corresponding increase of basal fetal heart rate and fetal heart rate accelerations.[20,47]

In general, measurements of the parameters of the profile were made as objective as possible. In the case of tone, assessment is made by sonographic observation of spontaneous fetal limb extension and flexion (Fig. 26-3). In an attempt to quantify the biophysical parameter of tone, Divon's group[17]

proposed using an electronic artificial larynx placed on the mother's abdomen to stimulate the fetus. With real-time ultrasound, it was observed that the startle response was elicited each time the stimulus was applied. This provoked response is felt to be less subjective than previous measures of fetal tone. Additionally, sound may stimulate fetal behavior from quietude to activity, thus increasing the likelihood of accurately identifying the fetal condition.

Kuhlman and associates[22] have used acoustic stimulation to evoke a startle response in fetuses, but they identified a facial startle reaction. All normal fetuses beyond 27 weeks' gestational age that were subjected to sound stimuli made startle responses. When a group of hydrocephalic fetuses were subjected to the sound stimuli, all those that failed to demonstrate startle responses died either in utero or within several months after birth, and this group had the most severe CNS defects.

Summary

The human fetus has completely developed its repertoire of motor behavior by 16 weeks' gestational age, including body movements and breathing movements. As the fetus matures, the frequency, nature, and relationship of each of the movements change, owing to CNS maturation. Diagnosis of fetal condition must be made in relation to the particular gestational age of that fetus, keeping in mind that there are wide variations in normal patterns of fetal motor behavior.

The fetal biophysical profile is an important tool for diagnosing fetal well-being. It is less predictive of fetal jeopardy. Analysis of additional variables (such as the acoustically stimulated startle response) or refinement of existing measures may increase the sensitivity of the profile.

References

1. Ahlfeld F. Uber bisher noch nicht beschriebene intrauterine Bewegungen des Kindes. Verh Dtsch Ges Gynakol. 1888; 2:203–210.
2. Baskett TF. Gestational age and fetal biophysical assessment. Am J Obstet Gynecol. 1988; 158:332–334.
3. Birnholz JC, Stephens JC, Faria M. Fetal movement patterns: A possible means of defining neurologic developmental milestones in utero. Am J Roentgenol. 1978; 130:537–540.
4. Boddy K, Dawes GS. Fetal breathing. Br Med Bull. 1975; 31:3–7.
5. Carmichael L, Campbell K, Patrick J. Fetal breathing, gross fetal body movements, and maternal fetal heart rates before spontaneous labor at term. Am J Obstet Gynecol. 1984; 148:675–679.
6. Connors G, Hunse C, Carmichael L, et al. The role of carbon dioxide in the generation of human fetal breathing movements. Am J Obstet Gynecol. 1988; 158:322–327.
7. Connors G, Natalie R, Nasello-Paterson C. Maternally perceived fetal activity from twenty-four weeks' gestation to term in normal and at risk pregnancies. Am J Obstet Gynecol. 1988; 158:294–299.
8. Dawes GS. Breathing before birth in animals and man. N Engl J Med. 1974; 290:557–559.
9. Dawes GS, Fox HE, Leduc BM, et al. Respiratory movements and rapid–eye movement sleep in the foetal lamb. J Physiol. 1972; 220:119–143.
10. DeVoe LD, Castillo RA, Searle N, et al. Prognostic components of computerized fetal biophysical testing. Am J Obstet Gynecol. 1988; 158:1144–1148.
11. deVries JIP, Visser GHA, Mulder EJH, et al. Diurnal and other variations in fetal movement and heart rate patterns at 20-22 weeks. Early Human Develop. 1987; 15:333–348.
12. deVries JIP, Visser GHA, Prechtl HFR. The emergence of fetal behaviour. I. Qualitative aspects. Early Human Develop. 1982; 7:301–322.
13. deVries JIP, Visser GH, Prechtl HFR. Fetal motility in the first half of pregnancy. Clin Develop Med. 1984; 94:46–64.
14. deVries JIP, Visser GHA, Prechtl HFR. The emergence of fetal behavior. III. Individual differences and consistencies. Early Human Develop. 1988; 16:85–103.
15. Dierker LJ, Pillay S, Sorokin Y, et al. The change in fetal activity periods in diabetic and nondiabetic pregnancies. Am J Obstet Gynecol. 1982; 143:181–185.
16. Dierker LJ, Rosen MG, Pillay S, et al. The correlation between gestational age and fetal activity periods. Biol Neonate. 1982; 42:66–72.
17. Divon MY, Platt LD, Cantrell CJ. Evoked fetal startle response: A possible intrauterine neurological examination. Am J Obstet Gynecol. 1985; 154:454–456.
18. Dobbing J, Sands J. Quantitative growth and development of human brain. Arch Dis Child. 1973; 48:757.
19. Granat M, Lavie P, Adar D, et al. Short-term cycles in human fetal activity. I. Normal pregnancies. Am J Obstet Gynecol. 1979; 134:696–701.
20. Grimwade JC, Walker DW, Bartlett M, et al. Human fetal heart rate changes and movement in response to sound and vibration. Am J Obstet Gynecol. 1971; 109:86–90.
21. Ianniruberto A, Tajani E. Ultrasonographic study of fetal movements. Semin Perinatol. 1981; 5:175–181.
22. Kuhlman K, Burns K, Sabbagha R, et al. Real-time ultrasonographic imaging of fetal response decrement to external acoustic stimulation. Presented at Society of Perinatal Obstetricians, San Antonio, TX; 1986.
23. Maloney JE, Alcorn D, Bowes G, et al. Development of the future respiratory system before birth. Semin Perinatol. 1980; 4:251–260.
24. McLeod W, Brien J, Loomis C, et al. Effect of maternal ethanol ingestion on fetal breathing movements, gross body movements, and heart rate at 37 to 40 weeks gestational age. Am J Obstet Gynecol. 1983; 145:251–257.
25. Manning FA, Platt LD. Maternal hypoxemia and fetal breathing movements. Obstet Gynecol. 1977; 53:758–760.
26. Manning FM, Platt LD. Fetal breathing movements: Antepartum monitoring of fetal condition. Clin Obstet Gynecol. 1979; 6:335–349.
27. Manning FH, Platt LD, LeMay M. Effect of amniocentesis on fetal breathing movements. Br Med J. 1972; 2:1582–1583.
28. Manning FA, Platt LD, Sipos L. Antepartum fetal evaluation: Development of fetal biophysical profile. Am J Obstet Gynecol. 1980; 136:787–795.

29. Manning FA, Baskett TF, Morrison I, et al. Fetal biophysical profile scoring: A prospective study in 1,184 high-risk patients. Am J Obstet Gynecol. 1981; 140: 289–294.

30. Manning FA, Morrison MB, Harman CR, et al. Fetal assessment based on fetal biophysical profile scoring: Experience in 19,221 referred high-risk pregnancies. Am J Obstet Gynecol. 1987; 157:880–884.

31. Manning FA, Platt LD, Sipos L, et al. Fetal breathing movements and the nonstress test in high-risk pregnancies. Am J Obstet Gynecol. 1979; 135:511–515.

32. Nasello-Paterson C, Natale R, Connors G. Ultrasonic evaluation of fetal body movements over twenty-four hours in the human fetus at twenty-four to twenty-eight weeks gestation. Am J Obstet Gynecol. 1988; 158:312–316.

33. Natale R, Nasello C, Turliuk R. The relationship between movements and accelerations in fetal heart rate at twenty-four to thirty-two weeks gestation. Am J Obstet Gynecol. 1984; 148:591–595.

34. Natale R, Nasello-Paterson C, Turliuk R. Longitudinal measurements of fetal breathing, body movements, heart rate, and heart rate accelerations at 24 to 32 weeks of gestation. Am J Obstet Gynecol. 1985; 151:256–263.

35. Natale R, Nasello-Paterson C, Connors G, et al. Patterns of fetal breathing activity in the human fetus at 24 to 28 weeks of gestation. Am J Obstet Gynecol. 1988; 158:317–321.

36. Patrick J, Campbell K, Carmichael L, et al. Patterns of human fetal breathing during the last 10 weeks of pregnancy. Obstet Gynecol. 1980; 56:24–30.

37. Patrick J, Campbell K, Carmichael L, et al. Patterns of gross fetal body movements over 24-hour observation intervals during the last 10 weeks of pregnancy. Am J Obstet Gynecol. 1982; 142:363–371.

38. Patrick J, Fetherston W, Vick H, et al. Human fetal breathing movements and gross fetal body movements at weeks 34 to 35 gestation. Am J Obstet Gynecol. 1978; 130:693–699.

39. Phelan JP, Smith CV, Broussard P, et al. Amniotic fluid volume assessment with the four-quadrant technique at 36-42 weeks' gestation. J Reprod Med. 1987; 32:540–542.

40. Phelan JP, Ahn MO, Smith CV, et al. Amniotic fluid index measurements during pregnancy. J Reprod Med. 1987; 32:601–604.

41. Platt LD, Manning FA, Lemay M, et al. Human fetal breathing: Relationship to fetal condition. Am J Obstet Gynecol. 1978; 132:514–518.

42. Platt LD, Walla CA, Paul RH, et al. A prospective trial of the fetal biophysical profile versus the nonstress test in the management of high-risk pregnancies. Am J Obstet Gynecol. 1985; 153:624–633.

43. Prechtl HFR. Continuity and changes in early neural development. Clin Develop Med. 1984; 94:1–15.

44. Preyer W. Spezielle Physiologie des Embryo. Leipzig: Greiben; 1885.

45. Rayburn WF, Barr M. Activity patterns in malformed fetuses. Am J Obstet Gynecol. 1982; 142: 1045–1048.

46. Rayburn WF, Motley ME, Stempel LE, et al. Antepartum prediction of the postmature infant. Obstet Gynecol. 1982;60:148–153.

47. Read JA, Miller JC. Fetal heart rate acceleration in response to acoustic stimulation as a measure of fetal well-being. Am J Obstet Gynecol. 1977; 129:512–517.

48. Richardson B, Natale R, Patrick J. Human fetal breathing activity during electively induced labor at term. Am J Obstet Gynecol. 1979; 133:247–255.

49. Roberts AB, Little D, Cooper D, et al. Normal patterns of fetal activity in the third trimester. Br J Obstet Gynaecol. 1979; 86:4–9.

50. Rutherford SE, Smith CV, Jacobs N, et al. The four-quadrant assessment of amniotic fluid "volume": An adjunct to antepartum fetal heart rate testing. Presented at The Society of Perinatal Obstetricians, San Antonio, TX; 1986.

51. Sadovsky E, Polishuk WZ. Fetal movements in utero. Obstet Gynecol. 1977; 50:49–55.

52. Sadovsky E, Polishuk WZ, Mahler Y, et al. Fetal movements recorder, use and indications. Int J Gynaecol Obstet. 1977; 15:20–24.

53. Schifrin BS, Guntes V, Gergely RC, et al. The role of real-time scanning in antenatal fetal surveillance. Am J Obstet Gynecol. 1981; 140:525–530.

54. Timor-Tritsch IE, Dierker LJ, Hertz RH, et al. Regular and irregular human fetal respiratory movement. Early Hum Dev. 1980; 4:315–324.

55. Valentin L, Marsal K. Fetal movement in the third trimester of normal pregnancy. Early Human Dev. 1986; 14:295–306.

56. Valentin L, Lofgren O, Marsal K, et al. Subjective recording of fetal movements. I. Limits and acceptability in normal pregnancies. Acta Obstet Gynecol Scand. 1984; 68:223–228.

57. Vintzileos AM, Bors-Koefoed R, Pelegaro JF, et al. The use of the fetal biophysical profile improves pregnancy outcome in premature rupture of the membranes. Am J Obstet Gynecol. 1987; 157:236–240.

58. Vintzileos AM, Campbell WA, Ingardia CJ, et al. The fetal biophysical profile and its predictive value. Obstet Gynecol. 1983; 62:271–278.

59. Vintzileos AM, Campbell WA, Nochimson DJ, et al. The fetal biophysical profile in patients with premature rupture of the membranes—An early predictor of fetal infection. Am J Obstet Gynecol. 1985; 152: 510–516.

60. Vintzileos AM, Campbell WA, Nochimson DJ, et al. Fetal biophysical profile versus amniocentesis in predicting infection in preterm premature rupture of the membranes. Obstet Gynecol. 1986; 68:488–494.

61. Vintzileos AM, Gaffney SE, Salinger LM, et al. The relationships among the fetal biophysical profile, umbilical cord pH, and Apgar scores. Am J Obstet Gynecol. 1987; 157:627–631.

62. Vintzileos AM, Gaffney SE, Salinger LM, et al. The relationship between fetal biophysical profile and cord pH in patients undergoing Cesarean section before the onset of labor. Obstet Gynecol. 1987; 70:196–201.

63. Wheeler T, Roberts K, Peters J, et al. Detection of fetal movements using Doppler ultrasound. Obstet Gynecol. 1987; 70:251–254.

CHAPTER 27

Intrauterine Growth Retardation

SHARON DALCOMPO, RUDY E. SABBAGHA

Intrauterine growth retardation (IUGR) occurs in 5 to 10% of fetuses and is directly related to the increase in their perinatal morbidity and mortality. Additionally, IUGR is responsible for long-term neurologic deficits noted in approximately 25% of such fetuses. Presently, the diagnosis of IUGR is best made using various modalities of ultrasound. In this chapter we define IUGR and discuss its etiology, morphology, and pathophysiology. Subsequently, we list the essential ultrasound parameters that the sonographer should obtain to make the diagnosis of IUGR and discuss the rationale for using these data. Finally, we outline a protocol for reporting the key fetal findings to the health professional managing the patient.

Definitions

The diagnosis of IUGR can be made when the estimated fetal weight (EFW) for a given pregnancy week falls at or below the 10th percentile. A list of the birth weight percentiles from the 23rd to the 44th weeks of pregnancy is shown in Table 1.[3] This table shows, for example, that IUGR fetuses weigh approximately 2510 g and 2750 g at the 38th and 40th weeks of pregnancy, respectively. It should be noted that the birth weights listed in Table 27-1 are derived from pregnant women residing at or near sea level. A different table is used for fetuses of pregnant women living at altitudes as high as 6000 feet above sea level because such fetuses are lighter in weight than those growing at or near sea level.[1]

Whereas the above-mentioned definition of IUGR is generally accepted, in many centers, a fetus' growth is considered to be retarded only when the estimated fetal weight is no greater than the 3rd or the 5th percentile, ranks that fall approximately 2 standard deviations below the mean weight.[10,21,30]

Further, the diagnosis of IUGR can also be made in neonates who are "skinny but long." These neonates have the same external appearance as all IUGR infants; that is, they exhibit loss of subcutaneous tissue, wrinkled skin, and a wizened look (Fig. 27-1). They are different from other IUGR infants in two respects: their crown-heel length (CHL) is long, exceeding the 90th percentile rank for dates, and their birth weight frequently exceeds the 10th percentile rank noted in fetuses with normal CHLs. The increase in birth weight is attributed to their long bones. In such infants the correct diagnosis of IUGR can be made when the ponderal index, that is, the birth weight/(CHL)[3] falls at or below the 10th percentile rank, for that index.[25] Alternatively, the diagnosis of IUGR can be made by comparing birth weights to a chart listing expected weights for different CHLs (Table 27-2).[16] For example, examination of Table 27-2 will show the marked difference in the 10th percentile birth

Table 27-1. Fetal weight percentiles throughout pregnancy

Gestational Age (Menstrual Weeks)	Smoothed Percentiles				
	10	25	50	75	90
23	370	460	550	690	990
24	420	530	640	780	1,080
25	490	630	740	890	1,180
26	570	730	860	1,020	1,320
27	660	840	990	1,160	1,470
28	770	980	1,150	1,350	1,660
29	890	1,100	1,310	1,530	1,890
30	1,030	1,260	1,460	1,710	2,100
31	1,180	1,410	1,630	1,880	2,290
32	1,310	1,570	1,810	2,090	2,500
33	1,480	1,720	2,010	2,280	2,690
34	1,670	1,910	2,220	2,510	2,880
35	1,870	2,130	2,430	2,730	3,090
36	2,190	2,470	2,650	2,950	3,290
37	2,310	2,580	2,870	3,160	3,470
38	2,510	2,770	3,030	3,320	3,610
39	2,680	2,910	3,170	3,470	3,750
40	2,750	3,010	3,280	3,590	3,870
41	2,800	3,070	3,360	3,680	3,980
42	2,830	3,110	3,410	3,740	4,060
43	2,840	3,110	3,420	3,780	4,100
44	2,790	3,050	3,390	3,770	4,110

(Adapted from Brenner WE, Edelman DA, Hendricks CH. A standard of fetal growth for the United States of America. Am J Obstet Gynecol. 1976; 126:555.)

weight of two 38-week neonates, one with an average CHL and the other with a long CHL:

IUGR neonate 1: CHL 48 cm, term birth weight (10th %) = 2560 g.
IUGR neonate 2: CHL 51 cm, term birth weight (10th %) = 3008 g.

Thus, for the neonate with a long CHL, the 10th percentile of birth weight exceeds the value expected for a fetus with a normal CHL. Thus, if no attention is paid to the CHL the weight of that fetus might pass for normal.

Ponderal index charts for the fetus are not completely developed yet. Presently, the most reliable method of diagnosing the skinny but long fetus is by comparing the abdominal circumference (AC) and femur length (FL) measurements. Characteristically, these fetuses have a small AC ($\leq$ 5th percentile), a long femur ($\geq$ 90th percentile), and their weight frequently exceeds the 10th percentile rank of fetuses with average femur length.

Perinatal Outcome

The perinatal period is defined as the interval between onset of fetal viability (approximately the 24th–26th menstrual weeks) and the end of the neonatal period (28th day of life). In the absence of high-risk factors the perinatal mortality is approximately 10 in 1000 live births. Perinatal mortality associated with IUGR is increased 6- to 10-fold, depending on the severity of the condition.[35]

Further, physical, metabolic, and neurologic complications are frequently noted in IUGR infants. As a result, the neonatal morbidity rate is increased and hospitalization is prolonged. These events are not only emotionally burdensome to the families of these affected infants but are also costly to society. Fitzhardinge and Steven have shown that approximately 25% of IUGR fetuses have

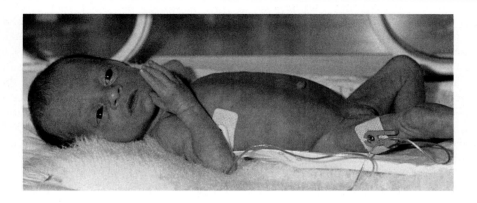

FIGURE 27-1. Symmetric growth retardation in a neonate weighing 1400 g at 36 weeks' gestation. The photograph was made 12 days after birth. Note the wrinkling of the skin in the lower extremities and in the right arm secondary to loss of subcutaneous tissue. Additionally, the infant has a wizened look, which was more prominent in the first few days of life.

TABLE 27-2. Birth weights for given percentiles in babies of different crown-heel lengths

BIRTH WEIGHT PERCENTILES	CROWN-HEEL LENGTH (CM)		
	48.0	51.0	55.0
95	3.16 kg	3.79 kg	4.76 kg
90	3.05	3.66	4.59
75	2.95	3.54	4.45
50	2.81	3.37	4.21
25	2.67	3.19	4.04
10	2.56	3.08	3.86
5	2.45	2.94	3.69

(Adapted from Miller HC, Merritt T. Fetal Growth in Humans. Chicago: Year Book Medical Publishers; 1979.)

long-term neurologic deficits and remain handicapped for life.[7]

Causes

The cause of IUGR remains idiopathic in approximately 50% of cases, but a number of fetal and maternal factors[26] are known to adversely influence fetal growth, including genetic and chromosomal causes, chronic fetal infections, maternal use of drugs (alcohol, narcotics, nicotine, dilantin, propranolol, steroids), maternal disease (cardiovascular, renal, metabolic), poor maternal nutrition or pregnancy weight gain, poor prepregnancy weight (<50 kg), high altitude, and irradiation.

Morphology and Pathophysiology

It is generally agreed that three types of IUGR are observed clinically: asymmetric, symmetric, and fetuses with abnormal ponderal indexes (abnormal weight-length ratios).

ASYMMETRIC IUGR

In asymmetric IUGR adverse factors such as hypertension or maternal renal disease exert their growth-retarding stimuli in the last 8 to 10 weeks of pregnancy, an interval during which the total number of cells required for the full development of organ size has been completely formed. Consequently, the "insult" only reduces cell size, not cell number.[31,33,34] The asymmetry refers to the disproportion between the size of the head and abdomen, a result of brain sparing. Thus, in such fetuses the head circumference (HC) is not only larger than the AC, but it also falls in a normal or nearly normal percentile rank. The reason for "head sparing" is related to the unique fetal circulation, in which blood rich in oxygen and nutrients is preferentially channeled from the placenta to the brain before it is available to other organs. The preferential channeling from the placenta to the brain—and subsequently to the rest of the body—is summarized in the following fetal blood flow schema: *Placenta* → umbilical vein → liver → inferior vena cava → right atrium → foramen ovale → left atrium → left ventricle → aorta → *brain* → superior vena cava → right atrium → right ventricle → pulmonary artery → ductus arteriosus → and descending branch of the aorta for distribution to the *rest of the body*.

Symmetric IUGR
In symmetric IUGR the etiology is usually a genetic, infectious, or environmental factor. These adverse factors exert their effect from early pregnancy. As a result, there is an externally apparent reduction in the size of both the head and trunk (i.e., IUGR is symmetric in appearance). In other words, the insult is of such long duration that the brain is not spared as in asymmetric IUGR. Additionally, there is microscopic reduction in both cell number and cell size, because the "insult" occurs early on, during the interval of cell division or hyperplasia.[34]

Abnormal Ponderal Indexes
Fetuses with long femurs (≥90th percentile) and small ACs (≤5th percentile) may be nutritionally deprived even though their estimated fetal weight falls at least in the 10th percentile. In other words, their ponderal index is abnormally low.

Ultrasound Diagnostic Criteria
Biparietal Diameter
The method of measuring biparietal diameter (BPD) and the precise anatomic plane used for the

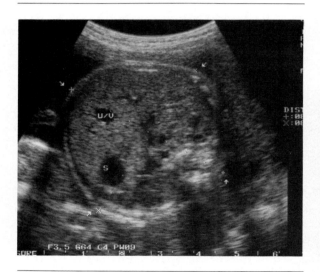

Figure 27-2. Sonogram depicts a transverse section of the fetal abdomen at the level of the stomach (s) and the umbilical vein (u/v). This is the section used to measure abdominal circumference. Note that the calipers (+) used for measuring the first diameter are placed at the outer aspects of the spine and anterior abdominal wall. The second set of calipers (×) are placed at the outer aspects of the lateral abdominal walls. The two diameters are perpendicular. The average diameter is 8.05 cm, and the calculated abdominal circumference is 8.05 × 3.14, or 25.3 cm.

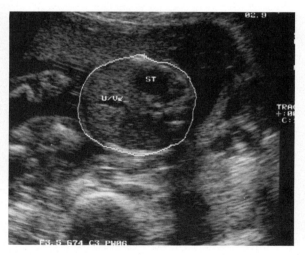

Figure 27-3. Sonogram of the fetal abdomen at the same level shown in Figure 27-2. The actual AC is traced on the screen rather than estimated by formula, as in Figure 27-2. Traced measurements are generally larger than those calculated from two diameters. U/V, umbilical vein; St, stomach.

Table 27-3. Percentile ranks of fetal head circumference measurements*

Gestational Age (LMP Weeks)	10th %ile HC (cm)	25th %ile HC (cm)	50th %ile HC (cm)	75th %ile HC (cm)	90th %ile HC (cm)
18	13.6	14.9	15.4	16.6	17.1
19	14.9	15.8	16.6	17.0	17.5
20	16.4	17.1	17.8	18.3	18.9
21	17.3	18.0	18.8	19.3	19.8
22	18.1	19.0	19.8	20.3	20.8
23	19.5	20.0	20.7	21.1	21.9
24	21.0	21.4	21.8	22.3	22.8
25	21.8	22.2	22.6	23.1	23.8
26	22.8	23.2	23.7	24.3	24.6
27	23.4	24.3	25.2	25.7	26.5
28	24.3	25.0	26.0	26.8	27.6
29	26.3	26.6	27.7	28.6	29.4
30	26.9	27.3	28.3	29.1	30.1
31	27.0	27.8	28.7	29.8	30.5
32	27.4	28.0	29.0	30.0	31.0
33	27.7	28.3	29.3	30.3	31.3
34	28.1	28.7	30.0	30.8	31.9
35	28.9	29.9	31.1	31.9	32.5
36	29.5	30.6	31.4	32.5	33.3
37	30.0	31.0	32.1	33.1	34.0
38	30.3	31.3	32.2	33.4	34.3
39	30.6	31.8	32.6	33.8	34.6
40	31.4	32.3	33.0	34.0	35.4
41	31.9	32.8	33.4	34.1	35.7

*Percentile Ranks derived from the average of direct head circumference measurements and circumference measurements calculated from diameters: (Biparietal diameter + Occipitofrontal diameter/2) × 3.14. All diameter measurements are obtained from outer edge to outer edge of fetal cephalic sonograms.

measurement are discussed in Chapter 17. The BPD is very useful for dating pregnancy and evaluating growth of the fetus[23]; however, it is subject to an artificial decrease or increase in size by normally occurring changes in head shape, such as dolichocephaly and brachycephaly; although these changes alter the BPD they do not change the HC measurement.

For example, although the BPD is actually reduced in microcephaly and in symmetric IUGR, both these conditions are better diagnosed by evaluation of HC in conjunction with AC. The diagnosis of asymmetric IUGR is also best made by comparing the fetal HC and AC measurements.[23] Finally, the BPD measurement is not utilized in many of the formulas designed for estimation of fetal weight (EFW).[12,24]

MEASUREMENTS OF HEAD AND ABDOMINAL CIRCUMFERENCE AND FEMUR LENGTH

To diagnose IUGR the sonographer should obtain HC, AC, and FL measurements[12] (see Chapters 17 and 25). It should be remembered that an error of approximately 6% is introduced when HC or AC is derived by formula (mean diameter × 3.14) and, subsequently, the respective percentile ranks obtained from charts based on traced measurements (Figs. 27-2, 27-3).[29] To reduce this error we have developed HC and AC charts based on the average of both methods, that is, the formula and direct-trace methods (Tables 27-3, 27-4).

Finally, the FL should be obtained because it correlates with the neonatal CHL, so it is used for estimating fetal weight and for calculating the ponderal index.[11,17,32]

Table 27-4. Percentile ranks of fetal abdominal circumference measurements*

Gestational Age (LMP Weeks)	10th %ile AC (cm)	25th %ile AC (cm)	50th %ile AC (cm)	75th %ile AC (cm)	90th %ile AC (cm)
18	11.0	12.1	13.5	14.3	15.9
19	13.0	13.6	14.5	15.4	16.9
20	13.6	14.4	15.2	16.1	17.6
21	14.7	15.6	16.4	17.5	18.8
22	15.7	16.4	17.6	18.8	19.9
23	17.1	18.0	19.0	19.8	20.7
24	18.0	19.4	20.1	20.8	22.1
25	18.8	19.9	20.7	21.7	22.9
26	19.7	20.8	21.7	22.6	23.6
27	20.7	22.3	23.0	24.0	26.0
28	21.7	23.7	24.7	25.5	27.3
29	23.6	24.9	26.1	27.4	28.8
30	24.5	25.5	26.8	27.9	29.2
31	25.6	26.4	27.7	28.7	29.9
32	26.0	27.2	28.5	29.8	30.9
33	26.4	27.6	28.7	30.3	31.3
34	27.5	28.8	30.0	31.2	32.6
35	29.7	30.6	31.6	33.5	34.8
36	31.1	31.8	32.8	34.3	35.8
37	31.7	33.0	33.8	35.5	36.7
38	32.5	34.0	34.9	36.4	37.5
39	33.0	34.6	35.3	37.1	37.9
40	33.2	35.0	36.5	37.7	38.4
41	33.8	35.7	37.5	38.2	39.0

*Percentile ranks derived from the average of direct circumference measurements and circumference measurements calculated from diameters: (Anteroposterior + Transverse abdominal diameters/2) × 3.14. All diameter measurements are obtained from outer edge to outer edge of fetal abdominal circumference sonograms.

Head Circumference to Abdominal Circumference Ratio

In some fetuses the HC/AC ratio may be useful to further substantiate the possibility of asymmetric IUGR. This is based on the fact that the HC/AC ratio is at least 2 SD above the mean in approximately 70% of asymmetric IUGR (Table 27-5).[4] It should be remembered, however, that in symmetric or nearly symmetric IUGR the size of the fetal head and abdomen are both reduced; as a result, the HC/AC ratio remains unchanged and, so, is not a useful parameter for diagnosing this condition. Another complicating factor is the fact that in *preterm* fetuses whose growth is not altered, the HC/AC ratio is normally high, similar to the level observed in asymmetric IUGR. As a result, the latter two entities can be differentiated only if gestational age is well-defined.

Table 27-5. Mean head/abdomen (H/A) circumference ratio at gestational age (GA)

GA (weeks)	Mean HA Ratio	+2 SD
28	1.13	1.21
32	1.075	1.17
34	1.04	1.13
36	1.02	1.12
38	0.99	1.06
40	0.97	1.05

(Adapted from Campbell S, Thoms A. Ultrasound measurement of fetal head to abdomen circumference ratio in the assessment of growth retardation. Br J Obstet Gynaecol. 1977; 84:165.)

Formulas for Estimating Fetal Weight

Having correctly derived the HC, AC, and FL measurements, it is possible to enter them into one of many formulas designed for EFW. In this chapter we discuss only the approaches used in three formulas.

Formula by MJ Shepard et al.[27] This formula incorporates only BPD and AC, and its predictive error is high (±20%).[12] There are two limiting factors to this formula. The first is use of the BPD, a parameter that can be altered secondary to "normal" changes in head shape such as dolichocephaly and brachycephaly. The second is exclusion of the HC and FL, both of which are important contributors to weight.

Formula by FP Hadlock et al.[12] This formula incorporates all three basic measurements, HC, AC, FL.[24] With this approach the 2-SD variation in the prediction of birth weight has been reduced from ±20.0% to ±15.0%.[12] However, by using this formula the authors have reported a wide error (± 19.4%) in estimating the size of fetuses that weigh less than 1500 g. Further, this formula is not targeted to specific fetal populations such as those that are large, appropriate, or small for gestational age. As a result, it does not take into account the proportional contributions of HC and AC to birth weight, contributions that are in a dynamic state of change. In other words, the HC/AC ratio is a variable dimension and depends on whether fetal growth is normal or altered and on whether the pregnancy is preterm or term. The following examples illustrate the dynamic differences that exist in the HC/AC ratios:

1. Prior to the 36th pregnancy week the HC/AC ratio is >1.0.
2. Following the 36th pregnancy week the HC/AC ratio is <1.0.
3. In the macrosomic fetus the HC/AC ratio is <1.0.
4. In symmetric IUGR the HC/AC ratio is not altered.
5. In asymmetric IUGR, the HC/AC ratio is markedly increased, even at term, when the ratio is normally <1.0.

Formulas by RE Sabbagha et al.[24] To account for the dynamically varying proportional contributions of the HC and the AC, these investigators derived three formulas, one from each of three fetal groups: large, appropriate, and small for gestational age; each of the three formulas is targeted to a specific group of fetuses. All three targeted formulas incorporate the following four parameters: gestational age in weeks, HC, AC (multiplied by 2), and FL. The accuracy of the assigned gestational age should be within ±2 weeks, and preferably determined by one of the following criteria: (1) early CRL or BPD (measurements obtained prior to 13 and 26 weeks' gestation, respectively); (2) known ovulation dates or certain last menstrual period; (3) confirmation of menstrual dates by early CRL or BPD, as defined in criterion 1; (4) the average of different dates estimated by early CRL and/or BPD, and FL, provided that the estimates do not differ from each other by more than 1 week; (5) the average of different dates provided by early CRL, and/or HC, or AC, and FL, again, provided that the estimates do not differ from each other by more than 1 week.

In estimating fetal weight by the targeted formulas, the percentile rank of the AC determines which of the three formulas should be employed. For example, if the AC is at least in the 90th percentile, the formula for the large-for-dates fetus is used. On the other hand, if the AC is average (between 5th and 90th percentile), the formula for the appropriate-for-dates fetus is used. Finally, if the AC is below the 5th percentile, the formula for the small-for-dates fetus is used.

In comparison to Hadlock's formula, the targeted formulas reduce the cumulative 2-SD variation by 8.4%. On the other hand, the cumulative *absolute* 2-SD variation of the targeted formulas is 12%, versus 15.6% for Hadlock's formula, a reduction of 23%.[24] It should be emphasized that the advantage of reduction in the 2-SD variation achieved by the targeted formulas may be lost if gestational age cannot be determined within a range of ±2 weeks.

The format of deriving estimates of fetal weight by the sum of four variables allows the sonographer the choice of reading the estimated fetal weight directly from a concise chart (Table 27-6) or entering all three formulas (Table 27-7) into a computer for automatic calculation of the estimated fetal weight.

Table 27-6. Estimates of fetal weight derived from formulas targeted to SGA, AGA, and LGA fetuses

Formula 1† Use When Abdominal Perimeter ≥90% Large-for-Gestational Age Group (LGA)			Formula 2† Use When Abdominal Perimeter >5% <90% Appropriate-for-Gestational Age Group (AGA)			Formula 3† Use When Abdominal Perimeter ≤5% Small-for-Gestational Age Group (SGA)		
SUM*	EFW	Diff	SUM*	EFW	Diff	SUM*	EFW	Diff
102	1385		88	506		81	507	
103	1401	16	89	536	30	82	521	14
104	1418	17	90	566	30	83	536	15
105	1437	19	91	596	30	84	552	16
106	1456	19	92	627	31	85	569	17
107	1477	21	93	659	32	86	586	17
108	1498	21	94	690	31	87	604	18
109	1521	23	95	723	33	88	623	19
110	1545	24	96	756	33	89	643	20
111	1570	25	97	789	33	90	663	20
112	1596	26	98	824	35	91	684	21
113	1623	27	99	858	34	92	706	22
114	1651	28	100	893	35	93	729	23
115	1681	30	101	929	36	94	752	23
116	1711	30	102	965	36	95	776	24
117	1742	31	103	1001	36	96	801	25
118	1775	33	104	1039	38	97	827	26
119	1809	34	105	1076	37	98	853	26
120	1843	34	106	1114	38	99	881	28
121	1879	36	107	1153	39	100	909	28
122	1916	37	108	1192	39	101	937	28
123	1954	38	109	1232	40	102	967	30
124	1993	39	110	1272	40	103	997	30
125	2033	40	111	1313	41	104	1028	31
126	2074	41	112	1354	41	105	1060	32
127	2117	43	113	1396	42	106	1092	32
128	2160	63	114	1438	42	107	1125	33
129	2205	45	115	1481	43	108	1159	34
130	2250	45	116	1524	43	109	1194	35
131	2297	47	117	1568	44	110	1229	35
132	2345	48	118	1613	45	111	1266	37
133	2393	48	119	1658	46	112	1303	37
134	2443	50	120	1703	45	113	1340	37
135	2494	51	121	1749	46	114	1379	39
136	2546	52	122	1795	46	115	1418	39
137	2599	53	123	1842	47	116	1458	40
138	2654	55	124	1890	48	117	1499	41
139	2709	55	125	1938	48	118	1540	41
140	2765	56	126	1986	48	119	1583	43
141	2823	58	127	2035	49	120	1626	43
142	2882	59	128	2085	50	121	1670	44
143	2941	59	129	2135	50	122	1714	44
144	3002	61	130	2185	50	123	1759	45
145	3064	62	131	2236	51	124	1805	46

TABLE 27-6. (continued)

Formula 1† Use When Abdominal Perimeter ≥90% LARGE-FOR-GESTATIONAL AGE GROUP (LGA)			Formula 2† Use When Abdominal Perimeter >5% <90% APPROPRIATE-FOR-GESTATIONAL AGE GROUP (AGA)			Formula 3† Use When Abdominal Perimeter ≤5% SMALL-FOR-GESTATIONAL AGE GROUP (SGA)		
SUM*	EFW	Diff	SUM*	EFW	Diff	SUM*	EFW	Diff
146	3127	63	132	2288	52	125	1852	47
147	3191	64	133	2340	52	126	1900	48
148	3256	65	134	2393	53	127	1948	48
149	3322	66	135	2446	53	128	1997	49
150	3389	67	136	2500	54	129	2047	50
151	3458	69	137	2554	54	130	2097	51
152	3527	69	138	2608	54	131	2149	52
153	3598	71	139	2664	56	132	2201	52
154	3669	64	140	2719	55	133	2254	53
155	3742	73	141	2776	57	134	2307	53
156	3816	74	142	2832	56	135	2362	55
157	3891	75	143	2890	58	136	2417	55
158	3966	75	144	2948	58	137	2473	56
159	4044	78	145	3006	58	138	2529	56
160	4122	78	146	3065	59	139	2587	58
161	4201	79	147	3124	59	140	2645	58
162	4281	80	148	3184	60	141	2704	59
163	4363	82	149	3244	60	142	2763	59
164	4445	82	150	3305	62	143	2824	61
165	4529	84	151	3367	62	144	2885	61
166	4613	84	152	3429	62	145	2947	62
167	4699	86	153	3491	62	146	3009	62
168	4786	87	154	3554	63	147	3073	64
169	4874	88	155	3617	63	148	3137	64
170	4963	89	156	3681	64	149	3202	65
171	5053	90	157	3746	65	150	3267	65
172	5144	91	158	3811	65			
173	5236	92	159	3877	66			
174	5329	93						
175	5424	95						
176	5519	95						
177	5616	97						
178	5713	97						
179	5812	99						
180	5912	100						
181	6013	101						

*SUM, sum of fetal parameters constituting independent variables: GA (weeks or weeks plus fractions thereof, e.g., 22.7 wks) + HC (cm) + (2 AC [cm]) + FL (cm)
†The equations used to generate the EFW in each subgroup are listed in Table 27-7.
Note: If sum of parameters falls between two numbers, e.g., 82.5, the estimated fetal weight may be extrapolated from the difference (Diff) between the upper and lower numbers (i.e., 521 and 636). Additionally, the accuracy of the assigned gestational age should be within ± 2 weeks. (From Sabbagha RE, Minogue J, Tamura RK, et al. Estimation of birth weight by the use of ultrasound formulas targeted to large, appropriate, and small for gestational age fetuses. Am J Obstet Gynecol. 1989; 160:854.)

Table 27-7. Formulas used in the prospective evaluation of 381 pregnancies

Groups	Formulas
Large for gestational age (LGA)	$5426.9 - (94.98 \times SUM)* + (0.54262 \times SUM^2)$ $(r = 0.93, r^2 = 0.87)$
Appropriate for gestational age (AGA)	$-55.3 - (16.35 \times SUM) + (0.25838 \times SUM^2)$ $(r = 0.97, r^2 = 0.94)$
Small for gestational age (SGA)	$1849.4 - (47.13 \times SUM) + (0.37721 \times SUM^2)$ $(r = .96, r^2 = .92)$

LGA, Fetuses with AC ≥90th percentile; AGA, fetuses with AC >5% and <90%; SGA, fetuses with AC ≤5th percentile, for dates. EFW, Estimated fetal weight; AC, abdominal circumference; HC, head circumference; FL, femur length.
*SUM = GA (wk) + (2 AC) (cm) + HC (cm) + FL (cm).
(From Sabbagha RE, Minogue J, Tamura RK, et al. Estimation of birth weight by the use of ultrasound formulas targeted to large-, appropriate-, and small–for–gestational age fetuses. Am J Obstet Gynecol. 1989; 160:854.)

Amniotic Fluid

Source. Amniotic fluid is derived from fetal and maternal sources. The exchange occurs in two directions within each of three compartments[13]:

Compartment 1, Mother and Amniotic fluid. The bidirectional flow takes place across the decidua and fetal membranes; at term, the normal net hourly exchange is approximately 135 ml in the direction of amniotic fluid.

Compartment 2, Mother and Fetus. The bidirectional flow takes place across the intervillous space; at term, the normal net hourly exchange is approximately 50 to 90 ml in the direction of the fetus.

Compartment 3, Fetus and Amniotic fluid. The flow mainly occurs through the respiratory, gastrointestinal, and urinary tracts. At term, the normal net hourly exchange is approximately 150 to 225 ml in the direction of the amniotic fluid compartment.

Amniotic Fluid Index. Recently, Phelan and coworkers developed a new ultrasound method that allows quantification of normal amniotic fluid volume at different intervals in pregnancy.[18] They divided the uterine cavity into four quadrants by two imaginary lines, one running transversely across the umbilicus and the other vertically across the linea nigra (Fig. 27-4). The vertical diameter of the largest pocket in each quadrant was measured and the sum of the four pockets was determined. This sum is called the amniotic fluid index (AFI). The mean values ($\pm$ 2-SD) of the AFI throughout pregnancy were then determined (Fig. 27-5). It became clear that, in the third trimester of pregnancy, the 2-SD variation about the mean AFI is very wide. Additionally, a progressive increase in the amniotic fluid volume (AFV) is noted until the 28th to 30th pregnancy weeks. Subsequently, a minimal but gradual decrease is observed until term (see Fig. 27-5).

Oligohydramnios.

Diagnosis. Most observers agree that, in the third trimester of pregnancy, oligohydramnios exists when: (1) the diameter of the largest pocket of amniotic fluid is less than 2 cm or 3 cm (depending on the guidelines adopted by each institution)[6]; (2) the AFI is no more than 8 cm, approximately 2 SD below the mean (however, until recently a statistically significant increase in poor perinatal outcome has been observed only when the AFI is 5 or less)[22]; (3) the experienced sonographer subjectively observes an overall diminution in AFV.

Clinical usefulness. Using the subjective method of assessing AFV in a large unselected population of pregnant women, Philipson, Sokol, and Williams showed that the prevalence of oligohydramnios is 3.9%.[20] Analysis of these data also showed that the predictive value of oligohydramnios in the diagnosis of IUGR was only 40%. Worse still, in another study the presence of oligohydramnios was shown to predict IUGR in only 19% of such cases.[2] The sensitivity of the test (that is, presence of oligohydramnios) is also low, 16%.[20] The fact that only 16% of all IUGR is associated with oligohydramnios may be related to the marked variation in AFV noted in different pregnancies. In other words, the AFV may be low in many normal pregnancies.

Despite the poor positive predictive value, it has become apparent that oligohydramnios is a clinically useful predictor of IUGR in complicated or high-risk pregnancies. For example, Phelan and colleagues have shown that in postterm pregnancies with severe oligohydramnios (largest vertical

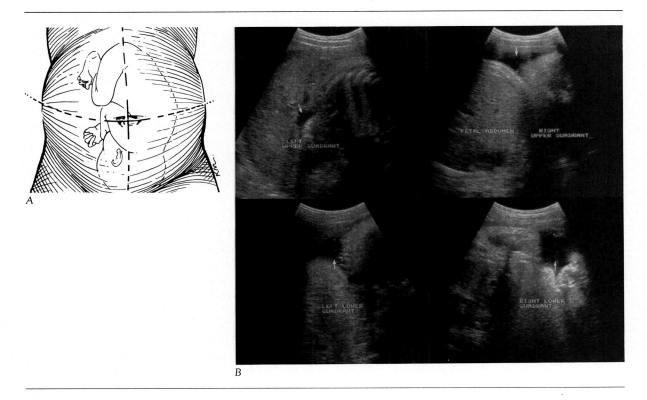

FIGURE 27-4 (A) Photograph shows division of the pregnant abdomen into four quadrants for obtaining the AFI. (B) Sonograms depicting amniotic fluid volume (*arrows*) in all four quadrants. The AFI is approximately 5 cm, since there is no measurable pocket in the left upper quadrant. The AFI is diagnostic of oligohydramnios.

FIGURE 27-5. The black area on the graph depicts the mean values (± 2SD variation) of the AFI, from the 12th to the 42nd weeks of pregnancy. Note that at 40 weeks' gestation an AFI of 8 cm falls at the critical 2SD level below the mean. (Phelan JP, Ahn MO, Smith CV, et al. Amniotic fluid index measurements during pregnancy. Reproductive Med 1987;32:602.)

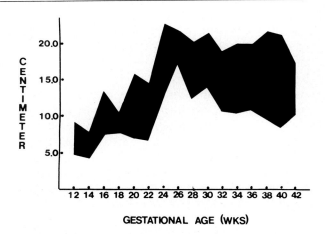

AF pocket <1 cm) the incidence of abnormal fetal heart tracings requiring cesarean section was 16.7%.[19] By comparison in postterm pregnancies with normal AFV the incidence of abnormal fetal heart tracings requiring cesarean section was only 1.05%.[19] Thus, the presence of oligohydramnios in postterm pregnancy is an ominous finding and points to the need to deliver the fetus. Similarly, the presence of oligohydramnios in a fetus whose EFW is below the 10th percentile is more likely to predict a worse outcome and is an indication for strict surveillance of the fetus to determine the most appropriate time for delivery.

Testing Protocols

Antenatal detection of IUGR is important because it increases the antenatal surveillance of this population. In this way, the most suitable time for delivering the affected fetus can be better delineated—the point in pregnancy when the fetus has attained maximum pulmonary maturity but has not yet developed central nervous system compromise. Once the diagnosis of IUGR is made the exact mode of surveillance followed by different clinical departments varies. Nonetheless, the basic modalities include the nonstress test (NST), the contraction stress test (CST), and the biophysical profile score (BPS). Importantly, when results of these tests are normal they accurately predict fetal well-being. On the other hand, abnormal test results do not have a high correlation with poor outcome or fetal hypoxia; in other words, the false positive rate of these tests is high (see below). Since the NST is part of the BPS and is frequently employed before other tests, it is discussed first.

NONSTRESS TEST

Although NSTs are usually conducted by a nurse-specialist, knowledge of the method of interpreting the test is important for sonographers. The NST is frequently referred to as a bioelectric test. It involves computation of the baseline fetal heart rate (FHR) and any changes that occur in response to fetal movement. A normal (or reactive) test depends on detection of at least two FHR accelerations above the baseline. Normally, in a 20-minute interval or window the FHR should accelerate by 15 beats per minute (bpm) for at least 15 seconds

(see Fig. 27-6).[14] Indicators of well-being also include a baseline FHR falling between 120 and 160 bpm and absence of any decelerations, that is, decrease in the FHR below baseline. A normal or reactive result implies good fetal outcome; that is, absence of asphyxia for 7 days in the preterm and term fetus and for 3 days in the postterm fetus. A reactive test correctly predicts fetal well-being in 62 to 89% of cases.

An abnormal or nonreactive NST is defined by absence of fetal movements or by FHR accelerations less than 15 bpm. Additionally, the presence of spontaneous heart rate decelerations and/or loss of beat-to-beat heart rate variability (a characteristic of normal fetuses, Fig. 27-6) may be associated with poor outcome. A nonreactive test correctly predicts fetal death (within 1 week of testing) in only 3 to 29% of cases; in other words, the predictive value of an abnormal test is poor. The reason may be partly related to the *normal periodicity* that characterizes biophysical functions; lack of motion during the 20-minute window may be an indication that the fetus is in a sleep cycle rather than in a state of flaccidity caused by hypoxia. In conclusion, the NST is more useful for predicting fetal well-being than fetal hypoxia because its false abnormal rate is high; to reduce the number of false nonreactive NST results many investigators are using the fetal acoustic stimulation test (FAS-Test) to awaken the fetus and make it reactive.

FETAL ACOUSTIC STIMULATION TEST (FAS-TEST)

In this test an artificial larynx (EAL Bell Telephone) is used to generate an acoustic-vibratory stimulus lasting 2 to 5 seconds.[28] The average sound energy produced at 1 meter of air equals 82 dB.[14] The frequency of the emitted sound is 80 Hz, with harmonics ranging from 20 to 9000 Hz.[28] The stimulus or buzz produced by the artificial larynx changes the fetal biologic cycle from sleep to awakening and, thus, reduces the number of false positive NSTs.[28]

There is concern about possible detrimental effects of externally applied acoustic-vibratory stimuli on fetuses.[28] Studies in mice have shown susceptibility to audiogenic seizures after exposure to a loud bell at 21 days of age.[9] Growth retardation has also been noted in mothers living near jet airports.[28] Long-term follow-up studies are necessary before the FAS-Test is routinely adopted.

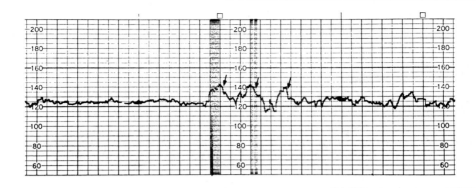

FIGURE 27-6. Bioelectric tracing shows a reactive nonstress test. The vertical line (*y* axis) delineates the FHR per minute. The horizontal (*x* axis) delineates time, approximately 10 seconds per small box (20 small boxes are placed between the vertical printed FHR numbers and are run through the NST machine at a rate of 1 box per 10 seconds or 20 boxes every 3.33 minutes, approximately 200 seconds). Note the following characteristics of a reactive test: (1) baseline is normal, ranging from 120 to 125 beats per minute, (2) beat-to-beat variability is clearly seen as the baseline heart rate has a jagged appearance, (3) no decelerations are recorded, and (4) three heart rate accelerations are recorded (*arrows*), each exceeding 15 beats per minute.

CONTRACTION STRESS TEST (CST)

In the CST three uterine contractions are induced during a 10-minute interval, either by controlled intravenous pitocin drip or by nipple stimulation. A hypoxic or compromised fetus will not tolerate the low intervillous blood flow and oxygen level brought about by the stress of the induced uterine contractions. As a result, fetal myocardial hypoxia is manifested as repetitive, uniform, and late heart rate decelerations (decelerations which occur at the end of a uterine contraction). The CST, like the NST, is much better at predicting the normal uncompromised fetus and its false negative rate is very low. Its false positive rate, noted in different studies, ranges from 30 to 60%.[5,8]

BIOPHYSICAL PROFILE

The biophysical profile is presented in detail in Chapter 26. In this discussion the reader is reminded that the BPS is based on the evaluation of five biophysical functions: fetal breathing movement (FBM), fetal motion (FM), fetal tone (FT), AFV, and NST. The reactivity of the biophysical variables is dependent on an intact central nervous system (CNS). A score of 2 is assigned for each normal variable and a score of 0 when the biophysical function is absent. All observations are made within an interval of 30 minutes.

Like the NST and the CST, the biophysical profile is a better predictor of normalcy than of fetal hypoxia. First, the result is likely to be negative in 97.5% of tested fetuses, and the predictive value of a normal test is quite high.[15] It would be extremely unlikely for a preterm or term fetus to die within 7 days if the biophysical profile result was negative and for a postterm fetus to die within 3 days of such a result. The biophysical profile can be equivocal in 1.72% of fetuses. Under such circumstances it should be repeated or a CST performed, depending on the management protocol of the particular institution.

The biophysical profile is clearly abnormal in a very small number (0.76%) of tested fetuses,[15] but the subsequent management of such fetuses is not uniform. In some centers delivery of the fetus may be effected, particularly if it is pulmonically mature. In other centers a CST is performed first to confirm fetal hypoxia, or, alternatively, fetal biophysical functions are continuously observed for 2 or 3 hours before decisive action is taken. The rationale for the latter thinking is the fact that absence of some biophysical functions may reflect normal periodicity rather than hypoxia. The absence of some biophysical functions for periods of 20 minutes to 2 hours or longer can be normal.

Absence of some biologic function may also be related to the time of testing or to medication used by the mother. FBMs follow a circadian rhythm (i.e., appear more frequently at specific times of the night), are more common 2 hours after meals, and can be suppressed by medication used to sedate the mother or treat her hypertension. There is no doubt, then, that the accuracy of the BPS will be enhanced if the mother is tested 2 hours after meals and is not using medication known to depress the fetal CNS.

Presently, the protocols used by various centers in the antenatal management of IUGR are not uniform. Some investigators argue that there is no need to spend a long time waiting to evaluate all the components of the biophysical profile and that adherence to the results of both the NST and AFV suffice. The rationale is as follows: (1) A reactive NST implies that fetal motion is indeed present and indirectly tests for this important function of fetal motion. (2) An NST should always be part of the antenatal testing schema because it may show variable decelerations, a finding that may be missed completely if one relies only on the other four functions of the biophysical profile. (3) Oligohydramnios may be a significant indicator of chronic hypoxia, particularly in the IUGR or postdate fetus, and should always be taken into consideration. Because specific management protocols are not universally adhered to, sonographers should follow the guidelines established by their respective institutions.

Protocol for Reporting Ultrasound Findings

The sonographer in possession of the background information discussed in this chapter is in a position to present the data to the referring physician in the most effective and practical way. The referring physician would like to have specific information regarding the following areas:

1. The *final assigned menstrual age* and the method used to assign these dates. An example of important comments would be:

   a. Dates are assigned by concurrence between early ultrasound (prior to 26 weeks' gestation) and menstrual dates, or, menstrual dates are confirmed by known ovulation day.

   b. Dates are assigned by CRL.

2. The *estimated fetal weight* and the 2-SD variation of the formula used.

3. The *birth weight percentile*, as outlined in Table 27-1. For example, it should be stated that an EFW of 2120 g at 36 weeks' gestation falls below the 10th percentile rank. The sonographer should specify which table was used.

4. The *fetal growth pattern*, as defined by the size of the AC. Usually, the percentile rank of the AC is similar to the percentile rank of the EFW. On some occasions, however, the AC percentile rank may be small but the fetal growth as judged by the EFW may be normal, or vice versa. Our studies in this area show that although the latter group of fetuses remain at risk for altered fetal growth, the majority will be normal. Nonetheless, it is important for the referring health professional to be aware of the discrepancy that can exist between the assigned percentile ranks of the AC and the EFW. Our studies also show that the predictive value of the EFW in correctly identifying IUGR is approximately 75%. Once the diagnosis of IUGR is suspected (by an EFW that falls below the 10th percentile), other ultrasound data should be carefully examined and follow-up examinations may be appropriate. The interval between these examinations should be agreed upon by the physician and the sonographer.

5. *Unusually small or large HC, AC, or FL in fetuses with normal EFW.* In such cases the sonographer should include this information on the report because it will help improve the interpretation of growth events. The information will also alert the physician to the need for follow-up examinations of these parameters at specific intervals.

6. *Ponderal index or AC/FL ratio.* Information regarding the ponderal index is significant. By definition the index is abnormal when the FL is at least in the 90th percentile and the AC is not higher than the 10th percentile. Such fetuses will have growth retardation even if their birth weight exceeds the 10th percentile rank. The combination of a small AC and a long femur occurs in less than 1% of cases, but it is precisely in

TABLE 27-8. Example of diagnostic ultrasound report of a fetus with symmetric IUGR*

---

1. Assigned dates = 35 menstrual weeks
   Dates assigned by early BPD, prior to 26 weeks
2. EFW = 1850 g
   EFW by the formula of Sabbagha et al. for the small fetus
3. EFW falls <10th %ile for 35 weeks
   Percentile by the chart of Brenner et al.
4. Fetal growth: AC falls <5th %ile for 35 weeks
   EFW and AC percentile rank, concordant
5. Other small or large parameters: HC <5th %ile for 35 weeks
   IUGR is symmetric
6. Ponderal index: normal
7. Amniotic fluid index: <5 cm
8. Placental grade: II
9. Biophysical profile score: 8
   FBM - 2, FM - 2, FT - 2, AFV - 0, NST - 2
10. Velocimetry: 2.8 (borderline)

---

*Note: Fetal biometry indicates symmetric IUGR and there is evidence of: 1. decreased AFV or oligohydramnios. However, the NST is still normal. Velocimetry and placental grade are also normal. Management will depend upon status of pulmonary maturity, obstetric history, and results of continued frequent surveillance.

such cases that IUGR may go undetected because the EFW may fall within normal limits.

7. *Amniotic fluid volume.* The sonographer should enter one or more of the following diagnostic criteria for oligohydramnios:
   a. Diagnosis of oligohydramnios is based on the subjective evaluation of AFV.
   b. Diagnosis of oligohydramnios is based on the fact that the largest vertical pocket of AF is less than 2 cm or than 3 cm (depending on the accepted threshold for oligohydramnios in the ultrasound department).
   c. Diagnosis of oligohydramnios is based on the fact that the amniotic fluid index is not more than 5 cm.
8. *Placental grade.* A grade 3 placenta may be associated with IUGR if it is noted prior to 36 weeks' gestation; this should be described here.
9. *Biophysical profile score.* The biophysical profile score should be reported when a specific request for this fetal evaluation is made. The results can be entered on one line, as in the following example: FBM = 0, FM = 2, FT = 2, AFV = 2, NST = 2; total score = 8.
10. *Velocimetry.* The systolic/diastolic (or S/D) ratio reflects blood velocity in the umbilical or cere-bral circulation. It should be reported, particularly in specific high-risk situations (see Chapter 19).

An example of a report describing an IUGR fetus is shown in Table 27-8.

References

1. Battaglia FC, Lubchenco LO. A practical classification of newborn infants by weight and gestational age. J Pediatr. 1967; 71:159.
2. Bottoms SF, Welch RA, Zador IE, et al. Limitations of using maximum vertical pocket and other sonographic evaluations of amniotic fluid volume to predict fetal growth: Technical or physiologic. Am J Obstet Gynecol. 1986; 155:154.
3. Brenner WE, Edelman DA, Hendricks CH. A standard of fetal growth for the United States of America. Am J Obstet Gynecol. 1976; 126:155.
4. Campbell S, Thoms A. Ultrasound measurement of the fetal head to abdomen circumference ratio in the assessment of growth retardation. Br J Obstet Gynaecol. 1977; 84:165.
5. Collea JV, Holls WM. The contraction stress test. Clin Obstet Gynecol. 1982; 4:707.
6. Crowley P, O'Herlihy C, Boylan P. The value of ultrasound measurement of amniotic fluid volume in the management of prolonged pregnancies. Br J Obstet Gynaecol. 1984; 91:444.
7. Fitzhardinge PM, Steven EM. The small-for-dates infant II. Neurological and intellectual sequelae. Pediatrics. 1972; 50:50.
8. Freeman RE, Anderson G, Dorcester W. A prospective multi-institutional study of antepartum fetal heart rate monitoring. I. Risk of perinatal mortality and morbidity according to antepartum fetal heart rate test results. Am J Obstet Gynecol. 1982; 143:771.
9. Goodlin RC. Possible deleterious effects of sound or vibratory fetal stimuli. Letter to the editors. Am J Obstet Gynecol. 1988; 159:1016.
10. Gruenwald P. Infants of low birth weight among 5000 deliveries. Pediatrics. 1964; 34:157.
11. Hadlock FP, Deter RL, Foecher E, et al. Relation of fetal femur length to neonatal crown-heel length. J Ultrasound Med. 1984; 3:1.
12. Hadlock FP, Harrist RB, Sharman RS, et al. Estimation of fetal weight with the use of head, body, and femur measurements—A prospective study. Am J Obstet Gynecol. 1985; 151:333-337.
13. Hutchinson DL, Gray MJ, Plentl AA, et al. The role of the fetus in the water exchange of the amniotic fluid in normal and hydramniotic patients. J Clin Invest. 1959; 38:971.

14. Lavery PJ. Nonstress fetal heart rate testing. Clin Obstet Gynecol. 1982; 25:689.

15. Manning FA, Morrison I, Lange MB, et al. Fetal assessment based on fetal biophysical profile scoring: Experience in 12,620 referred high-risk pregnancies. Perinatal mortality by frequency and etiology. Am J Obstet Gynecol. 1985; 151:343-350.

16. Miller HC, Merritt T. Fetal Growth in Humans. Chicago: Year Book Medical Publishers; 1979.

17. O'Brien GD, Queenan JT. Ultrasound fetal femur length in relation to intrauterine growth retardation. Am J Obstet Gynecol. 1982; 144:35.

18. Phelan JP, Ahn MO, Smith CV, et al. Amniotic fluid index measurements during pregnancy. J Reprod Med. 1987; 32:601.

19. Phelan JP, Platt LD, Yeh SY, et al. The role of ultrasound assessment of amniotic fluid volume in the management of the postdate pregnancy. Am J Obstet Gynecol. 1985; 151:304-308.

20. Philipson EH, Sokol RJ, Williams T. Oligohydramnios: Clinical associations and predictive value for intrauterine growth retardation. Am Obstet Gynecol. 1983; 146:271.

21. Rosenberg K. Grant J, Hepburn M. Antenatal detection of growth retardation: Actual practice in a large maternity hospital. Br J Obstet Gynaecol. 1982; 89:12.

22. Rutherford SE, Phelan JP, Smith CV, et al. The four-quadrant assessment of amniotic fluid volume: An adjunct to antepartum fetal heart rate testing. Obstet Gynecol. 1987; 70:353.

23. Sabbagha RE. Intrauterine growth retardation: avenues of future research in diagnosis and management by ultrasound. Sem Perinatol. 1984; 8:31.

24. Sabbagha RE, Minogue J, Tamura RK, et al. Estimation of birth weight by the use of ultrasound formulas targeted to large, appropriate, and small-for-gestational age fetuses. Am J Obstet Gynecol. 1989; 160:854.

25. Scott KE, Usher R. Fetal malnutrition: Its incidence, causes, and effects. Am J Obstet Gynecol. 1966; 94:951.

26. Scott A, Moar V, Ounsted M. The relative contributions of different maternal factors in small-for–gestational age pregnancies. Eur J Obstet Gynecol. 1981; 12:157.

27. Shepard MJ, Richards VA, Berkowitz RL, et al. An evaluation of two equations for predicting fetal weight by ultrasound. Am J Obstet Gynecol. 1982; 142:47.

28. Smith CV, Phelan JP, Paul RH, et al. Fetal acoustic stimulation testing: A retrospective experience with the fetal acoustic stimulation test. Am J Obstet Gynecol. 1985; 153:567.

29. Tamura RK, Sabbagha RE, Pan WH, et al. Ultrasonic fetal abdominal circumference: Comparison of direct versus calculated measurement. Obstet Gynecol. 1986; 67:833.

30. Tejani N, Mann LI, Weiss RR. Antenatal diagnosis and management of the small-for–gestational age fetus. Obstet Gynecol. 1976; 47:31.

31. Villar J, Belizan JM. The timing factor in the pathophysiology of the intrauterine growth retardation syndrome. Obstet Gynecol. 1982; 37:499.

32. Vintzileos AM, Campbell WA, Neckles S, et al. The ultrasound femur length as a predictor of femur length. Obstet Gynecol. 1984; 64:779.

33. Winick M. Fetal malnutrition. Clin Obstet Gynecol. 1970; 13:3,527.

34. Winick M, Brasel JA, Velasco EG. Effects of prenatal nutrition upon pregnancy. Clin Obstet Gynecol. 1973; 16:1,185.

35. Yerushalmy J. Relation of birth weight, gestational age, and rate of intrauterine growth to perinatal mortality. Clin Obstet Gynecol. 1970; 13:107.

CHAPTER 28

The Effect of Maternal Disease on Pregnancy

Dunstan Abraham, William Greenhut, Mordecai Koenigsberg

Maternal disease may have a wide spectrum of effects on pregnancy, ranging from destruction of the early zygote or embryo to major malformation and demise of the developing fetus. The mechanisms through which maternal disease can affect the fetus are varied; however, it has been clearly established that the placenta can play a crucial role in preventing or facilitating the transmission process.[61]

The major physiologic function of the placenta is to exchange gas, nutrients, and waste products between the maternal and fetal circulations. This is achieved by various methods, including diffusion, active transport, and pinocytosis. For example, blood gases move or diffuse speedily and easily across the placenta from maternal to fetal circulation, but larger molecules, such as carbohydrates, must be assisted or actively transported across the placental membranes.

Some substances, usually those that have larger molecules, are unable to cross the placenta and are thus effectively barred from entering the fetal circulation by the "placental barrier." This barrier prevents the mixing of the maternal and fetal circulations. Nevertheless, a variety of substances and agents are able to move across this barrier and harm the developing fetus. Examples include infectious agents, drugs, and antibodies.

In addition, maternal diseases may indirectly harm the fetus via the placenta. Maternal vascular disease such as hypertension decreases uteroplacental blood flow and compromises the placenta's function of providing nutrients for the fetus. Intrauterine growth retardation (IUGR) is not uncommonly encountered in these cases.

Sonography has a valuable role in evaluating pregnancies complicated by maternal disease. Generally, a fetus at risk can be screened for gross malformations and IUGR. In addition, sonography can assess placental maturation and amniotic fluid volume and can date pregnancies to determine the best date for cesarean section. In diagnostic procedures such as amniocentesis and percutaneous umbilical blood sampling (PUBS), in which fetal blood is obtained from the umbilical vein, ultrasound is used for needle guidance.[13,46]

More recently, information about the fetoplacental circulatory unit has been obtained with Doppler ultrasound. Technically, this is performed by recording the flow velocity waveform (FVW) of the umbilical artery—and, less frequently, the uterine artery. From this waveform a systolic to diastolic (S/D) ratio can be calculated, and abnormal values, indicating disease, can be detected.[15]

Doppler velocity waveform monitoring of the umbilical artery has proven to be a useful indicator of fetal well-being. Normally, as pregnancy progresses, increased diastolic flow is observed, representing reduced resistance to flow. High resistance to flow has been found in complicated pregnancies such as premature rupture of membranes, toxemia, IUGR, sickle cell disease, and diabetes mellitus.[15,23,67]

In this chapter we discuss some of the more commonly encountered maternal diseases and conditions that may adversely affect fetal outcome. These include infectious disease, endocrine and metabolic disorders, hematologic disorders, toxemia, drug addiction, and malnutrition. The specific role of sonography in these various situations is also discussed.

Infections

Fetal infection from maternal disease can occur at various times during gestation and can have a variety of clinical outcomes. Maternal infection even before conception may also have an adverse effect on future pregnancies.

The extent of damage to the fetus depends on several factors, including the virulence of the agent and the route of transmission. The gestational age at the time of infection is also of major importance, as in many cases this determines the susceptibility of the fetus to the agent. Since organogenesis occurs during the first trimester, the fetus is particularly susceptible at this time, but infection can occur before conception, before implantation, after implantation, and in the puerperium.[74]

Infection before conception has been studied in mouse systems by researchers using retroviruses. Results have demonstrated that these viruses can infect the embryo, integrate into the germ line, and cause disease in future generations.[37] Retroviruses have not yet been implicated in human disease, although their presence in human species has been established.

Infection before implantation may result from local infection of the maternal reproductive tract. The most likely routes of transmission are through the genital tract and through the circulation. At this early stage infection may destroy the zygote or embryo, although local barriers such as the zona pellucida prevent most agents from causing damage.

Infection after implantation, particularly during organogenesis, accounts for the largest number of adverse fetal effects. The disruption of normal development at this stage may lead to serious fetal ab-

normalities. Generally, after the infectious agent enters the mother, she develops viremia, bacteremia, or parasitemia. The agent then reaches and infects the placenta via the hematogenous route. Organisms cross the placenta, enter the fetal circulation, and spread throughout the fetus' body. The fetus is harmed as these agents destroy parenchymal cells and blood vessels. They replicate in fetal tissue, changing growth patterns and eliciting autoimmune responses. Fetal damage may be less severe if the mother has been immunized through prior exposure to the agent.

VIRAL INFECTIONS

Herpesvirus. The human herpesviruses (cytomegalovirus {CMV}, *Herpesvirus hominis* types I and II {herpes simplex viruses}, varicella zoster virus, Epstein-Barr virus {EBV}) infect most persons at some time during life. They usually remain latent in the body but may reactivate periodically to produce diseases. Gestational herpesvirus infections may reach the embryo or fetus via the placenta, by ascending through the cervix or through fetal contact with the birth canal during vaginal delivery.

Cytomegalovirus. CMV is the most common known cause of congenital infections in humans. Reports indicate that 6 to 19% of infants infected in utero develop the disease.[57] Features of CMV disease include hepatosplenomegaly, jaundice, thrombocytopenia, chorioretinitis, cerebral calcifications, and microcephaly (Fig. 28-1).

Congenital defects may include microcephaly, inguinal hernia, anomalies in the first bronchial arch, and central nervous system damage. Other reported fetal effects include ascites, splenomegaly, IUGR, hydrocephaly, and polyhydramnios.[16,49]

Herpesvirus hominis. Herpes simplex virus infection occurs in an estimated one to six newborns per 10,000 deliveries per year.[39] Primary infection during the first half of pregnancy has been associated with an increased frequency of spontaneous abortions and stillbirths.[40] Congenital malformations include microcephaly, hydranencephaly, intracranial calcifications, microphthalmia, and hepatosplenomegaly.

If the virus is present in the maternal genital tract at the time of delivery there is a 50% chance that the infant will be infected as it passes through the birth canal, so cesarean section is indicated.

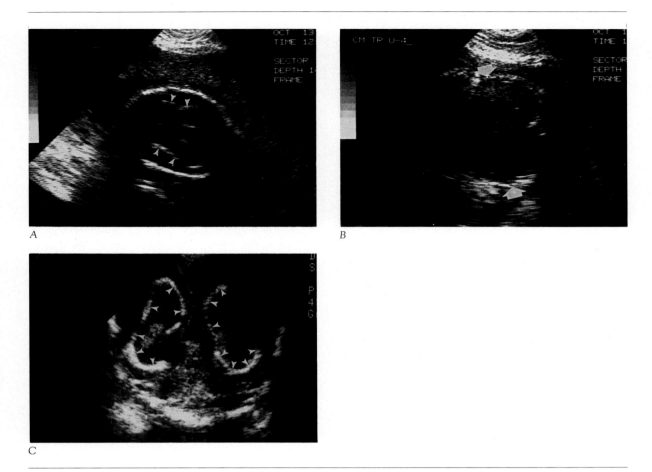

FIGURE 28-1. Fetal cytomegalovirus infection. (*A*) Cephalic sonogram of a fetus that appeared smaller on clinical examination than was expected by maternal dates. On a sonogram 8 weeks prior to this examination a fetal biparietal diameter of 44 mm was measured, consistent with 18.5 weeks' gestation on average. Femoral length was 33 mm, consistent with 20.5 weeks on average. On this axial sonogram there is evidence of microcephaly. A biparietal diameter of 62 mm is obtained, consistent with 24 weeks on average. A head circumference of 225 mm was calculated, consistent with 24.5 weeks' gestation on average. In comparison, a femoral length of 55 mm was measured at this time, consistent with 29 weeks' gestation on average. Hydrocephaly is also evident with a ventricular-hemispheric (VH) ratio of 0.52. Note the thick echogenic margin of the ventricular wall (*arrowheads*), due to diffuse periventricular calcification. (*B*) Transverse abdominal sonogram using the same image scale as in A. Abdominal diameter from side-to-side (*arrows*) measures 81 mm. The circumference is calculated at 250 mm, consistent with 30.5 weeks' gestation on average. (*C*) Postnatal coronal neurosonogram confirmed the presence of hydrocephaly and periventricular calcification (*arrowheads*). The cerebral tissue in the periphery shows a paucity of echogenic sulci, due to failure of normal migration of fetal ventricular lining cells to the periphery as a result of the periventriculitis. Cytomegalovirus was cultured from the neonatal nasopharynx and urine, and markedly elevated viral antibody titers were measured in the serum of mother and infant.

Varicella Zoster virus (Chickenpox). It is estimated that 95% of women of childbearing age in the United States have serologic evidence of past varicella infection. Three outcomes have been described in pregnancies infected with the varicella virus: congenital abnormalities, postnatal newborn disease ranging from benign to fatal, and zoster (shingles), which may appear months or years after birth.[57]

Congenital abnormalities, which were identified as early as 1947, include IUGR, limb aplasia, microphthalmia, and brain calcifications.[74] These abnormalities are observed when the virus is transmitted to the fetus during weeks 8 to 20 of pregnancy.

Epstein-Barr virus. While EBV infection is very common during childhood, primary EBV infection in pregnancy is not. In one study only three of more than 12,000 pregnant women tested positive.[21] EBV infection, which causes mononucleosis, has been linked to congenital heart anomalies, spontaneous abortions, stillbirths, low birth weight, and microphthalmia.[20,30] Since the available studies have been criticized for poor technique, further research is required to determine the extent of the correlation between EBV and fetal and congenital abnormalities.

Other Viruses. Other viruses such as rubella, influenza, and human immunodeficiency virus (HIV) also may be transmitted from mother to fetus. The rubella virus occurs in 30% of pregnant women, according to one study.[22] Infection during pregnancy may result in spontaneous abortion, stillbirth, or congenital defects. Congenital defects include microcephaly, hydrocephaly, cephalocele (Fig. 28-2), and cardiac anomalies. The evidence linking influenza to adverse pregnancy outcome has been inconsistent. Early reports have not been confirmed by later studies, but congenital malformation of the heart and central nervous system have been reported.[57] The effects of HIV, the agent of AIDS, are not fully known. Long-term studies of affected infants are needed. Nearly all infants with AIDS have been small for gestational age and premature, and have failed to thrive. They also have hepatomegaly and lymphadenopathy.[1,74]

BACTERIAL INFECTIONS
Syphilis and Gonorrhea. Syphilis infection in early

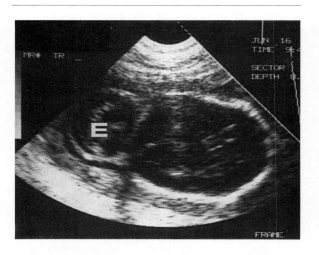

FIGURE 28-2. Cephalocele in 22-week fetus with rubella. Axial sonogram of the fetal head demonstrates a large occipital encephalocele (E) containing fluid and echogenic brain tissue.

pregnancy may result in spontaneous abortion. At a later stage, the fetus may be stillborn or may die in the neonatal period of congenital disease. If infection occurs very late in pregnancy, the clinical signs of congenital syphilis may not be apparent for 2 to 4 weeks.[57] Syphilis in neonates is characterized by hepatosplenomegaly, hyperbilirubinemia, evidence of hemolysis, and generalized lymphadenopathy.

Gonorrhea has been reported by Handsfield and colleagues[28] to be implicated in increased incidences of prematurity, prolonged rupture of fetal membranes, chorioamnionitis, sepsis, and IUGR. Gonococcal infections in neonates can result in meningitis and arthritis. Syphilis and gonorrhea can be treated successfully with penicillin, or with other antibiotics in patients who are allergic to penicillin.

Urinary Tract Infections. Urinary tract infections (UTIs) represent one of the most common medical complications of pregnancy. If not managed properly they may cause considerable adverse effects to both mother and fetus. UTIs include asymptomatic bacteriuria, acute cystitis, and acute pyelonephritis. Asymptomatic bacterial infection has been implicated in an increase in premature delivery and low birth weight, although some studies do not support this finding.[65] Pyelonephrosis in pregnancy has been associated with low birth weight, increased perinatal mortality, anemia, toxemia, and premature rupture of membranes.[62] Mental and motor development of children of pyelonephrotic mothers have been found to be impaired. Patients with UTIs during pregnancy are treated with antibiotics and monitored by frequent urine cultures.

Parasitic Infection

Parasitic infection during pregnancy may not always pose a risk to the fetus or mother. The clinical manifestations of parasitic disease are determined by several factors: the life cycle in the human host; the quantity and location of the parasite; and the host-parasite interaction.[33]

Parasites that penetrate and invade the host's viscera are a threat to the fetus. These organisms may directly penetrate and infect the uterus and placenta or may infect the fetus via the blood. Moreover, they are clearly a threat to both mother and fetus if they multiply within the human host. Malaria and toxoplasmosis are two of the more common parasitic diseases of humans.

In the United States, the incidence of congenital toxoplasmosis is approximately 1 per 1000 live births. Toxoplasmosis infection occurring early in pregnancy is less frequently transmitted to the fetus than infection acquired during the last trimester. In early pregnancy the small placenta usually protects the fetus from parasites. In late pregnancy this barrier is not as effective, owing to the expanded maternal-placental interface and the aging placenta. Fetal effects are usually devastating. These include severe IUGR, hydrocephaly, microcephaly, cerebral calcifications, hepatosplenomegaly, and fetal demise.

Malaria is transmitted by the bite of the female Anopheles mosquito. The incidence of congenital malaria in immune mothers residing in areas with high incidence of this disease is 0.3%. Maternal malaria promotes placental insufficiency, which causes IUGR, low birth weight, abortion, and stillbirth.[33] Antiparasitic drug therapy has been used successfully to treat toxoplasmosis and malaria infections during pregnancy, but some effective types of medication are potential teratogens.

Ultrasound has a useful role in evaluating fe-

tuses exposed to infectious diseases. For example, fetal echocardiography should be performed to exclude cardiac abnormalities in patients exposed to various viral diseases such as cytomegalovirus and rubella. IUGR, seen in some bacterial infections, can be diagnosed by serial scans and measurements of the fetal growth parameters. Fetuses who require delivery by cesarean section because of infections such as herpes or syphilis can be accurately dated by sonography.

Endocrine and Metabolic Disorders

Diabetes Mellitus

Diabetes mellitus is perhaps the most common maternal disorder the obstetric sonographer encounters. It has been estimated that it occurs in one of every 324 to 350 pregnancies in the United States.[4] The condition is a disorder of carbohydrate metabolism related to insulin deficiency and characterized by hyperglycemia.

Diabetes mellitus is classified as type I (insulin-dependent formerly known as juvenile-onset diabetes), type II (non-insulin dependent formerly known as adult onset), and other, or secondary, diabetes. Causes of secondary diabetes include pancreatic disease or pancreatectomy, hormones, drugs, or chemicals, and certain genetic syndromes. Additional classes of diabetes mellitus are impaired glucose tolerance and gestational diabetes, a condition manifested only during pregnancy.[41]

The association between diabetes mellitus and fetal congenital anomalies was recognized as early as 1885. Today, the frequency of anomalies among offspring of diabetic mothers is estimated at 3 to 6%.[51] The pathogenesis of these anomalies is ascribed to the hyperglycemia of diabetes, which disrupts organogenesis. Early diabetes control has been found to reduce the incidence of congenital malformations.[47]

Congenital anomalies in infants of diabetic mothers include skeletal, central nervous system (Fig. 28-3), cardiac, renal, and gastrointestinal types (Table 28-1). In addition, a single umbilical artery has been found in about 6.4% of diabetic mothers' pregnancies. This has been associated with various malformations: inguinal hernias, polydactyly, vertebral anomalies, talipes (clubfoot), cardiac and great vessel anomalies, pulmonary hypoplasia, and genitourinary tract anomalies.[51] The finding of a

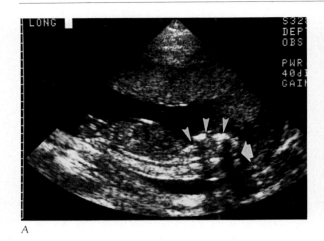
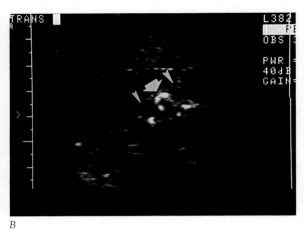

A   B

FIGURE 28-3. Anencephaly in the fetus of a diabetic mother. (A) Longitudinal sonogram demonstrates the fetal trunk and the facial structures (*small arrowheads*). No cranial vault is discerned (*large arrowhead*). The fetus was 15 weeks size by femoral length. (B) Sonographic section of the fetal orbits in a semiaxial plane. Note the nasal bridge (*large arrowhead*) separating the echopenic globes of the eyes (*small arrowheads*). A lens is seen anterolaterally in the globe on the right side of the image.

TABLE 28-1. Congenital anomalies in infants of diabetic mothers

Skeletal and central nervous system
    Caudal regression syndrome
    Anencephaly
    Other neural tube defects
    Microcephaly
Cardiac
    Transposition of the great vessels
    Ventricular septal defects
    Coarctation of the aorta
    Patent ductus arteriosus
    Atrial septal defects
    Cardiomegaly
Renal anomalies
    Hydronephrosis
    Renal agenesis
    Ureteral duplication
Gastrointestinal
    Duodenal atresia
    Anorectal atresia
    Small left colon syndrome
Other
    Single umbilical artery

(Adapted from Reece EA, Hobbins JC. Ultrasonography and diabetes mellitus in pregnancy. In: Sanders RC, James AE Jr, eds. Ultrasonography in Obstetrics and Gynecology. 3rd ed. Norwalk, CT: Appleton-Century-Crofts, 1985:299.)

single umbilical artery, therefore, warrants a complete examination of the fetus to exclude the above malformations.

In addition to malformations, fetuses of diabetic mothers may also experience growth disturbance problems such as IUGR or macrosomia (increased body tissues and fat). Growth retardation of a fetus of a mother with severe diabetes is attributed to uteroplacental vascular insufficiency, which results in less nutrients being transferred to the fetus. Fetal hyperinsulinemia is thought to be responsible for the development of macrosomia, as continuous maternal hyperglycemia gains access to the fetal circulatory system. Macrosomia is described as fetal weight in excess of 4000 g or a birth weight above the 90th percentile for gestational age, which predisposes the fetus to complications such as stillbirth and intrapartum trauma. In addition, both maternal and perinatal morbidity and mortality increase in relation to fetal birth weight.[25,72]

Several growth parameters can be examined with ultrasound to monitor the diabetic mother's pregnancy. These include the biparietal diameter (BPD), the abdominal circumference (AC), and the estimated fetal weight (EFW). Less commonly

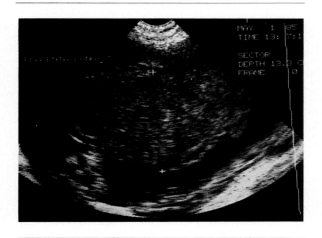

Figure 28-4. Placenta in a 29-week fetus of a diabetic mother. The placenta measures 7 cm in maximal thickness (between markers).

used parameters are chest size determination and the assessment of fetal breathing movements.[7,26,29,43,53]

In the sonographic evaluation of the diabetic mother's pregnancy it is recommended that an initial first-trimester examination be done to establish dates, followed by an examination between 18 and 22 weeks to screen for neural tube defects, caudal regression, and cardiac defects, and to exclude other gross malformations.[51]

Follow-up examinations should then be done every 4 to 6 weeks for fetal growth and estimated weight. Attention should be paid to placental size, since chronic hyperglycemia can cause placental enlargement (Fig. 28-4). Macrosomic and growth-retarded fetuses should be examined more frequently (Fig. 28-5). Umbilical artery flow tracings, specifically high-resistance Doppler velocity patterns, have also proven significant.[67]

Gestational diabetes—diabetes that occurs only during pregnancy—affects about 25 out of 1000 pregnant women. Risk factors for this condition include previous stillbirth or a baby with congenital anomalies, a previous macrosomic infant, and a family history of diabetes.[44]

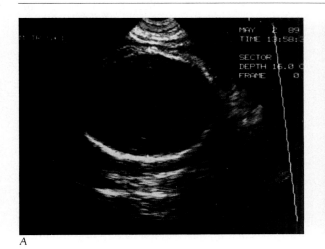

A

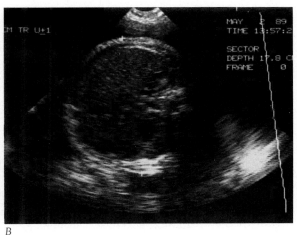

B

Figure 28-5. Macrosomia in the fetus of an insulin-dependent diabetic mother. (A) Axial cephalic sonogram demonstrates a biparietal diameter of 87 mm, consistent with 34 weeks' gestation on average. A head circumference (HC) of 320 mm is calculated. (B) Transverse abdominal sonogram using a depth scale greater than that in A shows a larger fetal abdomen. An abdominal circumference (AC) of 356 mm is calculated. HC-to-AC ratio equals 0.90, which is markedly small for a 34-week fetus. The fetal abdominal integument is thickened to 1 cm.

Gestational diabetes can affect the fetus in the same way that pregestational diabetes can but the later its onset occurs in pregnancy the less likely the fetus is to be affected during organogenesis. Because onset of clinical symptoms may lag behind maternal metabolic changes, there is no certainty that the fetus has gone through organogenesis unaffected, no matter how late in pregnancy the clinical diagnosis is established. A common-sense approach, such as examining all fetuses whose mothers develop symptoms before 24 weeks' gestation, generally prevails.

Hyperthyroidism

Hyperthyroidism, also known as thyrotoxicosis, occurs in approximately two of every 1000 pregnancies.[6] The additional thyroid stimulation produces thyroxine, which disrupts normal cell development, causing a significant increase in the incidence of low birth weight infants and a slight increase in the neonatal mortality rate.

The most common cause of clinical hyperthyroidism is Grave's disease (toxic diffuse goiter). Plummer's disease (toxic nodular goiter), trophoblastic tumors, and hydatidiform mole also cause hyperthyroidism.[6]

Hypothyroidism

The incidence of hypothyroidism is very low in pregnant women, because the absence of normal hormone stimulation makes a woman unlikely to conceive. When pregnancy does occur incidence of stillbirth is high.[6] The most common causes of hypothyroidism are thyroidectomy and radioactive iodine therapy.[12]

Hyperparathyroidism

The incidence of hyperparathyroidism is very low, the most common cause being parathyroid adenoma. An increase in spontaneous abortions, fetal demise in late pregnancy, and hypocalcemic tetany in newborns can be seen with hyperparathyroidism.[12]

Phenylketonuria

Phenylketonuria (PKU) is a genetic disorder that exposes the developing fetus of an affected mother who is not following a low-phenylalanine, low-protein diet to potentially toxic levels of otherwise important metabolic products. The risks of sponta-neous abortion, microcephaly, mental retardation, and congenital heart disease are increased.[34] Dietary restriction of phenylalanine should be started before conception to maximize the chances of producing a normal fetus. Maternal dietary adjustments reinstated after inception of pregnancy have been unsuccessful in preventing abnormalities.

Hematologic Disorders

Rh Isoimmunization

Also known as Rhesus incompatibility, Rh isoimmunization refers to the destructive nature of surface antigens on fetal red blood cells that are incompatible with maternal antibodies. The maternal antibodies perceive fetal antigens as invaders and they attack and destroy them. Erythroblastosis fetalis, a condition characterized by rapid destruction of fetal red blood cells and hepatosplenomegaly, may occur when an Rh-positive fetus is carried by an Rh-negative mother who has been sensitized to Rh antigen in a previous pregnancy. In its most severe form a fluid overload condition known as hydrops fetalis results (Fig. 28-6).

However, hydrops can also be caused by factors other than Rh incompatibility. Termed nonimmunologic hydrops (NIH) this condition may be caused by over 40 conditions.[17] Most commonly, NIH may be a result of fetal problems such as cardiovascular conditions (hypoplastic left heart, dysrhythmias), infections (toxoplasmosis, herpes simplex), obstructive vascular problems (umbilical vein thrombosis), pulmonary diseases (cystic adenomatoid malformation), neoplasms (neuroblastoma, teratoma), chromosomal anomalies (trisomy 18 or 21), and congenital nephrosis. Maternal causes include diabetes mellitus and toxemia.[50]

The ultrasound findings associated with hydrops include polyhydramnios or oligohydramnios, fetal ascites, pleural and pericardial effusions, fetal anasarca (subcutaneous edema with skin thickness greater than 5 mm), abnormally thickened placenta (greater than 6 cm), fetal hepatosplenomegaly and cardiomegaly, and umbilical vein dilatation.[19,48,70] The sonographically detectable structural anomalies associated with fetal hydrops are numerous and varied (Table 28-2).

Amniocentesis is an important procedure for monitoring the bilirubin concentration in amniotic fluid; the severity of hemolytic disease is re-

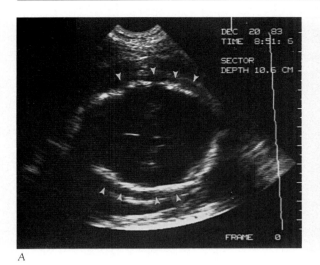

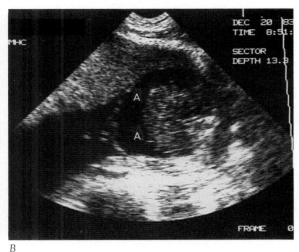

FIGURE 28-6. Hydrops fetalis in 24-week fetus of a mother with Rh sensitization. (A) Cephalic sonogram in axial view shows scalp edema (*arrowheads*) measuring 7 to 8 mm in thickness. (B) Transverse abdominal sonogram demonstrates fetal ascites (A). There is also hydramnios, especially evident when it is estimated what the net abdominal circumference would be without the fetal ascites.

lated to the bilirubin level. Ultrasound, therefore, is not only helpful in detecting changes in extra- and intrafetal fluid and growth rate abnormalities, but also in establishing accurate dates for timely amniocentesis and delivery and for conducting a safe amniocentesis, particularly when serial procedures may be indicated. The availability of percutaneous umbilical blood sampling (PUBS) now allows direct sampling of fetal blood from which antibody titers can be determined and a prompt diagnosis rendered. In many cases this may spare the patient the danger and expense of multiple high-risk tests. In recent years, isoimmunized pregnancies have been treated successfully by transfusing blood into the umbilical vein, through the cord near the insertion into the placenta or into the peritoneal cavity under ultrasound guidance.[5,58]

Doppler equipment can also be helpful in assessing the well-being of potentially affected fetuses. A correlation between increasing speed of blood flow to the fetus compensating for decreasing hemoglobin carried in the blood implies that periodic Doppler examinations may reveal timely information pertaining to intervention.[24,69]

SICKLE CELL ANEMIA

Sickle cell anemia is an inherited disorder that affects the black population predominantly. Normally round, the red blood cells are, instead, sickle shaped. This leads to abnormally high red cell destruction and occlusion of arterioles. Incidences of spontaneous abortion, prematurity, and stillbirth are increased. Perinatal morbidity and mortality have also been reported.[59] Short femurs may be present and low birth weight may occur.[54]

Fetuses should be followed sonographically for growth retardation and increased placental resistance to umbilical artery and uterine artery flow. The systolic-diastolic (S/D) pressure ratio can be monitored using Doppler techniques. An S/D ratio of 3.0 or higher after 30 weeks' gestation has been reported as predictive of fetal distress when detected in both umbilical and uterine artery flow. The same study recorded at least one artery with abnormal flow in 88% of pregnant women with sickle cell disease, as opposed to 4 to 7% of normal pregnant women.[2]

Management of sickle cell patients during pregnancy includes dietary supplementation of iron

TABLE 28-2. Structural anomalies associated with hydrops fetalis that may have sonographic manifestation

STRUCTURE	SONOGRAPHIC FINDING	ABNORMALITY
Head	Intracranial mass, associated with congestive heart failure and microcephaly	Arteriovenous malformation, vein of Galen aneurysm, cytomegalovirus or toxoplasmosis infection
Neck	Cystic neck masses	Lymphatic dysplasias
Thorax	Poorly contracting heart	Congestive heart failure
	Pericardial effusion, tachycardia	Cardiac anomaly
	Asystole	Demise
	Mediastinal mass	Tumor
	Chest mass	Cystic adenomatoid malformation
	Small thorax	Dwarfism
	Cystic masses crossing diaphragm	Diaphragmatic hernias
Abdomen	Tubular sonolucent structures	Gastrointestinal obstruction, atresia, or volvulus
	Abdominal masses	Tumors, neurofibromatosis
Retroperitoneum	Retroperitoneal mass	Neurogenic mass
	Hydronephrotic kidney	Hydronephrosis, posterior urethral valves
Extremities	Short arms, legs	Dwarfism
	Contractures	Arthrogryoposis
	Fractures	Osteogenesis imperfecta
Placenta	Thick placenta	Infection, extramedullary hematopoiesis, anemia
	Mass	Chorioangioma
Amniotic cavity	Number of fetuses, relative size, amniotic membrane	Twin-twin transfusion
	Umbilical cord anomalies	Single umbilical artery, umbilical cord torsion

(Adapted from Fleisher AC, Killam AP, et al. Hydrops fetalis. Radiology. 1981;141:163.)

and folic acid.[14,35] Prophylactic transfusions have been reported to improve both maternal and fetal morbidity and mortality, although this procedure carries the risk of blood-borne infection and the formation of alloantibodies which affect future transfusions.[38]

THALASSEMIA

Thalassemia has been cited as the most common maternal genetic abnormality associated with pregnancy worldwide.[71] It is a form of anemia, a reduction of red blood cell production, with multiple variations, the most common of which is referred to as Cooley's anemia or thalassemia major. Thalassemia often shortens the life span of an affected individual, because of the iron overload that develops from the necessary multiple transfusions.

Most women with thalassemia major die before reproductive age. In cases of successful pregnancy, effects on the fetus range from hydrops and death to no effect at all.[27,31]

Toxemia and Hypertension

Toxemia of pregnancy is a disease occurring in the third trimester characterized by maternal edema, hypertension, proteinuria, and central nervous system irritability. The disease has been classified into two stages, preeclampsia and eclampsia. The preeclamptic stage is marked by development of hypertension with proteinuria or edema, or both. In the eclamptic stage one or more convulsions will occur, significantly increasing the risk of maternal and fetal mortality.[18]

Preeclampsia affects less than 1.5% of all pregnancies, but when it occurs a prenatal mortality rate as high as 20% has been reported when the condition develops before 36 weeks' gestation. The disease has been found to occur most commonly in young primigravidas and in older multiparas. While the etiology of preeclampsia remains unclear, immunologic, hormonal, and nutritional factors are thought to be responsible. It has been postulated that the reduction in prostaglandin synthesis seen in preeclamptic patients promotes placental vascular disease and decreased uteroplacental blood flow. Low birth weight, fetal distress, and placental abruption are all associated with toxemia.[18] Treatment of this condition is dependent on the severity of the disease. Antihypertensive drugs can be used to control blood pressure and anticonvulsant medication for seizures in severe disease. Immediate delivery of the fetus is indicated in most cases of toxemia.

Hypertension during pregnancy may also occur without the development of toxemia. Hypertension preceding or persisting after pregnancy is diagnosed as essential hypertension whereas hypertension that occurs during pregnancy and disappears after parturition is considered to be pregnancy-induced hypertension. Hypertension during pregnancy, regardless of the type, always poses a risk to both mother and fetus. In a prospective study of 14,833 women Page and Christianson[45] reported that a mean arterial pressure of 90 mm Hg or more during the middle trimester of pregnancy significantly increased the risk of stillbirth, preeclampsia, and IUGR. Other reports have concluded that the maternal risk of mild chronic hypertension is small unless preeclampsia develops.[60]

Sonography can reliably monitor preeclamptic pregnancies and detect abnormalities early. A spectrum of ultrasound findings has been described in these patients: IUGR, oligohydramnios, decreased placental volume, accelerated placental maturation, and fetal demise.[8] In addition, S/D ratios can be followed serially to detect the development of increased placental vascular resistance.

A protocol for evaluating patients with hypertension has been described by Zuspan.[75] He advises that at least three ultrasound examinations be done. The first examination should be performed at 10 to 14 weeks, to date the preganancy; the second, at 20 to 26 weeks; and the third, at 32 weeks' gestational age. The later examinations should focus on detecting early evidence of IUGR and on documenting the amount of amniotic fluid, since this is a good index of fetal well-being.

In addition, women with chronic hypertension and complaints of abdominal pain should raise the clinical suspicion of placental abruption. These patients should be carefully monitored by ultrasound and clinical observation.

Drug Use and Nutritional Disorders

Drug use during pregnancy may affect its outcome by promoting fetal addiction, teratogenesis, altered uteroplacental blood flow, or IUGR.[52] It is estimated that drug exposure accounts for approximately 2 to 3% of birth defects in humans.[42] This teratogenic effect is dependent on several factors, including dosage, time of exposure, host susceptibility, genetic differences in the host, and interactions with other agents in the environment.[42] Generally, in the early period of gestation teratogens affect organs that develop first, such as the heart. Structures such as the palate may be affected when the insult occurs about 10 weeks into the gestation period.

While many drugs and chemicals have been sporadically associated with various fetal malformations, only a few are proven teratogens (Table 28-3). Some, unfortunately, are important medications whose use during pregnancy must be restricted.

Drugs used abusively include alcohol, amphetamines, barbiturates, and narcotics (heroine, methadone, and cocaine). These agents have reportedly been associated with a variety of effects in the fetus, ranging from mild to severe, but in other than proven teratogens, the main effect appears to be IUGR as a result of poor nutrition associated with drug use (Fig. 28-7).

Excessive consumption of alcohol, a known teratogen, during pregnancy can result in the fetal alcohol syndrome (FAS). This syndrome includes features of gross physical retardation, central nervous system dysfunction, and facial dysmorphology, including microcephaly and microphthalmia. Additional effects of alcohol on reproduction include cardiac anomalies, such as ventricular septal defects, increased risks of infections, placental

Table 28-3. Proven teratogens and their fetal effects

Teratogen	Fetal Effects
Aminopterin	Meningoencephalocele, hydrocephalus, clubfoot, hypoplasia of fibula
Antithyroid drugs	Polydactyly, goiter
Azathioprine	Pulmonary valvular stenosis
Carbon monoxide	Cerebral atrophy, hydrocephalus, cleft lip
Coumadin	Encephalocele, anencephaly, spina bifida, congenital heart disease, skeletal deformities, growth retardation
Cyclophosphamide	Tetralogy of Fallot, syndactyly, missing digits
Daunorubicin	Anencephaly, cardiac defects
Ethanol	Microcephaly, cardiac defects, growth retardation
Heparin	Absence of thumbs
Methotrexate	Oxycephaly, absence of frontal bone, dextrocardia, growth retardation
Methyl mercury	Microcephaly, head asymmetry
Phenytoin	Microcephaly, cardiac malformations, hypertelorism, cleft palate or lip, growth retardation
PCB	Growth retardation
Procarbazine	Cerebral hemorrhage
Retinoic acid	Hydrocephalus, microcephaly, congenital heart defects, malformation of cranium, face, and ribs, limb deformities
Thalidomide	Congenital heart malformations, spine malformations, limb reduction, duodenal stenosis or atresia, pyloric stenosis, microtia
Trimethadione	Microcephaly, cardiac defects, club foot, esophageal atresia, growth deficiency
Valproic acid	Meningomyelocele, microcephaly, growth deficiency, tetralogy of Fallot, oral cleft

(Adapted from Koren A, Edwards MB, Miskin M. Antenatal sonography of fetal malformation associated with drugs and chemicals: A guide. Am J Obstet Gynecol. 1987;156:79–85.)

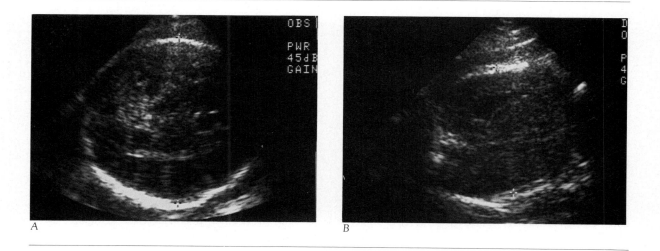

Figure 28-7. Serve intrauterine growth retardation in the fetus of a drug abuser. (A) Axial cephalic sonogram demonstrates a biparietal diameter (BPD) of 74 mm. HC was calculated at 245 mm. BPD and HC are both 4 to 5 weeks less than expected for this fetus, which should be 32 weeks, based on a sonogram at 17 weeks' gestation. (B) Transverse abdominal sonogram using the same scale as in A shows a much smaller fetal abdomen. The abdominal contour is not optimal owing to compression by the uterine wall as a result of severe oligohydramnios. AC is estimated at 190 mm. HC/AC ratio is 1.29, markedly increased for a 32-week fetus.

abruption, and spontaneous abortion.[52,55,63] Estimates indicate that 11% of pregnant women are problem drinkers and about 5 to 10% of this group's offspring demonstrate full-blown FAS. FAS occurs at a rate of 1 in 1500 to 2000 live births.[52]

The role of street drugs (amphetamines, barbiturates, narcotics) in the development of congenital anomalies has been difficult to define because of complicating factors such as drug potency and purity, multiple drug use, and the high incidence of perinatal infection and malnutrition among drug abusers.[3] Amphetamines have been implicated in causing cleft palate and IUGR. Barbiturate use has been reported to carry an increased risk for cardiac anomalies and cleft lip and palate.[52,73] The major effects of narcotics are drug dependency in both mother and fetus and IUGR. In addition, cocaine use has been associated with an increased risk of abruptio placenta, GU malformations, limb reduction, and cardiac defects.[9–11,52]

Nicotine and caffeine have also been assoicated with adverse fetal outcome. Nicotine use has been linked to an increased risk of perinatal mortality and low birth weight. Light smoking (<1 pack per day) was found to increase this risk by 20%; heavy smoking (>1 pack per day) increased the risk by 35%.[36] Excessive caffeine consumption (150 mg/day) has been associated with an increased rate of spontaneous abortion.[64]

Closely associated with drug abuse is the problem of malnutrition. Drug abuse not uncommonly leads to neglect of personal care, including nutrition. Mild degrees of maternal malnutrition have been associated with prematurity, low birth weight, and IUGR.[32] Maternal starvation in early gestation

TABLE 28-4. Sonographic findings in fetuses of mothers with disease

MATERNAL DISEASE	SONOGRAPHIC AND ASSOCIATED FINDINGS
Viral infection	
Cytomegalovirus	Microcephaly, hydrocephaly, cardiac abnormality, IUGR, splenomegaly, ascites, polyhydramnios, hydrops
Herpes simplex	Microcephaly, hydranencephaly, intracranial calcifications, microphthalmia, hepatosplenomegaly, hydrops
Varicella zoster	IUGR, limb aplasia, microphthalmia, intracranial calcifications
Epstein-Barr	Cardiac, IUGR, microphthalmia
Rubella	Microcephaly, cardiac, hydrocephaly, cephalocele, agenesis of the corpus callosum
Inlfuenza	Cardiac anomalies
HIV	IUGR, hepatomegaly
Bacterial Infection	
Syphilis	Hydrocephaly, iniencephaly, thick placenta, hydrops, osteitis, fetal demise
Gonorrhea	IUGR, oligohydramnios
UTI	IUGR, oligohydramnios
Parasitic Infection	
Toxoplasmosis	IUGR, hydrocephaly, microcephaly, cerebral calcification, agenesis of the corpus callosum, hepatosplenomegaly, hydrops
Malaria	IUGR
Endocrine and Metabolic	
Diabetes mellitus	Thickened placenta (see Table 28-1)
Hyperthyroidism	IUGR
Hypothyroidism	Fetal demise, goiter
Hyperparathyroidism	Fetal demise, goiter
PKU	Microcephaly, cardiac disease
Hematologic	
Isoimmunization	Pleural and pericardial effusion, ascites, skin thickening, polyhydramnios
Sickle cell anemia	Short femurs, IUGR
Thalassemia	Hydrops
Toxemia	IUGR, oligohydramnios, abruptio placenta, decreased placental volume, early placental maturation, fetal demise
Malnutrition	IUGR, oligohydramnios, decreased placental volume

has been reported to be associated with CNS abnormalities (spina bifida and hydrocephalus). In late gestation, famine can result in IUGR.

The most common nutritional disorder in developed countries is obesity. This is defined as weight 20% above standard for height at the onset of pregnancy.[68] Three major antenatal complications of moderate obesity are hypertension, preeclampsia, and gestational diabetes.[56,66] Massive obesity is a major problem, particularly when cesarean section is indicated.

Sonography has an important role in evaluating fetuses of drug-addicted, malnourished, and obese mothers. A considerable number of fetal structural anomalies can be detected in fetuses exposed to teratogenic agents. Careful sonography with high-resolution equipment can rule out malformations such as hydrocephalus, limb reduction defects, and cardiac anomalies as early as 17 to 18 weeks' gestation. In the malnourished pregnancy serial scans should be performed to follow growth patterns and to detect IUGR and macrosomia. Pregnancies of obese patients who require cesarean section can be dated accurately with sonography for correct planning of this procedure.

Summary

Pregnancies complicated by maternal disease represent a difficult and challenging problem for the obstetrician. Diagnostic sonography offers a safe and reliable modality for evaluating fetuses at risk for growth retardation and malformations produced by maternal disease (Table 28-4). Developments and advancements in the technology, such as Doppler systems, have enhanced our ability to collect more information about the fetus and to make better diagnoses. Moreover, as invasive obstetric procedures such as PUBS are performed more frequently sonography will assume a broader and more significant role in fetal surveillance.

References

1. Ammana AJ. Is there an acquired immune deficiency syndrome in infants and children? Pediatrics. 1983; 72:430.

2. Anyaegbunam A, Langer O, Brustman L, et al. The application of uterine and umbilical artery velocimetry to the antenatal supervision of pregnancies complicated by maternal disease. Am J Obstet Gynecol. 1988; 159:544–547.

3. Beckman DA, Brent RL. Mechanism of known environmental teratogens: Drugs and chemicals. Clin Perinatol. 1986; 13:649–687.

4. Benson RC. Handbook of Obstetrics and Gynecology. 8th ed. Los Altos, CA: Lange Medical Publications; 1983:365.

5. Berkowitz RL, Chitkara U, Goldberg JD, et al. Intravascular transfusion in utero: The percutaneous approach. Am J Obstet Gynecol. 1986; 154:622–623.

6. Burrow GN. Thyroid diseases. In: Burrow GN, Ferris TF, eds. Medical Complications During Pregnancy. 3rd ed. Philadelphia: WB Saunders; 1988.

7. Campbell S, Wilkin D. Ultrasonic measurement of fetal abdomen circumference in the estimation of fetal weight. Br J Obstet Gynaecol. 1975; 82:689.

8. Carroll B. Ultrasound features of preeclampsia. J Clin Ultrasound. 1980; 8:483–488.

9. Chasnoff IJ, Burns WJ, Schnolls, H, et al. Cocaine use in pregnancy. N Engl J Med. 1985; 313:666.

10. Chavez GF, Mulinare J, Cordero JF. Maternal cocaine use and the risk for genitourinary tract defects: An epidemiologic approach. Am J Human Genetics. (Suppl) 1988; 43:A43.

11. Cherukuri R, Minkoff H, Feldman J, et al. A cohort study of alkaloidal cocaine ("crack") in pregnancy. Obstet Gynecol. 1988; 72:147–151.

12. Creasy RK, Resnick R. Maternal-Fetal Medicine: Principles and Practice. Philadelphia: WB Saunders; 1984:926.

13. Daffos F, Capella-Pavlovsky M, Forestier F. A new procedure for fetal blood sampling in utero: Preliminary results of fifty-three cases. Am J Obstet Gynecol. 1985; 146:985–987.

14. Desforges JF, Warth J. The management of sickle cell disease in pregnancy. Clin Perinatol. 1974; 1:385–394.

15. De Vore GR, Brar HS, Platt LD. Doppler ultrasound in the fetus: A review of current applications. J Clin Ultrasound. 1987; 15:687–703.

16. Eliezer S, Ester F, Ehud W, et al. Fetal splenomegaly, ultrasound diagnosis of cytomegalovirus infection: A case report. J Clin Ultrasound. 1984; 12:520–521.

17. Etches PC, Lemons JA. Nonimmune hydrops fetalis: Report of 22 cases including three siblings. Pediatrics. 1979; 64:326–332.

18. Ferris TF. Toxemia and Hypertension. In: Burrow GM, Ferris TF, eds. Medical Complications During Pregnancy. 3rd ed. Philadelphia: WB Saunders; 1988.

19. Fleischer AC, Killam AP, Boehm FH, et al. Hydrops fetalis: Sonographic evaluation and clinical implications. Radiology. 1981; 141:163–168.

20. Fleischer G, Bolognese R. EBV infection in preg-

nancy: A prospective study. J Pediatr. 1984; 104:374.

21. Freij BJ, Sever JL. Herpesvirus infection in pregnancy: Risks to embryo, fetus and neonate. Clin Perinatol. 1988; 15:203–231.

22. Freij BJ, South M, Sever JL. Maternal rubella and the congenital rubella syndrome. Clin Perinatol 1988; 15:247–257.

23. Friedman DM, Rutkowski M, Synder JR, et al. Doppler blood velocity waveforms in the umbilical artery as an indicator of fetal well-being. J Clin Ultrasound. 1985; 13:161–165.

24. Gill RW. Doppler assessment in obstetrics and fetal physiology. Clin Diagn Ultrasound 1984; 13:131–147.

25. Golditch IM, Kirkman K. The large fetus. Management and outcome. Obstet Gynecol. 1978; 52:26–30.

26. Grandjean SH, Saraman MF, DeMouzo J, et al. Detection of gestational diabetes by means of excessive fetal growth. Am J Obstet Gynecol. 1980; 138:790–792.

27. Guy G, Coady DJ, Jansen V, et al. Alpha-thalassemia hydrops fetalis: Clinical and ultrasonographic considerations. Am J Obstet Gynecol. 1985; 153:500–504.

28. Handsfield HH, Hodson WA, Holmes KK. Neonatal gonococcal infections. 1. Orogastric contamination with Neisseria gonorrhoeae. JAMA. 1973; 225:697.

29. Houchang D, Modanlou ND, Komatsu G, et al. Large-for-gestational-age neonates: Antropometric reasons for shoulder dystocia. Obstet Gynecol. 1982; 60:417–423.

30. Icarf J, Didier J, Dalens M, et al. Prospective study of EBV infection during pregnancy. Biomedicine. 1981; 34:160.

31. Kelton JG, Cruickshauk M. Hematologic disorders of pregnancy. In: Burrows GN, Ferris TF, eds. Medical Complications During Pregnancy. 3rd ed. Philadelphia: WB Saunders; 1988.

32. Landon MB, Gabbe SG, Mullen JL. Total parenteral nutrition during pregnancy. Clin Perinatol. 1986; 13:57–72.

33. Lee RV. Parasites and pregnancy: The problems of malaria and toxoplasmosis. Clin Perinatol. 1988; 15:351–363.

34. Lenke RR, Levy HC. Maternal pheylketonuria and hyperphenylalaninemia. An internatioanl survey of the outcome of untreated and treated pregnancies. N Engl J Med. 1980; 303:1202.

35. Lindenbaum J, Klipstein FA. Folic acid deficiency in sickle cell anemia. N Engl J Med. 1963; 269:875.

36. Meyer MB, Tonascia JA. Maternal smoking, pregnancy complications and perinatal mortality. Am J Obstet Gynecol. 1977; 128:494–502.

37. Michalides R, Vantlie R, Nusse R, et al. Mammary tumor induction loci in GR and DBA mice contain one provirus of the mouse mammary tumor virus. Cell. 1981; 23:165–173.

38. Morrison JC, Blake PG, Reed CD. Therapy for the pregnant patient with sickle hemoglobinopathies: A national focus. Am J Obstet Gynecol. 1982; 144:268–269.

39. Nahmias AJ, Josey WE, Naib WE, et al. Perinatal risk associated with maternal genital herpes simplex virus infection. Am J Obstet Gynecol. 1971; 110:825–837.

40. Naib ZM, Nahmias AJ, Josey WE, et al. Association of maternal herpetic infection with spontaneous abortion. Obstet Gynecol. 1970; 35:260–263.

41. National Diabetes Data Group. Classification and diagnosis of diabetes mellitus and other categories of glucose intolerance. Diabetes. 1979; 28:1039.

42. Niebyl JR. Genetics and teratology, drug use in pregnancy. In: Pitkin R, Zlatnik F, eds. 1984 Year Book of Obstetrics and Gynecology. Chicago: Year Book Medical Publishers; 1984.

43. Ogata ES, Sabbagha R, Metzger BE, et al. Serial ultrasonography to assess evolving fetal macrosomia JAMA. 1980; 243:2405.

44. Olson C. Diagnosis and Management of Diabetes Mellitus. 2nd ed. New York: Raven Press; 1985:181.

45. Page EW, Christianson R. The impact of mean arterial pressure in the middle trimester upon the outcome of pregnancy. Am J Obstet Gynecol. 1976; 125:740–746.

46. Pearce JM, Chamberlain GV. Ultrasonically guided percutaneous umbilical blood sampling in the management of intrauterine growth retardation. Br J Obstet Gynaecol. 1987; 94:318–321.

47. Pedersen J, Molsted-Pedersen L, Andersen B. Assessors of fetal perinatal mortality in diabetic pregnancy. Analysis of 1,332 pregnancies in the Copenhagen series 1946-1972. Diabetes. 1974; 23:302.

48. Perlin BM, Pomerance JJ, Schifrin BS. Nonimmunologic hydrops fetalis. Obstet Gynecol. 1981; 57:584–588.

49. Price JM, Fisch AE, Jacobson J. Ultrasound findings in fetal cytomegalovirus infection. J Clin Ultrasound. 1978; 6:268.

50. Queenan JT, O'Brien GD. Diagnostic ultrasound in erythroblastosis fetalis. In: Sanders RC, James AE Jr, eds. Ultrasonography in Obstetrics and Gynecology. 3rd ed. Norwalk, CT: Appleton-Century-Crofts; 1985.

51. Reece AE, Hobbins JC. Ultrasonography and diabetes mellitus in pregnancy. In: Sanders RC, James AE Jr, eds. Ultrasonography in Obstetrics and Gynecology. 3rd ed. Norwalk, CT: Appleton-Century-Crofts; 1985.

52. Rodgers BD, Lee RV. Drug abuse. In: Burrow GN,

Ferris TF, eds. Medical Complications During Pregnancy. 3rd ed. Philadelphia: WB Saunders; 1988.

53. Romero R, Chervenak FA, Berkowitz RL, et al. Intrauterine fetal tachypnea. Am J Obstet Gynecol. 1982; 144:356–357.

54. Roopnarinesingh S, Ramsewaks S. Decreased birth weight and femur length in fetuses of patients with the sickle-cell trait. Obstet Gynecol. 1986; 68:46–48.

55. Rosett HL, Weinger L. Alcohol and the Fetus. A Clinical Perspective. New York: Oxford University Press; 1984.

56. Ruges S, Anderson T. Obstetric risks in obesity. An analysis of the literature. Obstet Gynecol Surv. 1985; 40:57.

57. Saltzman RL, Jordan MC. Viral infections. In: Burrow GN, Ferris TF, eds. Medical Complication During Pregnancy. 3rd ed. Philadelphia; WB Saunders; 1988.

58. Seeds JW, Watson AB. Ultrasound-guided fetal intravascular transfusion in severe rhesus immunization. Am J Obstet Gynecol. 1986; 154:1105–1107.

59. Serjeant GR. Sickle haemoglobin and pregnancy. Br Med J. 1983; 287:628.

60. Sibai BM, Abdella TM, Anderson DG. Pregnancy outcome in 211 patients with mild chronic hypertension. Obstet Gynecol. 1983; 61:571–576.

61. Simmons MA, Battaglia FC, Quilligan EJ. The fetus and newborn. In: Romney SL, Gray JM, Little AB, et al, eds. Gynecology and Obstetrics—The Health Care of Women. New York: McGraw-Hill; 1975:315.

62. Simpson ML, Graziano EP, Lupo VR, et al. Bacterial infections during pregnancy. In: Burrow GN, Ferris TF, eds. Medical Complications During Pregnancy. 3rd ed. Philadelphia: WB Saunders; 1988.

63. Sokol RJ, Miller SI. Identifying the alcohol abusing obstetric/gynecologic patient: A practical approach. Alcohol Health Res World. 1980; 4:3.

64. Srisuphan W, Braken MB. Caffeine consumption during pregnancy and association with late spontaneous abortion. Am J Obstet Gynecol. 1986; 154:14–20.

65. Sweet RL. Bacteriuria and pyelonephritis during pregnancy. Semin Perinatol. 1977; 1:25.

66. Treharne L. Obesity in pregnancy. In: Studd J, ed. Progress in Obstetrics and Gynecology. Edinburgh: Churchill Livingstone; 1984; 4:127–138.

67. Trudinger BJ. The umbilical circulation. Semin Perinatol. 1987; 11:311–321.

68. Wall RE. Nutritional problems during pregnancy. In: Abrams RS, Waxler P, eds. Medical Care of the Pregnant Patient. Boston: Little, Brown; 1983.

69. Warren PS, Gill RW, Fisher CC. Doppler flow studies in rhesus isoimmunization. Semin Perinatol. 1987; 11:375.

70. Weiner S, Bolognese RJ, Librizzi, DO. Ultrasound in the evaluation and management of the isoimmunized pregnancy. J Clin Ultrasound. 1981; 9:315–323.

71. White JM, Richards B, Byrne M, et al. Thalassemia trait and pregnancy. J Clin Pathol 1985; 38:810.

72. Wladimiroff JW, Bloemsma CA, Wallenburg HCS. Ultrasonic diagnosis of the large-for-dates infant. Obstet Gynecol. 1978; 52:285–288.

73. Wladimiroff JW, Stewart PA, Reuss A, et al. The role of ultrasound in the early diagnosis of fetal structural defects following maternal anticonvulsant therapy. Ultrasound Med Biol. 1988; 14:657–660.

74. Zeichner SL, Plotkin SA. Mechanisms and pathways of congenital infections. Clin Perinatol. 1988; 15:163–188.

75. Zuspan FP. Hypertensive disorders of pregnancy. In: Pauerstein CJ, ed. Clin Obstetrics. New York: John Wiley and Sons; 1987:645.

CHAPTER 29

Pelvic Masses in Pregnancy

JOHN YAGHOOBIAN

Sonography is the most commonly used modality for evaluating maternal disorders that occur during pregnancy. The absence of any significant biologic effects of ultrasound at the diagnostic range, its portability, and its relatively low cost make this examination a preferred method not only for making a diagnosis but also for serial follow-up. Since the advent of ultrasound, pelvic and abdominal masses occurring with pregnancy are recognized more frequently and at an earlier stage of gestation. The reliability of ultrasound in the diagnosis of pelvic masses in pregnancy is approximately 95%.[2] The size, location, internal consistency, and sometimes the origin of the pelvic mass can be evaluated. As in nongravid patients, the specificity of the sonographic appearance of a pelvic mass is relatively low, owing to the similarity of findings in the different types of pelvic masses and to variations of sonographic features seen in a given entity. In some cases, such as a dermoid cyst, the echogenic characteristics of the mass make a specific diagnosis more likely.

Indications for Ultrasound Examination

A large-for-date uterus is often the first clue to the presence of a pelvic mass. Some patients are referred for ultrasound examination because of pain associated with complications of the pelvic masses, such as torsion or hemorrhage. Some existing pelvic masses become clinically palpable for the first time during pregnancy because enlargement of the uterus makes them easier to palpate. As pregnancy progresses and the uterus enlarges, a mass that originated in the pelvis may be displaced into the abdomen.

Clinical Considerations

The patient who is seen during pregnancy with a pelvic mass presents a special problem for the obstetrician. It is difficult, if not impossible, to evaluate the mass that occurs during pregnancy by physical examination alone. Simultaneous evaluation of gestational age with an ultrasound examination will assist the obstetrician, who usually prefers to explore patients with pelvic masses during the second trimester, when there is the least likelihood of inducing premature labor by surgical intervention.

Potential complications of a pelvic mass during pregnancy include torsion, rupture of the mass, and interference with the progression of labor. The possibility of torsion is greater with pedunculated masses, and torsion of the mass causes hemorrhagic engorgement, which leads to rupture. Peritonitis may follow.

During vaginal delivery a cystic mass may rupture.[19] Some masses (such as cervical fibroids), because of their location near the birth canal, prevent normal vaginal delivery. In these instances delivery by cesarean section may be necessary to avert the complications.

491

In general, in a pregnant patient with a pelvic mass, if the possibility of ectopic gestation is excluded, conservative management, including close observation and follow-up sonograms, are an acceptable protocol to follow. This is because of the high incidence of spontaneous disappearance of the pelvic mass during pregnancy, the lower risk of malignancy, and the high risk of spontaneous abortion from surgery during early pregnancy.[5] When the patient's symptoms become severe due to complications of the mass, or when the mass persists into the second trimester and appears to be enlarging, surgical intervention is usually indicated. The procedure is performed between 16 and 20 weeks' gestation. If a mass that appears to be malignant is discovered in the third trimester, treatment is postponed until the viable fetus can be delivered. A benign mass is observed until term delivery, after which it is treated.

Sonographic Examination, Technique, and Protocols

Sonography is usually the first diagnostic examination in pregnant patients suspected of having a pelvic mass. The general techniques of scanning for pelvic masses apply to scanning the pregnant patient but with some special considerations.

It is essential that the patient have a full urinary bladder for a proper study, especially in the first trimester or when the mass is deep in the pelvis. In addition to displacing the bowel out of the pelvis, the bladder serves as an organ of reference for proper gain setting and as a reference for cystic masses. A pelvic mass is easier to evaluate in the first trimester of pregnancy, when the gravid uterus is clearly identified and the relationship to it of the mass in question can be seen. In late second- and third-trimester pregnancies, when most masses have been displaced into the abdomen, it is not necessary for the patient to have a full urinary bladder, but the examination must extend to the xyphoid. An unusual fetal position should also alert the examiner to the possibility of extrinsic pressure from a mass. In follow-up examinations, the mass may have changed position and location, so a complete search for it may be required and, of course, precise measurements must be taken because some masses (cystadenoma) tend to grow during pregnancy. Careful characterization of the echogenicity of the mass must be provided, to help narrow the diagnosis.

Rarely, a cystic pelvic mass may be confused with a distended urinary bladder (Fig. 29-1). In such instances, a repeat study after voiding or catheterization of the urinary bladder should solve the problem. Surveying the abdomen for associated disorders such as renal anomalies, obstructive uropathy, loculated ascites, or liver metastases should be a routine part of the examination of any pregnancy associated with a pelvic mass.

Classification

Because the origin of pelvic masses seen during pregnancy is usually uncertain, classification on the basis of sonographic characteristics (cystic, solid, or complex) rather than origin is preferred. It should be emphasized that many of these masses, especially when complicated, have variable sonographic characteristics and, therefore, may be included in many differential diagnoses.

CYSTIC MASSES

Cystic-appearing masses encountered during pregnancy are usually ovarian. Common cystic pelvic masses are corpus luteum cysts of pregnancy, theca lutein cysts, parovarian cysts, cystadenomas, cystadenocarcinomas, dermoids, and hydrosalpinges. Cystic masses arising from the adjacent structures such as bowel and mesentery are difficult to distinguish from ovarian masses, if not impossible. Cystic ovarian masses can be seen at any stage of gestation, but the majority are discovered before 16 weeks' gestation.[13] The prevalence of ovarian cysts in pregnancy is about 1.1%.[13] The higher frequency of association of cystic pelvic masses and pregnancy is due to more frequent sonographic detection of them in asymptomatic patients. In 80% of patients, the cyst resolves spontaneously. Most of the cystic lesions that persist and require surgery are larger than 8 cm.

Corpus Luteum Cysts. Corpus luteum cysts, the most common adnexal masses seen in pregnancy (Fig. 29-2), may reach a size of 10 cm in diameter, but they seldom exceed 6 cm. They are usually unilocular. If some echogenic material is seen in these cys-

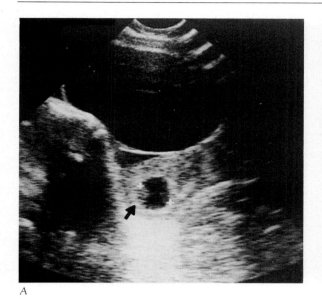

A

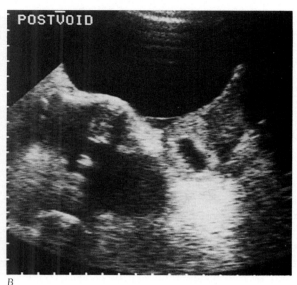

B

Figure 29-1. Ovarian cyst mimicking distended urinary bladder. (*A*) Cystic mass resembles a distended urinary bladder. Early IUP (*arrow*). (*B*) Postvoiding examination shows no change in the size of the cystic mass. (*C*) True nature of the mass is evident after urinary bladder (BL) is filled through a Foley catheter.

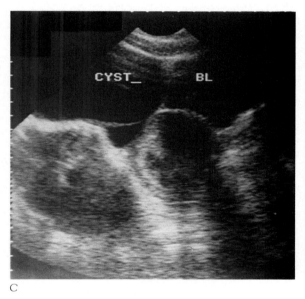

C

tic masses, it is most likely an organized clot. Corpus luteum cysts are expected to regress after 14 to 15 weeks' gestation. Those larger than 6 cm are prone to complications such as torsion (Fig. 29-3), rupture, third-trimester bleeding, and pelvic pain during pregnancy.[12] If a mass greater than 6 cm in diameter enlarges during pregnancy, surgical intervention is necessary to rule out the possibility of ovarian carcinoma.

Theca Lutein Cysts. Although they are seen in normal pregnancy, theca lutein cysts are usually associated with gestational trophoblastic disease, multiple gestations, or ovarian hyperstimulation syndrome. They are often bilateral and characteristically are multilocular. They are caused by elevated levels of human chorionic gonadotropin (HCG). Since this hormone level is elevated in a variety of conditions resulting in fetal hydrops, these cysts can also be seen with fetal hydrops. They regress spontaneously after termination of the pregnancy, so surgical removal should be avoided. Those associated with trophoblastic disease regress within several weeks after evacuation of the uterus.

Hyperreactio Luteinalis. Hyperreactio luteinalis is an association of large theca lutein cysts with intrauterine pregnancy. This is caused by HCG elevation, but is not associated with hydatidiform mole or choriocarcinoma. All mothers with such masses have presented with abdominal distension larger than that expected for gestational age. An ultrasound study is critical in showing a live intrauterine pregnancy and in excluding trophoblastic disease.[18] In a case report by Lawrence,[8] multilocular cysts filled the entire abdomen. In most of the reported cases the patient delivered a normal infant. Conservative management with careful sonographic and clinical evaluation is the most desirable procedure to follow unless complications such as torsion, rupture, obstructed labor, or severe maternal dyspnea due to abdominal distension occur.[8] The cysts resolve spontaneously following delivery.

Parovarian Cysts. Parovarian cysts arise from remnants of Gartner's duct in the mesovarium. They are separate from the ovary, but this separation is difficult to appreciate during pregnancy. Parovarian cysts range in size from a few centimeters to very large abdominopelvic masses.

Ovarian Neoplasms. The incidence of ovarian neoplasms is one in 1000 pregnancies[1]; the prevalence of malignancy in ovarian masses associated with pregnancy is 3 to 5%.[2] Cystadenoma is the most common pelvic mass to enlarge during pregnancy. As in nongravid patients, the mucinous variety of cystadenoma tends to be septate whereas the serous variety may be unilocular. Mucinous cystadenomas are rare in pregnancy and usually are unilateral. They can attain large sizes and if ruptured can lead to pseudomyxoma peritonei.[2] Sonographically,

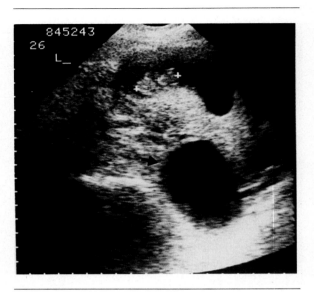

FIGURE 29-2. Nine-week IUP and corpus luteum cyst *(arrow)*.

they are seen as multilocular cysts. The malignant potential of these masses is related to the amount of solid tissue they contain.

Dermoid cysts have a wide variety of sonographic appearances, ranging from totally cystic to predominantly solid. Because they usually present as a complex mass they are discussed later.

Hydrosalpinx. Hydrosalpinx is a rare cause of cystic pelvic mass associated with pregnancy. During pregnancy, closure of the uterine cervix decreases the incidence of pelvic inflammatory disease (PID). Hydrosalpinx is also unlikely to occur because tubal stenosis, a complication of PID, reduces the chances of intrauterine pregnancy.

Mesenteric Cyst. A mesenteric cyst is another rare example of cystic pelvic mass during pregnancy. A case of a large mesenteric cyst containing numerous septations extending above the level of the umbilicus has been reported.[17]

Fluid-filled Bowel. Fluid-filled bowel loops can sometimes be confused with cystic pelvic masses. Real-

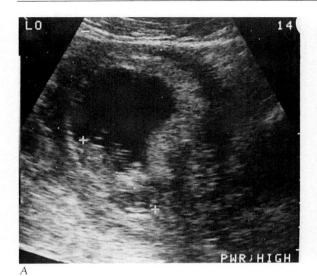

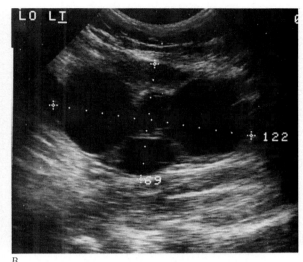

A

B

FIGURE 29-3. Twisted gangrenous corpus luteum cyst (CLC). (*A*) IUP is seen in the midline sagittal scan. (*B*) This parasagittal section on the left shows large multilocular predominantly cystic mass with thick septation. (*C*) Transverse section at the level of the umbilicus shows large solid component of the mass. A twisted gangrenous CLC was discovered at surgery, which was performed because of the patient's severe pain and the large size of the mass.

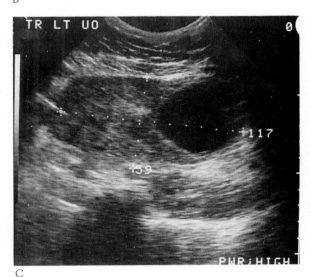

C

time imaging affords visualization of peristalsis, enabling differentiation.

SOLID MASSES

The most common solid pelvic masses seen during pregnancy are uterine myoma, congenital uterine anomalies, pelvic kidney, and solid ovarian tumors. Less common causes are cancer of adjacent organs, wandering spleen, and fecal impaction.

Uterine Leiomyoma. Uterine leiomyoma represents the solid mass most often encountered during pregnancy. Although most fibroids remain about the same size during pregnancy, some may enlarge as their growth is stimulated by estrogen.[6] Those that show rapid enlargement may outgrow their blood supply and undergo infarction and necrosis. This is manifested clinically by moderate to severe pelvic pain, sometimes resembling the pain of "acute

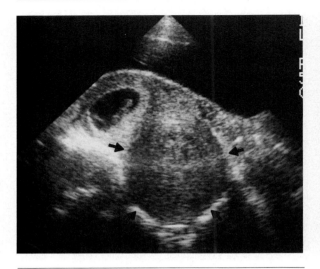

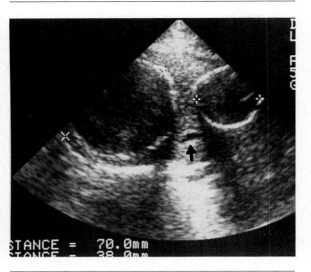

FIGURE 29-4. Midline sagittal section shows a large leiomyoma in the lower uterine segment (*arrows*).

FIGURE 29-5. This transverse scan shows two calcified uterine leiomyomas (xx and + +) associated with an early gestational sac (*arrow*).

abdomen." Ultrasound is capable of diagnosing myoma as a cause of pelvic pain. Once the diagnosis is established, treatment is generally directed to relieving the pain. A myoma seldom affects the outcome of pregnancy. A myomectomy is more hazardous than the myoma and is rarely performed during pregnancy.[21] Complications of pregnancy that have been reported in association with myoma include spontaneous abortion, intrauterine growth retardation, premature rupture of the membrane, uterine inertia, and postpartum bleeding. Ectopic pregnancy, disseminated intravascular coagulation, hemoperitoneum, extrusion of the myoma, and inversion of the uterus have also been reported.[21] A leiomyoma that lies in the lower uterine segment may prevent vaginal delivery (Fig. 29-4). Patients with the placenta near the myoma are at high risk for complications such as premature rupture of membranes, antepartum bleeding, and postpartum hemorrhage. The growth of the fetus and myoma, as well as the relationship of the placenta to the myoma, should be checked throughout the pregnancy.

Sonographic appearance. The sonographic appearance of uterine myomas during pregnancy is the same as in nonpregnant patients. The echogenicity of uterine myomas is usually less than that of the myometrium and placenta. Calcific degeneration may be observed as dense, echogenic areas with distal acoustic shadowing. Sometimes linear peripheral calcifications can resemble the fetal head (Fig. 29-5).

Demonstration of cystic areas within the myoma, when associated with pain, is suggestive of infarction and necrosis. A myoma followed during pregnancy may not always appear at the same location on subsequent scans, owing to the ability of the uterus to rotate.

Enlargement of the uterus due to the presence of a sizable myoma becomes a crucial matter in patients referred for termination of pregnancy who have a discrepancy between the estimated fetal age and uterine size. Ultrasound is useful for making the correct estimate of the fetal age and for demonstrating the associated uterine myoma. The subsequent management of these patients will be based on sonographic demonstration of gestational age rather than the uterine size. Demonstration of the location of the myoma and its relation to the placenta is helpful in selecting the ideal site for amniocentesis.

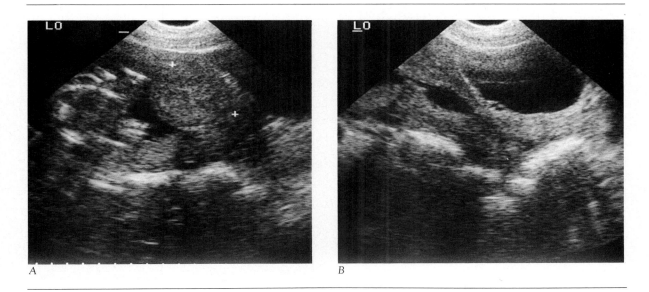

FIGURE 29-6. (A) Midline sagittal section shows a uterine contraction (+ +). (B) It disappeared later during the examination.

It may be difficult to distinguish a uterine myoma from common asymptomatic myometrial contractions. The latter appears as a transient, well-defined, diffusely echogenic area within the myometrium that usually disappears during the examination or within 20 to 30 minutes (Fig. 29-6). Its persistence is not always indicative of a myoma, as some contractions last longer. In addition, they typically extend toward the uterine cavity, unlike a myoma, which usually indents the outer margin of the uterus.

A degenerated, pedunculated, or subserosal myoma can easily be confused with an extrauterine mass, although sometimes its attachment to the uterus can be demonstrated. In these cases, it may be necessary to perform diagnostic surgical exploration in order to rule out the possibility of ovarian carcinoma.

Bicornuate uterus with a nongravid horn simulating a leiomyoma may be differentiated from leiomyoma if the nongravid horn has a similar texture to that of the uterus; leiomyomas tend to be less echogenic than normal myometrium. Decidual reaction within the nongravid horn may be another helpful sign.

Cervical carcinoma associated with pregnancy is rare.[10] Sonographically it is difficult to differentiate from enlargement of uterine cervix due to uterine myoma. The diagnosis can be confirmed by careful clinical examination and cervical biopsy.

Congenital Uterine Anomalies. Congenital uterine anomalies are very uncommon; their prevalence is approximately 0.1 to 0.5%. It is important to diagnose uterine anomalies associated with pregnancy for several reasons.[14] There is higher incidence of obstetric complications, such as spontaneous abortion, premature rupture of the membranes, premature delivery, abnormal fetal positions, and abruptio placentae, and of genitourinary anomalies.

Approximately one third of patients with uterine anomalies have entirely normal pregnancies; however, because of the high incidence of obstetric complications, it has been estimated that the overall pregnancy loss from bicornuate uterus approaches 50%. Therefore, this group of patients should be considered to have high-risk pregnancies. Close follow-up is in order, and cesarean section frequently becomes necessary.

Prior to performing a dilation and curettage the

obstetrician should be aware of any uterine anomalies and therefore avoid entering the nongravid horn.

Sonographic technique and appearance. A reliable indicator of a concurrent uterine anomaly is the identification of a bilobed uterine contour with an anterior or posterior indentation, eccentrically located gestational sac, and echogenic endometrium in the nongravid horn, which is probably due to blood and sloughed endometrial cellular material (Fig. 29-7). A bilobed uterine contour is best seen on high transverse images. In general, as the gestation progresses, the bilobed uterine contour becomes more difficult to recognize, owing to enlargement of the gravid horn with nearly complete effacement of the nongravid horn. A didelphic uterus is usually diagnosed during the physical examination, when two cervices are discovered.

In early gestation, the presence of an endometrial decidual response in the nongravid horn simulates an early twin gestation in a bicornuate uterus. A fibroid in a cornual location can be confused with a bicornuate uterus, but the increased attenuation of a leiomyoma and absence of a central decidual reaction should differentiate the two entities. The incidence of detection of uterine anomalies is related directly to the interest and index of suspicion of obstetrician and sonographer.

Pelvic Kidney. The diagnosis of ectopic pelvic kidney is important, as it may occasionally obstruct the birth canal or be injured during delivery. The gravid uterus may cause obstructive uropathy. The reniform appearance of a pelvic kidney is highly characteristic (Fig. 29-8). Careful examination of both renal fossas in a patient with suspected pelvic kidney is mandatory. Ectopic pelvic kidney is regarded as an indication for cesarean section.

Solid Ovarian Masses. Completely solid ovarian masses are relatively rare and can be either benign, such as fibroma or thecoma, or malignant. Sonographically, they appear solid, with a hypoechoic internal texture and poor sound transmission. They are often difficult to distinguish from subserous and pedunculated myomas.

Any organ in the vicinity of the uterus—such as ovaries, cervix, lymph nodes, urinary bladder, rectum—may be the site of neoplasia during preg-

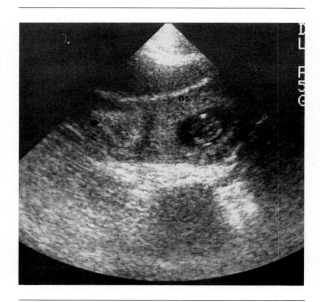

FIGURE 29-7. This transverse scan shows an eccentrically located gestational sac (GS) within a bicornuate uterus. Decidual reaction is seen in nongravid horn (*arrow*).

nancy. Although such lesions are rare, they may be considered in the differential diagnosis of a solid pelvic mass.

Cancer and Pregnancy. The incidence of cancer during pregnancy is one in 1000.[4] The cancers that are most likely to be seen in pregnancy are those of the breast, cervix, ovary, lymph nodes, and colon and rectum, in declining order of frequency. The frequency of cervical cancer is slightly less than one in 700 pregnancies.[4] The diagnosis of cervical cancer is similar to that in nonpregnant women. Vaginal bleeding as a sign of cervical carcinoma is infrequent in gravid women. Most cases are discovered by vaginal examination and Pap smear and by directed biopsy where indicated. Sonographically, it may appear as an enlarged, irregular cervix.

Management is determined by the stage of the disease and the trimester of pregnancy. In the absence of invasive carcinoma, conservative treatment with normal vaginal delivery has been adequate. Invasive carcinoma of the cervix diagnosed

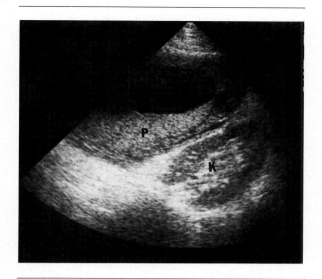

FIGURE 29-8. This transverse scan shows an ectopic pelvic kidney (K) at the region of the left lower quadrant, posterior to the gravid uterus (P, placenta).

during the first two trimesters of the pregnancy is managed as if the pregnancy did not exist. This includes total abdominal hysterectomy with or without pelvic lymph node dissection. In more advanced stages, the patient is treated with irradiation. In the third trimester, if the fetus has reached viability, it is delivered by cesarean section. The patient then undergoes surgical treatment or irradiation. If the fetus is not yet viable, a brief delay is considered acceptable. Vaginal delivery through an involved cervix is considered unwise as cancer cells may be spread by the process of cervical dilatation.[4]

Coexistence of endometrial carcinoma and pregnancy is very rare. Only 8% of endometrial carcinomas occur in women younger than 40 years. There are few case reports of patients treated for endometrial carcinoma who later became pregnant.[4]

All colorectal cancers associated with pregnancy have been reported to be adenocarcinoma. The symptoms are those associated with tumors of the large bowel, such as abdominal pain, nausea, vomiting, constipation, and rectal bleeding. Too often,

these symptoms are dismissed as the side effects of pregnancy or hemorrhoids. Digital rectal examination, testing of the stool for occult blood, and proctosigmoidoscopic examination can be performed safely at any stage of pregnancy and will detect more than 75% of carcinomas in the rectosigmoid region.[4]

The appropriate treatment during the first two trimesters of pregnancy is surgical resection without delay and without regard to the pregnancy. Performing cesarean section after the 33rd week of gestation means that the infant will be viable and that the tumor can be resected at the same time.[4] If the pregnancy is near term and the tumor is not in a position to cause dystocia, a vaginal delivery is permitted. To date, the prognosis for pregnant women with colon cancer has been dismal, with no 5-year survival. In the past 10 years, we have seen two cases of colon carcinoma, both arising from the right side of the colon.

In the first case, a sonographic appearance of pseudokidney at the region of the right lower quadrant raised the possibility of colon tumor (Fig. 29-9); however, this was disregarded clinically. After delivery of a normal, healthy boy, barium enema examination for full evaluation of the patient's abdominal pain revealed a carcinoma of the right side of the colon. The patient is alive approximately 2½ years after diagnosis. In the second patient, the diagnosis was made by the demonstration of a large, irregular solid mass in the region of the right colon and of liver metastases (Fig. 29-10). Gestational age was approximately 23 to 24 weeks. The patient refused any treatment, to avoid any effect on the fetus. Unfortunately, premature labor in the early third trimester resulted in delivery of a baby that died after a few days. The patient also died a few months later from spread of her cancer.

It is reassuring, however, that the concern that a maternal cancer may metastasize to the fetus is largely unjustified.[4] Rare tumors can coexist with pregnancy; a case of schwannoma has been reported that was seen as a large solid mass with multiple echogenic foci[17] adjacent to the fundal portion of the uterus.

Wandering Spleen. Wandering spleen is a term used to describe an ectopic location of the spleen. This condition is rare but more common in multiparous

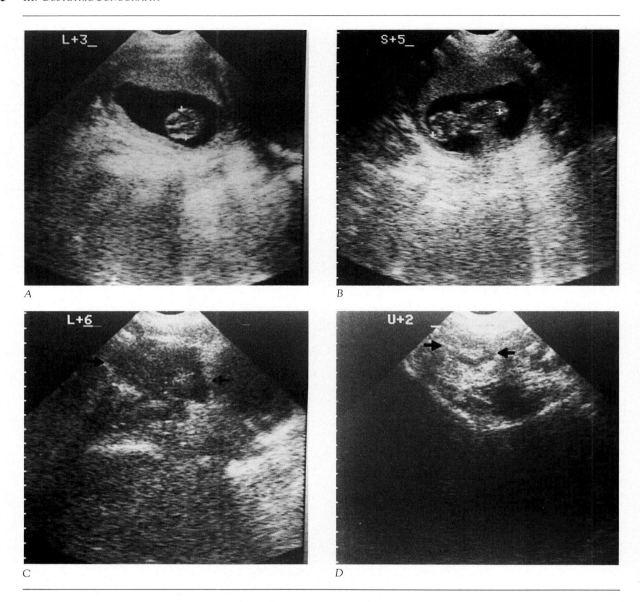

FIGURE 29-9. (A,B) Sagittal and transverse sections of pelvis demonstrating an IUP. (C,D) On right parasagittal and transverse sections a solid mass with a pseudokidney appearance is seen at the region of right lower quadrant. This proved to be colon carcinoma (arrows).

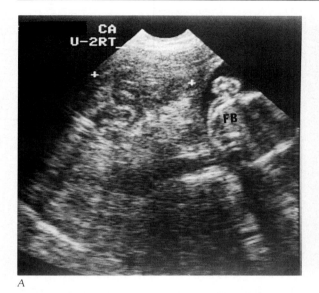

A

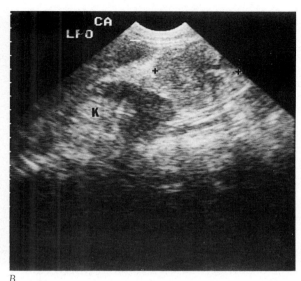

B

Figure 29-10. Colon carcinoma with liver metastases seen during pregnancy. (*A*) Transverse section at the level of the right lower quadrant. The solid mass (+ +) proved to be colon carcinoma (FB, fetal body). (*B*) This right parasagittal section shows the relation of the mass (+ +) to the right kidney (K). (*C*) Enlarged liver with multiple metastases (*arrowheads*).

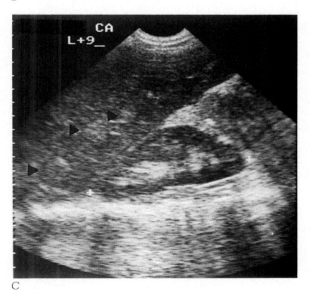

C

women,[6] and in Africa. The spleen may be located anywhere from the left upper quadrant to the left side of the pelvis. The spleen has been shown to prolapse into the pelvis and to present as a pelvic mass during pregnancy.[16] The clinical presentation varies from acute abdomen secondary to splenic volvulus to an incidental finding in an asymptomatic patient. When absence of the spleen in the left upper quadrant is documented, and provided it has not been surgically removed, the diagnosis can be strongly suggested if a solid mass with homogeneous fine echoes is found in the left side of the abdomen. In another case report of wandering spleen and pregnancy,[11] the patient presented with a palpable left-sided abdominal mass and pain, raising the possibility of hydronephrosis. The di-

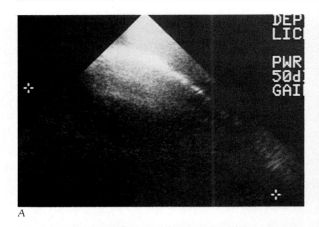

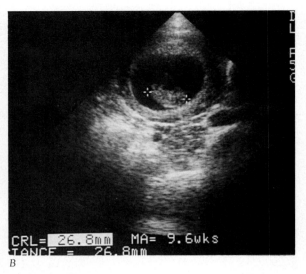

A

B

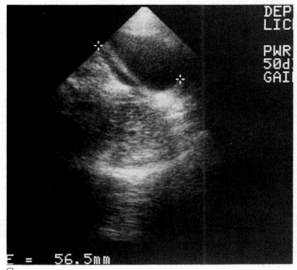

C

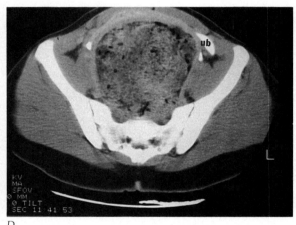

D

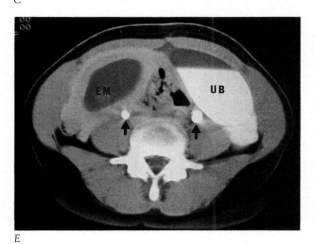

E

FIGURE 29-11. IUP and fecaloma. (A) Midline sagittal section shows a large solid mass with posterior acoustic shadowing. The urinary bladder is not seen. (B) Transverse section to the right of the umbilicus demonstrates an IUP. (C) Left parasagittal section at the level of the umbilicus demonstrates a cystic mass, which, after the patient voided, proved to be the urinary bladder. (D) Contrast-enhanced computed tomogram of the pelvis. Massively distended feces-filled bowel displaces urinary bladder (UB) to the left. (E) On axial computed tomographic section cephalad to scan in D the distended urinary bladder (UB) is displaced to the left. An embryo (EM) is seen within the displaced uterus. Arrows point to dilated ureters.

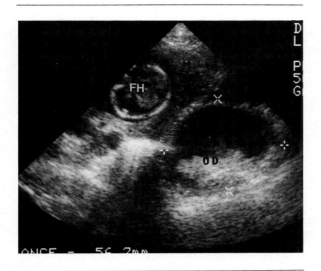

FIGURE 29-12. An ovarian dermoid (OD) was noted incidentally posterior to the gravid uterus (FH, fetal head).

agnosis in this case was made at the time of surgery. Wandering spleen is usually an enlarged spleen with a long pedicle. Because of the long pedicle, the primary complication is torsion, resulting in infarction and acute abdominal pain. Preoperatively the diagnosis is usually a twisted ovarian cyst. It has a high mortality rate (20 to 40%) in pregnancy. Because of the danger of torsion of the pedicle and predisposition to trauma, splenectomy is the treatment of choice.

Fecal Impaction. Fecal impaction is caused by incomplete evacuation of feces over an extended period. This may lead to formation of a fecaloma, which presents clinically as a large, firm mass. Sonographically, a fecaloma has a highly echogenic surface and posterior acoustic shadowing.[3] Recently we encountered a young patient referred to our institution for termination of pregnancy. A very large, solid abdominopelvic mass was seen displacing the urinary bladder to the left and the gravid uterus to the right (Fig. 29-11). The possibility of a solid ovarian mass was entertained, and because of the patient's willingness to terminate the pregnancy, body computed tomography was performed for full evaluation of the mass. This showed the mass to be a fecaloma. The diagnosis could be made with plain abdominal x-ray examination. There have been reports of patients who have undergone colon resection for suspected cancer in cases of fecaloma. The presence of tiny mixed air bubbles and dense solid surfaces of fecaloma may be the cause of acoustic shadowing on ultrasound examination. In most patients, a pelvic mass containing highly echogenic areas and acoustic shadowing is due to calcified uterine fibroids. Ovarian thecoma with a similar appearance has also been described.

COMPLEX MASSES

As a sonographic term, *complex* implies that a mass contains both cystic and solid components; either type may predominate. Coexistence of an intra-uterine pregnancy and a complex adnexal mass is rare (incidence about 1 in 800 pregnancies).[15] The primary concern about such masses includes malignancy, complications related to the mass itself, and possible ectopic gestation. The most common complex pelvic masses associated with pregnancy are benign cystic teratoma, ectopic gestation, endometrioma, ovarian carcinoma, pelvic abscesses, and hematoma. In addition, most if not all pelvic cysts, when complicated, appear sonographically as a complex mass.

Benign Cystic Teratoma. Benign cystic teratoma or dermoid cyst is the most common type of complex extrauterine mass associated with pregnancy (Fig. 29-12). Ovarian dermoid is usually seen for the first time during pregnancy in patients who have no symptoms, but they may come to the attention of the obstetrician because of the pain secondary to torsion. Benign cystic teratoma is often pedunculated and therefore is prone to torsion, causing acute abdomen and pelvic pain; sometimes rupture causes chemical peritonitis. The incidence of these complications increases among pregnant patients, and they often occur during or after vaginal delivery. Schaffer and coworkers[19] report a case of a complex, predominantly cystic mass during pregnancy that "disappeared" on the first postpartum day, with the development of free abdominal fluid. The patient's signs and symptoms allowed immediate recognition of the rupture of the cystic teratoma and appropriate treatment.

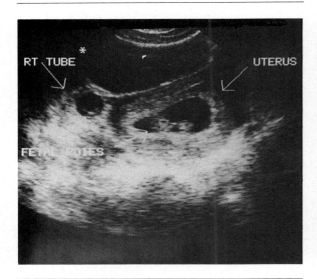

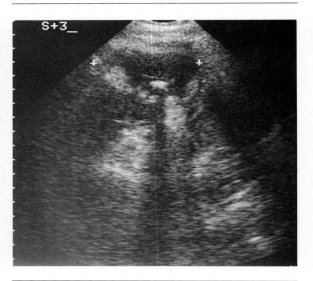

FIGURE 29-13. Live IUP with concomitant ectopic tubal gestation. (Yaghoobian J, Pinck RL, Ramanathan K, et al. Sonographic demonstration of simultaneous intrauterine and extrauterine gestation. J Ultrasound Med. 1986;5:309–312.)

FIGURE 29-14. Demonstration of an appendicolith (*arrow*) within an appendiceal abscess.

Ectopic Pregnancy. The incidence of ectopic pregnancy has recently increased. Simultaneous intrauterine and ectopic pregnancies are very rare (about 1 in 6000 pregnancies). These patients may be referred for ultrasound examination because of pain or adnexal mass (Fig. 29-13). In examining such patients, the sonographer should routinely search for an ectopic pregnancy, even in the presence of an intrauterine pregnancy.[20] The treatment is removal of the ectopic pregnancy.

Endometriosis. While approximately 40% of patients with endometriosis are infertile, the remainder can get pregnant. Endometrioma is rare during pregnancy. The hormonal changes of pregnancy cause atrophy of endometrial tissue so the symptoms often abate. Some of these patients' symptoms are controlled by creating pseudopregnancy after delivery.

Ovarian Carcinoma. The incidence of ovarian malignancy during pregnancy is 1 in 9000 to 25,000 deliveries.[4] This incidence is similar to that for a nonpregnant group of comparable age. Diagnosis of ovarian cancers is difficult, as they are obscured by the enlarged uterus. If they are found at an early stage and are of low-grade malignant potential, unilateral oophorectomy may be considered, allowing the pregnancy to proceed to term. This is not accepted uniformly, and some express reservations about treating a patient with carcinoma by unilateral oophorectomy.[4] The sonographic appearance of ovarian carcinoma is usually of a predominantly cystic mass with some septation and some solid components. The probability of malignancy is related to the amount of solid component and also to the thickness of the septa. The abdomen must be examined, with special attention to the possibility of ascites, hydronephrosis, and liver metastases.

Pelvic Abscess. Pregnancy is rarely associated with PID or with other intraabdominal abscesses that may follow appendicitis, bowel rupture, Crohn's disease, or rarely, preexisting inflammatory disease of the adnexa. The diagnosis of an abscess concomitant with pregnancy is of great importance because the spread of infection to the uterus may cause septicemia and shock. The ultrasound findings of an abscess depend on the extent of the inflammatory process and of abscess formation. An abscess usually has an irregular, moderately well-defined margin with a predominantly cystic appearance and some internal echoes. These echoes arise from debris, pus, or rarely from gas in the abscess. Rarely, the abscess may appear as an echogenic mass; however, it usually has good distal acoustic enhancement.

Diagnosis of acute appendicitis during pregnancy is a challenge because of the early signs and symptoms that may be altered by or attributed to the pregnant state. Delay in diagnosis is dangerous; maternal morbidity and fetal loss are increased owing to perforation and peritonitis. Demonstration of an appendicolith with acoustic shadowing within the abscess, when correlated with the patient's history, is almost pathognomonic (Fig. 29-14). Careful attention to history and physical examination combined with ultrasound findings can help to suggest the proper diagnosis in most cases. If diagnosis is in doubt, needle aspiration of the mass may be indicated. The treatment of choice is removal of the abscess.[21]

References

1. Barber HR. Diagnosing and managing the unilateral mass. Contemp Obstet Gynecol. 1976; 7:9.
2. Bezjian AA. Pelvic masses in pregnancy. Clin Obstet Gynecol. 1984; 27:402–415.
3. Derchi LE, Musante F, Biggi E, et al. Sonographic appearance of fecal masses. J Ultrasound Med. 1985; 4:573–575.
4. Donegan WL. Cancer and pregnancy. Cancer. 1983; 33:194–214.
5. Fleischer AC, Boehm FH, James AE Jr. Sonography and radiology of pelvic masses and other maternal disorders. Semin Roentgenol. 1982; 17:172–181.
6. Fleischer AC, Boehm FH, James AE Jr. Sonographic evaluation of pelvic masses and maternal disorders occurring during pregnancy. In: Sanders RC, James AE Jr, eds. The Principles and Practices of Ultrasonography in Obstetrics and Gynecology. 3rd ed. Norwalk, CT: Appleton-Century-Crofts; 1985.
7. Kinori I, Rifkin MD. A truly wandering spleen. J Ultrasound Med. 1988; 7:101–105.
8. Lawrence PH, Lyons EA, Levi CS. Hyperreactio luteinalis. J Ultrasound Med. 1983; 2:375–376.
9. McGahan JP, Phillips HE, Oi RH. Coexistent endometriomas in pregnancy: Sonographic appearance. J Clin Ultrasound. 1982; 10:180–182.
10. Mack LA, Gottesfeld K, Johnson ML. Ultrasonic evaluation of a cervical mass in pregnancy. J Clin Ultrasound. 1981; 9:49–50.
11. Miller EI. Wandering spleen and pregnancy: Case report. J Clin Ultrasound. 1975; 3:281–282.
12. Miller EI, Thomas RH, Applegate JW. Persistent corpus luteum cyst of pregnancy: Sonographic evaluation of cause of third-trimester bleeding. J Clin Ultrasound. 1978; 6:187–188.
13. Nelson MJ, Cavalieri R, Graham D, et al. Cysts in pregnancy discovered by sonography. J Clin Ultrasound. 1986; 14:509–512.
14. Pennes DR, Bowerman RA, Silver TM. Congenital uterine anomalies and associated pregnancies: Findings and pitfalls of sonographic diagnosis. J Ultrasound Med. 1985; 4:531–538.
15. Pennes DR, Bowerman RA, Silver TM. Echogenic adnexal masses associated with first-trimester pregnancy: Sonographic appearance and clinical significance. J Clin Ultrasound. 1985; 13:391–396.
16. Pritchard JA, MacDonald PC. Williams' Obstetrics. 16th ed. New York: Appleton-Century-Crofts; 1980:847–857.
17. Rahatzad MT, Adamson D. A pictorial essay of pelvic and abdominal masses seen during pregnancy. J Clin Ultrasound. 1986; 14:255–267. (Published erratum in J Clin Ultrasound 1986; 14:493.)
18. Rowlands JB. Hyperreactio luteinalis: A case report. J Clin Ultrasound. 1978; 6:327–329.
19. Schaffer RM, Cataldi GA, Shih YH. Sonographic demonstration of rupture of a cystic teratoma during pregnancy. J Ultrasound Med. 1984; 3:425–427.
20. Yaghoobian J, Pinck RL, Ramanathan K, et al. Sonographic demonstration of simultaneous intrauterine and extrauterine gestation. J Ultrasound Med. 1986; 5:309–312.
21. Zymlyn S. Ultrasonographic evaluation of the large-for-date uterus. In: Sarti D, ed. Diagnostic Ultrasound Text and Cases. 2nd ed. Chicago: Year Book Medical Publishers; 1987.

CHAPTER 30

Multiple Gestations

Julia A. Drose, Mark A. Dennis

As sonologists we have seen many an unsuspecting couple react with excitement at the discovery of a twin pregnancy. Members of the medical community respond in a tempered fashion, being aware of the numerous problems and complications that may accompany multiple gestation. For example, although multiple gestations account for approximately 1% of all live births, the associated perinatal mortality rate may be as much as 5 to 10 times higher than in singleton births, principally secondary to prematurity. That 1% also accounts for 10 to 13% of all neonatal deaths.[8,18] These alarming statistics may be altered through early diagnosis and ultrasound monitoring. Although in prospectively screened populations ultrasound is 98% sensitive in diagnosing multiple gestations, because ultrasound screening in the community is not performed routinely on all pregnancies, many multiple gestations still go undiagnosed until late. Late diagnosis is associated with elevated mortality and morbidity rates. Once it is diagnosed and followed with monitoring, the probability of an unfavorable outcome in multiple gestations may actually be reduced from 60 to 25%.[20] The role of the sonographer therefore is to accurately diagnose multiple gestation when given the opportunity to examine a pregnant patient and to observe the pregnancy regularly to detect associated fetal complications.

Clinical Information

The most common reason for suspecting a multiple gestation is the physical finding of "large for gestational age." The differential diagnosis for this clinical presentation includes polyhydramnios, uterine fibroids, molar pregnancy, erroneous dates, macrosomic fetus, and ovarian masses. On physical examination, the diagnosis of multiple gestations also may be suspected through the palpation of two or more fetuses or when two or more fetal heart tones varying in location and by more than 10 beats per minute in rate are discovered by auscultation or Doppler examination. Early increases in maternal blood pressure and anemia, greater than would be expected with a singleton gestation, may also be found.

Laboratory values may indicate multiple gestations as well. Routine maternal serum α-fetoprotein (MSAFP) determination is performed in many centers today. Twenty to thirty percent of pregnant women have an MSAFP greater than the 95th percentile.[27] About 10% of these pregnancies are multiple gestations. Quantitation of human serum placental lactogen (HPL) is a less common but more sensitive test for detecting multiple gestations. Ninety-five percent of twin pregnancies fall within the group of HPL levels greater than 1 standard deviation (SD) above the mean for gestational age in singleton pregnancies.[13] A combined increase in

MSAFP and HPL can raise the twin detection rate to approximately 80% without imaging. The maternal serum human chorionic gonadotropin (HCG) level may also be higher in multiple gestation.[14]

The level of clinical suspicion for multiple gestation is elevated by maternal history. Briefly, the two major types of twinning are monozygotic (MZ) and dizygotic (DZ). Thirty percent of all twins are of the MZ type, in which a single embryo divides after fertilization. This type of event appears to be random and independent of clinical and epidemiologic factors except in rare instances.[8] Nearly 70% of all twin gestations are dizygotic, the result of the fertilization of two ova. This type of event depends upon polyovulation, which in turn is related to maternal medical history and environmental factors. DZ twinning is increased if there is a history of DZ twinning on the maternal side of the family, and women who are themselves DZ twins have 1 chance in 58 of delivering twins. Women who have borne dizygotic twins previously have 1 chance in 40 of repeating this in a subsequent pregnancy. The incidence of multiple births appears to increase with advancing maternal age as well, peaking at 35 to 39 years. There is an overall twinning rate in the United States of approximately 1 in 90 births. Blacks have the highest incidence of multiple births (1/76), orientals the lowest rate (1/92), and the probability of whites bearing DZ twins is 1 in 86. As far as geographic differences, the highest global DZ twinning rate is in Chile (1/51) and the lowest is in Venezuela (1/294). Finally, pharmacologic ovulation induction variably increases the probability of multiple births.[8]

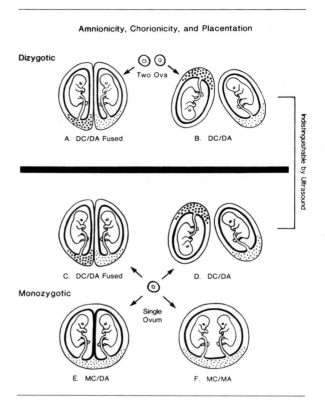

FIGURE 30-1. Dizygotic twinning is depicted above the horizontal bar and monozygotic twinning, below. *A-D* are dichorionic-diamniotic twins; monozygosity and dizygosity cannot be differentiated by evaluation of placentation or membranes alone. The appearance of a single placenta results from fusion of separate placentas and may be distinguished from *E* and *F* (monochorionic pregnancies with diamnionic and monoamnionic membranes, respectively) by the presence of a thick membrane. Note the thick membranes in *A* and *C* and the thin membrane in *E*.

Anatomy and Physiology

The placental membranes are composed of two layers, the outer layer (chorion) and the inner layer (amnion). Three types of placentation or combinations of the membranes and placentas are possible with twin gestations (Fig. 30-1). In dichorionic-diamnionic gestations the fetuses have separate placentas and chorions, and therefore, their own separate amniotic sacs. As pregnancy progresses the placentas may fuse, giving the ultrasonographic appearance of a single placenta. Monochorionic-diamnionic fetuses are enclosed in separate amnionic sacs but share one placenta and one chorion. In the third category, the monochorionic-monoamnionic pregnancy, both fetuses share the same placenta, chorion, and amniotic sac. All DZ twins are of the dichorionic-diamnionic variety, but the type of placentation in MZ twins depends on the stage of embryonic development at which separation occurs (Table 30-1). In MZ gestations, the mortality rate can range from 9% in dichorionic

TABLE 30-1. Association of placentation of MZ twins with timing of zygote division

TIME OF ZYGOTE DIVISION (DAYS)	MZ PLACENTATION*	APPROXIMATE FREQUENCY
3	DC/DA	33%
4–7	MC/DA	66%
8–13	MC/MA	3%
13 +	Conjoined (MC/MA)	1/50,000–1/100,000

*Key: DC, dichorionic; DA, diamniotic; MC, monochorionic; MA, monoamniotic. (Adapted from Crane JP. Sonographic evaluation of multiple pregnancy. Semin Ultrasound CT MR. 1984;5:144.)

cases to 50% in monoamniotic placentation.[2] Because of the differing risks associated with different types of MZ placentation, it is desirable that amnionicity and chorionicity be determined, if possible, through ultrasound examination (Table 30-2).[19]

Examination Techniques and Imaging
SCANNING PROTOCOL
When scanning multiple gestations, it is of utmost importance to be thorough by giving each fetus a completely separate examination, thereby avoiding oversights (Table 30-3). The sonographer should resist the tendency to condense the multiple gestation examination into the time normally allotted for a singleton examination, and if possible appropriate time should be reserved in advance. The examination should begin with scanning of the uterus in either a transverse or a longitudinal plane, from one side to the other, to determine the number of fetuses. Next, the lower uterine segment is scanned again to identify the presenting fetus. The fetus with the lowest presenting part should be labeled fetus A. Unusually, two fetuses may coexist at the same level, in which case they should be labeled "left fetus" or "right fetus." It may also be helpful to identify the fetus' sex. If the twins are dizygotic, 50% will be of opposite sexes. In this situation, should the fetuses change in relative posi-

TABLE 30-2. Association of placentation and complications

ULTRASOUND FINDINGS	PLACENTATION	SIGNIFICANCE
Single placenta, thin membrane	MC/DA	Intrapartum jeopardy of second twin after first twin delivered Only necessary to aspirate one sac on amniocentesis Twin-twin transfusion is possible and periodic US is recommended beginning 25 wks Contraindication to selective termination of one twin Complications possible in surviving twin if one twin dies
Single placenta, no membrane	MC/MA	High mortality rate if MC/MA due to entanglement or twin-twin transfusion
	Fused DC/DA or MC/DA	Always rescan later if no membrane is detected early
Entangled fetuses or cords	MC/MA	Extremely high risk
No membrane with stuck twin	MC/DA with one placenta	Both fetuses at risk due to vascular communications
	DC/DA with two placentas	Lower risk for nonstuck twin (excludes TTS as a cause)
Single placenta, thick membrane	MZ or DZ, DC/DA	Low risk
Two placentas with or without membrane	DZ, DC/DA	Low risk
Two fetal sexes	DC/DA	Low risk

Table 30-3. Sonographic protocol for examination of multiple gestation

Identify number of fetuses present
Identify fetal positions
Label presenting fetus A
Identify presence and thickness of membrane
Identify number of placentas
Show similar fetal parts on same scan to demonstrate the number of fetuses and to prove those parts are not conjoined
Measure both fetuses': BPD, HC, AC, FL

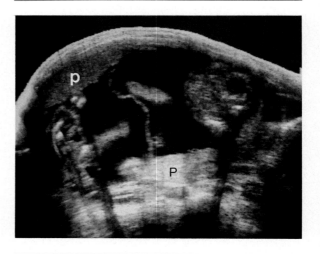

Figure 30-2. Longitudinal ultrasound image of a dichorionic diamniotic pregnancy as demonstrated by two fetuses separated by a membrane, and two separate placentas (P), one ventral and one dorsal.

tion (fetus A become fetus B), follow-up growth measurements will still be possible, if each fetus has been identified previously through sex determination. Because it is very rare for MZ twins to be of different sexes, if two separate fetal sexes are identified, this virtually guarantees dizygosity. Twins of the same sex may be DZ or MZ.

Once the presenting fetus (A) has been identified, the fetal spine should be followed to connect the appropriate head with its corresponding body. After fetus A's body parts have been identified and its position determined, a routine fetal anatomy examination and documentation, as set forth by the AIUM and the ACR, should be performed. After this is completed, fetus B should be identified and its head and body connected in the manner described above. The anatomy of this fetus should then be documented. Also, when multiple pregnancies are documented both heads should be recorded on one scan and both bodies on another, if possible, to prove that it is a multiple gestation and that the fetuses are not conjoined.

Next, it is important to identify the number of placentas, to identify a membrane, if there is one, and to characterize the membrane. In the classic articles by Mahony[25] and Hertzberg,[19] ultrasonographic differentiation of placentation was first described in some detail. Essentially, if two placentas are identified, the pregnancy is dichorionic-diamnionic, and the fetuses are in the lowest risk category for complications (Fig. 30-2). The dividing membrane in this instance is thick early on, and at times all four layers of membranes may be seen (two amnions and two chorions). If only one placenta is identified and the membrane appears thick, again, the pregnancy is dichorionic-diam-

nionic with fused placentas (Fig. 30-3). In either of these two situations, the appearance may be associated with DZ or MZ twins. In the event that only one placenta is identified, if the dividing membrane is wispy or hairlike, is seen over only a short segment, and has only two layers (two amnions), the pregnancy is monochorionic-diamnionic (Fig. 30-4) and is at higher risk for fetal complications. If no membrane is readily visualized, it is important to search for one thoroughly and carefully as membranes may be difficult to find later in gestation, even when they are present. In general, membranes are seen in 90% of all twins at some point in pregnancy, and only 10% of the remainder are actually monoamnionic gestations (Fig. 30-5). Therefore, although failure to identify a membrane late in the third trimester when a single placenta is present cannot be considered strong evidence of a monochorionic-monoamnionic pregnancy, it must be suspected, and other signs of monoamnionic-monochorionic twinning, such as fetal entanglement or cord entanglement, should be sought. The highest fetal morbidity and mortality rates are associated with these findings in a twin gestation. Finally, intrauterine bands, synechiae, amniotic

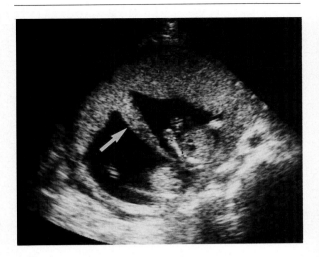

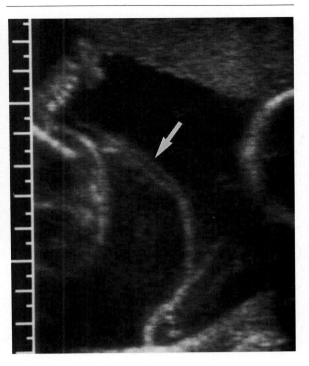

FIGURE 30-3. Real-time image of early twin diamniotic dichorionic pregnancy as demonstrated by a thick membrane (white arrow) separating two fetuses. It should be noted that it is difficult to separate the two placentas, and in this instance, the thickness of the membrane differentiates a dichorionic pregnancy with a fused placenta from a monochorionic pregnancy and only one placenta, since in the latter case, the membrane would be thin.

FIGURE 30-4. Image demonstrates a monochorionic diamniotic twin gestation with a thin membrane composed of two layers separating the fetuses. (The *white arrow* points to two layers in the diamniotic membrane.)

"sheets,"[34] or uterine septa should not be mistaken for membranes. Usually the distinction is straightforward: A free edge is visible in the aforementioned entities, whereas a membrane separating fetuses is uninterrupted.

As in routine singleton scans, the amount of amniotic fluid should be determined. A previously held concept that polyhydramnios is common in twin gestations has not been confirmed in recent studies; actually it occurs in only 5 to 10% of twin gestations.[17] Although two amniotic cavities with normal amounts of amniotic fluid may initially give the impression of increased fluid on ultrasound, true polyhydramnios is not a common finding, as these statistics reflect.[17] So it is important to assess amniotic fluid quantity as objectively as possible. Some centers utilize articulated-arm scanners for a more objective estimation of the total amniotic fluid volume, although in the hands of an experienced sonographer, real-time examination of

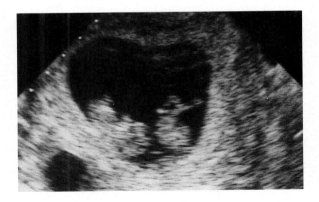

FIGURE 30-5. Real-time image of early monochorionic monoamniotic gestation shows two fetuses in close proximity with no separating membrane.

the intrauterine volume may be accurate as well. When articulated-arm scanning is available it is of use especially after 16 weeks, when the intrauterine contents outgrow the real-time field of view. At this gestational age, the uterus is scanned in 1-cm increments in both longitudinal and transverse planes. As the overall uterine size increases, longitudinal scanning is performed at 1-cm increments with 2-cm incremental transverse scanning. In higher order multiple gestations, static scanning may diminish the possibility of error in determining the total number of gestations and provides a basis for orientation and comparison in follow-up examinations.

In uncomplicated twin and high-order multiple gestations interval scanning should be planned every 3 to 4 weeks in the third trimester, to detect complications as they arise and to allow appropriate management. If the placentation is monochorionic, even more frequent scanning may be necessary, since these fetuses are at high risk for complications of discordance (twin-twin transfusion) or entanglement.

The Vanishing Twin

The actual prediction of fetal number at term by the ultrasonologist depends on technical factors as well as the probability of fetal survival. Interestingly, a significant number of pregnancies that begin with ultrasound-demonstrated multiple sacs end as singleton gestations at term. In a study by Jeanty and coworkers,[12] 23 multiple pregnancies were identified in a total of 300 prospectively examined women. Three out of the 21 women carrying early twin pregnancies ultimately delivered twins, and of the two remaining multiple gestations, one triplet pregnancy resulted in normal twins, and a quadruplet pregnancy resulted in a normal singleton birth. One explanation for this phenomenon is that the nonviable gestation represents an anembryonic gestation, which is proposed to be the cause of 50 to 90% of early spontaneous abortions.[3] Histopathologic examination of these anembryonic gestations reveals autosomal trisomies (52%), triploidies (20%), and monosomy X (15%), among other disorders. Gestational sac growth early on can suggest the diagnosis of an anembryonic gestation, since a normal sac grows at a rate of approximately 0.12 cm per day and a nonviable pregnancy at 0.025 cm per day. Later on, the nonviable gestational sac may begin to involute. Ultrasonographic criteria for this vanishing sac include a smaller gestational sac than expected for menstrual age, an irregular margin of the sac, and a crescent-shaped sac with incomplete trophoblastic ring.[12] A small echogenic spot may be seen even later, corresponding to a totally involuted gestational sac. In cases where an anembryonic gestation or vanishing sac is suspected, vaginal probe examination may be helpful in excluding the possibility of a viable gestation, which is difficult to see (i.e., it may aid in visualizing a yolk sac or small fetal pole where none was seen on transabdominal scanning).

Members of multiple pregnancies have been seen to vanish even later in pregnancy, when fetal poles are identified. An interesting article in the recent literature prospectively studied pregnancies and early on documented a group in which twins were identified with fetal cardiac activity but subsequent scans revealed a singleton.[22] This occurred in approximately 21% of twins prospectively diagnosed; this rate of spontaneous demise is actually very similar to that of spontaneous singleton demise. In the situations in which one live twin has vanished, the remaining fetuses were found to have a normal prognosis for survival.

In the second or third trimesters and in MZ twin gestations fetal demise may result in the formation of a fetus papyraceus (Fig. 30-6).[10] Instead of the usual complete decomposition and absorption of the fetus, it is preserved in a distorted form. In twins, the postulated mechanism is transient polyhydramnios of one fetus in a monochorionic-diamniotic pregnancy exerting a lethal compressive effect on the other nonhydropic twin. Fetal papyraceus occurs in 1 of 12,000 live births but is more common in the subgroup of twin gestations (1 in 184 twin births).[22]

Technical Pitfalls

Technical pitfalls, the other factor in accurately determining fetal number, should be kept in mind when diagnosing multiple gestations or abnormal sacs in multiple gestations. Crescentic implantational hemorrhage or amnionic-chorionic separation should not be mistaken for second pregnancies or nonviable pregnancies (Fig. 30-7). The

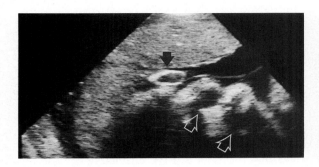

FIGURE 30-6. Sector real-time image demonstrates a thin membrane (monochorionic) separating the small distorted skull of a fetus papyraceous (*black arrow*) and the normal face of the surviving, large twin (*open white arrows* indicate orbits in transaxial scan with fetus looking upward and to the right in the illustration).

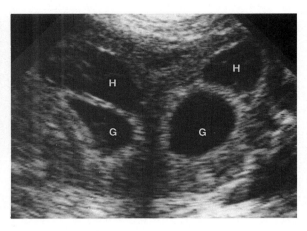

FIGURE 30-7. Sector scan demonstrating two normal gestational sacs (G). Above each of the sacs is noted an implantational hemorrhage (H) with ill-defined margins and low-level echoes within.

distinction is usually obvious by the configuration of the fluid collections and the lack of a well-defined decidual rind. A ghosting artifact[6] may be seen in transverse scans of the pelvis, where small anatomic areas such as early gestations are being investigated; this creates the illusion of two sacs where there is only one (Fig. 30-8). The effect is most pronounced in muscular patients, although it can occur in any patient; the phenomenon is secondary to the rectus muscle acting as a lens, refracting the ultrasound beam. Examining the patient in the longitudinal plane will expunge this artifact and prevent misdiagnosis. The same artifact may also duplicate ovarian follicles or the uterus, may overestimate crown-rump length, and may even mimic fetal omphalocele.

Although intuitively this seems unlikely, late in pregnancy a second fetus may be completely overlooked because the nondependent fetus obscures the underlying one. Sonographers should be alerted to this possibility if the visualized fetus is situated more anteriorly than would be expected and if there are more fetal parts in the image than seems appropriate. Later in pregnancy, owing to relative decrease in amniotic fluid with respect to the fetal volume, important areas of fetal anatomy may be hidden, and an effort must be made to evaluate obscured anatomy by scanning at multiple an-

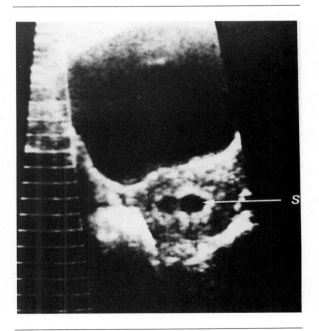

FIGURE 30-8. Ghosting artifact. S = gestational sac. (Buttery B, Davison G. The ghost artifact. J Ultrasound Med. 1984;3:49–52.)

gles and with the mother in different positions. Finally, there is a tendency to overdiagnose increased amniotic fluid in multiple gestations, so when this is suspected, anteroposterior distance measurements of amniotic fluid should be obtained so that the diagnosis may be made according to the criteria of the specific institution.

Multiple Gestations Other Than Twins

SPONTANEOUS HIGHER-ORDER GESTATIONS

The number of fetuses in a multiple gestation is inversely related to the probability of that particular higher-order gestation arising. While the average incidence of twins is 1 in 100 pregnancies, triplets occur in only approximately 1 in 7600 pregnancies (Fig. 30-9), and the spontaneous rates for quadruplet and quintuplet pregnancies are 1 in 729,000 and 1 in 65,610,000, respectively.[8] Interestingly, triplet pregnancies—and even quadruplet pregnancies—may be MZ. For example, 60% of triplet pregnancies are secondary to the fertilization of two ova (Fig. 30-10), 30% arise from the fertilization of three ova, and 10% arise from the fertilization of a single ovum.[16]

FERTILITY AUGMENTATION

Fertility drugs alter the rate of higher-order gestations. Three are currently used in fertility augmentation.[37] The first is clomiphine citrate; its use in ovulation induction results in an 8 to 13% rate of multiple gestation, most being twins. Although this drug has several mechanisms of action, the predominant one is most widely believed to be displacement of estrogen from hypothalamic receptors, which augments release of gonadotropin-releasing hormone (GRH), ultimately causing follicular maturation and ovulation. The second agent, human menopausal gonadotropin (HMG), is a combination of follicle-stimulating hormone (FSH) and lutenizing hormone (LH). When ultrasound demonstrates follicles measuring 2.0 to 2.5 cm, HMG is administered to simulate the LH surge, resulting in ovulation. The rate of multiple gestations when this type of stimulation is employed has approached 42% in some series; however, if estrogen level is monitored closely it is possible to decrease this to a more acceptable rate of 10%. It also should be noted that higher-order multiple gesta-

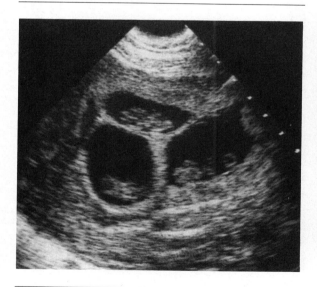

FIGURE 30-9. Real-time scan of early triplet gestation demonstrates three separate gestational sacs with small fetal poles within.

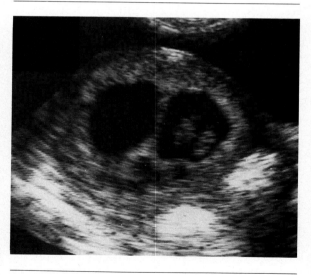

FIGURE 30-10. Triplet pregnancy resulting from the fertilization of two ova with one gestational sac on the left without the fetus in the field of view, and two monoamnionic twins in the gestational sac to the right with no dividing membrane.

cause the ovaries to attain huge proportions (Fig. 30-11). These changes may lead to ascites from cyst rupture, pleural effusion, and ovarian torsion. Rarely in twins and higher-order gestations, ovarian hyperstimulation may occur spontaneously when no fertility drug was administered.

Abnormal Twinning

A variety of unusual abnormal twin types may occur. The most commonly thought of abnormal twins are conjoined (approximately 1 in 50,000 to 1 in 100,000 live births).[38] Thoracopagus (joined at the thorax), omphalopagus (joined at the abdominal wall), or a combination of the two constitute approximately 70% of all conjoined twins (Figs. 30-12, 30-13). Other varieties (Figs. 30-14, 30-15) are craniopagus (joined at the head), pygopagus (joined at the buttocks), ischiopagus (joined at the

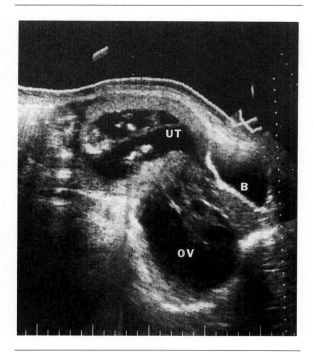

FIGURE 30-11. Longitudinal articulated arm scan in a patient who received HMG ovulation induction. A large hyperstimulated ovary (OV) is identified in the cul-de-sac posterior to the uterus (UT). The maternal urinary bladder is identified for reference on this longitudinal scan (B).

tions are more frequent with HMG than with clomiphine: Triplets occur in as many as 5 to 6% of HMG-induced pregnancies. Bromocriptine, the third agent, acts directly on the pituitary, decreasing the production of prolactin in patients with hyperprolactinemia. This diminishes the inhibition of the release of hypothalamic GRH by prolactin, allowing the return of the hypothalamic-pituitary-gonadal axis to nearly normal function. Because this is more or less the restoration of a physiologic situation, the incidence of twinning is not much greater than normal. Approximately 1.2 to 1.8% of these pregnancies are multiple, mostly twins.

Finally, there are extrauterine complications of the ovulation induction technique, especially with HMG. Specifically the ovarian hyperstimulation syndrome may occur, in which multiple large cysts

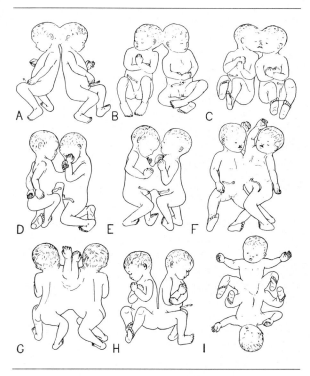

FIGURE 30-12. Possibilities for partial fusion of fetuses: (A–C) craniopagus; (D–G) thoracopagus; (H–I) pygopagus. (From Patten BM: Human Embryology. New York: McGraw Hill; 1968.)

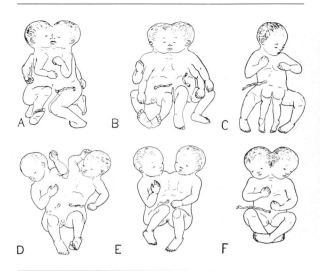

FIGURE 30-13. Images demonstrate more complete forms of conjoined twinning. (From Patten BM: Human Embyrology. New York; McGraw Hill; 1968.)

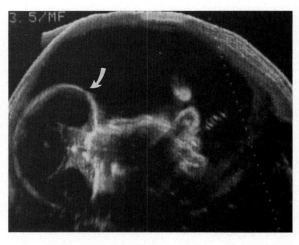

FIGURE 30-14. Transverse static scan demonstrates fused crania (curved arrow) in cephalothoracoomphalopagus (conjoined twins) with grossly abnormal intracranial contents.

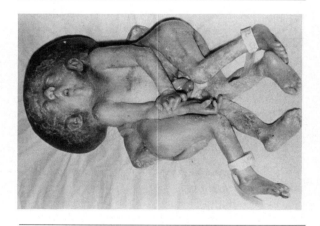

FIGURE 30-15. Photograph of fetus in Figure 30-14 after cesarean section delivery demonstrates the fusion at the level of the heads, thoraces, and abdomens. Note the associated gastroschisis.

ischia), and cephalothoracopagus.[16,24,39] An interesting variation on the theme of conjoined twinning is the localized anatomic duplication anomaly, termed diprosopus, which consists of duplication of the nose, at one end of the spectrum, and of two complete faces with partial duplication of the intracranial structures, on the other. This anomaly may be especially challenging to diagnose by ultrasound.[30,38]

Developmentally, conjoined twins arise from monochorionic-monoamnionic gestations in which division of the embryo occurs after the 13th day of conception. They are always of the same sex, and 70% are female. Sonographic findings in conjoined twins include lack of visualization of a separating membrane between the twins, inability to separate the fetal bodies (Fig. 30-16) or heads despite changes in fetal position, more than three vessels in a single umbilical cord, and complex fetal structural anomalies.[21] Polyhydramnios is more common in conjoined twins, occurring in approximately 50% of cases (in contrast to 5 to 10% of normal twins).[38] It is important to make the diagnosis of conjoined twins, because approximately one third are stillborn and an additional third die on day 1. Because the relationship of the heart to each fetus is a critical determinant of survival, fetal echocardiography is essential for all conjoined twins. Conjoined twins also may occur in higher-order gestations. In one series, without ultrasound planning of delivery, five of nine extra fetuses co-existing with conjoined twins died in the perinatal period.[20]

Another variation on abnormal twinning is the parasitic twin found within the abdomen of its sibling. This is referred to as fetus in fetu[23] and should not be confused with a teratoma. Although the distinction between parasitic twin and teratoma may be difficult, it is important to establish, as teratomas have a definite malignant potential whereas the fetus in fetu is technically a hamartoma and entirely benign. Fetus in fetu occurs more commonly in the upper retroperitoneum whereas teratomas usually arise in the lower abdomen, most commonly in the ovaries or the sacrococcygeal region. Also, there is usually radiographic or at least microscopic evidence of a vertebral column in fetus in fetu.

One type of parabiotic twinning, termed the *twin reversed arterial perfusion* (TRAP) syndrome,[11] leads to the development of a grossly malformed twin, referred to as an acardiac monster or acardiac anomaly (Fig. 30-17). The syndrome may arise whenever there is the potential for vascular communication between twins through the placenta (i.e., in monochorionic pregnancies) and re-

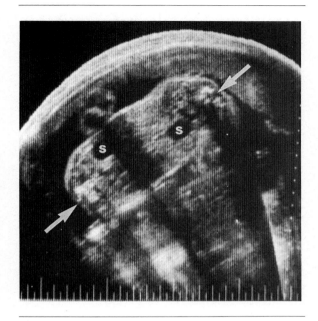

FIGURE 30-16. Image of thoracoomphalopagus demonstrates opposing spines (*white arrows*) and fetal stomachs (s). In this case, the fetuses were obviously conjoined and could not be identified as separate fetuses despite multiple maneuvers.

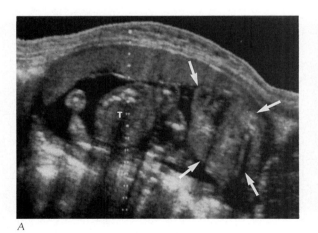
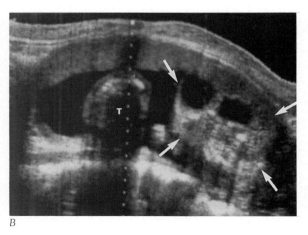

A   B

FIGURE 30-17. Two different longitudinal static scans demonstrate a normal twin (T) and a disorganized mass of tissue (*white arrows*) in the lower uterine segment representing an amorphus, acardiac twin. An umbilical cord was identified on other images entering the acardiac monster.

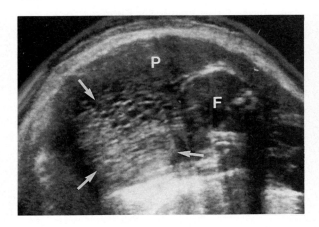

Figure 30-18. Transverse sonogram demonstrates a normal fetus (F) to the right, the placenta associated with the normal fetus (P), and the adjacent complete mole to the left (*arrows*).

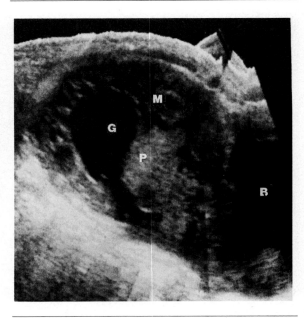

Figure 30-19. Longitudinal scan shows bladder (B) as reference, remnant portion of normal placenta (P), molar tissue (M), and the gestational sac (G). Note the small amount of shadowing in the dependent portion of the gestational sac from fetal parts.

sults from one large arterial-arterial and one large venous-venous anastomosis between the twins. The acardiac twin, which possesses either no heart of its own or a grossly malformed heart, is completely perfused by the donor twin through the arterial-arterial communication. Because the blood perfusing the parasitic twin is not well oxygenated and enters through the abdominal aorta, preferential development of the lower extremities and body occurs, with frequent sacrifice of the fetus' upper thorax, head, and upper extremities. If this anomaly is detected, close monitoring should be considered during the third trimester, because there is a 20% mortality rate if the normal donor twin becomes hydropic owing to high-output cardiac failure. Fortunately the acardiac anomaly is rare, occurring in 1 in 35,000 live births. This anomaly occurs exclusively in MZ twin gestations or triplets, is most common with monochorionic-monoamnionic pregnancies, and carries with it no increased risk of recurrence.[11] In utero, occlusion of arterial and venous communications mark a promising form of antenatal therapy, with select termination of the anomalous twins.

Another example of abnormal twinning is a nor-mal twin coexisting with a complete hydatidiform mole (Fig. 30-18). This is a rare occurrence, and more commonly a partial mole occurs where a chromosomally abnormal (triploid) fetus is present with molar tissue replacing most of the placenta (Figs. 30-19, 30-20). Early fetal demise is the rule in cases of partial mole. The appearance of fetal parts within or adjacent to molar tissue may establish the diagnosis of partial mole, which has less malignant potential than a complete mole. Also when fetal parts and tissue that appear to represent a hydatidiform mole coexist, the possibility of a singleton demise with hydropic degeneration of the placenta should be suspected. It is interesting that the serum β-HCG level cannot be used reliably to distinguish between missed abortion and complete or partial mole.[40]

Heterotopic pregnancies may even be considered a type of twinning when single or multiple intra-

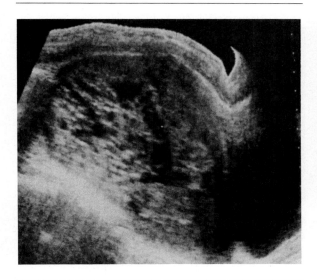

FIGURE 30-20. Longitudinal scan adjacent to Figure 30-19 more clearly demonstrates the abnormal inhomogeneous molar placental tissue with sonolucent areas.

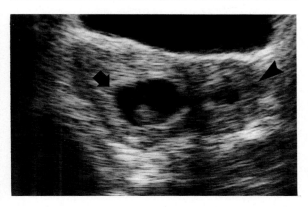

FIGURE 30-21. Transverse sector scan shows the two horns of a bicornuate uterus with a fetal pole in the gestational sac in the right horn (*black arrow*), and the "pseudogestational sac" in the left horn (*black arrowhead*) caused by vicarious stimulation of the endometrium in the left horn.

uterine pregnancies coexist with an ectopic pregnancy.[36] The incidence of this was once thought to be 1 in 30,000 pregnancies, but owing to the increase in ectopic pregnancies it is now thought to be 1 in 6000 or lower.[15] Predisposing conditions include ovulation induction, pelvic inflammatory disease, endometriosis, and in vitro implantation of multiple embryos.[36] Heterotopic pregnancy or heterotopic twinning should not be confused with two pregnancies each within a horn of a bicornuate uterus or with an early singleton, unicornuate gestation within a bicornuate uterus and a pseudogestational sac in the contralateral horn (Fig. 30-21). The differentiation may be quite difficult to make using ultrasound.

Finally, other twinning abnormalities include superfetation, in which there is fertilization of two separate ova months apart, (i.e., ovulation occurs after conception), and superfecundation, in which two ova are fertilized at different times by the sperm of two different fathers or by the same father within a shorter period.[32,33]

Complications

MATERNAL COMPLICATIONS

Both maternal and fetal complications may occur in multiple gestations. Premature labor is the most common fetal and maternal complication. At least 52% of multiple fetuses are delivered before term, and 18% before 35 weeks.[8] Premature labor may ensue because the large fetoplacental mass causes uterine overdistention and subsequent contractions or because of premature rupture of the membranes resulting from increased intraamnionic pressure.[27] There is also an increase in third-trimester bleeding, possibly related to the increased prevalence of placenta previa, abruption, and velamentous insertion of the cord with placenta previa. Miscellaneous maternal complications that occur with increased frequency in multiple gestations include hypertension of pregnancy, anemia, pyelonephritis, hepatic cholestasis, preeclampsia, and eclampsia.[18]

FETAL COMPLICATIONS

All fetuses in multiple gestations are at risk. Fetal complications in multiple pregnancies are extensive, and because ultrasound can have a significant impact on the high rate of mortality and morbidity due to these complications, it should be used routinely to monitor these fetuses at risk. Discordancy or intrauterine growth retardation (IUGR) in one fetus is a major fetal complication, second only to prematurity of all of the fetuses in the pregnancy due to early labor. The smaller fetus in the discordant pair is at risk for perinatal anoxia. Normal intrauterine growth of twins parallels that of singleton pregnancies until approximately 31 or 32 weeks.[14] After that point, the head and abdominal growth rates are thought by some authors to slow down while the femurs continue to grow normally.[14] Abnormal intrauterine growth or discordancy results in a weight difference greater than 15 to 20% of the larger twin's weight,[1,5] or an overall weight differential of 500 g at birth.

To identify these fetuses at risk, several sonographic criteria have been used, including a difference in biparietal diameter (BPD) of at least 5 mm. The BPD alone, however, is a poor indicator of fetal growth and a poor standard for comparison in twin gestations, because there is an inherent problem in accurately measuring normal fetal heads in unusual positions or when they are obscured by fetal superimposition. Second, normal fetuses not uncommonly become dolichocephalic secondary to uterine crowding or breech presentation.

Recently, a more sensitive measurement to identify discordant fetuses was found to be an abdominal circumference (AC) differential greater than 20 mm.[1] This is a sensitive indicator because the fetal liver mass, as reflected in the AC, is the first parameter to become abnormal in fetuses with asymmetric IUGR. It is important to realize, however, that the sensitivity and specificity is not 100% for detecting IUGR in any one fetus using multiple criteria, and the sonographer is encouraged to be vigilant for other signs associated with IUGR, such as oligohydramnios (Fig. 30-22) or abnormal Doppler waveforms.

Discordancy may be secondary to either idiopathic IUGR of one fetus with the other fetus growing normally as discussed above, or to the parabiotic syndrome of which twin-twin transfusion and the previously mentioned acardiac anomaly are manifestations. To date, the twin-twin transfusion syndrome (TTS) has been found to

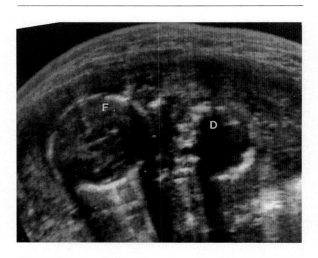

FIGURE 30-22. Transverse sonogram demonstrates a normal-appearing fetal head (F), a somewhat distorted cranial vault in the adjacent nonviable twin (D), and oligohydramnios. Although both fetuses' growth was retarded, this demonstrates the ultimate form of discordancy—one live fetus and one nonviable fetus.

occur only with monochorionic twins, whether they be diamnionic or monoamnionic, and has not been definitely demonstrated with separate placentas in close proximity or after fusion. Again, this underscores the importance of determining the amnionicity and chorionicity of a gestation.

In TTS the sharing of a common placenta allows anastomoses to develop between arterial and venous circulations, resulting in abnormal shunting of blood from one fetus to the other. Approximately 15 to 20% of all monochorionic twins have TTS to some extent. The sonographic criteria for TTS include disparity of fetal size, disparity in size of the two amnionic sacs when the pregnancy is diamnionic and not monoamnionic, separate umbilical cords with disparity in size or number of vessels, a single placenta (monochorionic) with areas of inhomogeneity of the villi supplying the two cords, and hydrops of either fetus (Fig. 30-23).[4,31]

A "stuck" twin[25] is a discordant twin located in an oligohydramniotic sac whose fetal movements are restricted by the closely applied membrane. This is easily diagnosed when the restricted fetus is in the nondependent portion of the uterine cavity

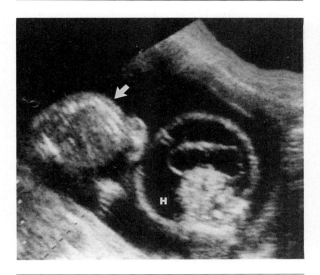

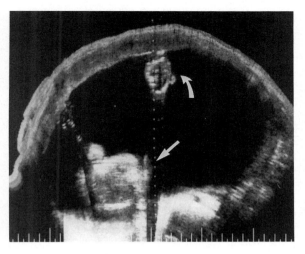

FIGURE 30-23. Obstetric static scan shows a normal (*white arrow*) fetus adjacent to a grossly hydropic (H) fetus with a large amount of ascites. This appearance was secondary to TTS, and the relatively normal-looking fetus actually measured small for gestational age.

FIGURE 30-24. Curved arrow demonstrates a "stuck" twin in the nondependent portion of the uterine cavity due to oligohydramnios and a restrictive membrane. Gross polyhydramnios surrounds the more normal-looking fetus (*straight arrow*) in the dependent portion of the uterine cavity.

(Fig. 30-24). The finding of a stuck twin may be helpful in the diagnosis of TTS; however, the stuck twin appearance is not peculiar to this syndrome. Any cause of oligohydramnios, such as IUGR or genitourinary anomaly affecting one of the twins, may give the same appearance. Also a pregnancy with a stuck twin need not be monochorionic, since it sometimes occurs with dichorionic-diamnionic twins.[24] Although usually the "recipient" fetus in TTS is the large, hydropic fetus, and the "donor" fetus is the small, oligohydramniotic fetus, the presence of hydrops is not a reliable sign for identifying the recipient, as it has been reported in both donor and recipient twins. Unfortunately, TTS carries a very poor prognosis for both twins: the mortality rate approaches 70 to 80%.[2,31] Recently, reversal of the oligohydramnios and hydrops present in TTS has been documented by performing a therapeutic amniocentesis to remove excess fluid from the polyhydramniotic sac.

Whether the problem is TTS or discordancy secondary to IUGR of indeterminant cause, pulsed Doppler examination can evaluate hemodynamic changes in the fetoplacental unit and may eventu-

ally be a useful tool for assessing fetal well-being. Because it may be technically difficult in cases of multiple gestations to identify with certainty which fetus is associated with which umbilical cord, attempts have been made to evaluate fetal aortic flow as an indicator of the status of the fetoplacental unit.[28] Usually the cord-fetus association is clear, though, and the umbilical artery is investigated. Increased vascular resistance resulting from placental insufficiency may cause a decrease in diastolic blood flow resulting in an abnormally high peak systolic–to–end diastolic waveform ratio. Some authors advocate the addition of fetal carotid artery Doppler to umbilical artery measurements to increase the sensitivity and specificity of Doppler for IUGR. This is because with asymmetric IUGR, the brain is preferentially perfused, or spared, and the diastolic flow increases when this occurs. Increasing diastolic flow from decreasing cerebrovascular resistance, secondary to loss of autoregulatory mechanisms stemming from hypoxic metabolic abnormalities, may be the explaining mechanism. Doppler wave forms also reflect shunting of blood in TTS through absolute decreases in the diastolic waveform (Fig. 30-25). Umbilical arterial pulsed Doppler studies in TTS have identified the fetus in which placental vascular resistance is greater, but neither the identification of hydrops nor abnormal Doppler waveforms can differentiate donor from recipient fetus or provide consistently useful prognostic information for fetal outcome.

The biophysical profile has also established itself as an important way of estimating fetal well-being in complicated pregnancies. It involves the quantitation of fetal movement, tone, breathing, amniotic fluid volume, and in some cases placental grading, in conjunction with nonstress testing (the test for normal increases in fetal heart rate associated with fetal movement).[23] The biophysical profile appears to be able to identify fetuses at risk for perinatal anoxia and is more accurate than nonstress testing alone.

Aside from discordancy and its deleterious effects, genetic and developmental abnormalities are also more common in twins. Genetically similar MZ twins are nearly 100% concordant for genetic defects (e.g., Down's syndrome). The most common discordant genetic defect in an MZ twin pair is a normal fetus paired with one that has Turner's syndrome. MZ twins are only 2 to 10% concordant for isolated developmental defects.[27] Because dizygotic twins are not genetically identical, they have a very low concordance for both genetic and developmental abnormalities.

Approximately 5 to 10% of twin pregnancies are complicated by polyhydramnios. When polyhydramnios does occur, it may be either chronic or acute. The chronic form usually develops over a period of weeks in the third trimester and is associated with an increased mortality rate (45%).[8] The even more ominous acute form usually develops over a period of days between 20 and 26 weeks, primarily among dizygotic twins, and carries with it a mortality rate of nearly 100%. This mortality figure is most likely secondary to fetal prematurity when the polyhydramnios causes early labor.

For several reasons the highest morbidity and mortality rates are associated with monochorionic-monoamnionic twins. These pregnancies are associated with cord accidents, including prolapse, entanglement, and nuchal cord, as well as malpresentation and interlocking twin phenomenon. The interlocking of fetal anatomy where one twin is breech and the second vertex may prevent normal vaginal delivery. The possibility of these compli-

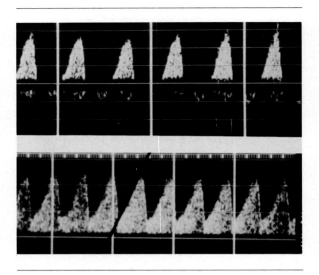

FIGURE 30-25. Umbilical artery waveform in a fetus with TTS demonstrates an absence of diastolic flow.

cations is so worrisome that in some centers all monochorionic-monoamnionic MZ pregnancies are delivered via cesarean section.[8]

Invasive Fetal Evaluation

As a preface to amniocentesis, ultrasound is utilized to determine that the gestational age is appropriate for the procedure, to verify viability and the number and location of fetuses and placentas, and to identify the presence of membranes. Safe needle placement is ensured with intraoperative ultrasound monitoring. If separate fetal compartments are identified, the needle is inserted into the first sac, samples are obtained, and 1 to 2 ml of indigo carmine dye is deposited in the sac before the needle is withdrawn.

Next, the second compartment is punctured, and if the fluid is clear, the operator may be assured that the second sac has indeed been aspirated. If the fluid is blue, the first sac has been reentered; another attempt must be made. Sampling of both fetal sacs in twin gestations is successful in approximately 88% of cases; however, if amnionic fluid from the second sac cannot be successfully aspirated, ultrasound demonstration of a monochorionic-diamnionic gestation reassures the operator that the pregnancy is monozygotic and therefore the fetuses would undoubtedly possess the same chromosomal complement. In cases where no membrane can be identified and there are two fetuses, two punctures should be performed as far apart as possible and as close to each fetus as possible to maximize the possibility of obtaining appropriate samples, in the event that the pregnancy is not monoamnionic (i.e., that a membrane was present but could not be visualized).[9]

When amniocentesis is performed to determine the lecithin-sphingomyelin (LS) ratio for lung maturity, and if the fetuses' growth is concordant, it may not be necessary to tap both sacs. If only one sac is sampled, the use of an LS ratio of 2.5:1 instead of 2:1 is recommended, to predict lung maturity at a greater confidence level. If the twins' growth is discordant and the operator elects to tap only one sac or can gain entry to only one sac, the sac associated with the larger normal twin should be selected. The pulmonary maturity of the pair may not be accurately reflected in the smaller fetus' amniotic fluid because of accelerated pulmonary maturity secondary to antenatal stress. Therefore, the smaller twin may be assumed to have an LS ratio that is at least as mature as that of its normal sibling.[9]

Early in pregnancy, chorionic villus sampling can be performed as an alternative to genetic amniocentesis. This is feasible in twins, as it is often possible to determine the number of placentas present at 10 to 12 weeks' gestation. If two placental sites are identified, a separate sample is taken from each as close to the cord insertion as possible. Ultrasound is used continuously throughout the procedure to locate the placenta(s) and to guide the sampling catheter through the cervix or transabdominally into the placental site(s). In higher-order gestations this procedure may not be practical because it becomes more difficult to identify the correct number of placentas.[7,26]

Selective Termination

Should serious complications or anomalies occur in multiple gestations, selective termination may be offered to the parents as an option. In cases where only one twin is affected with a serious chromosomal or congenital anomaly, or when decreasing the number of fetuses in a multifetal pregnancy might improve the perinatal result, selective termination of fetuses may be a reasonable alternative. This procedure usually involves the direct injection of air into the fetal heart or umbilical vein or fetal exsanguination via cardiac puncture. It is important to realize that selective termination should be performed only in dichorionic pregnancies (i.e., those which the placentas are visualized in different locations or where there appears to be one placenta {fused placentas} and the dividing membrane is thick).

If selective termination is performed on a monochorionic pregnancy or if spontaneous fetal demise occurs in a monochorionic pregnancy, the potential exists for a thromboplastic substance to be released from the dead twin, passing into the surviving twin, and causing intrauterine disseminated intravascular coagulation with potential brain and multiorgan damage or death.[35] Since MZ twins are rarely discordant for genetic defects, selective termination in monozygotic pregnancies would involve cases of isolated congenital anomalies or would be performed to reduce the number of fetuses. The role of ultrasound in the procedure includes locating the appropriate fetus, guiding the needle for puncture, and monitoring the well-being of surviving fetuses. Hysterotomy may also be an option to correct defects instead of terminating the pregnancy.

Conclusion

With the use of ultrasound, increased morbidity and mortality associated with multiple gestations can be dramatically reduced through early detection and through serial scanning, which will identify associated abnormalities of growth and structure.

References

1. Barnea ER, Romero R, Scott D, et al. The value of biparietal diameter and abdominal perimeter in the diagnosis of growth retardation in twin gestation. Am J Perinatol. 1985; 2:221–222.
2. Benirschke K, Kim CK. Multiple pregnancy. N Engl J Med. 1973; 288:1276–1336.
3. Bernard KG, Cooperberg PL. Sonographic differentiation between blighted ovum and early viable pregnancy. AJR 1985; 144:597–602.
4. Brennan JN, Diwan RV, Rosen MG, et al. Fetal-fetal transfusion syndrome: Prenatal ultrasonographic diagnosis. Radiology. 1982; 143:535–536.
5. Brown CEL, Guzick DS, Levino KJ, et al. Prediction

of discordant twins using ultrasound measurement of biparietel diameter and abdominal perimeter. Obstet Gynecol. 1987; 70:677–681.

6. Buttery B, Davison G. The ghost artifact. J Ultrasound Med. 1984; 3:49–52.

7. Cadikin AV, Ginsberg NA, Pergament E, et al. Chorionic villi sampling: A new technique for detection of genetic abnormalities in the first trimester. Radiology. 1984; 151:159–162.

8. Crane JP. Sonographic evaluation of multiple pregnancy. Semin Ultrasound CT MR. 1984; 5:144–156.

9. D'Alton ME, Alton ME, Dudley DKL. Ultrasound in the antenatal management of twin gestation. Semin Perinatol. 1986; 10:30–38.

10. Gericke GS. Genetic and teratological considerations in the analysis of concordant and discordant abnormalities in twins. S Afr Med J. 1986; 69:111–114.

11. Gibson JY, D'Cruz CA, Patel RB, et al. Acardiac anomaly: Review of the subject with case report and emphasis on practical sonography. J Clin Ultrasound. 1986; 14:541–545.

12. Gindoff PR, Yeh MN, Jewelewicz R. The vanishing sac syndrome. Ultrasound evidence of pregnancy failure in multiple gestations, induced and spontaneous. J Reproductive Med. 1986; 31:322–325.

13. Grennert L, Persson PH, Gennser G, et al. Ultrasound and human placental lactogen screening for early detection of twin pregnancies. Lancet 1976; 1:4–6.

14. Grumbach K, Coleman BG, Arger PH, et al. Twin and singleton growth patterns compared using ultrasound. Radiology. 1986; 158:237–241.

15. Hann LE, Bachman DM, McArdle CR. Coexistent intrauterine and ectopic pregnancy: A reevaluation. Radiology. 1984; 152:151–154.

16. Hartung RW, Yiu-Chiu V, Aschenbrener CA. Sonographic diagnosis of cephalothoracopagus in a triplet pregnancy. J Ultrasound Med. 1984; 3:139–141.

17. Hashimoto B, Callen PW, Filly RA, et al. Ultrasound evaluation of polyhydramnios and twin pregnancy. Am J Obstet Gynecol. 1986; 154:1069–1072.

18. Hays PM, Smeltzer JS. Multiple gestation. Clin Obstet Gynecol. 1986; 29:264–285.

19. Hertzberg BS, Kurtz AB, Choi HY, et al. Significance of membrane thickness in sonographic evaluation of twin gestations. AJR. 1987; 148:151–153.

20. Hughey MJ, Olive DL. Routine ultrasound scanning for the detection and management of twin pregnancies. J Reprod Med. 1985; 30:427–430.

21. Koontz WL, Layman L, Adams A, et al. Antenatal sonographic diagnosis of conjoined twins in a triplet pregnancy. Am J Obstet Gynecol. 1985; 153:230–231.

22. Landy HJ, Weiner S, Corson SL, et al. The "vanishing twin": Ultrasonographic assessment of fetal dis-

appearance in the first trimester. Am J Obstet Gynecol. 1986; 155:14–19.

23. Loderio JG, Vintzileos AM, Feinstein SJ, et al. Fetal biophysical profile in twin gestations. Obstet Gynecol. 1986; 67:824–827.

24. McLeod K, Tan PA, DeLange M, et al. Conjoined twins in a triplet pregnancy: Sonographic findings. J Diagn Med Sonogr. 1988; 4:9–12.

25. Mahony BS, Filly RA, Callen PW. Amnionicity and chorionicity in twin pregnancies: Prediction using ultrasound. Radiology. 1985; 155:205–209.

26. Mulcahy MT, Roberman B, Reid SE. Chorion biopsy, cytogenetic diagnosis, and selected termination in a twin pregnancy at risk of haemophila. Lancet. 1984; 2:866–867.

27. Newton ER. Antepartum care in multiple gestation. Semin Perinatol. 1986; 10:19–29.

28. Nimrod C, Davies D, Harder J, et al. Doppler ultrasound prediction of fetal outcome in twin pregnancies. Am J Obstet Gynecol. 1987; 156:402–406.

29. Nocera RM, Davis M, Hayden CK, et al. Fetus-infetu. AJR. 1982; 138:762–764.

30. Okazaki JR, Wilson JL, Holmes SM, et al. Diprosopus: Diagnosis in utero. AJR. 1987; 149:147–148.

31. Pretorius DH, Manchester D, Barkin S, et al. Doppler ultrasound of twin transfusion syndrome. J Ultrasound Med. 1988; 7:117–124.

32. Pritchard JA. Multiple pregnancies. In: Pritchard JA, MacDonald PC, eds. Williams Obstetrics. 12th ed. New York: Appleton-Century-Crofts; 1961; 687–688.

33. Pritchard JA. Multifetal pregnancy. In: Pritchard JA, MacDonald PC, eds. Williams Obstetrics. 16th ed. New York: Appleton-Century-Crofts; 1980; 655–656.

34. Randel SB, Filly RA, Callen PW. Amniotic sheets. Radiology. 1988; 166:633–636.

35. Redwine FO, Hays PM. Selective birth. Semin Perinatol. 1986; 10:73–81.

36. Rowland DM, Geagan MB, Paul DA. Sonographic demonstration of combined quadruplet gestation, with viable ectopic and concomitant intrauterine triplet pregnancies. J Ultrasound Med. 1987; 6:89–91.

37. Scialli AR. The reproductive toxicity of ovulation induction. Fertil Steril. 1986; 45:315–323.

38. Strauss S, Tamarkin M, Engleberg S, et al. Prenatal sonographic appearance of diprosopus. J Ultrasound Med. 1987; 6:93–95.

39. Wilson DA, Young GZ, Crumley CS. Antepartum ultrasonographic diagnosis of ischiopagus: A rare variety of conjoined twins. J Ultrasound Med. 1983; 2:281–282.

40. Woo JSK, Wong LC, Hsu C, et al. Sonographic appearances of the partial hydatidiform mole. J Ultrasound Med. 1983; 2:261–264.

CHAPTER 31

Sonography of the Postpartum Uterus

DIANE M. KAWAMURA

The puerperium is the postpartum period (after parturition), commencing with the expulsion of the placenta and extending to the time when the maternal physiology and anatomy is restored to its approximate prepregnant state.[21,30] A sonographic examination during the puerperium may be indicated to (1) examine the uterine cavity for the cause of postpartum hemorrhage; (2) evaluate complications such as puerperal infection; (3) determine the extent of postpartum ovarian vein thrombophlebitis; and (4) survey cesarean section incision sites of the uterine and abdominal wall for complications such as hematomas and abscesses.

Normal Postpartum Anatomy and Physiology

The postpartum period lasts 6 to 8 weeks and involves both biochemical and physiologic changes.[33] These changes are a consequence of the withdrawal of luteal and placental estrogen and progesterone, which reverses the morphologic and functional changes of pregnancy, resulting in involution of the uterus.[13,14,33] Lactation begins at this time and when it is discontinued the normal reproductive organ functions, such as ovulation and menstruation, resume.[2,13,14,16,22,28,31,33]

Immediately after delivery the uterus is heavy, and retrodisplacement occurs when the patient lies supine.[35] As involution or contraction progresses, the uterus assumes its normal prepregnant shape and position unless pelvic supports have undergone extensive damage.[33,35] The fundus descends from its subxyphoid location to a level just above the umbilicus, assuming a slightly dextroverted position referred to as "physiologic right torsion of the uterus."[21,33] Within 1 week after delivery, rapid uterine involution results in a change in uterine size from approximately 1100 g to 500 g.[13,21,33] This event also restores the uterus to a position between the symphysis pubis and umbilicus.[13,21,33]

Under normal conditions, uterine involution is assessed by clinical examination, consisting of external or bimanual palpation.[21,33] In obese patients, patients who are in pain, or have recently undergone surgery (e.g., cesarean section, cholecystectomy) sonography provides a complementary noninvasive way to follow uterine involution.

Scanning Technique

Sector real-time transducers are preferred to linear-array real-time transducers as the latter are less effective in visualizing the nonperpendicular interfaces of the pelvic structures postpartum.[6,12,19] A sector real-time transducer, either mechanical-pulsed or annular-array type, with the capability of scanning cephalad, caudad, and from side to side, is preferred for optimal demonstration of the entire pelvis.[6,12,19]

A 3.5- or 5-MHz transducer with a long internal focus (8 to 12 cm) is appropriate for scanning the uterus transabdominally.[9,19] Distension of the urinary bladder is necessary for the transabdominal examination of the ovoid puerperal uterus and the pelvic cavity.[21] The time gain compensation (TGC) or slope should be decreased in recognition of the enhanced sound transmission qualities of the urine-filled bladder.[6]

Visualization of the entire puerperal uterus requires examination of the pelvis in both transverse and sagittal plane sections.[9] For accurate measurements, it may be necessary to turn the transducer from the sagittal and transverse body planes to accommodate for the physiologic right torsion of the uterus.[9,19,21]

Sonographic Appearance of Normal Postpartum Anatomy

UTERUS

Bimanual examination alone may not be sufficient to precisely determine uterine size postpartum.[32] Sonography not only permits reliable measurement of uterine dimensions but also provides a noninvasive method for making repetitive clinical studies to establish physiologic and pathologic changes.[10,25,32]

Uterine involution has been assessed with sonography by several investigators.[10,15–17,25,32] Postpartum the uterus can assume varying shapes from long and narrow to short and wide and can produce a wide range of measurements in each dimension. The cavity shape, however, remains the same, eventually appearing as an inverted triangle in all patients.[25] On day 1, the internal os may be open and ill-defined compared to its appearance on subsequent days.[25]

In the anteroposterior (AP) dimension, the uterine myometrium has homogeneous echogenicity and averages 3 to 6.5 cm in thickness, with a range of 7 to 10 cm for total uterine thickness.[17] Prominent myometrial vessels can be sonographically visualized within the normal uterine wall.[16] The endometrial cavity appears as a linear echo with an AP thickness measurement of 5 to 13 mm initially, involuting to 0.3 to 0.6 mm within 10 days postpartum.[17,33] An anechoic separation of the internal endometrial walls (representing residual blood or serous fluid[9]) normally measures 0.4 to 1.3 cm; focal

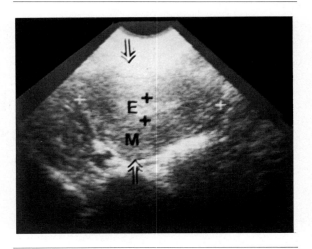

FIGURE 31-1. Transverse sonogram of a normal uterus 2 days postpartum demonstrates the location for the AP dimension (*black arrows*) and the endometrial cavity (*black crosses*; M, myometrium; E, endometrium). (Courtesy Tamara Salsgiver, Ogden, UT.)

areas of greater separation are considered abnormal (Fig. 31-1).[21]

The length of the uterus after delivery ranges from 14.5 to 25 cm, decreasing as the puerperium advances.[16,17,25,32] Errors in uterine length measurements are associated with the degree of bladder filling, which influences the cavity distance between the fundus and the internal os (Fig. 31-2).[25]

The width measurement is made at right angles to the longitudinal measurement at the widest uterine segment. The maximum width measurement of the uterus has been reported as 7 to 14 cm.[16,17,25,32] A variability of this measurement can be associated with uterine contractions and the location of the measurement (Fig. 31-3).[25]

Three studies indicate no correlation in regression size between breast-feeding and bottle-feeding mothers.[16,21,32] Table 31-1 provides the normal range of postpartum sonographic measurements presented in the literature.[10,15,16,25,32]

LIGAMENTS

The eight ligaments supporting the uterus are flaccid following delivery but assume normal prepregnancy firmness within a few weeks.[33] In the puer-

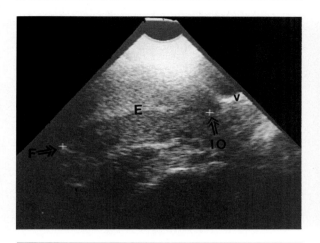

FIGURE 31-2. Longitudinal sonogram of a normal uterus 2 days postpartum demonstrates a cavity distance of 12.5 cm (between crosses) between the fundus (F) and the internal os (IO). (Courtesy Tamara Salsgiver, Ogden, UT.)

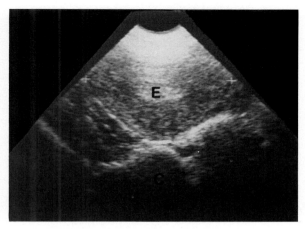

FIGURE 31-3. Transverse sonogram of a normal uterus 2 days postpartum demonstrates the widest transverse measurement of 10.7 cm (between crosses; E, endometrium; C, colon). (Courtesy Tamara Salsgiver, Ogden, UT.)

TABLE 31-1. Ranges of normal sonographic postpartum uterine measurements

STRUCTURE	DIMENSIONS (CM)
AP Thickness	
Endometrium	0.4–1.3
Myometrium	3.0–6.5
Uterus	7.0–10.0
Length	14.5–25.0
Width	7.0–14.0

peral patient, initially only the broad ligaments and their components can occasionally be visualized sonographically. In order to avoid any confusion with an abnormality, it is important to recognize the broad ligaments and their components when they are imaged.[21] As the uterus regresses, the adnexa become more readily identifiable.[16]

Postpartum Pathology

POSTPARTUM HEMORRHAGE

Postpartum hemorrhage is defined as blood loss exceeding 500 ml[33]; it occurs after less than 5% of all deliveries but is potentially the most lethal compli-

cation of the puerperium and accounts for 35% of maternal deaths.[21,34,35] Death can be prevented with immediate blood replacement.[35] Acute postpartum hemorrhage occurs within the first 24 hours; delayed postpartum hemorrhage occurs between days 2 and 31 of the puerperium.[33]

Predisposing Factors. Uterine muscles must contract rapidly and firmly following delivery to occlude the vessels at the point of placental separation. Factors that delay contraction and interfere with the normal mechanism that controls the amount of bleeding are listed in Table 31-2.

Etiology. The most common causes of acute hemorrhage are uterine atony and soft tissue damage. Delayed hemorrhage is most commonly caused by retained secundines (products of conception such as the placenta, umbilical cord, and fetal membranes) or subinvolution (local endometritis) of the former placental site.

Acute Hemorrhage. After the placenta separates from the maternal decidua spongiosa, uterine bleeding is initially controlled by uterine contraction and compression of blood vessels at the site of

TABLE 31-2. Predisposing factors for postpartum complications

COMPLICATION	PREDISPOSING FACTORS	COMPLICATION	PREDISPOSING FACTORS
Postpartum hemorrhage	Delayed contraction if the uterus (1) emptied very rapidly; (2) has been overdistended (large infant, multiple gestation, or hydramnios), stretching muscle fibers excessively; (3) does not contract normally because the patient received deep inhalation anesthesia; (4) was manipulated or massaged in an attempt to expel the placenta before it was completely separated; (5) retains a large fragment or a succenturiate lobe of the placenta; and when there is a history of postpartum bleeding of unknown cause in a multipara[35]		(10) lacerations resulting from spontaneous or operative vaginal delivery; (11) manual removal of the placenta; (12) cesarian section; (13) retention of secundines[23,33,35]
		Puerperal ovarian vein thrombophlebitis	(1) Metritis; (2) increased age or parity; (3) obesity; (4) history of thromboembolism; (5) administration of high-dose estrogen to suppress lactation; (6) heart disease; (7) anemia[20,22,32]
Postpartum infection	(1) Poor nutrition and hygiene; (2) prepartum and postpartum anemia; (3) vaginitis and/or cervicitis; (4) coitus late in pregnancy; (5) toxemia; (6) prolonged labor; (7) delayed rupture of membranes; (8) frequent internal examination during labor; (9) use of invasive (intrapartum) fetal and maternal monitoring devices;	Cesarean section infection	(1) Protracted operation time; (2) amniotic fluid bacterial contamination before surgery or other preexisting infection; (3) duration of labor; (4) number of vaginal examinations; (5) length of internal fetal monitoring; (6) estimated blood loss; (7) obesity; (8) surgery as a result of labor dystocia (difficult labor associated with either a large fetus or a small maternal pelvis[29,30])[11]

separation. The healing process produces lochia, a copious (dark red-brown) exudate, which is discharged through the vagina. Uterine atony is the failure of the uterus to contract following delivery. Treatment for acute postpartum hemorrhage due to uterine atony includes intravenous oxytocin, manual uterine massage, and keeping the patient in a supine position.[33]

Sonographically, there is no significant difference in the size or shape of the uterus of patients with uterine atony and of those with a normal postpartum uterus.[17,21] Consequently, the sonogram is representative of a normal postpartum uterus and no retained products of conception are identified, uterine atony is considered the most likely cause for the hemorrhage.[21] Acute postpartum hemorrhage can also result from torn blood vessels in soft tissue lacerations located in the cervix, vagina, or perineum or from hematomas located in the uterus or adnexa.[35] If bleeding continues after treatment, sonography can be utilized to investigate the cause of this prolonged hemorrhage.

Delayed Hemorrhage. Retention of secundines and subinvolution are the leading causes of delayed postpartum hemorrhage. Uterine subinvolution is a localized form of endometritis which contributes to continued delay in the normal regression of the uterus. The treatment and sonographic appearance are the same as for uterine atony.

With retained secundines, the uterine cavity remains expanded and bleeding continues at the pre-

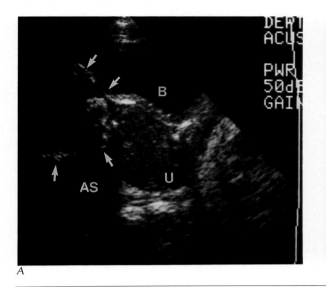
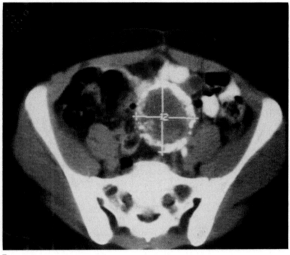

A *B*

FIGURE 31-4. (*A*) This longitudinal section demonstrates a large mass with peripheral calcification casting acoustic shadows (AS) present in the body and fundus (*arrows*) of the uterus of a patient 2 months after normal vaginal delivery. She had a clinical history of slight bleeding and spotting. The patient was referred for CT (U, uterus; B, bladder). (*B*) The CT scan disclosed the uterine mass to be retained placenta rather than a calcified fibroid. Surgery confirmed the diagnosis. (Courtesy Jim Baun, San Francisco, CA.)

vious placental attachment site. Retained products of conception produce variable sonographic appearances, depending on the type of tissue retained and its degree of necrosis at the time of the examination (Fig. 31-4).[17]

In cases of postpartum hemorrhage, sonography provides valuable information for narrowing the differential diagnoses. Even though sonographic appearances are not tissue specific, the sonographic examination can delineate normal and abnormal structures, determine the presence of a mass, its organ of origin, and its internal consistency. The sonographic appearance of lesions that can cause hemorrhage is listed in Table 31-3.

PUERPERAL INFECTION
Puerperal infection occurs in 6 to 8 mothers per 100,000 and accounts for approximately 20% of maternal deaths.[34] It is suspected when the patient experiences elevated body temperatures of 38°C

(100.4°F) or greater on any two of the first 10 postpartum days (not including the first day of fever).[34]

Predisposing Factors. Certain factors (Table 31-2) increase the risk of infection, but they do so inconsistently.[35]

Etiology. The vagina is the most common route of infection into the uterine cavity. The normal acidity of the vagina prevents many pathogens from proliferating within the uterus, but after the rupture of membranes and parturition, the amniotic fluid, blood, and lochia have a neutralizing effect and the vagina becomes alkaline, providing an environment conducive to growth of bacteria and other microorganisms.[34] Vaginal bacteria and microorganisms readily enter the uterine cavity and can develop into pathogens. Seventy percent of puerperal infections are caused by anaerobic bacteria, and the remaining 30 percent are caused by aerobic

Table 31-3 Sonographic appearance of postpartum complications

Complication	Sonographic Appearance
Hemorrhage due to:	
Retained products	Endometrial cavity echogenic and expanded with round, oval or lobulated intracavitary tissues; stippled echo pattern; may have hyperechoic foci, with or without associated acoustic shadowing; may have fluid within the uterine cavity
Local endometritis	Normal postpartum appearance except for size; uterus fails to return to normal postpartum size owing to imperfect involution
Uterine atony	Appearance of normal postpartum uterus with expanded and echogenic endometrial cavity
Endometritis	In advanced stages, separation of uterine cavity walls by anechoic space with smooth or irregular margins; may have echogenic shadows due to gas formation
Puerperal ovarian vein thrombophlebitis	Anechoic to hypoechoic round to oval mass in mid- to upper retroperitoneal cavity; Doppler shows limited blood flow
Bladder flap hematoma	Complex mass, poorly defined borders, primarily anechoic with internal septations or debris located at junction of uterus and bladder measuring 2.5 to 15 cm
Cesarean section hematoma	Anechoic to hypoechoic, smooth or irregular masses in the incision site areas
Cesarean section abscess	Echogenic, smooth or irregular masses; may have hyperechoic areas with shadowing, indicating gas formation

microorganisms. The devitalized intrauterine tissues, especially the thrombosed uteroplacental vessels, provide a congenial culture site that can result in the spread of infections outside the uterus such as parametritis, septic pelvic thrombophlebitis, femoral thrombophlebitis, peritonitis, and pulmonary infarct or abscess (septic embolus).[24,34]

In most cases, treatment for puerperal infections involves antibiotic therapy. Clinically, it is difficult to distinguish between urinary tract infections and endometritis because the blood cultures are usually negative.[21] In the event of further complications resulting from the puerperal infection, a curettage procedure is performed. If no improvement is observed with curettage following antibiotic treatment, the findings suggest myometrial infectious necrosis (gangrene), and a hysterectomy may be performed.[34]

Endometritis. Following delivery, endometritis develops in 3 to 4% of all women and in 13 to 27% of those who are delivered by cesarean.[34] Endometritis results from retention of secundines or from vaginal microorganisms contaminating the uterine cavity with a mixed flora of both anaerobic and aerobic pathogens.[21,34]

The sonographic representation of retained secundines and endometritis can overlap.[21] In mild to moderate intrauterine infections, endometritis is not detectable sonographically. In the advanced stages, sonographic examination should demonstrate separation of the uterine cavity walls if inflammation and exudation are present.[18] The endometrial cavity can be separated by an anechoic space that has either smooth or irregular margins (Fig. 31-5).[3] Without clinical evidence of endometritis, the normal postpartum uterus can also present with an anechoic separation representing blood or serous fluid in the endometrial cavity.[3] When presented with endometrial separation, the sonographer can make a substantial contribution to the diagnostic process by knowing the normal range of postpartum endometrial cavity measurements (see Table 31-1).

Prior to any surgical manipulations, the presence of gas in the endometrial cavity of a patient suspected of puerperal infections is most commonly caused by gas-forming microorganisms. The sonographic examination to rule out endometritis should be performed prior to curettage, as air can be introduced into the uterine cavity during surgical manipulation.[21] Air produces echogenic streaks on ultrasound (see Table 31-3).

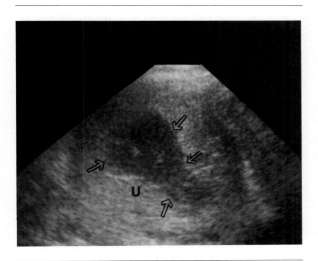

FIGURE 31-5. The uterine cavity (U) is filled with an irregular collection of fluid (M), measuring approximately 3 cm in diameter by approximately 7 cm in length (*arrows*), and echogenic material. This mass represents either blood or pus. (Courtesy Susan Olson, Salt Lake City, UT.)

OVARIAN VEIN THROMBOPHLEBITIS

Thrombophlebitis is inflammation of a vein secondary to formation of a thrombus.[30] Puerperal ovarian vein thrombophlebitis (POVT) is an uncommon complication of the puerperium. The prevalence is 0.2% for vaginal deliveries and 1 to 2% following cesarean section.[7,26]

Etiology and Predisposing Factors. The pathogenesis of POVT is related to Virchow's triad: (1) the natural hypercoagulability of blood during pregnancy and the puerperium; (2) venous stasis of blood; and (3) alterations in the vein walls.[21,23,27,33] The incidence in patients delivered by cesarean is probably increased because they are immobilized longer and the risk of thrombus is thus greater.[33] POVT is a significant life-threatening postpartum sequela to metritis.[1,7,23,26,29,33,35,36] Before the onset of POVT symptoms, uterine infection and anaerobic streptococci are present or are suspected in most cases.[21,23,33,35]

Thrombus formation can be secondary to injury during delivery or to bacterial inflammation and bacterial toxins to the endothelium of the blood vessels in the pelvis, vagina, perineum, and superficial muscle of the legs. Other predisposing factors are listed in Table 31-2.

The ovarian veins are predominantly involved in puerperal pelvic thrombophlebitis, but the disease process can extend into or be isolated to the pelvic and femoral veins.[1] The right ovarian vein is involved more often than the left, probably because of compression from the normal uterine dextrorotation during pregnancy and early postpartum.[7,23,27]

Symptoms. The POVT syndrome is difficult to diagnose clinically because findings are consistent in only about half of the patients.[7,23] The most remarkable and dependable physical finding is a palpable lower abdominal mass. Unilateral lower abdominal pain, tenderness, fever, and an elevated pulse rate related to the fever are the most frequent symptoms.[23,35] Nausea, vomiting, and ileus are less common.[23] These symptoms are usually experienced within the first few days after delivery, and the pain can radiate to the groin, flank, or the costophrenic angle.[35]

Diagnosis. Sectional plane imaging contributes significantly to the diagnosis of POVT. Prior to the availability of sonography, computed tomography (CT), and magnetic resonance imaging (MRI), POVT was diagnosed indirectly by intravenous pyelography (IVP) or venography.

It has been recommended that CT be the method of choice because of its sensitivity and specificity for the diagnosis of POVT (Fig. 31-6).[26,27,29] Factors that need to be considered in determining the benefits of the CT examinations should include the cost effectiveness of the examination as the initial evaluation of a febrile postpartum woman, the use of radiation on women with childbearing potential, and the sensitivity of some patients to the contrast material that is used to enhance the vascular structures.[26,27,29]

With current and future equipment improvements, sonographic evaluation has great potential for becoming the imaging modality of choice.[23] On sonography a thrombosed ovarian vein would have

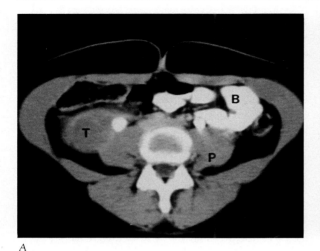
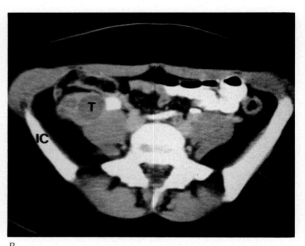

A

B

FIGURE 31-6. (A) A CT scan demonstrates an extremely dilated, thrombosed (T) right ovarian vein. The tortuous right ovarian vein has a maximum diameter of 2.8 cm and was seen to be thrombosed throughout its distance (approximately 4 cm) from the right ovary to its entrance into the inferior vena cava (B, bowel; P, psoas muscle). (B) On the same patient, a CT scan more superior demonstrates the extension of the thrombus (T); (IC, iliac crest). (Courtesy Sandra Bringhurst, Centerville, UT.)

an appearance of an anechoic to hypoechoic, round to oval mass in the middle to upper retroperitoneal cavity (Table 31-3).[27] The scanning technique must include an effort to demonstrate the phlebitic vein from the adnexal area to the suprarenal inferior vena cava.[26,27] The examination can be limited in the presence of ileus.

Doppler evaluation of deep abdominal vessels documents vessel flow and can be used adjunctively to make the diagnosis and to follow flow restoration after treatment.[27]

At present, MRI is used as an adjunct to sonography or CT. MRI in the coronal plane demonstrates the full extent of ovarian vein involvement.[27]

Sonographically, the differential diagnoses can include appendicitis, ovarian torsion, tubo-ovarian abscess, pelvic abscess, broad ligament hematoma, and volvulus of the bowel.[21,26,27,29,36]

Treatment. Currently, a conservative approach is employed in the treatment of POVT. The patient

is given antibiotics and anticoagulation therapy. Surgical intervention is associated with significant mortality and is indicated in some cases after failure of conservative therapy.[36] One third of patients with POVT develop septic pulmonary emboli.[7]

EVALUATION OF CESAREAN SECTION INCISIONS

In many high-risk centers in the United States, 15 to 20% of deliveries are by cesarean section.[5,20] In an effort to reduce this number and allow patients to deliver vaginally in the future, the lower–uterine segment transverse incision is commonly used.[4,20] The sonographic appearance of the incision is variable and is related to local tissue reaction and to the type of suture material utilized.[5,8,21] Interposed between the lower uterine segment and the posterior urinary bladder wall, it is normal to see (1) a symmetric region of distinct echogenicity generated by the suture material; (2) medium-intensity echoes, relative to the myometrium, surrounding the suture material; (3) anechoic areas anterior to the wound between the uterus and

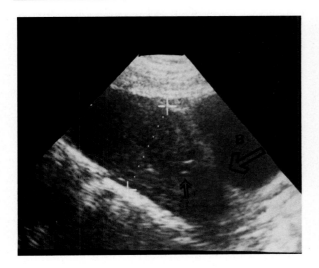

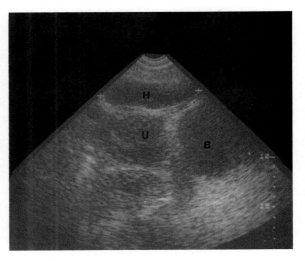

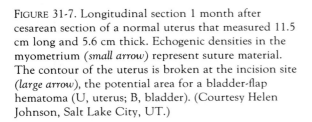

FIGURE 31-7. Longitudinal section 1 month after cesarean section of a normal uterus that measured 11.5 cm long and 5.6 cm thick. Echogenic densities in the myometrium (*small arrow*) represent suture material. The contour of the uterus is broken at the incision site (*large arrow*), the potential area for a bladder-flap hematoma (U, uterus; B, bladder). (Courtesy Helen Johnson, Salt Lake City, UT.)

FIGURE 31-8. A mass (H) measuring 9.7 × 3.5 cm is identified on this patient 4 days after cesarean and is most consistent with a bladder-flap hematoma. Uterine measurements were within the normal postpartum range (U, uterus; B, bladder). (Courtesy sonographers, Kings County Hospital, Brooklyn, NY.)

bladder; and (4) anechoic areas both at the wound site and anterior to it.[3,5,21]

Hematomas. During a cesarian section, the surgeon incises the vesicouterine reflection of the peritoneum to obtain access to the lower uterine segment. This creates a potential space between the bladder and uterus, commonly described as the bladder flap (Fig. 31-7).[37] If hemostasis is not obtained after closure of the uterine incision, a hematoma forms between the lower uterine segment and the urinary bladder[4] or at the abdominal incision site.

A patient with a bladder flap hematoma can present with an elevated temperature, a mass, or dropping hematocrit. An infected hematoma can manifest itself with the same symptoms, but the patient can additionally have leukocytosis and more pain. The elevated temperature can be caused by postsurgical complications such as endometritis, septic thrombophlebitis, abscess, hematoma, or wound infection.[37]

The incidence of bladder flap hematoma is unknown and the sonographic appearance described in the literature varies from a mass 2.5 cm in diameter to a mass measuring 15 × 12 × 9 cm (length × width × height) (Fig. 31-8).[4,37] The majority of the bladder flap hematomas identified show a complex mass with poorly defined borders that are primarily anechoic with internal septations or debris (Table 31-3).[37]

Since it is not possible to differentiate sonographically between a hematoma, an infected hematoma, and an abscess, the patient's clinical presentation is important.[4,21,37] A symptomatic patient with symptoms and a clinical history of leukocytosis suggests an abscess; a dropping hematocrit, a hematoma; and a dropping hematocrit with leukocytosis, an infected hematoma. Figure 31-9 and Figure 31-10 demonstrate the importance of obtaining laboratory values and of having the patient's clinical history.

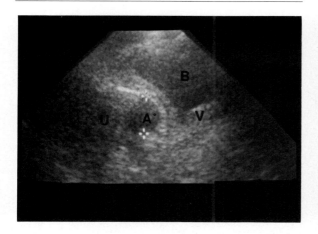

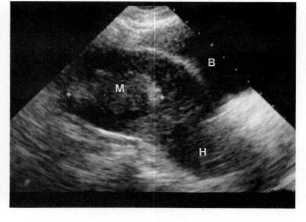

FIGURE 31-9. Between the uterus (U) and the urinary bladder (B) is an anechoic mass, which could represent a local abscess (A) if correlated with a patient finding of leukocytosis. Without having the patient's laboratory values, a hematoma cannot be excluded entirely and would be included in the differential diagnosis. (V, vagina). (Courtesy Susan Olson, Salt Lake City, UT.)

FIGURE 31-10. The uterus (U) is slightly prominent, compatible with the patient's clinical history of cesarean section, and measures 10.8 cm long, 4.6 cm AP thickness, and 5.8 cm transversely. The endometrial cavity is markedly hyperechoic, expanded, and occupied by a lobulated mass (M) seen with endometritis, infected or noninfected hematoma, or even retained secundines. A small amount of fluid in the pelvis surrounds the uterus. A large solid mass is seen posterior, probably representing intrapelvic hematomas (H), but an infected hematoma may appear similar (B, bladder). Correlating these findings to the patient's laboratory values aids in the differential diagnosis of a hematoma (dropping hematocrit) or an infected hematoma (dropping hematocrit with leukocytosis). (Courtesy Susan Olson, Salt Lake City, UT.)

Wound Infections. Approximately 5% of patients develop a wound infection after cesarean section.[11] Factors that contribute to wound infection are included in Table 31-2.

Hypoechoic masses in the area of the incision in afebrile patients probably represent small seromas or hematomas that develop as a normal surgical complication (Fig. 31-11).[21] In febrile patients, fluid collections suggest abscess, especially if strong echoes with associated acoustic shadowing are seen. These are indicative of an abscess with gas formation (Table 31-3).[21]

Wound infection can develop in the uterine incision and in the abdominal wall incision from the same vaginal microorganisms that cause infected endometritis.[11] Abdominal wall disorders can be difficult to detect clinically because of tenderness and induration due to edema.[21] At various stages, seromas, hematomas, and abscesses can have a similar sonographic appearance.

Conclusion

A noninvasive ultrasound examination during the postpartum period can be indicated for a number of reasons. Even though the sonographic findings are not tissue specific, correlating these findings with the patient's clinical history and laboratory values greatly assists in the diagnostic process and makes a substantive contribution to the management of postpartum complications.

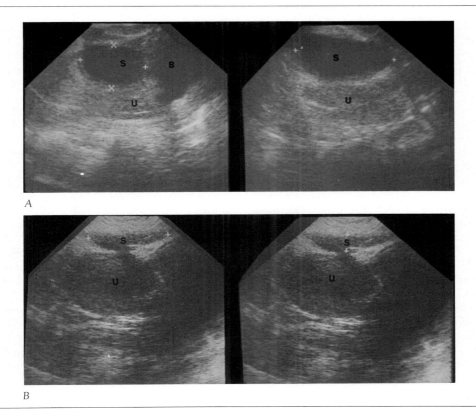

FIGURE 31-11. (*A*) The longitudinal (*left*) and transverse (*right*) sections on a 21-year-old cesarean patient with a clinical history of fever and anemia demonstrates an anechoic mass representing a bladder-flap seroma (S) measuring 5.6 cm long, 3.9 cm thick, and 8.7 cm wide. Aspiration was performed on both the seroma and on a subfascial (abdominal wall) wound abscess (U, uterus; B, bladder). (*B*) The sonographic findings in the same patient at an 18-day follow-up examination demonstrates that the seroma (S) is a more heterogenous collection and measures 6.6 cm long (left) and 1.5 cm thick (right). (Courtesy sonographers, Kings County Hospital, Brooklyn, NY.)

References

1. Allan TR, Miller GC, Wabrek AJ, et al. Postpartum and postabortal ovarian vein thrombophlebitis. Obstet Gynecol. 1976; 47:525–528.
2. Anthony CP, Thibodeau GA. Textbook of Anatomy and Physiology. 10th ed. St. Louis: CV Mosby; 1979.
3. Athey PA. Uterus: Abnormalities of the endometrial cavity. In: Athey PA, Hadlock FP, eds. Ultrasound in Obstetrics and Gynecology. 2nd ed. St. Louis: CV Mosby; 1985.
4. Baker ME, Bowie JD, Killam AP. Sonography of post-cesarean-section bladder-flap hematoma. AJR. 1985; 144:757–759.
5. Baker ME, Kay H, Mahony BS, et al. Sonography of the low transverse incision, cesarean section: A prospective study. J Ultrasound Med. 1988; 7:389–393.
6. Bowie JD. Sonography of the uterus. In: Sabbagha RD, ed. Diagnostic Ultrasound: Applied to Obstetrics and Gynecology. 2nd ed. Philadelphia: JB Lippincott; 1987.
7. Brown TK, Munsick RA. Puerperal ovarian vein

thrombophlebitis: A syndrome. Am J Obstet Gynecol. 1971; 109:263–273.

8. Burger NF, Darazs B, Boes EGM. An echographic evaluation during the early puerperium of the uterine wound after cesarean section. J Clin Ultrasound. 1982; 10:271–274.

9. Cooperberg PL, Kidney MR. Ultrasound evaluation of the uterus. In: Callen PW, ed. Ultrasonography in Obstetrics and Gynecology. 2nd ed. Philadelphia: WB Saunders; 1988.

10. Defoort P, Benijts G, Thiery M, et al. Ultrasound assessment of puerperal uterine involution. Eur J Obstet Gynecol Reprod Biol. 1978; 8:95–97.

11. Emmons SL, Krohn M, Jackson M, et al. Development of wound infections among women undergoing cesarean section. Obstet Gynecol. 1988; 72:559–564.

12. Fleischer AC. Gynecologic sonography. In: Fleischer AC, James AE, eds. Diagnostic Sonography: Principles and Clinical Applications. Philadelphia: WB Saunders; 1989.

13. Guyton AC. Textbook of Medical Physiology. 6th ed. Philadelphia: WB Saunders; 1981.

14. Henry G. Gray's Anatomy of the Human Body. 29th ed. (American edition, Edited by Charles Mayo Goss.) Philadelphia: Lea & Febiger; 1973.

15. Land JA, Stoot JE, Evers JL. Puerperal ultrasonic hysterography. Gynecol Obstet Invest. 1984; 18:165–168.

16. Lavery JP, Shaw LA. Sonography of the puerperal uterus. J Ultrasound Med. 1989; 8:481–486.

17. Lee CY, Madrazo B, Drukker BH. Ultrasound evaluation of the postpartum uterus in the management of postpartum bleeding. Obstet Gynecol. 1981; 58:227–232.

18. Lee CY, Madrazo BL, Parks S, et al. Ultrasonic evaluation in the management of postpartum infection. Henry Ford Hosp Med J. 1987; 35:58–62.

19. Leopold GR. Pelvic ultrasonography. In: Sarti DA, ed. Diagnostic Ultrasound: Text and Cases. 2nd ed. Chicago: Year Book Medical Publishers; 1987.

20. Lonky NM, Worthen N, Ross MG. Prediction of cesarean section scars with ultrasound imaging during pregnancy. J Ultrasound Med. 1989; 8:15–19.

21. Madrazo B. Postpartum sonography. In: Saunders RC, James AE, eds. The Principles and Practice of Ultrasonography in Obstetrics and Gynecology. 3rd ed. Norwalk, CT: Appleton-Century-Crofts; 1985.

22. Marieb EN. Human Anatomy and Physiology. Redwood City, CA: The Benjamin/Cummings Publishing Company; 1989.

23. Munsick RA, Gillanders LA. A review of the syndrome of puerperal ovarian vein thrombophlebitis. Obstet Gynecol Survey. 1981; 36:57–66.

24. Netter FH. The Reproductive System. The CIBA Collection of Medical Illustrations. Rochester: The Case-Hoyt Corporation; 1978; 2.

25. Rodeck CH, Newton JR. Study of the uterine cavity by ultrasound in the early puerperium. Br J Obstet Gynaecol. 1976; 83:795–801.

26. Rudoff JM, Astrauskas LJ, Rudoff JC, et al. Ultrasonographic diagnosis of septic pelvic thrombophlebitis. J Ultrasound Med. 1988; 7:287–291.

27. Savader SJ, Otero PR, Savader BL. Puerperal ovarian vein thrombosis: Evaluation with CT, US, and MR imaging. Radiology. 1988; 167:637–639.

28. Seeley RR, Stephens TD, Tate P. Anatomy and Physiology. St. Louis: Mosby College Publishing; 1989.

29. Shaffer PB, Johnson JC, Bryan D, et al. Diagnosis of ovarian vein thrombophlebitis of the ovarian vein. J Comput Assist Tomogr. 1981; 4:436–439.

30. Thomas CL, ed. Taber's Cyclopedic Medical Dictionary. 15th ed. Philadelphia: FA Davis; 1985.

31. Tortora GJ, Anagnastakos NP. Principles of Anatomy and Physiology. 5th ed. New York: Harper and Row; 1987.

32. VanRees D, Bernstine RL, Crawford W. Involution of the postpartum uterus: An ultrasonic study. J Clin Ultrasound. 1981; 9:55–57.

33. Vorherr H. Puerperium: Maternal involutional changes—management of puerperal problems and complications. In: Sciarra JJ, ed. Gynecology and Obstetrics. Philadelphia: Harper and Row; 1982.

34. Vorherr H. Puerperium: Puerperal genitourinary infection. In: Sciarra JJ, ed. Gynecology and Obstetrics. Philadelphia: Harper and Row; 1982.

35. Willson JR, Carrington ER. Obstetrics and Gynecology. 7th ed. St. Louis: CV Mobsy; 1983.

36. Wilson PC, Lerner RM. Diagnosis of ovarian vein thrombophlebitis by ultrasonography. J Ultrasound Med. 1983; 2:187–190.

37. Winsett MZ, Fagan CJ, Bedi DG. Sonographic demonstration of bladder-flap hematoma. J Ultrasound Med. 1986; 5:483–487.

CHAPTER 32

Amniocentesis and Chorionic Villus Sampling

GEORGE I. SOLISH

Amniocentesis and chorionic villus sampling (CVS) are but two of several clinical techniques designed to obtain living fetal cells or fetal cell products from the pregnant uterus for prenatal diagnosis that rely heavily on high-resolution diagnostic ultrasound. Percutaneous umbilical vein sampling (PUBS) or cordocentesis[11] and fetoscopy,[18] for example, are similar techniques designed for the same purpose, but they are reserved for more special indications and carry a higher procedure-related risk than amniocentesis and CVS.

The revolution in biotechnology in both the diagnosis and management of an increasing number of genetic disorders, procedures that use amniocentesis and CVS, has brought these techniques more prominently into the realm of everyday practice. Because these new modalities are invasive procedures they carry a certain risk. It is important that the patient be made aware of all possible complications, the risks as well as the benefits, and the limitations as well as the indications. This information is communicated to the patient in genetic counseling sessions.

Genetic counseling has been described as a communication process concerning the occurrence and the risks of recurrence of genetic disorders within a family.[27] In fact it is more than this. The genetic counselor also has the responsibility of providing a person or family with the most recent relevant information regarding a genetic disorder, the risks involved in diagnosis, and available treatment options.[32,33]

Manipulations that involve the pregnant uterus and the developing fetus within are always highly charged emotional issues with moral and ethical overtones that must be addressed in dealing with patients today. Patients ask legitimate questions, and to meet present day standards of care in prenatal diagnosis, as in general medical care, these questions must be appropriately answered. A team approach is useful; generally this involves not only the obstetrician but a genetic counselor, a sonographer, and surgical and medical specialists. Professional opinions are very often needed to help the patient in the decision-making process and to provide the necessary treatment, based on the results of diagnostic procedures. In most medical centers when genetic diseases are involved, the responsibility of overseeing the referrals for these services is assumed by the genetic counselor and the medical genetics center.

Amniocentesis

Amniocentesis, derived from the Greek, means puncture of the amniotic sac. The amnion and the chorion are the two major membranous structures surrounding and protecting the developing fetus within the uterus throughout pregnancy. The amniotic and chorionic sacs develop from the same fertilized ovum as does the fetus, serve their function during pregnancy, and are then discarded with expulsion of the placenta after the birth of the child.

History

The technique of amniocentesis was first described in the last century by Lambl (1881)[23] and by Schatz (1882)[34] as a method of relieving the intrauterine pressure resulting from abnormal accumulation of amniotic fluid, which in turn was due to interference with the normal amniotic fluid circulation. Parvey (1933),[28] who was one of the first to report successful management of acute hydramnios treated by abdominal puncture in this country, credits Bumm with having actually attempted this procedure in 1900. The same theoretic objections to the blind insertion of a needle into the pregnant uterus were voiced by prominent physicians of that day as were raised by modern-day critics. Objections included possible injury to the fetus, damage to the placenta, uterine hemorrhage, infection, and interruption of the pregnancy. These objections were apparently sufficient to discourage further progress until Bevis (1950)[4] showed that certain characteristics of amniotic fluid had diagnostic and prognostic value for hemolytic disease of the newborn. Walker (1957)[38] and later Liley (1961)[24] were able to demonstrate the relative safety of the procedure by performing serial amnioceneses on one patient without incident.

Originally, prenatal diagnostic amniocentesis was recommended for patients who were at risk for congenital malformations because of advanced maternal age or a child with a specific birth defect. However, the President's Commission for Study of Ethical Problems in Medicine and Biomedical and Behavioral Science, convened in 1983,[30] recommended that the criteria for eligibility for genetic amniocentesis be reexamined so that this procedure could be offered more equitably to pregnant women of all ages.

The increasing diagnostic accuracy, the decreasing risk of complications, and publicity on television and in other mass media have increased the acceptability of amniocentesis among most populations of the world. The risk of complications has been variously reported to be 0.5% and higher; in many centers where this procedure is performed regularly and by well-trained personnel, the actual procedure-related complication rate seems to be less than 3 per 1000 examinations.

The number of requests for amniocentesis and for CVS can be expected to escalate significantly in the next few years, with the advent of newer DNA technology and the identification of an increasing number of genetic defects by these molecular biologic techniques. Both procedures use sonographic guidance to obtain fetal DNA.

Indications for Genetic Amniocentesis

The most frequent requests for genetic amniocentesis come from women 35 years or older, because of the maternal age-related increase in the risk of fetal Down's syndrome. This category accounts for about 65% of requests in some studies[10] and as many as 80% in others.[15]

The next largest category is usually women with abnormal screening results for maternal serum α-fetoprotein (msAFP) level, either too high[25] or too low,[26] and those whose previous infants were born with neural tube defects. An association between abnormally high levels of this protein and neural tube defects was first described by Leek and colleagues.[25]

AFP is a serum protein found normally in the fetal circulatory system and produced by the fetal liver. If the circulation of amniotic fluid is obstructed, protein accumulates in the amniotic fluid and subsequently appears in the mother's serum. AFP is also elevated in serum of mothers carrying a multiple pregnancy, a dead fetus, or a fetus with any of a number of other abnormal conditions.[27] The msAFP levels in blood and in amniotic fluid (afAFP) differ at different weeks of gestation. The level of AFP must therefore be evaluated in relation to the normal level for a particular gestational age. An msAFP value in excess of 2.5 times the mean for that gestational age is generally considered to be suspect. The usual protocol followed in the screening procedure is to repeat the AFP test if the first result is elevated. A second positive result is followed by an ultrasound examination to confirm gestational age and to determine whether multiple pregnancies or other ultrasound-detectable factors are responsible for the apparently elevated AFP value. Failure to correctly determine the gestational age may lead to incorrect interpretation of

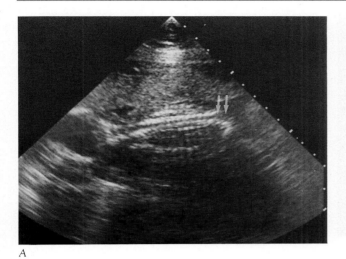

A

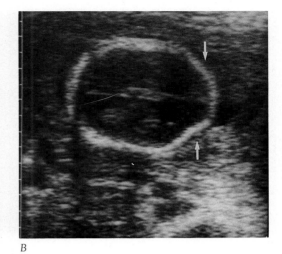

B

FIGURE 32-1. A pregnant 36-year-old woman had a routine amniocentesis for prenatal diagnosis because of advanced maternal age. A markedly elevated level of α-fetoprotein in the amniotic fluid led to reexamination of the fetus in utero, which disclosed (A) splaying of the distal sacral vertebral column (*arrows*); (B) a positive "lemon" sign of the fetal skull (*arrows*). (C) These findings were the basis for the termination of this pregnancy. Spina bifida was seen after abortion.

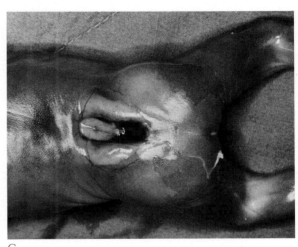

C

the AFP results. At this point careful ultrasound examination in most instances detects the presence of a neural tube defect or other anatomical cause of the AFP elevation (Figs. 32-1, 32-2).

An abnormally low msAFP (i.e., 0.4 times the mean value for that gestational age) is used to screen for fetuses at risk of having chromosomal trisomy. These AFP problems account for 10 to 15% of the total requests for amniocentesis.

A varying but steadily growing number of well-informed patients who are in no specific risk cate-gory but are overly concerned about the possibility of abnormal pregnancy outcome are asking to be tested. Maternal anxiety has therefore become a recognized indication for prenatal genetic diagno-sis regardless of maternal age. Some may be seeking relief from a variety of feelings and anxieties re-garding pregnancy outcome that arise from their social, moral, and ethical behavior (e.g., drug abuse, out-of-wedlock pregnancy, mixed ethnic un-ions).

Amniocentesis is also advisable for mothers who

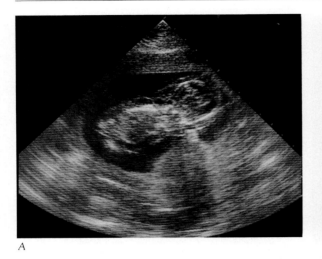
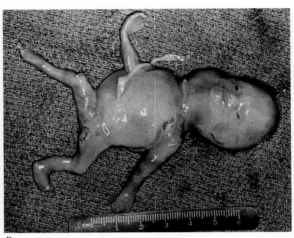

A   *B*

FIGURE 32-2. A cystic hygroma identified on sonographic examination (*A*) prior to amniocentesis was confirmed after abortion (*B*). The chromosomes and α-fetoprotein value were normal.

have borne children with chromosomal defects or metabolic disorders. More than 100 metabolic disorders are now detectable biochemically in the prenatal period. The chance of recurrence of a genetic condition depends on its inheritance pattern. The risk may range from less than 1% in the case of a previous child with a chromosomal defect not found in the parents, to 25% in the case of an autosomal-recessive biochemical defect such as Tay-Sachs disease, to 50% (for males) in sex-linked muscular dystrophy.

Timing of Amniocentesis

Amniocentesis is usually performed between the 16th and 18th gestational weeks. The fluid volume is adequate at this time for obtaining a good sample with minimal threat to the fetus, and the ratio of viable to nonviable cells is optimal. Furthermore, sonographic visualization at this gestational age defines more of the fetal anatomy than it could have earlier and therefore permits easier detection of abnormalities.

Prenatal diagnosis attempts to obtain results as early in pregnancy as possible, but to date, the safety of the procedure earlier than 14 to 15 weeks has not been clearly established. The deadline for performing amniocentesis is frequently related to individual state legal restrictions for pregnancy termination rather than to other factors. Amniocentesis for determining fetal maturity (by the ratio of lecithin to sphingomyelin {LS ratio}) and severity of erythroblastosis (by optical density measurements of the amniotic fluid) are safely performed much later in pregnancy.

The legal limit for elective termination of pregnancy in New York State is 24 weeks; in other states it may be 20 weeks. The timing of genetic amniocentesis must therefore allow for completion of all laboratory testing so that the option of pregnancy termination is not denied to those who might choose this alternative. The average waiting period for results of chromosome studies is 7 to 14 days, although in some instances because of slow cell growth it may require 3 weeks for a result.

Many institutions have appointed ethics committees composed of laymen, clergy, and nonmedical and medical professionals. These committees evaluate individual cases and make recommendations regarding such critical issues as terminating a pregnancy with a severely malformed fetus after

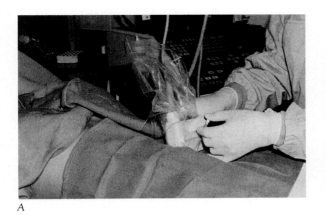
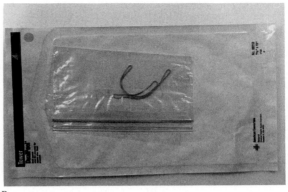

A   *B*

FIGURE 32-3. (A) Insertion of amniocentesis needle under direct ultrasonic visualization. The abdomen has been prepared and draped with sterile towels. The ultrasound transducer is encased in a sterile plastic bag. (B) Plastic bag is gas sterilized along with rubber bands for covering ultrasound scanner for amniocentesis.

the legal 24-week limit has passed. In some institutions anencephalic fetuses have been aborted after 28 weeks of pregnancy.[9]

PROCEDURE FOR ULTRASOUND-GUIDED AMNIOCENTESIS

Following genetic counseling and completion of the informed consent process, which usually occurs days or weeks prior to the procedure, an appointment is made for simultaneous ultrasound and amniocentesis. Amniocentesis is an outpatient procedure and is performed in the ultrasound laboratory in accordance with the guidelines of the American Institute of Ultrasound in Medicine.[1]

At our institution the following information was found useful and is therefore routinely obtained by the sonographer prior to amniocentesis.

1. Pregnancy, number of fetuses, fetal position, and viability are confirmed.
2. Amniotic fluid volume is estimated as normal, decreased, or increased.
3. Placental location is recorded.
4. Gestational age is determined using the following measurements: biparietal diameter, femur length, humoral length, abdominal circumference, head circumference, and binocular distance.
5. The following anatomic structures are identified and recorded: lateral horns of the cerebral ventricles, fetal heart (four-chamber view), stomach, urinary bladder, umbilical cord insertion, kidneys.
6. The optimal fluid pocket for amniocentesis is determined.
7. Fetal heart rate is estimated and recorded before and after the procedure.

Amniocentesis Technique. The abdominal surface is prepared with povidone iodine solution, after the gel used for ultrasound examination is removed. Strict sterile precautions are observed—sterile drapes, handwashing, sterile gloves, and instruments. Because some of the complications following amniocentesis have been related to infection,[14] it seems prudent therefore that all possible precautions to avoid this complication be observed (Figs. 32-3, 32-4).

The ultrasound transducer is coated with regular transmission gel and held by an assistant as the

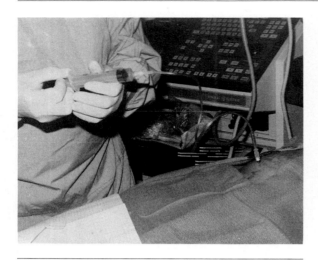

Figure 32-4. The amniotic fluid specimen is withdrawn under sterile conditions by means of a sterile plastic catheter attached at one end to the amniocentesis needle and to a 20-ml syringe at the other.

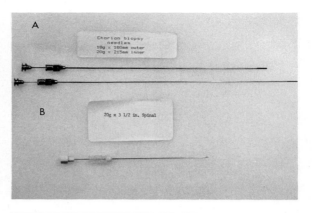

Figure 32-5. (A) Double needle set with stylets for transabdominal CVS. The larger-bore needle is inserted first through the abdominal wall to just proximal to the target site. The stylet is withdrawn and the second smaller (20-gauge) needle is inserted through the first one to the site of sampling and the specimen obtained as described in the text. (B) Spinal needle with stylet partially withdrawn. This needle can be used for both amniocentesis and for transabdominal CVS.

physician covers the transducer with a sterile plastic bag obtained from the local supermarket and individually gas-sterilized (Fig. 32-3).[12] The plastic bag over the functional surface of the transducer is, in turn, coated with sterile gel. Under sonographic visualization a 3½-inch, 20-gauge, sterile, disposable, spinal needle with a stylet is used to enter the amniotic sac (Figs. 32-3, 32-5). Progress of the needle through the tissue layers is followed easily on the ultrasound screen. With a little practice, ultrasound monitoring and amniocentesis can be performed simultaneously by one operator. It must be remembered, however, that the ultrasound image of the needle direction is distorted somewhat when both procedures are performed simultaneously.[36] The beveled tip of the needle is seen as a bright spot on the ultrasound screen, described as a "flare" by Simpson and Elias. (Fig. 32-6).[36] The amniocentesis site is thus documented on film.

The stylet is removed and the first 1 or 2 ml of fluid is discarded, to avoid contaminating the specimen with the mother's cells.[2,3] A 20-inch length of sterile, flexible, extension tubing is attached to the Luer-lok needle hub, the other end of which has a sterile, 20-ml syringe attached (see Fig. 32-4). From 20 to 40 ml of amniotic fluid is withdrawn and transferred to sterile, properly labelled, 15-ml conical tubes for transport to the laboratory. Following removal of the fluid sample, the needle is withdrawn. Although needle injuries to the fetus have been reported, using the above described technique none has been noted in our experience of 15 years.

The amniocentesis site is massaged gently for a few moments after the needle is removed, in an attempt to stimulate a normal uterine contraction, which would aid in obliterating the puncture site and prevent amniotic fluid seepage. The skin wound is covered with a bandaid to prevent adherence of clothing to the site. A final check of the fetal heart is made before the patient is discharged.

The amniocytes are separated from the amniotic fluid by centrifugation in the laboratory. The fluid is assayed for AFP or other biochemical substances, as indicated, and the cells are cultured for karyotyping.

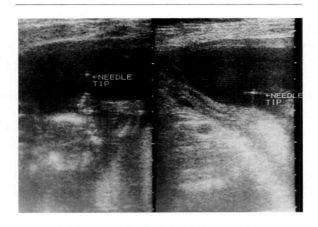

FIGURE 32-6. The beveled tip of the needle is easily identified in the amniotic sac as a "flare."

Multiple gestation. In the event of diamniotic twins, each sac is identified sonographically and labelled according to its position in the mother's abdomen. In most instances the amniotic membrane separating the diamniotic twin sacs can be recognized. This is helpful in the planning strategy for tapping each sac separately. Each fetus is scanned, measured, and treated as if it were a singleton.

After tapping the first sac (twin A), 20 to 25 ml of fluid is removed. Into a separate syringe prepared with 1 to 2 ml of indigo carmine dye, 5 to 10 ml of amniotic fluid is aspirated. The diluted dye then is instilled into sac A. The second sac is then similarly entered. Blue-stained fluid withdrawn from the second sac indicates either that a communication exists between the sacs, such as occurs in monoamniotic twins, or that the first sac was inadvertently reentered. Direct simultaneous visualization of the inserted needle's progress with ultrasound helps to avoid reentry. If triplets are encountered, the blue dye procedure is repeated after successful tapping of the second sac.

Chorionic Villus Sampling (CVS)

HISTORY

CVS is one of the more recently developed techniques for effectively and safely obtaining living trophoblastic tissue for genetic diagnosis in the first trimester of pregnancy. The tissue thus obtained can be tested for a rapidly increasing number of biochemical disorders of the fetus and for fetal chromosomal abnormalities. The trophoblast, one of the extraembryonic structures that develop from the fertilized egg, becomes the placenta as the pregnancy progresses.

Working in the preultrasound era the earliest investigators[16,22] passed a rigid endoscope called a hysteroscope through the uterine cervix to obtain trophoblastic tissue for analysis. A blind approach was used by the Chinese,[17] with a metal cannula without ultrasound monitoring, to aspirate tissue for sex determination.

Kazy and colleagues[21] were the first to use ultrasound to guide a flexible biopsy forceps into the uterus to obtain tissue under direct vision, but it is an Italian group[33] that deserves most of the credit for defining the risks and the benefits of the procedure and for demonstrating the value of CVS in biochemical fetal tissue diagnoses. Their results served to popularize the method and to stimulate others to further develop and expand it.

TRANSCERVICAL VERSUS TRANSABDOMINAL TECHNIQUE

Until recently the most universally accepted method of CVS was the transcervical technique introduced by Brambati and his coworkers.[5] This method uses a flexible plastic catheter with a malleable inner obturator that is inserted into the cervix *per vaginum,* guided by an abdominally placed transducer (Fig. 32-7). On the other hand, the transabdominal route first introduced by Smidt-Jensen and Hahnemann in 1984[37] is rapidly gaining acceptance owing to the reported decreased chance of procedure-related risk of infection and the greater success rate of obtaining specimens. The transabdominal approach has occasionally been successful when the transcervical approach failed, as for example, in the case of the anteriorly implanted placenta. Figure 32-8 shows the instruments used for transcervical CVS. Figure 32-5 shows two different types of needles used in the transabdominal method.

ADVANTAGES AND DISADVANTAGES

The desire for earlier diagnosis of fetal genetic disorders and inherited metabolic derangements in

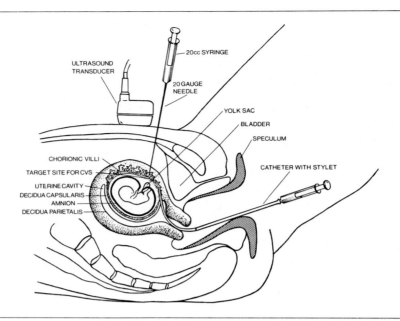

FIGURE 32-7. Diagram of the target area for CVS. (A) The vaginal approach uses a pliable plastic catheter. (B) The abdominal approach uses a spinal needle introduced transabdominally.

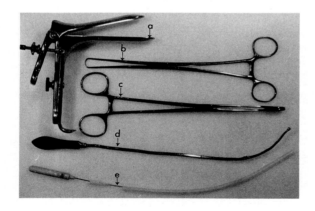

FIGURE 32-8. Instruments used in transvaginal chorionic villus sampling: (a) vaginal speculum, (b) tenaculum, (c) ring forceps, (d) uterine sound, (e) plastic catheter enclosed in plastic sleeve with the malleable obturator withdrawn slightly from the catheter.

pregnancy was, and continues to be, the impetus for further development of this mode of diagnosis. The attraction of the no-needle transcervical technique, the earlier diagnosis, and shorter waiting period for results (24 to 48 hours rather than the 2 or 3 weeks for amniocentesis) are especially appealing to patients. A diagnosis can therefore be forthcoming even before any body changes are detected by the patient or any deep psychological attachment to the growing fetus is established.

CVS is performed between the 8th and 12th weeks after the last menstrual period rather than at 15 to 18 weeks as with amniocentesis. Laboratory results are obtainable within 48 hours by the short-term culture method.[35] This is backed by the long-term culture method, which provides results in 4 to 7 days.[29]

The possibility of a diagnosis of a severely affected fetus before the 40th day of pregnancy makes termination a more acceptable option to some orthodox Jewish religious groups. CVS therefore may be more appropriate than amniocentesis for them.[13]

Balanced by these favorable aspects of CVS are some drawbacks:

Safety. There are still lingering doubts and uncertainties about the safety of the procedure. Until recently the fetal loss rate following CVS was 4%, compared to the 0.3 to 1.0% loss rate reported following amniocentesis.[19] More recent data from a compilation of the CVS registry data[20] indicate a significant reduction in fetal loss in centers with the largest experience, making the risk for this procedure comparable to that of amniocentesis.[39,40]

Reliability. The problem of discordance of chromosome results among cells obtained from the chorion, from the amniotic fluid, and from the newborn has yet to be resolved. A recent report by Callen and coworkers,[8] for example, noted a discordance of 22 karyotypes out of 1312 diagnostic CVSs, a 20-fold higher incidence than that reported for amniocentesis. Chorionic cells may not always be a true representation of the fetus.

Timing. The optimal time for CVS may be before the patient recognizes that she is pregnant and customarily seeks obstetric prenatal care. She may be ineligible for this procedure when she does in fact register for prenatal care. This is particularly likely to occur when the pregnancy is unplanned.

Bleeding. Vaginal bleeding following CVS has variously been reported to occur in 10 to 20% of patients. While generally this is of no serious import, it can be somewhat frightening to the patient.

Two additional recent developments should be mentioned. First, the transabdominal approach, which requires a needle of the same size as that used in amniocentesis, is rapidly gaining favor. This negates the appeal of "no needle." Second, studies of feasibility of amniocentesis earlier than 15 weeks have yielded promising results. If early amniocentesis becomes an established procedure, it would nicely fill the gap between CVS (performed at 8 to 12 weeks) and the current standard for amniocentesis (15 weeks or later) and would make prenatal diagnosis available before 15 weeks to late CVS registrants.

It is becoming abundantly clear that any center offering prenatal genetic testing will need to be able to provide all of the above accepted techniques so that individual situations can be accommodated.

PROCEDURE FOR ULTRASOUND-GUIDED SAMPLING

In all methods of prenatal fetal evaluation ultrasound visualization has become a *sine qua non* whether the prenatal procedure is for diagnostic or operative guidance purposes. More important than the equipment used is the training and experience of the sonographer, who must be able to work in consort with and in coordination with the operator obtaining the tissue sample. For CVS, the type of real-time equipment used does not seem to matter.[31] Scanning and sampling can be performed simultaneously by the same person, or one person can scan while the other obtains the tissue. A third alternative is for the obstetrician to scan while manipulating the cannula and then to hand the transducer to the sonographer, leaving both of the obstetrician's hands free to obtain the specimen.

Transcervical Technique. Like amniocentesis, CVS is considered to be an outpatient procedure performed in an ultrasound laboratory. The aim is to obtain a small sample of viable chorionic tissue without contamination with maternal cells and without injuring the pregnancy. The patient at risk for a genetic problem must be identified early in pregnancy, properly counseled, and scheduled for the procedure between the 8th and 11th gestational weeks.

A careful obstetric and gynecologic history should be taken before scheduling the patient for testing. Among the contraindications to CVS are active infection of the vagina or any part of the genital tract, the presence of an intrauterine device, and stenosis of the cervical os. The patient's bladder may be full or empty, depending on which affords a better view of the pelvic organs. A distended bladder at times can cause undesirable distortion of the uterine contents.

In the face of an abnormal appearance of the gestational sac on sonography or absence of fetal heart tones, the patient must be so informed before proceeding. Missed abortion or blighted ovum was found in as many as 15 to 20% of patients scanned between 6 and 8 weeks. For diagnostic purposes this would be a desirable time to obtain tissue samples anyway, but proper informed consent must be obtained before proceeding.

Ultrasound examination prior to CVS is essential, not only to confirm pregnancy and the presence of a viable fetus in the uterus but also to evaluate the gestational age, condition, and location of the placenta and to identify the intended biopsy site.

Vaginal and cervical smears are usually taken for culture to rule out *Neisseria gonorrhoeae* and other pathogens prior to preparing the vagina and cervix with povidone iodine solution. A vaginal speculum is inserted; the cervix is visualized and carefully grasped with a tenaculum. A uterine sound may be used to confirm the patency and the location of the internal os on the ultrasound screen (Fig. 32-8).

A variety of rigid instruments and an equal number of flexible catheters or cannulas are used by different operators. Whichever is used, its course into the uterus via the cervix is guided by ultrasound visualization. The thickest part of the placenta, the chorion frondosum, where the umbilical cord is attached, is the target area for obtaining samples (Figs. 32-7, 32-9). The crown-rump length is measured; the shape of the uterus and the direction of the uterine axis are then determined; and if a flexible catheter is used, its shape is adjusted to the shape of the uterus via the obturator, to match the direction it must traverse to reach the proposed biopsy site.

When the catheter tip has reached the proper site, the malleable aluminum obturator is removed. A 20-ml syringe, previously prepared and containing 3 to 5 ml of sterile culture medium and a small amount of heparin, is attached to the outer end of the catheter, and the specimen is obtained by aspiration, using negative pressure generated by withdrawing the barrel of the syringe either once, as recommended by some, or repeatedly, as recommended by others, as the catheter is slowly withdrawn. This is done under constant ultrasound visualization.

An average of 20 to 30 mg of tissue is obtained and transferred to a sterile Petri dish containing culture medium. The specimen is then washed and examined under a low-power dissecting microscope, to verify the presence of chorionic villi. The specimen is separated from possible maternal cell contamination with a dissecting needle under the

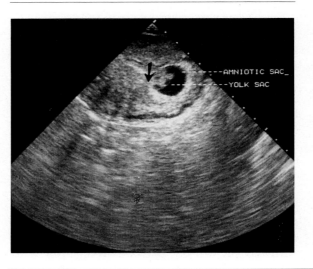

FIGURE 32-9. A vaginal ultrasound scan of the target area for CVS.

dissecting microscope. The washed chorionic tissue specimen is then taken to the tissue culture laboratory for processing.

Following the collection of the specimen the instruments are removed and the patient is reexamined sonographically before being released. The examiner looks for evidence of hematoma formation or other complications that may have occurred as a result of the procedure. Follow-up ultrasound examinations are often scheduled at intervals, a few days to a week later.

Transabdominal Technique. The transabdominal approach differs from the transcervical only in the anatomic access route and the instrument used to obtain the specimen (see Fig. 32-7). The preparation of the patient, the treatment place, and goals are the same in both approaches.

In this procedure the patient is in the supine rather than the lithotomy position. The placenta is identified and its thickness measured. The abdomen, at the elected site, is cleansed with povidone iodine solution. A 20-gauge, 3½-inch spinal needle with stylet, like that used with amniocentesis, is introduced into the placenta (see Fig. 32-5).

The transducer is held by the sonographer while the physician removes the stylet, attaches a 20-ml Luer-lok syringe containing 3 ml of Hanks culture medium mixed with a few drops of heparin, and collects the specimen. By intermittent vigorous withdrawal of the barrel of the syringe, negative pressure is created as the needle tip is slowly moved back and forth until a specimen of about 30 mg of tissue is obtained. The needle is then removed and the patient is treated as described above for amniocentesis and transcervical CVS. In both transcervical and transabdominal CVS the patient is informed that amniocentesis may be necessary if results are equivocal.

Conclusion

The rapid development that has marked the progress of these methods of detecting fetal abnormalities is noteworthy. Within a few short years these techniques have established a route of access to the developing fetus in utero that has already proved its value by the results obtained. Rapid acceptance by populations in all parts of the world has further affirmed their effectiveness and safety. In many countries of the world both amniocentesis and CVS have become standard medical practice. The rapid progress of these prenatal diagnostic methods is due in no small measure to the availability of high-resolution ultrasound. The machinery that has been developed for viewing the fetus in utero forms the essential element that has made all of this possible. Furthermore, ultrasound techniques have demonstrated a potential greater utility that promises to be even more valuable in the future for intrauterine fetal manipulation and treatment of a great number of developmental and genetic defects of the fetus.

References

1. American Institute of Ultrasound. Guidelines for Second- and Third-Trimester Sonography. AIUM. 1985; 2–5.
2. Benn PA, Hsu LYF: Maternal cell contamination of amniotic fluid cell cultures: Results of a U.S. nationwide survey. Am J Med Genet. 1983; 15:297.
3. Benn PA, Schonhaut AG, Hsu LYF. A high incidence of maternal cell contamination of amniotic fluid cell cultures. Am J Med Genet. 1983; 14:361.
4. Bevis DCA. Composition of liquor amnii in hemolytic disease of newborn. Lancet. 1950; 2:443.
5. Brambati B, Simoni G. Fetal diagnosis of trisomy 21 in the first trimester of pregnancy. Lancet. 1983; 1:586.
6. Brock DJ, Sutcliffe R. Alpha-fetoprotein in the diagnosis of anencephaly and spina bifida. Lancet. 1972; 2:197.
7. Brock DJ, et al. Significance of elevated mid-trimester maternal plasma alpha-fetoprotein values. Lancet. 1979; 1:1281.
8. Callen DF, Korban G, Dawson G, et al. Extraembryonic/fetal karyotypic discordance during diagnostic chorionic villus sampling. Prenatal Diagn. 1988; 8:453–460.
9. Chervenak FA, Farley MA, Walter L, et al. When is termination of pregnancy during third trimester morally justifiable? N Engl J Med. 1984; 310:501.
10. Dacus JV, Wilroy RS, Summitt RL, et al. Genetic amniocentesis: A twelve years' experience. Am J Med Genet. 1985; 20:443.
11. Daffos F, Capella-Pavlosky M, Forestier F. A new procedure for fetal blood sampling in utero: Preliminary results of 53 cases. Am J Obstet Gynecol. 1983; 146:985.
12. Duff P, Brady WK, Robertson AW. An important medical use for the baggie. N Eng J Med. 1986; 315:1681.
13. Edelman C, Heimler A, Stamberg J. Acceptability of chorionic villus sampling in view of the orthodox Jewish views on abortion (unpublished); 1988.
14. Elias S, Simpson JL. Ultrasound and amniocentesis. In: Sabbagha RE, ed. Diagnostic Ultrasound Applied to Obstetrics and Gynecology. 2nd ed. Hagerstown, MD: Harper & Row; 1980.
15. Golbus MS, Loughman WD, Epstein CJ, et al. Prenatal diagnosis in 3000 amniocenteses. N Engl J. Med. 1979; 300:157.
16. Hahnemann N. Early prenatal diagnosis: A study of biopsy techniques and cell culturing from extrambryonic membranes. Clin Genet. 1974; 6:294–306.
17. Han A, Zhou B, Wang H. Long-term follow-up results after aspiration of chorionic villi during early pregnancy. In: Fraccaro M, Simoni G, Brambati B, eds. First-Trimester Fetal Diagnosis. Berlin: Springer-Verlag; 1985.
18. Hobbins J, Mahoney M. In utero diagnosis of hemoglobinopathies: Technique for obtaining fetal blood. N Engl J Med. 1974; 290:1065.
19. Jackson LG. Pregnancy outcome and the need for centralized data collection in chorion villus sampling. In: Liu DTY, Symonds EM, Golbus MS, eds. Chorionic Villus Sampling. Chicago: Year Book Medical Publishers; 1987.

20. Jackson LG. CVS Newsletter No. 26. Philadelphia: Jefferson Medical College; 1988.

21. Kazy Z, Rozovsky IS, Bakharev VA. Chorion biopsy in early prenatal diagnosis of inherited disorders. Prenat Diagn. 1982; 2:39.

22. Kullander S, Sandahl B. Fetal chromosome analysis after transcervical placental biopsies during early pregnancy. Acta Obstet Gynecol Scand. 1973; 52:355–359.

23. Lambl D. Ein seltener Fall von Hydramnios. Zentralbl Gynaekol. 1881; 5:329.

24. Liley AW. Liquor amnii analysis in the management of the pregnancy complicated by Rhesus sensitization. Am J Obstet Gynecol. 1961; 82:1359.

25. Leek AF, et al. Raised alpha-fetoprotein maternal serum with anencephalic pregnancy. Lancet. 1972; 2:385.

26. Merkatz IR, Nitowsky HM, Macri JN, et al. An association between maternal serum alpha-fetoprotein and fetal chromosome abnormalities. Am J Obstet Gynecol. 1984; 148:1331–1334.

27. Milunsky A. Genetic counseling. In: Milansky A, ed. Genetic Disorders and the Fetus. Diagnosis, Prevention, and Treatment. 2nd ed. New York: Plenum Press; 1986.

28. Parvey B. Report of a case of acute hydramnion treated by abdominal puncture. N Engl J Med. 1933; 208:683–685.

29. Pergament E, Verlinsky Y. Fetal karyotyping by chorionic tissue culture. In: Brambati B, Simoni G, Fabro S, eds. Chorionic Villus Sampling. Fetal Diagnosis of Genetic Disease in the First Trimester. New York: Marcel Dekker; 1986.

30. President's Commission for the Study of Ethical Problems in Medicine and Biomedical and Behavioral Science. Screening and Counseling for Genetic Conditions. Washington, DC: US Government Printing Office; 1983.

31. Richardson RE, Liu DTY. Ultrasound for transcervical chorionic villus sampling. In: Liu DTY, Symonds EM, Golbus MS, eds. Chicago: Year Book Medical Publishers; 1987.

32. Shaw MW. Review of published studies of genetic counseling: A critique. In: Lubs HA, de la Cruz F, eds. Genetic Counseling. New York: Raven Press; 1977.

33. Shaw MW. Genetic counseling. Science. 1974; 184:751.

34. Schatz F. Eine besondere Art von ein seitiger Polyhydramnic mit Oligohydramnie bei Zwillingen. Arch Gynaekol. 1882; 19:329.

35. Simoni G, Brambati B, Danesino C, et al. Diagnostic application of first-trimester trophoblast sampling in 100 pregnancies. Hum Genet. 1984; 66:252–259.

36. Simpson JL, Elias E. Genetic amniocentesis. In: Sabbagha RE, ed. Diagnostic Ultrasound. 2nd ed. Philadelphia: JB Lippincott; 1987.

37. Smidt-Jensen S, Hahnemann N. Transabdominal fine-needle biopsy from chorionic villi in the first trimester. Prenat Diagn. 1984; 4:163–169.

38. Walker AHC. Liquor amnii studies in the prediction of haemolytic disease of the newborn. Br Med J. 1957; 2:376.

39. Rhoads GG, Jackson LG, Schlesseiman SE, et al. The safety and efficacy of chorionic villus sampling for early prenatal diagnosis of cytogenetic abnormalities. N Engl J Med. 1989; 320:609–617.

40. ACOG Opinion Committee on Obstetrics. Maternal and fetal medicine chorionic villus sampling. Washington, D.C.: The American College of Obstetrician and Gynecologists. 1989; 69.

Technical and Psychosocial Topics in Gynecologic and Obstetric Sonography

CHAPTER **33**

Controversies in Obstetric and Gynecologic Ultrasound

MARVEEN CRAIG

Historically, it has been shown that technologic advances are achieved much faster than technical, legal, and ethical protocols are developed to guide them. In this chapter, I attempt to explore some of the major areas of controversy involving the use of diagnostic ultrasound in the practice of obstetrics and gynecology, and their impact on patients, fetuses, and sonologists and sonographers.

Obstetric Ultrasound

With diagnostic ultrasound we are able to follow the critical stages of fetal development. Little wonder, then, that ultrasound complements the practice of obstetrics. In addition, its safety and low cost make it the preferred tool for many obstetric applications. Its use has implications beyond diagnosis, for those who would unravel the mysteries of life in utero have an obligation to maintain the dignity of that life.

ROUTINE VERSUS SELECTIVE SCANNING
Continuing and sometimes heated debate often centers on the topic of routine scanning. Most proponents are members of the medical community who recognize the fetus as a patient, albeit one inaccessible to the traditional forms of clinical investigation such as palpation and inspection.[19]

Among the opponents of this concept are some physicians, policy makers, insurance carriers, and special-interest groups who decry even the notion of such a practice. Unfortunately, there is insufficient scientific proof of the efficacy of routine obstetric scanning in the eyes of the National Institutes of Health Consensus Panel, which deliberated for over a year before coming to this conclusion. A review of their document suggests that the findings of this panel were heavily weighted toward perinatal outcome rather than the positive contributions and attributes that diagnostic ultrasound can provide in pregnancy.[13,19]

It is interesting to note that scanning of pregnant patients is already routine in some countries. The primary reasons cited for the United States not adopting this practice are the question of safety, the cost, the lack of established standards or protocols, and the inconsistent quality of operators, interpreters, and equipment.

Benefits of Routine Scanning. The benefit of using diagnostic ultrasound routinely in pregnancy is its ability to answer basic questions about the embryo or fetus: Is it alive? Is it growing normally or is it malformed? What is its current age?

Because ultrasound is noninvasive and provides the earliest direct evidence of embryonic life, there is little disagreement about its value in this regard.

At least 70% of obstetric scans are performed for the purpose of dating a pregnancy.[19] Correct assessment of gestational age is the most important aspect of prenatal care—in normal and in complicated pregnancies.[23] Sonographic assessment of gestational age is easily achieved at a much earlier stage than by clinical examination on a single visit. It is less reliant upon the patient's body habitus, recall of the last normal menstrual period, early pelvic exam, fundal height measurements, listening for a fetal heart beat, or urine pregnancy testing. Recognizing the fact that preterm delivery is a major cause of perinatal mortality and that postmaturity syndromes are associated with fetal distress and long-term developmental disorders, it is easy to see what a boon to obstetrics ultrasound can be.[16,19]

The early recognition of fetal growth disorders is critical if appropriate changes in obstetric management are to be made to avoid further fetal compromise. The addition of ultrasonic dating to the clinical parameters of menstrual history, fundal height, and biochemical assays can only make each of them more sensitive. Early detection of multiple gestation is another advantage of routine scanning, although it is a benefit only if it results in an improved outcome for the fetuses and the mother.

Although the incidence of placenta previa is only a few in every thousand pregnancies, it is considered a common obstetric problem with serious consequences including perinatal mortality and maternal morbidity. When it is detected early the outcome is usually better. The detection of congenital malformations, which affect approximately 2 to 4% of all newborns,[19] is increasingly important in terms of mortality, and also because of the emotional and economic stresses that morbidity places on the family and society. Such information is also critical to patients who must decide whether to continue or terminate such a pregnancy.[15]

Although ultrasound cannot detect all anomalies, it does detect the major morphologic anomalies that produce the most profound effects. For patients who opt to continue such pregnancies, ultrasound can identify defects that are incompatible with life, decrease the potential for neonatal complications, eliminate unnecessary procedures such as cesarean section, and identify fetuses that will require operative correction after delivery or would benefit most from intrauterine surgery.

Because the usual clinical methods of menstrual history and physical examination are inadequate for prenatal identification of congenital anomalies, proponents of routine scanning urge screening for all patients at least once in the second trimester of pregnancy. Ideally, two studies should be done: one at 20 weeks to assess gestational age and to detect possible anomalies and the second one at 32 to 36 weeks, to assess fetal growth.[19]

Potential Disadvantages to Routine Scanning. Before ultrasound is adopted as a screening test in pregnancy the following considerations must be explored: (1) its rate of sensitivity and specificity (efficacy), (2) its potential risks (safety), (3) its cost, (4) patient acceptance, and (5) quality control. For our purposes in discussing the merits of diagnostic ultrasound, it is helpful to define the terms sensitivity and specificity. Sensitivity is the probability that a test demonstrates an abnormality or disease when it is in fact present. Specificity is the probability that test results will be negative when indeed a patient has no disease. Further discussion of these concepts can be found in Chapter 36. Frigoletto has commented on and questioned the efficacy of using ultrasound as a screening device.

Whether mass screening should be done for a medical condition depends on the properties of the screening test. For instance, a screening test with a sensitivity of 0.99 and a specificity of 0.999 for a condition that has a low prevalence (such as neural tube defects in the United States) has a high rate of false positive results. Frigoletto argued that a large number of false positive results is the strongest argument against routine scanning.[13] Other considerations about a screening test should include costs, risk, and acceptability to patients.

EFFICACY

The dramatic acceptance and increased use of ultrasound in obstetrics has resulted in numerous articles and claims of improved patient care and fetal outcome. None of the latter claims, however, have been scientifically documented and tested by random controlled clinical trials.[13,19]

SAFETY FACTOR

Although no adverse effects have been reported in patient populations scanned in the early 1960s and 1970s, and despite the fact that more than 10 million newborns have been scanned worldwide without evidence of ill effects due to ultrasound exposure, we in the United States are reluctant to surrender our concerns for safety.[19] Opponents to routine screening are quick to point out that follow-up of infants exposed to ultrasound in utero has been insufficient to test for delayed effects. The bitter lessons learned from thyroid and thymus irradiation and from diethylstilbestrol (DES) exposure exert a powerful influence. They also point out that there is no convincing evidence that increased detection of twins has reduced their mortality or morbidity.[13]

We know that theoretically energy can interfere with living systems through (1) tissue destruction, (2) induction of abnormal cell development, and (3) production of abnormal chemical reactions. Despite ongoing vigilance, there has been no evidence to date that any of these actions occurs, either in vitro or in animal models, when *diagnostic power levels* are used. The lingering concerns that ultrasound exposure may produce subtle effects in subsequent generations is the underlying force behind today's policy of using diagnostic ultrasound prudently or only when it is clinically indicated.

Cost Factor

The cost of diagnostic ultrasound is vastly different in America than in developed countries such as England, Germany, and France, where routine scanning is practiced more widely. In those areas, scanning costs range between $7 and $20. In America, costs are based on the time required to perform the examination, equipment costs, personnel, and miscellaneous institutional and insurance costs. Consequently, the cost of a single ultrasound scan in the U.S. is estimated to range from $60 to $450. Cost is a major deterrent to routine screening of pregnancy by ultrasound. It will continue to be so until caregivers agree to run efficient, high-volume services and to be content with modest profit margins.[19]

Unlike chemical screening tests, ultrasound examinations require special human skills that legitimately increase the cost of the study. A desperate need exists for an adequate cost-benefit analysis of routine ultrasound screening of pregnancy. Previous estimates were derived from very limited studies in which only one or two conditions were used as the topics of detection and only a few variables (length of hospital stay, improved quality of life, increased life span) were examined.[19]

Expanded studies are needed that will address the potential of ultrasound not only as a means of assessing gestational age and detecting congenital disorders, but also as a useful tool for evaluating fetal growth and providing care and management of pregnancies. We need statistics that quantify the benefits of delivering term versus preterm infants and of delivering fetuses with correctable defects in centers equipped to deal with such problems and the savings to be realized from interrupting nonviable or severely compromised pregnancies. In essence, cost-benefit analysis must also address more complicated issues than the purely financial ones—issues that involve ethical and philosophical factors.

National Institutes of Health Consensus Panel Findings

In 1984, after a year of deliberation, a consensus development conference, sponsored by the National Institutes of Child Health and Human Development, the Office of Medical Applications of Research, the Division of Research Resources, and the Food and Drug Administration issued their report, in which they concluded that diagnostic ultrasound could be of benefit in a variety of clinical situations. With specific regard to pregnancy, they agreed that where clinical questions existed, ultrasound could be extremely valuable. Citing (1) the absence of any well-controlled studies to prove that routine scanning of all pregnant patients would improve the outcome of pregnancy, (2) the lack of consensus among professionals that ultrasound should be used to examine all pregnant women, and (3) the inconclusive evidence about long-term effects, the decision reached was that ultrasound is indicated only in the presence of medically valid criteria.[13] The FDA reaffirmed its policy that, until risks are better defined, only prudent and judicious use of ultrasound should occur and exposure, duration, and ultrasound intensity should be limited to what is needed to produce the necessary diagnostic information.[13]

Conclusion. Routine scanning has been demonstrated to have tangible benefits in specific areas of pregnancy; however, data are insufficient to prove that such detection has routinely improved the outcome of those pregnancies. The costs of routine scanning in the U.S. are significant, but accurate cost-benefit evaluations have not been performed to determine whether routine scanning costs more than, as much as, or less than selective scanning, nor is it known whether additional costs are justified by improved outcome.

The studies performed to date that address the issues of safety do not allow any firm conclusions to be drawn.[16] The difficult task of judging a technology that has been widely embraced by both physicians and their patients is further compounded now that concerns for safety have lessened. Even while the debate about routine versus selective scanning continues, there is an increasing demand from physicians and their patients for ultrasound scans. The previous stumbling blocks— primitive technology, lack of skilled operators, and the need to prove the clinical value of the technique—have been overcome, so much so, that a form of routine scanning may actually be taking place, as progressively more and more pregnant patients are being scanned.

The Fetus As Patient

The concept of the fetus as a patient is a very modern one that owes much of its current status directly to the use of diagnostic ultrasound in pregnancy. Although the first direct view of ovulation was observed in 1930, followed in 1944 by the microscopic observation of fertilization, it was not until the 1960s that accurate and specific diagnosis and fetal therapy became a reality. That one instance was in Rh isoimmunization disease, treated with serial amniocentesis and intrauterine fetal transfusions. At about the same time, diagnostic ultrasound was being hailed as a promising tool for evaluating fetal response to this maternal condition.[15]

Since then, many ultrasound milestones have been passed:

1. The identification of the fetus during embryonic development.
2. The ability to demonstrate fetal physiology and fetal disease.
3. The ability to detect the need for fetal therapy and to guide or monitor such therapy.

4. Follow-up monitoring of fetal tolerance and response.

Prenatal ultrasound testing can actually produce a paradoxical effect. On one hand, its use in developing new tests and therapies for common disorders is very positive; on the other, its use to justify pregnancy termination can create moral dilemmas when one considers that the protection of life is medicine's highest calling. Along with the ability to detect and treat a variety of fetal problems comes the obligation to monitor the entire spectrum of responses to fetal diagnosis and therapy. Less attention has been given to the sudden emotional and economical difficulties such decisions create. Clearly, guidelines for what to do when defects are found do not exist.

Some opponents of fetal diagnosis and therapy think of it as a means of carrying out search-and-destroy missions, seeing it as a means for selective breeding and possible genocide (e.g., screening for sickle cell disease). It is doubtful that such fears can be eliminated solely by rhetoric. To those who embrace the concept, the goal is to provide deeper understanding of a wide range of fetal illnesses and to be able to offer brighter prospects than the present alternatives of neonatal death, abnormality, or abortion.[15]

FETAL THERAPY

Fetal therapy can be divided into several categories: indirect, specific, invasive, and surgical. *Indirect fetal therapy* involves the use of drugs to manipulate the fetus' physiologic status. Such agents as corticosteroids, thyroid hormones, and glucose solutions are only a few examples. These procedures are designed to stimulate fetal pulmonic maturity or to improve the condition of the fetus with a potential for fetal distress (J. C. Hobbins, personal communication).

Specific therapies may involve administering to the mother substances intended to control or correct fetal disease. Such agents as vitamins and heart medications can be used as noninvasive therapies to improve fetal life in utero. Sonography's roles in indirect and specific therapy are obviously detection and follow-up of therapeutic response.

The administration of agents such as hormones and red blood cells are considered *invasive therapies,* as they involve entering the uterus, amniotic cavity, or fetus. In such instances diagnostic ultrasound has an additional role, mapping the area of interest, monitoring the procedure, and in some cases guiding it.

Surgical intervention is clearly a more potentially dangerous form of fetal therapy. Decompression of cyst, shunt placement in fetal hydronephrosis or hydrocephaly, draining abnormal fluid collections—all have been greatly improved with the aid of diagnostic ultrasound, and that fact has contributed to its increasing use. Perhaps the most daring feat is intrauterine fetal surgery, in which the gravid uterus is exposed through a midline incision, a hysterotomy is performed, and the appropriate fetal part is exteriorized and subjected to corrective surgery. Successful fetal nephrostomy and ureterostomy have proven that open fetal surgery with continuation of pregnancy or delivery near term is feasible.[15] An unexpected finding has been that fetuses who undergo intrauterine surgery heal without scars. The work accomplished in this area has clearly been facilitated by the availability of diagnostic ultrasound. Proponents of fetal therapy point to these procedures as leading unexpectedly to a greater understanding of fetal problems and alternative solutions; however, they acknowledge that it will be many years before the benefits of these activities can be fully evaluated. Proper case selection and performance of procedures only in centers offering unusual diagnostic support services are key factors to successful treatment (J. C. Hobbins, personal communication).

Fetal Tissue Research

The magnificent medical advances of the past decade have also produced monstrous ethical problems. One such involves fetal tissue transplantation, which raises the ethical fear of fetal exploitation. Voices have already been raised demanding that this particular aspect of medical research be safeguarded from any possible commercial enterprise.[21]

Fetal tissue research holds important potential benefits for victims of major disease such as diabetes, Parkinson's disease, and other brain disorders and for medical research. Researchers have shown that implanted fetal tissue grows rapidly and is less likely than adult tissue to be rejected by the recipient's immune system. One promising study involves the transplantation of fetal tissues involved in the formation of blood and immune cells as a powerful new tool against AIDS and other immune-mediated diseases.[21]

Would sonography play a role in evaluating the living fetus prior to a selection process? Would its use extend to recipients as a means of detecting and demonstrating their abnormality? And once transplantation was completed, would it be used in follow-up studies to determine the positive or negative effects?

An advisory committee of the NIH has concluded that it is morally acceptable to use human fetal tissue obtained from legal abortions for therapy and research. Although fetal tissue can be obtained from miscarriages and stillbirths, the major available source of fetal tissue for research would be from elective abortions. This factor poses the most difficult ethical dilemma. Religious groups in particular are concerned that the routine use of fetal organs could result in a morally unacceptable collaboration with "the abortion industry." Would researchers be tempted to declare fetuses dead prematurely or to encourage more abortions? Would such practices result in one generation living off another by using fetuses as spare parts for a senescent population? To deter potential abuse, guidelines obviously are called for:

1. Remove all nonregenerative, nonrenewable tissues from commercial enterprise.
2. Prohibit purchase of organs for surgical transplant procedures.
3. Prohibit elective abortion patients from choosing the recipient of fetal tissue from their pregnancy.

Unless genetic engineering is perfected to the extent that fetal organs can be "grown" in the laboratory, the source of fetal tissue will be associated primarily with abortions.

Fetal Reduction

That multiple gestation can produce complications in pregnancy is well-known. This problem surfaces most often in women who have undergone ovulation induction or in vitro fertilization. Studies have shown that the risk of stillbirth and infant deaths are greater when a woman is carrying three or more fetuses.

To increase the chances of viable infants in such situations, reducing the number of fetuses has been suggested. This can be achieved by cardiac puncture, injection of formaldehyde into the fetal heart, or injection of filtered air into an umbilical vessel in fetuses targeted for selective feticide or abortion.[28] Because diagnostic ultrasound plays a pivotal role in the performance of such selective reduction therapies, many sonographers are confronted with a moral dilemma. Sonographers who view abortion as unacceptable under any circumstances would decline to be involved in such procedures. Those who think that abortion might be appropriate under special circumstances would be forced to wrestle with the concept of sacrificing some fetuses so that others might survive.

Pregnancy Termination

The practice of obstetrics was seriously affected by the proabortion rulings of the 1960s, and especially by the 1973 rulings of Roe versus Wade, and the most recent 1989 Webster Decision of the Supreme Court. The capability of diagnostic ultrasound to provide detailed images of the developing fetus and to determine its age has placed the technique front and center in this controversy. New screening techniques for the detection of genetic disease and ultrasound-assisted fetal tissue sampling add new dimensions to fetal testing. The detection of abnormality or serious disease forces parents to painfully review their options—continuing or terminating the pregnancy.

One of sonographers' biggest problems involving elective abortion centers around the fact that referring physicians often fail to disclose that the pregnancy is going to be terminated. The common practice of permitting patients to view the display screen during ultrasound studies and sonographers' willingness to point out fetal structures during routine scanning creates potential problems. Should women who are contemplating abortion watch their fetuses? Should sonographers freely answer questions that such patients may be prompted to ask as a result of seeing their fetus? Shouldn't such patients be clearly identified as potential or certain elective abortion patients prior to arriving in the ultrasound facility?

Obstetric sonographers often relate stories about patients who are considering abortion but change their minds after seeing their baby on the display screen. In such cases, perhaps the patient was not fully committed to proceeding with the abortion and the ultrasound experience made her realize that. Some suggest that all women who are considering abortion should undergo ultrasound examination expressly to witness the fetus and its activities, but we must also respect those women who reached the decision to abort after considerable thought and emotional stress.

Most sonographers feel it is unfair to expect them to determine which type of patient they are dealing with on the basis of their observations of the patient's moods or conversation. The failure of referring physicians to inform the ultrasound center that the patient being scheduled for sonography is also scheduled for abortion is unconscionable, yet, it happens daily and forces sonographers into compromising situations. Such problems could be eased if (1) clinicians fully explained the ultrasound procedure to patients prior to scheduling and communicated their combined wishes regarding patient viewing of the study, and (2) sonographers offered patients the option of viewing the screen during a study instead of assuming that all patients wish to do so. They could then adjust the position of the display screen and restrict their comments during the examination.

One fact about this issue is abundantly clear: the patient and her physician have considered her problem and have based their decision on multiple facts that may be unknown to the sonographer. It is not the province of diagnostic ultrasound and its purveyors to attempt to dissuade, encourage, or punish patients.

It is unlikely that there is a more divisive aspect of obstetric sonography than its use in pregnancy termination. A small but growing number of sonographers find themselves in direct conflict with their moral principles and the demands of their profession.[25,26] As the bitter drama of pro-life versus pro-choice advocates continues to unfold around them, sonographers are unlikely to escape the crossfire.

The best advice seems to be that sonographers must take a personal inventory of their feelings and beliefs regarding abortion and medical intervention procedures. Those who are unable to accept the current laws and medical practices regarding them must express their convictions and request to be relieved of the duty of working with patients destined to undergo such procedures. Depending on the type of patient population and the activities of the institution, this may not be easy to arrange. Nevertheless, sonographers should never be forced through fear of professional or economic reprisal to perform ultrasound procedures that conflict with their personal beliefs; and a sonographer who once accepts responsibility toward a patient must *never* refuse to carry out or complete a procedure.

Fetal Rights

What began as a physician dilemma has widened to take in fundamental moral questions: Does the fetus have a right to life? What are the mother's rights with respect to her fetus? What is the state's interest in a fetus?

The concept of the fetus as a patient in need of consideration, care, and sometimes corrective protection has been widely accepted. Thus far, however, all parties concerned have been unable to achieve emotional satisfaction and political clarity regarding the sanctity of life in this particular context. In light of the prevailing legal, ethical, and moral climate surrounding the issues, sonographers, sonologists, and their institutions must be aware of the assertion of fetal rights—aware that they are legally responsible for their actions and diagnosis until the fetal patient reaches the age of majority. This responsibility demands that they keep well-documented records of *all* studies involving pregnancy and fetuses and keep them for longer periods than other types of patient studies are kept.

The Obstetric and Gynecologic Sonographer's Role

Beside the moral issues that confront sonographers there are many ethical considerations to resolve. One leading area of controversy surrounds the role of sonographers in dispensing information to patients and to referring or interpreting physicians. Another is the proper degree of involvement of the patient's family and loved ones during sonography.

SONOGRAPHER-PATIENT INTERACTION

Pregnancy has become more of a social event than ever before. With the institution of childbirth classes, birthing rooms, rooming in, and similar innovations it is not surprising that today's pregnant women want to share the first views of their unborn child with family and friends. Close family members can experience bonding as a direct result of viewing fetal images on an ultrasound display (see Chapter 34). For whatever reason, the positive results of allowing family and friends into the examining room during obstetric scanning far outweigh the risk that problems or abnormalities will be encountered.

Sonographers should consider carefully not only *what* they say to patients but *how* they deliver the information. Often, patients do not fully understand what is said, misunderstand, or take statements out of context. Some patients hear only what they wish to hear. Is my baby normal? is obviously a loaded question but one that is frequently asked of sonographers. It is critically important to give a qualified answer before expanding further, such as, "Diagnostic ultrasound is limited in its ability to demonstrate *all* effects." Even though patients use terms such as placenta previa or breech position, their understanding of those terms may be distorted or incomplete.

Despite this warning, communicating with patients can be one of the most rewarding experiences available to sonographers. Considering the apprehension and concerns that patients bring to the scanning experience, one of our goals should be to prepare them psychologically by explaining the procedure and establishing realistic expectations.[5,10,20]

FAMILY-CENTERED SONOGRAPHY

Diagnostic ultrasound poses no harm to bystanders, and pregnancy is a family affair that produces anxiety as well as joy. These are two practical reasons for turning a diagnostic study into a family event.[5] Pregnancy differs from other medical situations because it springs from a partnership that creates a family as well as a fetus. This is a compelling reason to admit the mother's loved ones into the examination room. The chief argument against such a practice is the fear of discovering an abnormality. Many sonographers do not want to be placed in the position of handling the distress of the patient, let alone that of her support group. Another frequent objection is that it is distracting to the sonographer to have family members present and is likely to interfere with the complete concentration necessary to produce a diagnostic study, whether or not abnormalities are discovered.

If an institution wishes to encourage or permit family involvement, participation guidelines must be developed to prevent crowding and distractions that could compromise the diagnostic quality of the study. The following suggestions are relevant:

1. Admit only one or two people.
2. Have guests be seated.
3. Admit no small children.
4. Reserve for the sonographer the option of performing the study in private and then admitting guests for a review of selected highlights of the fetal examination.[5] A brief explanation of the policies of the department and of the actual ultrasound procedure establishes a professional tone and allows the sonographer to control the situation.

If an abnormality is discovered it will be necessary to extend scanning time to provide complete documentation of the problem. The interpreting physician should be contacted immediately and consulted on the further handling of the case. Ideally, the sonologist should become personally involved, as most patients can sense when something is wrong and expect to be informed of the result of the examination. In such settings, the physician acts as the sonographer's "supporter" and the patient's loved ones are there to support her at a time when she needs them most.

It is extremely important that an ultrasound facility's internal policies and procedures be developed in such a way that the sonographer's role is clearly defined. All parties involved in the delivery of diagnostic ultrasound should provide input to any policy-making session, so that a set of guidelines is developed that allows sonographers to discharge their duties without evading their responsibilities or breaking the patient's trust. The following list offers a practical approach to developing obstetric ultrasound scanning policies:

1. Review the patient's rights document adopted by your institution.
2. Establish what information (i.e., gender identification, number of fetuses, fetal viability) sonographers are permitted to deliver and what they should withhold.
3. Establish the number of family members permitted to view an examination and rules for their conduct.
4. Explain to the patient and family members how you plan to conduct the examination.
5. Inform the patient prior to commencing the examination that the privilege of delivering medical results belongs solely to the physician.
6. Treat family members with the same respect you accord the patient.
7. Describe the routine portions of the examination in a basic way, without referring to specific fetal or maternal abnormalities or results.
8. If an abnormality is discovered, contact the physician in charge as soon as possible and seek further instructions.

At times, anxious patients and relatives have presented various challenges to all members of the health care community, but in many instances patient care and procedures are carried out in the presence of family members without major upsets. Sonographers must realize and accept the fact that obstetric patients no longer submit passively to procedures. The general population, and this group in particular, are becoming increasingly aware of the options available to them. The concept of family-centered care is actively promoted by consumer groups, physicians, nurses, and administrations, and is changing attitudes toward the services provided by others in related fields.[5]

The issues of what constitutes a sonographer's professional relationship with patients and physicians is complex and still evolving. While we go about the task of recognizing the obligations, duties, benefits, and liabilities of being sonographers we must not diminish the potential for good that diagnostic ultrasound can provide.

SONOGRAPHER REPORTS

A sonographer's desire to generate preliminary impressions or reports in order to contribute to the patient's diagnosis in a professional way must be weighed against medical-legal implications and self-doubt. In the course of their daily practice sonographers are consulted by some persons, threatened by others, and must constantly avoid being manipulated. Although they are fully aware that rendering a diagnosis is not included in their professional or job descriptions, they are nevertheless frequently urged to "share their thoughts" about a case. This request may be made by the interpreting or referring physician, patients, or family members.[17,18]

Initially, when ultrasound was still a very new entity that was not yet included in physician training, sonographers were required to contribute written or verbal findings to their supervising physician. This concept developed either because the trained physician was not able to be present for the patient study or because the interpreting physician had less training and experience than the sonographer.

The practice of writing sonographer impressions evolved to provide sonographers a written document to which they could refer if a case were ever questioned.[6] These technical impressions were also invaluable to novice sonologists, reinforcing their impressions or alerting them to the need to consult with the sonographer and possibly rescan a patient if their findings did not concur. Unfortunately, in some instances sonographer impressions became a crutch for some physicians, who took them literally and even dictated them verbatim. Today, the increased number of physicians with ultrasound training and experience has limited such reliance on preliminary impressions.

Every health care worker knows the value, and sometimes urgent need, for an instant report. Because of economic pressures some sonographers are required to work in unsupervised settings, where they are frequently pressured by referring physicians to interpret a study.[17] Every ultrasound facility should draw up policies to guide sonographers in these situations, and when they are first established should circulate a letter to all house staff and referring physicians, stating the valid reasons for adopting such policies.

The basic problem of sonographers' rendering an impression seems to stem from misunderstanding on the part of referring physicians: Sonographers' impressions must be recognized not as diagnoses but as technical interpretations, and the final diagnosis must be rendered by the interpreting physician. When properly used, sonographers' impressions promote an open environment and offer an opportunity for their intellectual growth.[5] By continuing to strive for better definition of their roles, sonographers will find their proper place in the diagnostic process. Only when the community of sonographers establishes a national standard of care that requires documentation of sonographer input will oral or written reports or entries in patient charts be sanctioned.

VIDEOTAPING PRACTICES

Some patients arrive with blank tapes on which to take home a recording of the video portions of their ultrasound examination. This is strong evidence that the growing sophistication of ultrasound techniques and the commercial world of imaging have not eluded the patient. Today's patients are definitely more aware and want (at times demand) filmed or taped documentation of the time they spend in the ultrasound laboratory. Some even seek permission to bring home video cameras into the scanning environment to record the entire event.[8]

As in any controversial issue, there are pros and cons to these practices:

Pro: Satisfies patient/obstetrician request
Encourages family-centered sonography
Enhances family bonding
Enhances attractiveness of diagnostic
ultrasound

Con: Should not be provided for nonmedical or
official use
Distracts sonographer's concentration
Extends scanning time and patient exposure

If videotaping for the patient is offered, a specific time should be set aside for carrying out this service. Physicians should be aware of the examination results before any videotape is made for the patient. Nothing that was not visualized on the diagnostic recording should appear on the patient's copy.[8]

In obstetric office practices, Polaroid films are given to patients, and most, if not all, pregnant patients are scanned. Although families now press for tangible mementos of the examination, even in office practices these should not be given until a complete diagnostic study has been performed and reviewed.

Historically, obstetric ultrasound examinations have the highest percentage of happy endings. The rewards of parental bonding, patient education and cooperation, and the improved public image for diagnostic ultrasound and the sponsoring institution are strong incentives to share information with the patient. Experience has shown that this activity has negative sequelae when poorly trained sonographers or sonologists perform the study, when patients misunderstand the information they are given, or when unsuspected fetal anomalies surface, either during taping or afterward, at delivery. Along with being one of the most interesting and rewarding ultrasound experiences, obstetric sonography is an area in which oral, written, and sonographic statements may return to haunt a person.

Every department, clinic, or office practice must address this issue independently as there are no national standards. Common sense and experience would indicate the following considerations:

1. A written policy should be established for providing patients with hard-copy images of their ultrasound study.
2. Nothing should appear on a patient's hard copy that was not seen on the diagnostic study or survey.
3. The physician in charge of the imaging facility should view the tape or images before they are given to the patient and should retain the right to deny the tape or photos for patient use if an abnormality is found or suspected.

The legal representatives of some ultrasound facilities have indicated that providing a tape of the patient's ultrasound examination does not increase their liability but that to allow these practices without physician approval or preview might. Any existing department protocols should be viewed by the institution's or the physician's legal representative. All personnel involved should remember that, in the event of litigation, national, not local, standards, will apply.[11]

LEGAL CONSIDERATIONS

The 1980s trend toward medical malpractice litigation strikes most deeply in the area of obstetric ultrasound. In fact, ultrasound appears to have created new medical-legal corridors. Some areas can potentially lead to legal difficulties (those marked with an asterisk relate specifically to sonographers):

Failure to conform to a standard of care in performing or not performing an ultrasound examination.
Performing an incomplete study and "missing" a lesion.
Improper interpretation of the sonogram.
Failures and misdiagnoses due to instrumentation.
Complications from invasive ultrasound procedures.
Failure to adequately inform the referring physician.
*Professional misconduct.
*Misinterpreting and reporting a diagnosis.
*Failure to provide for patient safety during the ultrasound examination.[26]

In each diagnostic ultrasound study there are four important variables to consider: the knowledge and skill of the sonographer, the knowledge and skill of the sonologist, the quality of the ultrasound instrument, and the patient's unique sonographic characteristics.

It is clear that high standards offer the best protection against obstetric sonography claims. A critical component is the need for detailed documentation of all studies. The majority of ultrasound-related malpractice suits in the United States are the result of missed diagnosis.[18,26] The obvious causes of such misadventures are poor-quality images, poor documentation, and poor technical performance of the study. Many times, these factors result from failure to use state-of-the-art equipment and transducers. Sometimes they result from failure of the sonography service to communicate the limitations of ultrasound to the referring doctor and patient or from inappropriate use of ultrasound during a specific stage of pregnancy.

At the root of malpractice is the lack of quality control guidelines for obstetric sonography. Although the American Institute of Ultrasound in Medicine (AIUM) recently published guidelines for the use of ultrasound in obstetrics, there is still concern that they will not be widely circulated and adopted.[22]

EDUCATION AND COMPETENCY

Who should perform diagnostic ultrasound studies? Who should interpret them? Sadly, the lack of rules governing these aspects of diagnostic ultrasound has opened wide the potential for abuse of this noble profession. A sonologist must not only be skilled in interpreting images but must also be sure that images are obtained with optimal examination technique and equipment. Expert performance of ultrasound examinations is an art that cannot be learned from books alone but requires sonologists and sonographers to practice and to use intelligence, medical knowledge, and experience.[12,27]

Unfortunately, the deceptively simple appearance of the scanning technique, which is enhanced by the fact that anyone can purchase diagnostic ultrasound equipment and offer scanning services, has attracted some practitioners of questionable competency. The crux of the problem appears to be that there are no national standards. As the field of sonography advances in both years and experience, one would think that the number of incompetent or poorly trained practitioners would decline. This has not been the case, for two basic reasons: (1) enthusiastic patient acceptance and increasing demand for the technique and (2) the manufacture and sale of less expensive "basic" models to private offices, where a casual approach to the use of ultrasound may be adopted. In such settings many persons are asked to learn to perform ultrasound studies on their own who are entirely unaware of the educational demands on and resources available to professional sonographers.

Two levels of ultrasound are in use today. In a level 1 study, ultrasound is used as an everyday clinical tool by physicians with little skill to make immediate, crude decisions. In a level 2 study ultrasound is used to look at intricate intra-abdominal or fetal anatomy and pathology to make much more subtle decisions.[12,27]

Filly has pointed out that, for all intents and purposes, level 1 sonography is the standard second- or third-trimester obstetric examination as described in the American Institute of Ultrasound in Medicine/American College of Radiology guidelines, and although the specific purpose of the examination is not to detect fetal anomalies, there is a reasonable probability that, during the course of the data acquisition, many anomalies will be recognized and that a prudent effort should be made to this end.[12] He expressed concern that the term "level 1" might be used as a shield for incompetency and noted that patients have a right to expect that the person performing and interpreting their examination has the appropriate knowledge to do so. He calls for the elimination of level 1 and level 2 examinations, stressing that there should only be one level of ultrasound, that which is optimal.[12]

Unfortunately in the practice of ultrasound today there are instances of inept examinations performed by persons with inadequate skills and dedication. Legal suits involving ultrasound are primarily related to obstetric ultrasound, where it is evident that studies are performed by operators who are relatively inexperienced.[27]

Currently, training criteria are virtually nonexistent for all specialties that use diagnostic ultrasound. An oral segment of the radiology boards is devoted to obstetric ultrasound, but no period of practical training in ultrasound is mandated; it is merely suggested that 2 months is appropriate. Both the obstetric and cardiology boards contain a limited number of oral and written questions on diagnostic ultrasound, but no time requirements or minimum number of examinations are required.[23,27]

Until recently there has been no incentive for training programs to provide adequate ultrasound instruction to residents. The impetus for change has begun through the efforts of the Commission on Ultrasound of the American College of Radiology, the American College of Obstetrics and Gynecology, and the American Institute of Ultrasound in Medicine.[23]

In 1975, the American Registry of Diagnostic Medical Sonographers (ARDMS) conducted the first voluntary registry examinations for sonographers. Thus that test became not only the first but the only available yardstick for measuring minimum levels of competency of persons who perform a variety of diagnostic ultrasound studies. Since

1975, more than 14,000 sonographers have been registered through the ARDMS.[1] Among them are a small but growing number of physicians who have also seen the value of sitting for the examinations, to establish their competency. Perhaps the greatest contribution of the ARDMS, however, has been the mandatory continuing education requirements to maintain registered status.

Transvaginal Scanning

The application of transvaginal transducers to both obstetric and gynecologic examinations has exposed sonographers and sonologists to new areas of legal sensitivity. Laws governing the actions of health care providers toward patients vary greatly from state to state, making it impossible to be specific in suggesting guidelines for the use of transvaginal transducers. Therefore, a general approach is usually advocated that can be fashioned to fit a specific patient population and geographic location by trimming away any unnecessary components.

At this writing, no official guidelines have been adopted that can serve as a national standard. Both the SDMS and the AIUM are currently conducting surveys in preparation for publishing a position paper on this topic (R. Bree, personal communication).[2] It is important that institutions develop standards of practice. Such projects should not be limited solely to the imaging department but should be reviewed by the legal representatives of the institution, by referring and interpreting physicians, and by any available patients' rights representatives.[9,14]

Transvaginal Examination Precautions

1. The procedure must be explained to the patient, who has the right to refuse the examination.
2. Either male or female sonographers may perform the examination.
3. The examination should be performed with a third party assisting in the room as a chaperone. At no time should the chaperone be a relative or friend of the patient.
4. The probe can be inserted by the patient, the physician, or the sonographer, depending on hospital or laboratory policy.
5. Sonographers should be gloved during the procedure, should be responsive to patient complaints and requests, and should demonstrate a professional attitude at all times.[4,9,13]

Sonographers' Code of Conduct

Through the efforts of the Professional Status Committee of the SDMS a sonographer's code of conduct has been adopted.

Code of Professional Conduct for Diagnostic Medical Sonographers

Preamble The Code of Professional Conduct of the Society of Diagnostic Medical Sonographers is a statement of the high standards of conduct toward which sonographers are committed to strive. Sonographers, as members of a health care profession, acknowledge their responsibilities to their patients, to other health care professionals, and to each other.

I. Sonographers shall act in the best interests of the patient.
II. Sonographers shall provide sonographic services with compassion, respect for human dignity, honesty, and integrity.
III. Sonographers shall respect the patient's right to privacy, safeguarding confidential information within the constraints of the law.
IV. Sonographers shall maintain competence in their field.
V. Sonographers shall assume responsibility for their actions.

Conclusion

Sonography has had a profound impact on medicine, revolutionizing the evaluation and treatment of many clinical problems. The expanding role of diagnostic ultrasound, especially as applied to the practice of obstetrics, has simultaneously created questions and controversy.

In this chapter we have attempted to present the many divergent views and possible solutions to some of these perplexing issues. It is the duty of all sonographers to become familiar with the issues and to remain current with the medical, professional, and legal solutions regarding them.

References

1. American Registry of Diagnostic Medical Sonographers. Directory and Informational Booklet—1989. Cincinnati: American Registry of Diagnostic Medical Sonographers; 1989.
2. Anderhub B. Survey on endocavitary ultrasound. Soc Diagn Med Sonogr Newsletter. 1989; 10:1.
3. Berlin L. Proposed code of professional conduct for

diagnostic medical sonographers. Soc Diagn Med Sonogr Newsletter. 1989; 10:4.

4. Bernaschek G. Endosonography. In: Sabbagha RE, ed. Diagnostic Ultrasound Applied to Obstetrics and Gynecology. 2nd ed. Philadelphia: JB Lippincott; 1987:572–582.

5. Craig M. Family centered sonography. J Diagn Med Sonogr. 1986; 2:96–103.

6. Craig M. The eternal controversy: Sonographer's reports. J Diagn Med Sonogr. 1987; 3:244–248.

7. Craig M. The challenge of patient interaction. J Diagn Med Sonogr. 1987; 3:147–150.

8. Craig M. Baby videos: A boon or liability? J Diagn Med Sonogr. 1988; 4:19–22.

9. Craig M. Ethical implications of advanced technology. J Diagn Med Sonogr. 1989; 2:66–70.

10. Craig M. Treating patients with patience. J Diagn Med Sonogr. 1989; 1:16–18.

11. Everett SL. Ultrasound: Legal issues. Presented at Redwood Society of Sonographers, Santa Rosa, California, May 7, 1987.

12. Filly RA. Level 1, level 2, level 3 obstetric sonography: I'll see your level and raise you one. Radiology. 1989; 172:312.

13. Frigoletto FD. Obstetrical ultrasound: Selective use. In: McGahan JP, ed. Controversies in Ultrasound. New York: Churchill-Livingstone; 1987; 20:113–122.

14. Gosink G. Endovaginal scanning: Techniques and applications. Conference Proceedings of the Society of Diagnostic Medical Sonographers' 5th Annual Conference. March 1988, Anaheim, California.

15. Harrison MR, Golbus MS, Filly RA. The Unborn Patient: Prenatal Diagnosis and Treatment. Orlando, FL: Grune and Stratton; 1984.

16. Hughey MJ. Routine vs. indicated scans. In: Sabbagha RE, ed. Diagnostic Ultrasound Applied to Obstetrics and Gynecology. 2nd ed. Philadelphia: JB Lippincott; 1987:46–53.

17. James AE, Fleischer AC, et al. Diagnostic ultrasonography: Certain legal considerations. J Ultrasound Med. 1985; 4:427–431.

18. James AE, Bundy A, Fleischer AC, et al. Legal aspects of diagnostic medical sonography. Semin Ultrasound CT MRI. 1985; 5:207–216.

19. Jeanty P, Romero R, Hobbins JC. Obstetrical ultrasound: Routine use. In: McGahan JP, ed. Controversies in Ultrasound. New York: Churchill-Livingstone; 1987; 20:113–122.

20. Lea JH. Psychosocial progression through normal pregnancy. A model for sonographer-patient interaction. J Diagn Med Ultrasound. 1985; 1:55–58.

21. Leary WE. U.S. panel backs research use of fetal tissue from abortions. New York Times. September 17, 1988:1.

22. Leopold GR. Antepartum obstetrical ultrasound examination guidelines. J Ultrasound Med. 1986; 5:241–242.

23. Miller EI. Specialty certification in diagnostic ultrasound: Disadvantages. In: McGahan JP, ed. Controversies in Ultrasound. New York: Churchill-Livingstone; 1987; 20:47–51.

24. Platt LD. Assessment of Gestational Age. In: Queenan JT, Hobbins JC, eds. Protocols for High-Risk Pregnancies. Oradell, NJ: Medical Economics Books; 1982.

25. Ruiz MA, Murphy-Irwin K. Sonographer-fetus bonding. (In preparation.)

26. Sanders RC. Malpractice and ultrasound. In: Sanders RC, Hill MC. Ultrasound Annual—1986. New York: Raven Press; 1986.

27. Sanders RC. Specialty certification in diagnostic ultrasound: Advantages. In: McGahan HP, ed. Controversies in Ultrasound. New York: Churchill-Livingstone; 1987; 20:39–45.

28. Simpson JL, Sherman E. Genetic amniocentesis. In: Sabbagha RE, ed. Diagnostic Ultrasound Applied to Obstetrics and Gynecology. 2nd ed. Philadelphia: JB Lippincott; 1987:64–76.

CHAPTER 34

Sonographer Support of Maternal-Fetal Bonding

JEAN LEA SPITZ

Attachment and bonding are interactions between mother and infant that reinforce their relationship, which is vital for the survival and normal development of the infant. Extensive research on bonding during the postnatal period has shown that bonding is an ongoing process that is apparent immediately after birth and throughout infancy and childhood.[9] With the advent of ultrasound imaging in pregnancy, reactions of the mother to prenatal visualization of the baby have been described.[5,6,10,13,14,16] Although visualization is essentially a reaction in the mother, and not an interaction between the mother and fetus, many observers of ultrasound examinations have speculated that the visualization process facilitates earlier and stronger bonding with the child by increasing the mother's recognition of and attachment to the baby before birth.

The importance of a strong maternal-child bond cannot be overemphasized. According to Klaus, the bond that is formed between mother and baby is the "well-spring for all the infant's subsequent attachments and is the formative relationship in the course of which the child develops a sense of himself. Throughout his lifetime, the strength and character of this attachment will influence the quality of all future bonds to other individuals."[9] A weak or dysfunctional bond may be associated with emotional and physical child abuse, neglect, and abandonment, all of which are major problems in our society. It has recently been postulated that prenatal bonding may promote prenatal care and the mother's adherence to health regimens beneficial to the pregnancy.[16] For many reasons it is important for sonographers to encourage prenatal bonding and promote protocols that positively influence bonding.

Studies of Bonding and Ultrasound Fetal Imaging

Postnatal bonding has been measured by quantifying physical interactions and communication patterns between mother and child. A reliable measure of prenatal attachment has not been developed. In normal pregnancies, there is a body of studies and anecdotal information that suggests that the ultrasound examination at least transiently affects the mother's perception of the fetus. In a small sample of patients Holland found that the mother was less likely to characterize her baby as smaller or weaker than other babies and rated her baby as more active in postscan questionnaires than in prescan questionnaires.[6] Geisler found that 71% of the women in her survey indicated that being able to see the baby on the screen made them feel "closer to the baby or more maternal."[5] Milne and Rich have observed mothers during an examination and studied the process of recognizing the baby and the excitement of the mothers. The same researchers observed anecdotally that several women continued to mentally visualize their babies as they had been observed on the ultrasound instrument screen weeks after the examination.[13]

Kohn and colleagues observed a greater sense of attachment to the fetus among patients who received ultrasound examinations that included a good deal of feedback by the sonographer.[10] Reading and Cox assessed maternal attitudes toward pregnancy by adjective analysis. They found prescan and postscan differences and more positive attitudes in the group who received the greatest feedback from the sonographers.[14] In a later study, however, Reading and Cox could not confirm a relationship between ultrasound feedback conditions and attitudes toward the pregnancy or the baby.[15]

In another study of pregnant women, Reading and Cox document better adherence to health-related regimens, particularly the advice to stop smoking, when the advice is associated with an ultrasound examination.[16] A group of Swedish researchers found that women who had sonograms delivered larger babies, on average, and that the weight differences were most pronounced among women who at their first visit reported being smokers.[17] The inference is that the sonography enhanced adherence to smoking advice, which resulted in larger babies. This study is cited as evidence of a beneficial effect for routine scanning in all pregnancies.

Psychological Responses of Pregnant Patients

Knowledge of the normal psychological progression of pregnancy is not only interesting but very important to the development of communication strategies for sonographers. The optimal strategy may be one that serves to reduce patient anxiety and enhance attachment to the fetus. Since the major anxieties of pregnancy change during its course, it follows that appropriate and supportive interaction strategies may vary throughout the mother's pregnancy. Sonographers' ability to discern that stage and to adapt their communication to individual needs—or to the particular concerns of that pregnancy—may be heightened by attention to the psychological process of pregnancy.

In a previous review article a graphic model (Fig. 34-1) characterizing the psychological process of pregnancy was presented.[12] The base of the model represents conditions with which the mother enters pregnancy, variables such as age, parity, socioeconomic status, culture, previous mothering experience, and family support systems, which affect her adaptation to pregnancy. Major sources of anxiety during pregnancy are also listed. Activities typical of each trimester of pregnancy are within a triangular section of the model. The activities express the paths for resolving the underlying anxieties of pregnancy. It is hypothesized that through supportive activities, the anxieties of pregnancy are reduced and attachment to the fetus can grow. In the model anxieties, activities, and attachment typical of each trimester are listed.

FIRST TRIMESTER

During the first trimester of pregnancy, anxiety is related to acceptance of the reality of pregnancy and normal ambiguity toward the pregnancy. Teenagers have difficulty accepting the reality of pregnancy because they have not fully accepted their womanhood. Teenagers often perceive themselves more as children than as adults and so have difficulty acknowledging a pregnancy. Older patients generally are capable of accepting the reality of pregnancy but may deny ambiguous feelings toward it. Even under optimal conditions, when the pregnancy was planned and actively sought, women can expect to feel some ambiguity. Pregnancy entails a major commitment and life change for women and is therefore greeted with both positive and negative expectations. Psychologically healthy women accept, express, and share doubts and fears related to the pregnancy with support persons. Such women resolve their ambiguity by making a decision either to retain or terminate the pregnancy and then act on that decision.

Remarks that express disbelief, excitement, disappointment, and worry are typical during the first trimester. Sonographers working with these patients may encourage them to accept the reality of the pregnancy and openly explore their own feelings about the fetus. The ultrasound image, when it is seen by the patient, is powerful evidence of the reality of pregnancy. Connecting the image to the patient's body by verbally pointing out the area within which the fetus lies further emphasizes this

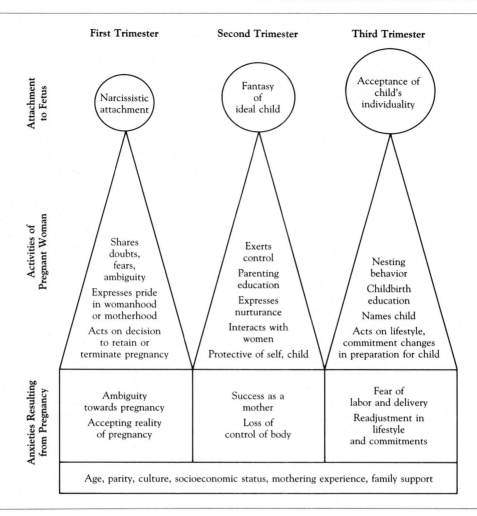

FIGURE 34-1. A model of the psychological process of pregnancy. Variables that may impact adaptation to pregnancy are presented at the base of the model. Anxieties common to pregnancy (squares) may be resolved by activities (triangles). Through such resolution maternal-fetal bonding processes (circles) are enhanced.

reality. The sonographer may be a supportive and nonjudgmental listener to positive or negative expressions concerning the pregnancy. Ambiguity is normal, and the more openly it is expressed, the more quickly it can be resolved.

Women initially attach to the fetus because it is part of themselves. They do not perceive of it as a separate person. Traditionally it has been assumed that recognition of the fetus as a separate individ-

ual begins at quickening, when the mother first perceives fetal motion. With ultrasound imaging it is possible that this recognition of individuality begins when the mother first sees the fetal movement within, which may occur before quickening.

SECOND TRIMESTER

Along with the perception of the fetus as a separate person anxiety related to the woman's ability to mother arises. Sonographers are often asked by patients about their own children or their own parenting experiences. This is a natural expression of the need to explore mothering alternatives. Parenting classes are often helpful at this stage. Along with concern about her mothering ability a strong protectiveness toward herself and toward the fetus develops in most women. This may be expressed to the sonographer as concern about the safety of the ultrasound procedure or concern about adequate visualization of all parts of the fetus. The continuing growth of the fetus creates in the woman a sense of a loss of control over her own body. Anxiety related to this loss of control may lead to activities that express the desire to control the environment, herself, or others. Rearranging furniture, changing diets, or beginning exercise programs are examples of external efforts to control.

Second trimester is the ideal time to talk with patients about changes in diets or habits that may benefit the fetus. The desire to control and the increasing sense of protection toward the fetus lead many women to incorporate advice regarding changes in diet or smoking habits. If a sonographer is uncomfortable providing this type of patient education, a poster in the ultrasound laboratory about healthy eating or other habits might be effective. Such posters are available from many sources, including March of Dimes, the American Lung Association, and the American Dietetics Association.

Attachment to the fetus may grow rapidly during the second trimester. The mother is generally feeling well, the sickness of early pregnancy has subsided, and the heaviness of later pregnancy has not yet begun. The mother perceives the fetus as a separate individual and often an individual endowed with characteristics of the mother's ideal child.

Third Trimester

During the third trimester anxiety is related to fear of labor and delivery. The need to readjust lifestyles or relationships with others in order to create more time for the new baby may cause anxiety as well. "Nesting," or nursery preparation, is undertaken and professional commitments may be reduced. Childbirth education classes taken at this time may alleviate some of the anxiety related to labor and delivery. It is helpful for obstetric sonographers to have some knowledge of labor alternatives in order to answer patients' questions.

Attachment to the fetus continues to grow but less rapidly than in the second trimester. The "ideal child" is by now kicking quite hard, making the mother feel heavy and uncomfortable, and often interrupting her sleep. The mother's perceptions of the fetus contain positive and negative elements, and the child is increasingly perceived as a separate individual with unique personal characteristics. Mothers who did not want to know the sex of the child earlier may change their minds during the third trimester. Others, of course, do not. Many mothers settle on a name or names at this point in pregnancy and if the sex is known may refer to the baby by name. The perception of separateness and fetal individuality that develops at this stage promotes the development of an optimal mother-child relationship after the birth.

Sonographer-Patient Interactions

It is apparent from the studies cited above that ultrasound scanning may have a positive effect on pregnancy and that this effect may be influenced by the communication style of the sonographer during the examination. It is also apparent that interactions that minimize anxiety and enhance attachment may vary somewhat from trimester to trimester. Communication may also differ depending on the specific needs of that pregnancy or the results of the examination.

Sonographers have been leaders in developing strategies to make the ultrasound examination a positive experience for expectant mothers. In the literature and at national meetings anecdotal and researched communication strategies to lessen maternal anxiety before the examination and improve maternal understanding of the examination have been shared. There remains widespread controversy and confusion about what feedback is appropriate for obstetric patients. Sonographers are caught between institutional needs to schedule more patients, marketers' demands to cater to patients' requests and produce videotapes and images for them to take home, and lawyers' warnings to be realistic and not overly reassuring. It is no wonder that in the midst of this complexity there is confusion.

COMMUNICATION BASICS

It is generally agreed that the approach of the sonographer working with obstetric patients at any stage of pregnancy should include but not necessarily be limited to the following:

Prior maternal knowledge of and consent to the presence of nonessential personnel, whose number is kept to a minimum.

An intent to share with parents, either during an examination or shortly thereafter, the information derived.

An offer of choice about viewing the fetus.

An offer of choice about learning the sex of the fetus if such information becomes available.[3]

Additional guidelines first suggested in *Medical Ultrasound*[11] and subsequently modified are listed at right. The International Childbirth Education Association (ICEA), in a position paper on diagnostic ultrasound, discusses "family-centered aspects" of ultrasound examinations and includes several suggestions for sonographer communication with the patient.[8]

In an article on legal malpractice risks in radiology,[4] Dr. Edward Bartlett, president of a consulting firm that specializes in finding communications solutions to the problem of malpractice risk, contends that most malpractice suits can be attributed to lack of communication and are thus preventable. "We have to look at that 79% of cases filed that were the result of temporary, emotional and minor injuries and ask why people go to the bother of filing that claim when the chances are they won't recover a penny through the litigation process." Anger resulting from misconceptions about what the procedure will yield or what it entails may prompt many malpractice claims, Bartlett suggests. Similarly if a patient is frustrated with one aspect of care and there is a negative outcome, the patient may blame the outcome on those who frustrated her.

Communication important to legally safeguarding sonographers is communication that facilitates the following ends:

COMMUNICATION GUIDELINES FOR OBSTETRIC ULTRASONOGRAPHY

Dos

Do try to maintain an easy flow of conversation throughout the examination.

Do encourage the patient to talk.

Do ask for the patient's version of the referral reason. This will give them the security of knowing that you are addressing their perceived need.

Do point out normal anatomy when asked.

Do discuss or clarify information that the patient has already been given by the physician.

Do be firm about information you will and will not discuss.

Do know laboratory guidelines relative to revealing obvious diagnoses.

Do be supportive and honest about invasive procedures.

Do strive to maintain a positive attitude. Since we do not know for certain the outcome during any examination, we should strive to think positively in order not to alarm the patient.

Don'ts

Don't be falsely reassuring.

Don't compare physicians or recommend other procedures.

Don't discuss the diagnosis of the current examination.

Don't play dumb.

Don't express negative feelings about your ability, your job, or your day.

Don't talk about other patients or other staff members.

Don't be afraid to touch the patient.

The patient leaves feeling that he or she has been treated in a competent, professional, and empathetic manner.

The patient is not surprised by any aspect of the ultrasound procedures, the sonographer's care, or the possible outcomes.

Pertinent patient communications shared with the sonographer are in turn shared with those on the medical team responsible for acting on that information.

ACTIVITIES THAT MAY PROMOTE BONDING

The goal of interactions between the sonographer and the patient is to reduce the patient's anxiety and promote fetal attachment. It can be assumed that pointing out fetal anatomy and allowing the mother to watch the fetus move enhance attachment. Connecting the image to the patient's body by pointing out where the fetus is enhances bonding to the fetus as part of oneself. Spending additional time to visualize the face and holding the transducer in one place to watch the fetus yawn, suck, or shift positions may be a very memorable experience for the mother. Linda Carter-Jessop has suggested teaching mothers in late pregnancy to rub their baby's back, talk to it, and otherwise interact with it when it is active.[2] This is a strategy that sonographers could adopt as well.

The careless use of terminology (i.e., *breech*, the placenta is not *right*, checking for intrauterine growth *retardation*) may increase anxiety.[1] Similarly, other interactions that alarm or anger the mother may interfere with the attachment process during the examination. It is essential that anxiety-provoking comments be carefully avoided during obstetric examinations.

ABNORMAL PREGNANCIES, ADOPTIONS, AND TERMINATIONS

Specific guidelines for communication during examinations involving abnormal fetuses have not been developed. The guidelines above relate to these examinations as well, however, and during the initial examination it is important for the sonographer to be firm about information that can and cannot be discussed without playing dumb or sowing doubts about his or her skill or the care the patient is receiving. A child who spends a lot of time in the hospital, who is handicapped, or who has special needs is a child at greater risk for neglect and abuse than are more typical children.[7] Once the mother has been informed of the diagnosis bonding activities during the examination may be more important than usual. In follow-up examinations, as in all examinations, it is important to ask the mother whether she wants to see the screen and to follow the mother's lead in determining how much information she is ready to accept. In general parents preparing for the birth of an abnormal child need every opportunity to acknowledge and accept that child. Unless the abnormality is unequivocally lethal the sonographer should not hesitate to point out portions of the baby if the mother seems interested and has been given basic information about the diagnosis. Allowing the mother to observe any normal activities of the baby may help her attach and better prepare her for the challenges she and the family will face after the birth.

Sonographers should ask each pregnant patient whether she wishes to see the screen before beginning the ultrasound examination. This is particularly important in situations in which the mother is giving up the child for adoption, a termination is planned, or a lethal anomaly is present. If the mother indicates that she wants to see the screen the sonographer should allow her to do so and should answer any questions that arise during the examination and that fall within these guidelines. Spending time on bonding activities, unless this is specifically requested by the mother, is inappropriate.

The evidence of prenatal bonding mandates continued development by sonographers of appropriate, realistic, and efficient communication during all obstetric examinations. Sonographers' interactions with pregnant patients are as varied as the individuals involved and often challenge the best instincts. Studying and optimizing the value of their communication and creating additional guidelines for patients who face adoptions, terminations, or abnormalities is an important role for obstetric sonographers.

Future Research

There is no evidence that the transient impact on the mother of the obstetric ultrasound examination relates to long-term beneficial effects. There may be negative psychological effects of ultrasound imaging in abnormal pregnancies or in mothers prior to termination of pregnancy. The present state of knowledge in these and other areas is largely speculative or anecdotal. Sonographers are in an optimal position to study prenatal bonding. Some of the questions that need to be answered are in the NIH Consensus Conference monograph[3]:

Are there incidences of deleterious effects of ultrasound imagery on maternal perception of the fetus?

Can ultrasound imaging produce a positive effect on patients who are highly anxious prenatally?

Would a positive effect on anxiety have clinical significance as measured by pregnancy outcome and child development?

How many women are receiving prenatal gender information through ultrasound imagery?

Does prenatal knowledge of fetal gender affect prenatal attachment or anxiety?

What is the appropriate role of sonography personnel in relation to patients' image perceptions?

Is attachment of the mother to the fetus enhanced by ultrasound imagery?

If enhancement occurs, should it be encouraged in special situations such as high-risk preganancies, terminations, or adoption?

The answers to these questions and others may be learned by careful observation and inquiry by sonographers.

Sonographers and consumers have long been aware that ultrasound imaging is not just another diagnostic tool used in pregnancy. The social and psychological ramifications of ultrasound imaging are enormous. The potential for its therapeutic use in stimulating bonding is largely unexplored. The possibility that sonographers may be able to use instruments not only to diagnose but to help mothers with a poor bonding history, teenagers who deny the reality of pregnancy, and others, carries with it an awesome responsibility to observe, to study, and to learn more about these complex interactions.

References

1. Boyce K. Patient's reactions to medical terminology. Student Research Paper, University of Oklahoma Department of Radiologic Technology. 1983.

2. Carter-Jessop L. Promoting maternal attachment through prenatal intervention. Maternal Child Nurs. 1981; 6:107–112.

3. Consensus Development Conference. The Use of Diagnostic Ultrasound Imaging in Pregnancy. NIH Publication No. 84-667. Washington, DC: US Government Printing Office; 1984; 173–174.

4. Dakins D. Radiologists at greater legal risk as role in patient care expands. Diagn Imaging. 1987; 9:8.75–83.

5. Geisler D. The effects of ultrasound examinations on maternal-infant bonding. Student Research Paper, State University of New York Health Science Center at Brooklyn Department of Radiologic Sciences and Technology, 1987.

6. Holland M. Evidence of bonding between a mother and fetus during an ultrasound examination. Student Research Paper, University of Oklahoma Department of Radiologic Technology, 1988.

7. Hunner R. Child abuse and the special-needs child. Presented at the 7th National Conference on Child Abuse and Neglect, Chicago, Illinois, 1985.

8. International Childbirth Education Association Position Paper. Diagnostic Ultrasound in Obstetrics. ICEA News, 1983; 22:2.

9. Klaus MH, Kennell JH. Maternal-Infant Bonding. St. Louis: CV Mosby; 1976:3.

10. Kohn CL, Nelson A, Weiner S. Gravidas responses to real time ultrasound fetal image. J ObGyn Nursing. 1980; 9:77–80.

11. Lea JH. Educationally speaking: The value of role playing in sonography education. Med Ultrasound. 1983; 7:81–82.

12. Lea JH. Psychosocial progression through normal pregnancy, a model for sonographer-patient interaction. J Diagn Med Sonogr. 1985; 1:2.

13. Milne LS, Rich OJ. Cognitive and affective aspects of the responses of pregnant women to sonography. Maternal Child Nurs. 1981; 10:15–39.

14. Reading AE, Cox DN. The effects of ultrasound examination on maternal anxiety levels. J Behavior Med. 1982; 5:237–247.

15. Reading AE, Cox DN. Psychological changes over the course of pregnancy: A study of attitudes toward the fetus/neonate. Health Psychol. 1984; 3:211–221.

16. Reading AE, Cambell S, Cox D, et al. Health beliefs and health care behavior in pregnancy. Psychol Med. 1982; 12:379–383.

17. Sonograms Are Eye-Openers. U.S. News and World Report. October 3, 1988.

CHAPTER 35

Computer Software
for Obstetric Sonography

TERRY J. DuBose

As sonographic evaluation of the human fetus has progressed over the past 20 years, the numbers of parameters studied and of calculations that use those parameters have steadily increased. Today sonographers can easily spend up to an hour doing calculations and charting the data from a single obstetric sonographic examination. The advantage of using a computer to automate these routine calculations and charts is obvious. Computers can perform very complex computations and allow easy comparison of multiple fetal parameters. Not only does a computer allow more complex calculations than are possible with a hand-held calculator, but the computer also produces more accurate results almost instantly. As an added advantage, computers can store and quickly recall results of prior sonographic examinations for easy comparison in serial growth studies.

Beyond making faster and more accurate sonographic calculations, computers are perfect for maintaining patient records, creating typewritten (word-processed) reports, and numerous other tedious tasks. This chapter is intended to help the sonographer or sonologist who is not familiar with personal computers (PCs) to begin using these labor-, energy-, and time-saving instruments in daily practice.

Hardware

Computer hardware, as the name implies, is any computer equipment that is "hard" (i.e., that can be physically touched or seen). A minimally configured PC usually consists of the following hardware:

1. The computer itself, which is a box containing various configurations of chips, wires, circuit boards, power supply (electrical transformer), electrical connectors, and disk drives.
2. The monitor is a cathode ray tube on which the user can observe what the computer is doing.
3. Of the many different input devices, the keyboard is most common, but many computers use a mouse (electromechanical pointing device) in addition to the keyboard.
4. Disk drives are of two basic types: with removable and nonremovable disks. On the disks the computer stores (and from them retrieves) the bits and bytes of information with which the computer works.
5. A printer allows the information processed by the computer to be printed on paper. (Printed information is called hard copy.)

These hardware items are not the only things that can be interfaced and used with a computer, but they are the basic components required for a PC. It should also be noted that all of these devices come in a variety of types and configurations. The various forms of hardware must be compatible with the computer with which they are to be used.

The computer contains a central processing unit (CPU), a chip that is the "brain" of the computer.

The CPU is almost invisible to the user. It is "almost invisible" because the CPU determines how fast the computer operates and how much data it can access. For the purpose of most novice users any CPU is fine as long as it works. As one becomes more sophisticated and starts doing complex numeric functions, graphics, and multitasking, larger, faster CPUs are more appropriate.

The computer also contains many other chips, most notably the memory chips, or random-access memory (RAM). The RAM is where the computer puts the information (programs and files) that it reads from the disks. It is in the RAM that the computer works on data. Some programs may require that the entire file be able to fit into the RAM in order for it to work. These RAM-based programs are usually very fast but can use only limited file sizes. As a general rule one should obtain as much RAM as possible when purchasing a new system. This is because memory chips are now relatively cheap and as a user becomes more experienced the tendency is to want more sophisticated and larger software programs, which require more RAM.

Other programs are able to read part of a file from disk into RAM, do some processing of the data, put the partially processed data back on the disk, and then read and process another batch of data. In this way these programs are able to use a relatively small RAM to work with very large files. These disk-based programs can work with huge files. They are limited only by the amount of disk memory available but are slower because they must read and copy each batch of data to a mechanical disk. This trade-off of file size and operation speed must be considered when planning a system.

Other chips in the computer with which the user must be concerned are usually on "boards," collections of chips and supporting electrical hardware on a printed circuit board that fits into the computer and enables the basic computer to do a variety of special tasks. The most common board is the video controller board, sometimes called the video card or video adaptor, into which the monitor and printer are plugged. The video board controls the computer output to the video monitor and printer; the cards must be compatible with both the computer and the monitor type. The basic video card allows the computer to use a mono-chrome monitor, usually white, amber, or green on black, in a text mode only. More advanced video controllers allow monochrome or color graphics of varying degrees of resolution and numbers of color selections. Some software programs require certain types of graphics cards to work properly. Many more expensive video cards allow input direct from video sources. This direct video input ability holds great potential for all medical imaging modalities that use video, especially sonography.

Some add-in cards allow the computer to communicate by telephone, do desk-top publishing, expand RAM, network with other computers, and even do voice translation for direct voice-typing functions. The coming years will give us a great many useful, new, and powerful functions from computers that are physically very small.

The computer keyboard, much like a typewriter with many additional keys, usually plugs into the back of the computer. I say usually, because some keyboards use infrared light to communicate with the computer instead of being plugged into it. (The IBM PC Junior is this type.) A mouse is another type of input device. Mice are usually associated with Apple Mackintosh PCs, but they are available for all types. Personal style determines whether a user will like a mouse. With a mouse the user does not type in commands but uses a cursor to point at desired commands on the monitor. Other types of input devices are track balls, light pens, touch pads, and many more too numerous (and infrequently used) to include in this discussion.

The most common computer drives use floppy diskettes. A vast majority of software programs and data files are sold and transported from one computer to another on these removable diskettes. Since IBM introduced the XT class of computer, nonremovable (hard) disks have become more common. Hard disks are precision, high-speed disks that can store huge amounts of data. Because of the great precision required by hard disks, most cannot be removed from the drive.

The hard drive should be used for software programs and frequently used data files such as permanent patient records, periodic, cumulative reports, and often-used form letters. Floppy diskettes should be used to store small, infrequently needed data files such as letters, memos, and temporary spread sheets. If a user makes a habit of storing all data files on the hard disk, it eventually fills up with unimportant memos and the like. As the hard drive becomes full it performs more slowly, making it difficult to find frequently used files. If letter files and the like are stored on floppies, it is easier to find old files by date, and the diskettes can be reused when desired. In the case of obstetric patient records, it is probably best to have two cross-referenced files. One would be the permanent patient files on hard disk (with backup), which would refer to individual pregnancy records on floppy disks. The pregnancy records are needed frequently only for about 9 months.

General Software

OPERATING SYSTEMS

The computer hardware is useless without a set of instructions to tell it when to receive data from the keyboard or from the disk drive, when to send data to the monitor or the printer, and when to do the myriad other tasks a computer does. These instructions are called software, or computer programs. Software in general is of two types, the operating system and application programs.

An operating system, or disk operating system (DOS), is a set of instructions that all computers must use to control the hardware. The DOS works directly with the hardware, whereas the applications programs use the DOS to control the hardware indirectly.

A user need not know a lot about the operating systems of PCs in order to do useful work. This can be compared to the carburetor of an automobile: Drivers don't have to know exactly how it works or how to fix the carburetor to drive a car, but they must be able to tell when the carburetor needs a new supply of gasoline and how to make that supply of gasoline available. The user must know how to load, or boot, the operating system into the computer; how to use certain rudimentary commands such as how to format a disk to make it usable; how to copy files from one disk to another; and how to backup their work. Backing up work is one of the first things a user should learn. A power failure, no matter how brief, can wipe out several hours' work, or a hard disk containing important data may fail, and return the message "Read fault error. Abort,

Retry, Ignore:."!! The system should also be protected against static electricity and electric line surges by proper grounding and a surge protector hooked between it and the power line.

Applications software is what most people refer to as a computer program; examples are word processors, spread sheets, and data bases. Word processors turn the computer into a sophisticated typewriter; spread sheets are displays of rows and columns for doing numeric functions and recording data; and data bases are rows and columns of textual information such as a medical record or phone book. These applications programs allow the user to work more efficiently and are very useful in medical office practices.

COMPUTER SYSTEM FOR OBSTETRIC ULTRASOUND PRACTICE

A good obstetric computer system consists of a large data base of all basic patient records. A hard disk with backup is recommended. This data base may include, as a minimum, identifying patient information such as name, date of birth, address, phone number, office file number, referring physician (last referral only), the last five examinations performed according to dates, and other pertinent information. All of the word-processed reports of each examination should be kept on floppy disks for 30 days, and archives maintained in standard film and paper files. After 5 years, all archives should be transferred to microfilm. Hopefully, within the not-too-far distant future, sonographic images as well as all other medical records can be digitized and saved on optical disks capable of storing larger quantities of data than the storage devices that are common today.

It is critically important to back up important changes to data files and programs that are kept on the hard drive. These important files should be saved on floppies or special back-up systems each time changes are made and before closing down the computer. It is helpful to use the same floppy to back up the same file each time, unless you need a record of changes, because eventually, the numbers of floppies becomes more difficult to manage than a full hard disk. Computers allow you to create huge numbers of files in a relatively short time. Managing these large electronic file systems requires some forethought and time.

Specific Hardware and Software for Sonographic Fetal Analysis

HISTORICAL PERSPECTIVE

Several computer programs are designed to analyze sonographic fetal measurements, and many sonography machines now contain limited software to do simple analysis. The following discussion should by no means be considered comprehensive. Since new software is being designed constantly it is almost impossible to keep up with all new developments.

One of the earliest public discussions of computer use for analysis of sonographic images was Brinkley, Moritz, and Baker's "A Technique for Imaging Three-Dimensional Structures and Computing Their Volumes Using Non-Parallel Ultrasonic Sector Scans,"[1] but the first presentation of the specific use of PCs for the analysis of obstetric sonographic data may have been the lectures by Dr. Christopher Merritt and the late Dr. Charles Hohler in 1983.[2,3] Hohler's great interest in computers was very encouraging to those working on programs for use in the field of diagnostic sonography. He provided a list of available programs for obstetric analysis, many of which have now been replaced by newer programs.

OBSTETRIC PROGRAMS FOR PERSONAL COMPUTERS

Software for fetal analysis can be thought of as two types: macro programs, which run under larger applications programs such as dBASE III+, FrameWork II, or Lotus 123. These are the control programs for the macro, not to be confused with the DOS. (All programs require the DOS.)

Macros are actually collections of individual commands that are executed automatically when certain keys are pressed. These can be quite large collections of commands, and very often macros are almost as large as or larger than the applications program under which they operate. Many macro-type programs are available to do many jobs: keeping appointment calendars, balancing checkbooks, analyzing fetal sonographic data.

Several factors should be considered before purchasing a macro program. Users should know they must also purchase and learn to use the applications program (a large data base, spread sheet, or word processing program or an integrated program that does all of these things). Such programs are complex and relatively expensive; most popular programs cost $200 to $700 (USA, 1988) in addition to the macro cost. The macro makes using the applications program easier for specific jobs such as entering fetal measurements, calculating circumferences, and estimating dates, but the user must learn to use the applications program as well as the macro. Many people feel that the user does not really need to learn the applications program to use the macro, but it is recommended that a user understand the applications program. If there is ever a problem, pressing the wrong key or wrong sequence of keys can cause the user to be "dropped out" of the macro back into the applications program. Only with an understanding of the applications program is the user able to recover or retrieve the data. Learning complex programs is time consuming, and the macro must also be learned. The advantages of macros are that once you have learned the applications program, it can be used for other jobs. Newer, more powerful ones are being released every day, but fetal analysis macros may not be available for all of them. It is usually safer to choose popular programs, because it is easier to obtain help with problems when using well-known programs. Eventually, the tried and proven programs from major software houses will be improved.

Stand-alone programs are applications programs designed to do a specific task, in this case analyze fetal measurements. They do not require another applications or control program to operate, only the DOS that all programs require. The advantage of stand-alone programs is their ease of use: there are no other applications programs to learn. The set of commands is small and very specific because the program does only the one job for which it was designed. Stand-alone programs are usually simpler and much faster than macros and should not drop information if the wrong key is pressed. There are also no hidden costs, such as purchasing and learning the applications program.

The disadvantages of stand-alone programs are that they do only one job and generally are not user modifiable. (Changes can be introduced only by the author in the source code {programming language version} and recompiled for the new version.)

The programs for sonographic fetal analysis, both stand-alones and macros, are being updated and changed continually, though not as fast as more general-purpose software. Some that are currently available are listed below:

ABACUS OB: Stand-alone application, programmable computer (comes with program).
Solomon Technology Corporation
2405 E. Southern Avenue, Suite #10
Tempe, AZ 85282

BASIC BABY II: Stand-alone application for IBM-type PCs.
Mind's Eyes Images
3606 Grooms Street
Austin, TX 78705

OB Scan System: Stand-alone application for Radio Shack pocket computers.
Orange Research & Development, Inc.
428 Gregory Avenue
Wilmette, IL 60091

Digisonics OB-110XD/OB-500XD: Stand-alone application for Apple IIe- and IBM-type PCs.

Digisonics, Inc.
3701 Kirby Drive
Houston, TX 77098

OBUS–OB Ultrasound: Stand-alone application for IBM-type PCs.
Decision Technology, Inc.
241 Perkins Street, Suite A601
Boston, MA 02130

OURS–OB Ultrasound Reporting Software: Lotus 123 macro on IBM-type PCs.
Mrs. I. Cunningham
Springer-Verlag
175 Fifth Avenue
New York, NY 10010

Because all software tends to go through a succession of changes or versions, details of the above programs are not provided. The reader can write to the addresses provided for complete information. The following worksheet is suggested for requesting information.

Worksheet for Evaluating Software for Obstetric Sonography

Program name: _____

Program cost? _____ Shipping? _____

Stand-alone application? _____ Macro? _____

If it is a macro, under what applications program does it work?
_____

Hardware requirements:
What type of personal computer? _____

Operating system? _____ Minimum RAM? _____

Number of disk drives? Floppies _____ Hard disks _____

Does it require special graphics adaptors? _____

Type of printer support? _____

Other special requirements? _____

_____

Integrating the PC and the Sonography Machine

Almost all PCs use a video display that looks like a television and is called a monitor (it is not a TV). Although a monitor is similar to a television video display, a television cannot be used as a PC display unless the computer has a special "composite" or TV-type video output and hookup.

If you have a computer that has a normal television video output, it can probably be plugged into your sonography machine and computer reports can then be recorded on a multiformat camera along with other sonographic images for documentation along with the patient's other medical records. The image of the BASIC BABY II reports in Figure 17-2 was recorded by this method.

Essentially, this method plugs the composite video from the computer into the sonography machine's video cassette recorder (VCR) input jack. Because most sonographic laboratories also want to use a VCR to record dynamic processes, such as the fetal heart beating, a video switching device is used to switch the video signal from the computer or VCR video output to the sonography video input. Either the computer or VCR video can then be viewed on the system's display monitor and recorded by multiformat camera. Using this system avoids the added expense of a printer if a paper copy of the computer output is not required.

Figure 35-1 is a schematic diagram of how this computer–VCR–sonography machine hookup was done to record the image in Figure 17-2. The video switches described are available from many electronic supply houses for under $10, but the buyer must be sure that the computer has an output for a standard television display. If it does not, some computer manufacturers offer an add-in graphics board or card that provides the composite video output. Such boards may cost $200 or more.

The interconnecting wires will cost a little more, and the purchaser must be sure that the connector types are matched to the type of jacks from each piece of equipment. These connectors may be RCA, BNC, or standard phono-type jacks, depending on the equipment. Those who feel uncomfortable making this type of electrical connection to an expensive piece of equipment should seek the advice of an electrician or their maintenance personnel.

Obstetrical Calculation Software Packages Available in Diagnostic Ultrasound Scanners

Many currently available sonography machines contain built-in, or on-board, software for fetal analysis. Most of this software consists of various fetal parameter tables (data bases) or linear regression formulas that calculate a fetal age from some fetal measurement. Some of these calculations are contained in "firmware" and cannot be changed by the user. Other machines contain both software and firmware, so that the user can enter her or his own measurements for various parameters or can use the machine's preset charts for determining fetal age. The number and sophistication of fetal parameters available in a sonographic system should be considered when purchasing new equipment.

Any machine to be used for obstetric work should possess, as a minimum, the following calculation capabilities:

A. Tables for making fetal age calculations from these parameters:
   1. Biparietal diameter (BPD)
   2. Transverse head circumference (HC)
   3. Femur length (FL)
   4. Abdominal circumference (AC)
   5. At least two tables into which the user may enter other fetal age calculation charts.
B. Ratio calculations to determine fetal proportionality:
   1. BPD/fronto-occipital diameter
   2. AC/transverse HC or transverse HC/AC. (Other ratios undoubtedly will be available in machines of the future.)
C. Estimation of fetal weight using either the Warsof-Shepard or the Hadlock formulas. At least 13 different sonographic methods for computing estimated fetal weight exist. The Hadlock formula, which uses FL, AC, and BPD or transverse HC, is slightly more accurate and is well-suited to computerization, but not to hand-held–calculator manipulation.

Machines that accept user-entered charts usually call for the user to enter the weeks (most often weeks from the last menstrual period) and the corresponding parameter measurement for each week. The machine's computer puts this chart into a

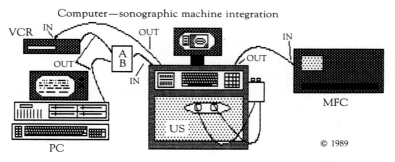

Computer—sonographic machine integration

IN and OUT refer to video connections.

© 1989

FIGURE 35-1. Integration of a PC and sonographic machine. In the above illustration the VCR, computer (PC), sonographic machine (US), and multiformat camera (MFC) are labeled. The video cables are labeled IN and OUT at the appropriate ends. In the above hook-up, if the A cable on the video switch is active (closed) then the VCR playback signal will be sent to the MFC via the US. If the B cable is active the PC video output will be sent to the MFC via the US.

memory; then, each time a measurement is taken the user can call up that chart to calculate the fetal age for a given parameter. The chart needs to be entered only once and can be changed at any time. The process of entering a chart usually takes about 15 minutes. User-entered charts are very useful for research or special populations.

If their sonography system has a built-in fetal dating capability, sonographers should be sure they understand how the measurements were taken to estimate the fetal age and should use the same methods to measure any fetuses that will be dated using that system. The manufacturer should supply this information with the machine.

If the sonographer has any questions or doubts about the accuracy of fetal ages from a system or from any fetal analysis software, both the measurement methods and the accuracy may be tested by using measurements from a standard chart. Most sonographers have a fetal age chart with which they are familiar, a BPD age chart for instance. When they get a new system that has a BPD age chart, or if there are questions about its accuracy, they should test their tried and true chart against the machine: The electronic calipers are used to measure a distance that is on the age chart. If the machine returns the same fetal age as the chart

shows, all is in order. In this way all fetal parameters for which the sonography machine contains age charts can be tested. If a different age is returned, the sonographer needs to investigate the source of the difference: whose chart is being used, how the measurements were taken (outer-to-inner or outer-to-outer edge). If this investigation does not reveal the source of the difference, then the machine should not be used to calculate fetal ages until the technical representative of the manufacturer is contacted for an answer or to make the appropriate data base changes.

Some machines are starting to do complex analysis of fetal parameters such as composite menstrual ages from multiple fetal parameters and ratios for the comparison of various parameters. These on-board fetal analysis programs are different from manufacturer to manufacturer and change with almost every new generation of machine.

THE FUTURE

One of the best new features is the ability to continuously save a sequence of the original digital images and replay them and take measurements. Although this does not relate directly to the measurement or computation of fetal size and age, it does make that process much easier. This save-replay feature constantly records the last 4 to 6 seconds of real-time ultrasound images. When the image is frozen operators can run the last few seconds of real-time backward or forward as slow or as fast as they wish, stopping at any time to take measurements or to obtain hard copy. This feature is important for difficult examinations of patients who cannot sustain suspended respiration or of active fetuses. The advantage of the save-replay feature in studying the fetal heart is obvious.

Another new feature allows one sonography machine to communicate images to another by telephone. This ability is already available for many PCs, and as it is added to more sonography machines it facilitates second opinions and consultations at great distances.

A feature that would be useful is a complete personal computer inside the sonography machine, which would allow users to select their own software package to be run for fetal analysis. These computers should have sufficient memory and capabilities for the user to do word processing beyond simple words and phrases and to be able to save data and images to disk or tape memories. Onboard PCs would also allow internal data bases for all patients, for quick entry and archiving. Such data bases would be extremely useful for case load counts by examination type, sonographer, and diagnosis, and for teaching files and follow-up examinations.

Suggestions and Recommendations for New PC Users

1. Learn something of the disk operating system (DOS or OS/2 for IBMs and clones, The System on Apples). At a minimum the user should know:
   a. How to start the computer and boot the system.
   b. How to format a new diskette (be careful, or you may wipe out data).
   c. How to copy or back up files from one disk to another so that when a disk goes bad all your work and data will not be lost.
   d. How to create, change, and use directories and subdirectories, if using a hard disk.

2. Be sure to establish a routine back-up procedure for your programs and files.
3. Purchase as much RAM as possible.
4. Consider getting a hard disk; they are fast and convenient to use.
5. If you have a hard disk, do not abandon diskettes for data files. Filling the hard disk with many, unimportant, small files is a mistake that wastes memory, and could result in loss of data and programs.
6. Give your computer filing system some forethought. Computers allow rapid creation of huge numbers of files, which can become very difficult to manage. Computer housekeeping takes some time.
7. If you have a problem, refer to the computer and software manuals. You cannot operate them by telepathy, and punching random keys will not solve the problem; it will usually make it far worse.
8. Do not be afraid of the computer. Pressing the wrong key will not break it (though it may waste a lot of time).
9. Treat your computer like a good friend and it will be one.

References

1. Brinkley JF, Moritz WE, Baker DW. A technique for imaging three-dimensional structures and computing their volumes using non-parallel ultrasonic sector scans. Proceedings of the 22nd annual conference, AIUM, Dallas. October 1977, pp. 471–474.
2. Merritt, CRB. Computers in OB/GYN ultrasound. 1983 AIUM/SDMS annual convention, October 18–21, New York City. Abstracts of the Categorical Courses.
3. Hohler CW, Krenick CJ, Warford SHS, et al. A new method for prediction of fetal weight from ultrasound measurement of fetal abdominal circumference, thigh circumference, and femur length. J Ultrasound Med Supplement. 1983; 2; 10:107.

Recommended Readings

Angus J, ed. Info World Consumer Product Guide. New York: Brady; 1989. (Collected reviews of hardware and software.)
Arnold DO, et al. Getting Started with PC's and Com-

patibles. New York: Brady; 1988. (IBM and Compatibles.)

Blodgett R, Rosenthol E. Hard Disk Management for IBM PCs and Compatibles. Portland, OR: Management Information Sources; 1988. (IBM and Compatibles.)

Duncan R. Advanced MS DOS. Redmond, WA: Microsoft Press; 1986. (IBM and Compatibles.)

Grauer R, Sugrue PK. Microcomputer Applications. 2nd ed. New York: McGraw-Hill; 1989. (Good reference for all users.)

Helms H, ed. The McGraw-Hill Computer Handbook. New York: McGraw-Hill; 1983. (Look for later edition.)

Juliussen E, Juliussen K. The Computer Industry Almanac. New York: Simon & Schuster; 1988. (Good reference for all users.)

Lu C, Chu EW. The Apple Macintosh Book. 3rd ed. Redmond, WA: Microsoft Press; 1988. (Apple Macintosh.)

McWilliams PA. The Personal Computer Book. Garden City, NY: Prelude Press; 1984. (Look for later edition.)

Naiman A. The Macintosh Bible. Berkeley, CA: Goldstein & Blair; 1989. (Apple Macintosh.)

Turley JL. PC's Made Easy. New York: OSBORN McGraw-Hill; 1989. (Very basic information.)

Wolverton D. Running MS DOS. Redmond, WA: Microsoft Press; 1985. (IBM and Compatibles.)

chapter 36

Statistical Methods
in Obstetric Ultrasound

H. J. KHAMIS, ROGER W. WARNER

The methods of applied statistics can be used to effectively and clearly formulate important problems in obstetric ultrasonography and to solve them. Specifically, statistical principles are used to formulate proper experimental designs and sampling techniques and to analyze and interpret the resulting data. In this chapter we discuss basic statistical concepts and terminology as well as many of the common techniques used in obstetric ultrasonography.

The need for statistical techniques in analyzing ultrasonographic data (or, for that matter, any other kind of data) is due to the basic inherent variability in the data; specifically, variation among the individuals being measured. For instance, if an investigator using real-time sonography takes fetal abdominal circumference measurements on several fetuses, it is unlikely that all of the measurements will be identical. The variation observed in such measurements is due to the natural differences among the fetuses. If more than one investigator takes the measurements, then additional variation will be observed in the data (interobserver variability[21]). It is the purpose of applied statistics to take this variation into account or to assess the reliability of the measurements, in order to facilitate description, analysis, and interpretation of the data.

In statistical terms, the set of measurements (from a group of subjects) that characterizes a phenomenon under study is called a *population*, and a

sample is some subset of the population. It is of paramount importance in ultrasound studies to define the sample that is obtained, the method of data collection, and the kinds of statistical analyses used to make inferences from the sample to the population. A sample should represent the population that is to be studied. If the sample consists of randomly selected measurements from the population of interest (random sampling), then the sample is said to be *representative* of the population; otherwise the sample is *biased*. For instance, if the study population is the set of all second-trimester femur lengths (FLs) of fetuses measured in the last 2 years at a given hospital, a random sample (using a random number table or a random number generator on a computer) of case records containing such measurements obtained from that hospital would be considered to be representative of the study population. If the study population is the set of all second-trimester FLs of fetuses measured in the last 2 years at all hospitals in the country, then the above sample would not be considered representative of the study population unless it could be argued that the hospital where the sample was obtained does not differ substantively from any other hospitals in the county with regard to any parameters that influence FL.

In addition to defining the sample and how it was obtained, the investigator must describe the measurement procedure fully. There is great potential in any study for the reliability and integrity of the measurements to be compromised. Such compromise can be due to an error on the part of the investigator or inexperience of the investigator with the measuring instrument, or to a measuring instrument that is not adjusted properly. A high degree of quality control must be maintained with regard to the measurements that are recorded, because the entire quantitative approach is based on these measurements (garbage in, garbage out!) The issues of proper experimental design, bias in sampling, and the overall integrity of the study protocol are discussed further in texts by Schefler[18] and Fleiss.[7]

Generally, two different kinds of measurements can be observed, those that are *discrete* and those that are *continuous*. Discrete measurements correspond to values that are finite in number (that can be counted). Examples of discrete measurements are: sex of the fetus (M, F), disease state (mild, intermediate, severe), and number of fetuses (1, 2, 3, 4, . . .). Such data is referred to as discrete data. Continuous measurements correspond to values that come from a continuum on the real number line. Examples of continuous measurements are fetal blood flow velocity in centimeters per second, biparietal diameter (BPD) of a fetal head in centimeters, and age of the fetus in weeks. This kind of data is referred to as continuous data. Different statistical techniques are used to describe and analyze data generated by these two different kinds of measurements.

Typically, the first thing that an investigator wishes to do upon obtaining the sample data is to summarize the findings in an efficient and useful manner. Second, the investigator may wish to make inferences about the study population based on the sample, such as prediction, estimation, and answering research questions about population characteristics. *Descriptive statistics* is that branch of statistics that deals with the description and summarization of data. Some techniques in descriptive statistics applied to ultrasonographic data are given in the next section of this chapter. *Inferential statistics* is the area of statistics that deals with making an inference or generalization about the study population based on information contained in a sample.

Descriptive Statistical Techniques in Medical Sonography

Generally, there are two different but related ways in which data can be summarized and described effectively. One is to use *graphic techniques* for data description; the other is to use *numerical measures* of important characteristics of the data. The use of graphic techniques for describing data is particularly effective: it provides a visual presentation of important characteristics of the data and typically the techniques are very simple.

BAR GRAPH

Suppose a set of discrete data is to be summarized graphically. A bar graph is constructed as follows: List the values of the discrete measurement on a horizontal axis, and for each of these values draw a rectangle whose height is equal to the frequency with which that value is observed in the data set. An example should clarify the technique.

Example 1. A sample of 85 pregnant women is taken, 15 of whom are less than 20 years of age, 50 are between 20 and 30 years, and 20 are more than 30 years of age. The bar graph of this discretized age variable is Figure 36-1.

Note that in the use of the bar graph, the vertical axis can designate the relative frequency, or percentage of the sample, that corresponds to each value on the horizontal axis (e.g., in Example 1, 17.7% of the women in the sample are under 20

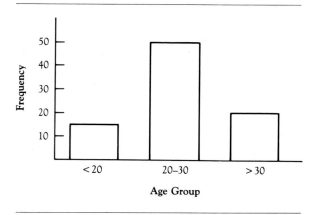

FIGURE 36-1. Bar graph of frequency of three age groups.

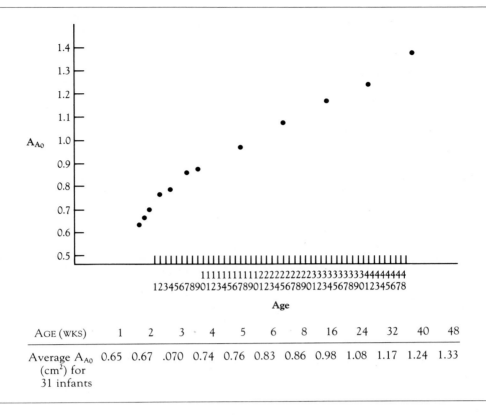

AGE (WKS)	1	2	3	4	5	6	8	16	24	32	40	48
Average A_{A_0} (cm^2) for 31 infants	0.65	0.67	.070	0.74	0.76	0.83	0.86	0.98	1.08	1.17	1.24	1.33

FIGURE 36-2. Plot of ascending aorta cross-sectional area by gestational age. (Data from Alverson, DC, Aldrich M, Angelus P, et al. Longitudinal trends in left ventricular cardiac output in healthy infants in the first year of life. J. Ultrasound Med. 1987;6:519–524.)

years of age, 58.8% are between 20 and 30 years, and 23.5% are over 30 years.

PLOTTING DATA

In order to investigate the relationship between two continuous variables it is useful to plot the paired observations on the x-y coordinate axis system. Consider the following example:

Example 2. A study was made of the ascending aortic cross-sectional area (A_{A_0}) longitudinally in 31 healthy infants from birth through the first year of life using M-mode echocardiography. The following data appear in an article by Alverson and coworkers[1]:

These data are plotted in Figure 36-2.

From this plot it is easy to see that the average

A_{A_0} increases with age in a nearly linear fashion, since the points fall approximately along a straight line. Such a relationship is referred to as a simple linear regression (see below).

Many other graphic techniques are used to summarize and describe data, including pie charts, boxplots, and histograms (see, for example, the text by McClave and Dietrich[15]).

In addition to graphically depicting important features of the data, certain key characteristics can be determined through numerical measures. Two particularly important characteristics of any set of numerical data are its *central tendency* and its *variability*.

MEASURES OF CENTRAL TENDENCY

The central tendency of a set of measurements is

the value about which the measurements tend to cluster or tend to be centered. The most common measure of central tendency is the mean. The *mean* of the sample, denoted by $\bar{x}$, is defined as the sum of the measurements divided by the number of measurements. Notationally, we write

$$\bar{x} = \Sigma x/n,$$

where n represents the sample size, and Σx represents the sum of the measurements in the sample.

Example 3. Consider the following set of measurements: 8, 12, 7, 10, 8, 6, 10, 8, 5, 9. The mean of this sample is computed as follows:

$$\Sigma x = 8 + 12 + 7 + 10 + 8 + 6$$
$$+ 10 + 8 + 5 + 9 = 83$$

and $n = 10$; so $\bar{x} = \Sigma x/n = 83/10 = 8.3$.

Another measure of central tendency is the median. The *median* of a sample of size n is obtained by first listing the measurements from smallest to largest. If n is an odd number, the median is defined as the middle measurement from this ordered list of measurements. If n is an even number, then the median is defined as the midpoint (or average) of the middle two measurements from the list.

Example 4. For the sample given in Example 3, the ordered list of measurements is: 5, 6, 7, 8, 8, 8, 9, 10, 10, 12. Since $n = 10$, the median of this sample is the average of the middle two measurements: median = ½(8 + 8) = 8.

MEASURES OF VARIABILITY

The *variability* of a set of measurements refers to how closely the measurements cluster about the central location or, alternatively, how spread out the measurements are. One very simple measure of variability is the range. The *range* of a sample is defined as the difference between the largest measurement and the smallest measurement.

Example 5. Consider the following sample: 3, 4, 2, 5, 1, 2.

The range of this sample is $5 - 1 = 4$. One might also say that these data range from 1 to 5.

Intuitively, the range is a very reasonable mea-sure of variability: the more spread out the measurements in a sample are, the larger the range will be. However, two very different data sets can give rise to the same range. For instance, the following two samples have the same range (49):

Sample 1: 1, 1, 1, 1, 50   Sample 2: 1, 10, 25, 35, 50

A measure of variability that is sensitive to distinctions of this kind is the *variance*. The variance of a sample, denoted by S^2, measures the average squared distance between the measurements and $\bar{x}$. The formula for S^2 is:

$$S^2 = \{n\Sigma x^2 - (\Sigma x)^2\}/n(n - 1),$$

where n is the sample size, Σx the sum of the measurements in the sample, and Σx^2 the sum of the squares of the measurements. For sample 1 above, $S^2 = 480.2$ and for sample 2, $S^2 = 380.7$; so the variance of sample 1 is greater (the measurements are more dispersed) than the variance of sample 2.

Example 6. For the sample of Example 5,

$$n = 6, \Sigma x = 3 + 4 + 2 + 5 + 1 + 2 = 17 \text{ and}$$
$$\Sigma x^2 = 9 + 16 + 4 + 25 + 1 + 4 = 59. \text{ So,}$$
$$S^2 = [6 \cdot 59 - (17)^2]/6 \cdot 5 = (354 - 289)/30$$
$$= 2.167.$$

Although the variance is more complicated to compute than the range, it is the most common measure of variability used in data description. Note, however, that the variance is expressed in terms of squared units. For instance, if the units of measurement are centimenters, then S^2 is expressed in square centimeters. In order to have a measure of variability that is in the same units as the original measurements, the *standard deviation* (SD) is used. The standard deviation of a sample is denoted by S and is defined as the positive square root of S^2; $S = \sqrt{S^2}$. For the data given in Example 5, the SD is $S = \sqrt{2.167} = 1.472$.

Example 7. Sonographic studies were performed on a random sample of 50 normal pregnant women whose fetuses' gestational ages ranged from 30 to 40 weeks. For each fetus the transverse cerebellar diameter was obtained. Suppose the diameters (in millimeters) are as follows:

44.4, 41.7, 41.4, 47.4, 42.0, 41.5, 39.5, 42.6, 36.8, 40.7, 36.8, 39.4, 41.2, 40.3, 45.1, 37.5, 43.4, 44.8, 38.5, 41.9, 43.2, 45.6, 35.4, 41.4, 42.4, 39.7, 37.3, 39.0, 40.3, 42.5, 40.2, 39.8, 36.4, 43.3, 39.4, 45.7, 38.7, 34.3, 38.8, 40.5, 38.2, 37.4, 38.4, 39.4, 44.5, 46.1, 40.5, 40.4, 42.3, 43.1.

For these data we have $n = 50$, $\Sigma x = 2{,}041.2$, and $\Sigma x^2 = 83{,}746.84$. Then, $\bar{x} = \Sigma x/n = 40.824$. From the ordered data values it is easy to count up to the 25th and 26th measurements (the middle two measurements); they are 40.5 and 40.5. The median is the average of these two values, 40.5. The variance is

$$S^2 = \{50 \cdot (83{,}746.84) - (2{,}041.2)^2\}/50 \cdot 49 = 8.508,$$

and the SD is $S = 2.917$. The range is $47.4 - 34.3 = 13.1$

INTERPRETATION OF THE STANDARD DEVIATION

We have seen that if one sample has a larger SD than another it is the more variable of the two. In order to see how the standard deviation provides a measure of variability of a data set, consider the following questions about the data: How many measurements are within 1 SD of the mean, $\bar{x}$? How many measurements are within 2 SDs of $\bar{x}$? How many measurements are within 3 SDs of $\bar{x}$? That is, how many measurements are between $\bar{x} - S$ and $\bar{x} + S$; how many are between $\bar{x} - 2S$ and $\bar{x} + 2S$; and how many are between $\bar{x} - 3S$ and $\bar{x} + 3S$? We will answer these questions and see what they mean for the data of

Example 7. The mean and SD have been computed to be $\bar{x} = 40.824$ and $S = 2.917$, respectively. Therefore,

$(\bar{x} - S, \bar{x} + S) = (37.91, 43.74),$
$(\bar{x} - 2S, \bar{x} + 2S) = (34.99, 46.66),$ and
$(\bar{x} - 3S, \bar{x} + 3S) = (32.07, 49.58).$

Now, referring to the data in Example 7, we can determine that 34 of the 50 measurements, or 68%, fall between $\bar{x} - S$ and $\bar{x} + S$; 48 of the 50 measurements, or 96%, fall between $\bar{x} - 2S$ and $\bar{x} + 2S$; and all 50 of the measurements, or 100%, fall between $\bar{x} - 3S$ and $\bar{x} + 3S$.

These conclusions illustrate criteria for interpreting a standard deviation for so-called *bell-shaped* or *normally distributed* data. A set of data is considered to have bell-shaped distribution if the mean is approximately the same as the median (so that the measurements are symmetric about the mean) and the measurements tend to cluster about the mean while becoming less and less frequent farther from the mean. For such data sets, the *empirical rule* provides criteria for interpreting the standard deviation, S:

1. About 68% of the measurements fall between $\bar{x} - S$ and $\bar{x} + S$,
2. About 95% of the measurements fall between $\bar{x} - 2S$ and $\bar{x} + 2S$, and
3. Almost 100% of the measurements fall between $\bar{x} - 3S$ and $\bar{x} + 3S$.

Note that the data set in Example 7 follow the empirical rule very closely, the 1-, 2-, and 3-SD percentages being 68%, 96%, and 100%, respectively.

The distribution of many measurements used in sonographic studies is bell shaped. In fact, many different kinds of data sets from all disciplines take on bell-shaped distributions; that is, most of the measurements tend to be close to the mean (95% within 2 SDs of the mean), with few that are distant from the mean (only 5% that are more than 2 SDs away). This is why a laboratory test result is often classified as normal when it falls within 2 SDs of the mean and abnormal when it falls outside this range.

Generally it is desirable to have a small SD for a given set of data because then the interval from $\bar{x} - 2S$ to $\bar{x} + 2S$, where about 95% of the measurements are located (by the empirical rule), is small. Consequently, the vast majority of the measurements are very close to the mean, $\bar{x}$. In this sense we would consider such measurements to be of *low variability*; that is, we would consider the measurements to be *reliable*.

OTHER NUMERICAL MEASURES

One is often interested in where a particular measurement falls in a given data set in relation to the other measurements. Is it the largest measurement? Is it the smallest measurement? Is it close to the largest or close to the smallest? One way to measure the *relative standing* of a measurement is to count the number of measurements in the data set that are smaller than that measurement. That number of measurements, expressed as a percentage of the total number of measurements in the data set, is referred to as the *percentile ranking* of the measurement of interest. For instance, in the data set presented in Example 7, the 10th percentile is 37.3 because 5 of the 50 measurements, or 10% of the measurements, are smaller than 37.3. The measurement 46.1 is the 96th percentile because 48 of the 50 measurements, or 96% of the measurements, are smaller than 46.1. Percentile rankings are of practical value only for large data sets. Note that the median is, by definition, the 50th percentile, since half, or 50%, of the measurements are smaller than the median. When using charts, one of the considerations sonographers should keep in mind is the percentile in which the fetus' measurement falls; this is especially true of fetal weight.

There are two numerical measures, the slope and the correlation coefficient, that are useful in helping to describe the linear relationship between two continuous variables, say x and y. In order to provide the formulas for these measures, some notation must be established that will make the formulas easier to write.

Let

$$S_{xx} = \Sigma x^2 - \frac{1}{n}(\Sigma x)^2, \; S_{yy} = \Sigma y^2 - \frac{1}{n}(\Sigma y)^2, \text{ and } S_{xy}$$
$$= \Sigma xy - \frac{1}{n}(\Sigma x)(\Sigma y),$$

where Σxy represents the sum of the products of the x measurements and the y measurements.

Example 8. Consider the following sample of (x,y) values: (1, 2), (1, 1), (3, 2), (2, 2), (2, 4). Computation of S_{xx}, S_{yy}, and S_{xy} can be effected through the use of Table 36.1.

Then, with $n = 5$, we have

$$S_{xx} = 19 - (9)^2/5 = 2.8, \; S_{yy} = 29 - (11)^2/5$$
$$= 4.8, \text{ and } S_{xy} = 21 - (9)(11)/5 = 1.2.$$

The *slope* for a sample of (x,y) measurements represents the change in the y measurement that corresponds to a 1-unit increase in the x measurement. The *slope* is denoted by b,

$$b = S_{xy}/S_{xx}.$$

If b is negative, then y decreases as x increases; if b is positive, then y increases as x increases. If b is 0, then y remains constant for all values of x. For the sample in Example 8, $b = 1.2/2.8 = 0.429$. This means that, on average, for every unit increase in x, y *increases* by 0.429.

The *correlation coefficient* is a measure of the strength of the linear relationship between the x measurements and the y measurements. The correlation coefficient is denoted by r, and

$$r = S_{xy}/\sqrt{S_{xx} \cdot S_{yy}}.$$

It can be proven that r always lies between -1 and $+1$. If r is positive, then the y measurements tend to increase as the x measurements increase; if r is negative, the y measurements tend to decrease as the x measurements increase. If r is 0, then the x measurements and y measurements are not linearly related. For the data given in Example 8, $r = 1.2/\sqrt{(2.8)(4.8)} = 0.327$, indicating that y increases as x increases in this sample. Because $r = 0.327$ is not very close to -1 or $+1$, this correlation is not considered to be strong.

In Example 2, the correlation coefficient $r = 0.982$ indicates a very strong, positive linear relationship between age and ascending aortic cross-

TABLE 36-1. Sample calculation for data (x,y) plotted on a graph

x	y	x^2	y^2	xy
1	2	1	4	2
1	1	1	1	1
3	2	9	4	6
2	2	4	4	4
2	4	4	16	8
$\Sigma x = 9$	$\Sigma y = 11$	$\Sigma x^2 = 19$	$\Sigma y^2 = 29$	$\Sigma xy = 21$

sectional area (A_{A_o}). The plot in Figure 36-2 confirms these conclusions: The dots tend to increase at the rate of 0.0142 cm^2 per week ($b = 0.0142$), and the dots fall very nearly along a straight line rising from left to right ($r = 0.982$).

It is important to emphasize that no causal relationships can be inferred from the value of b or r. So, although a value of r close to 1 or close to -1 establishes a linear relationship between x and y, it provides no information about the reason for that linear relationship, in particular, whether it is causal or not. For instance, it may be that x and y are highly correlated but that both are influenced by a third intervening variable.

SUMMARY TABLES

When presenting the descriptive statistics of a study, it is important to include all pertinent information in an effective format. For a discrete measurement, a bar graph is useful for visual purposes, and the frequencies and relative frequencies, or percentages, should be given for each level of the measurement (frequency table). For continuous measurements, sample means are usually recorded. Some investigators display $\bar{x} \pm 2S$, as this interval contains about 95% of all of the measurements in the sample, and so represents the interval within which "normal" values fall.

When the mean and median for a given set of data are about equal, then the distribution for those data is said to be *symmetric*. For instance, in the data of Example 7, $\bar{x} = 40.824$ and median = 40.5. However, for data having an *asymmetric* distribution these measures of central tendency differ. In these cases, it is important that both the mean and the median be presented. The more asymmetric the distribution is, the farther apart the mean and median will be.

Finally, when discussing the linear relationship between two continuous variables, plots of the type given in Figure 36-2 are useful, as well as the slope (b) and the correlation coefficient (r).

Testing in Medical Sonography

In addition to summarizing and describing experimental data in ultrasound studies, one typically wishes to make inferences about the study population based on information contained in a random sample for the population. Such inferences can be made by testing research hypotheses.

TESTING

Very often in a research paper, especially one involving the collection and analysis of data, a certain amount of statistical jargon and notation arises with respect to testing research hypotheses, and a familiarity with statistical concepts is helpful for fully understanding the research being presented. For instance, phrases such as the following are very often encountered: "significantly higher," "velocity did not change significantly," "a linear increase in the blood flow amount," "did not reach statistical significance at 0.05," "$0.05 < P < 0.1$." This section provides an intuitive understanding of the concept of significance testing and how it is used in research articles.

Certain elements occur in every statistical testing problem. They constitute a *five-step procedure for a test of hypothesis*.

1. The researcher begins by setting up two hypotheses, the *null* and the *alternative* hypotheses, keeping in mind that the data will be analyzed to determine how strongly they contradict the null hypothesis. Typically, the null hypothesis is the hypothesis of no change or status quo and the alternative hypothesis is the hypothesis of change. For instance, a researcher may be interested in knowing whether the average umbilical vein blood flow velocity is the same for women in the 33rd week of pregnancy as for women in the 39th week of pregnancy. The null hypothesis would be that the average blood flow velocity is the same for both groups of women; the alternative hypothesis would state that the average blood flow velocity differs between the two groups of women. Then the data would be collected and analyzed to determine how strongly they contradict the null hypothesis and support the alternative hypothesis.

2. The investigator must decide how strongly the data should contradict the null hypothesis before he or she will conclude that the null hypothesis is indeed false. This decision is made by choosing a *level of significance* for the test, namely, the probability that the null hypothesis will be rejected erroneously. The level of significance most commonly used in ultrasonographic studies is 0.05. So with a 0.05 level of significance in the test for deciding whether or not the null hypothesis is false, there will be only a 5% chance of rejecting a true null hypothesis.

In order to decide whether the null hypothesis is false or not, we compare a measure called the P value to our level of significance. The P value is calculated from the data and is a measure of how strongly the data contradict the null hypothesis (or, equivalently, how strongly the data support the alternative hypothesis); the smaller the P value, the more the data contradict the null hypothesis. So, we will reject the null hypothesis when the P value is small and will not reject the null hypothesis when the P value is large. Specifically, we will reject the null hypothesis when the P value is smaller than the chosen level of significance (say 0.05).

3. The data are collected. Again, the sample must be representative of the population being studied.

4. The P value that corresponds to the data is calculated. Generally, computation of the P value is based on mathematical properties of the measurement representing the characteristic being studied and the kind of statistical test being conducted; most statistical software programs provide the P value automatically.

5. Compare the P value to 0.05 (or whatever level of significance was chosen in step 2); if it is smaller, reject the null hypothesis, and if it is larger, do not reject the null hypothesis.

This five-step procedure can be generalized to handle an enormous variety of statistical testing problems, and for each one the *P value is the measure of the extent to which the null hypothesis is contradicted by the data*. A few of the more common tests of a hypothesis are presented in the following section.

Proportion. In the 1986 Society of Diagnostic Medical Sonographers Professional Profile Survey, Khamis and Warner[13] report that 377 of the 2479 respondents had a bachelor's degree or higher education. Assuming that the 2479 respondents form a representative sample of all U.S. sonographers, is it true that over 13% of all U.S. sonographers have a bachelor's degree or higher education? To answer this question, set up the null hypothesis as the claim that 13% or less of all U.S. songraphers have a bachelor's degree or higher education, and the alternative hypothesis as the claim that over 13% of U.S. sonographers have a bachelor's degree or higher education. Then, the P value corresponding to the sample proportion observed above, $377/2479 = 15.2\%$, is $P = 0.0011$. The test used to obtain this P value is the *binomial test*. More specifically, it is called an *upper-tail* binomial test because the alternative hypothesis specifies that the proportion under study exceeds 13%.

Since the computed P value is smaller than 0.05, our level of significance, we would reject the null hypothesis and conclude that over 13% of all U.S. songraphers have a bachelor's degree or higher education.

Mean. It is often of interest to test hypotheses concerning the mean of the population. Suppose we hypothesize that the mean velocity of umbilical venous blood flow for pregnant women in their 33rd week is 15 cm/sec, and a random sample of 30 normal pregnant women rendered a sample mean velocity of 13.9 cm/sec, as reported by Chen's group.[3]

In this problem, the null hypothesis is that the mean velocity of umbilical venous blood flow for pregnant women in their 33rd week is 15 cm/sec. The alternative hypothesis is that it is different from 15 cm/sec. Suppose the level of significance is set at 0.05. Does the sample value of 13.9 cm/sec differ from 15 cm/sec enough to enable us to reject the null hypothesis? Based on the so-called *t* test, the P value corresponding to 13.9 cm/sec turns out to be $P = 0.603$. This test is referred to as a *two-tailed t* test, because the alternative hypothesis specifies that the true mean velocity is either larger or smaller than the hypothesized value of 15 cm/sec.

Since the P value exceeds 0.05, we conclude that the null hypothesis cannot be rejected. The reason that the null hypothesis cannot be rejected: 13.9 cm/sec is not unusually far from 15 cm/sec, certainly not far enough away for us to doubt the null hypothesis.

Two Means. It is sometimes useful to compare two different means. For instance, suppose we wish to test the null hypothesis that the average umbilical venous blood flow velocity is the same for women in the 33rd week of pregnancy as for women in the

39th week. Suppose that a sample of 30 women in their 33rd week have an average velocity of 13.9 cm/sec and a sample of 26 women in their 39th week of pregnancy have an average velocity of 13.4 cm/sec.[3] Do these two sample means differ enough to enable us to reject the null hypothesis? The P value associated with the difference between these two sample means is 0.772 (two-tailed t test). This value far exceeds the 0.05 level of significance, so we fail to reject the null hypothesis and conclude that the average umbilical venous blood flow velocity does not differ significantly between the two groups of women.

The examples presented above should focus the logic behind the decision-making process involving a given parameter.

READING RESEARCH ARTICLES

In general, the following approach might be helpful in wading through the statistics in a research article:

1. Identify the parameter or parameters that are being studied. The most common parameters that are discussed are proportion, mean, variance, correlation coefficient, coefficient of variation, and slope of a linear regression. If you are unfamiliar with the meaning of a given parameter, refer to a statistics book. There are many good statistics books that require no more mathematic knowledge than high school algebra. [5,8,15] In addition, several statistics books emphasize only statistical ideas and concepts and present few, if any, mathematical formulas and equations.[2,9,10]

2. Determine the hypotheses concerning the parameter of interest.

3. Read the conclusion concerning the parameter of interest, and locate the P value to determine how strongly the data support the conclusion. The use and interpretation of the P value is developed and discussed more fully in an article by Khamis.[11]

Diagnostic Test Evaluation in Medical Sonography

A very important consideration among investigators in ultrasound is the ability to assess the comparative usefulness of diagnostic techniques such as sonography, CT, and MRI. The following discussion focuses on how to determine the diagnostic and predictive value of tests that are designed to make such assessments.

Consider a new test designed to discriminate between persons with a particular disease (or condition) and persons who are disease free. Two traditional measures of the diagnostic value of such a test are the *sensitivity* and the *specificity*. The *sensitivity* of a test, or *true positive ratio*, is defined to be the proportion of those having the disease whose test result is positive for it (i.e., for whom the test indicates presence of the disease). Hence, it is a measure of how sensitive the test is in detecting the disease. Analogously, the *specificity* of a test, or *true negative ratio*, is the proportion of persons who do not have the disease whose test result is negative.

In order to quantify these two measures, suppose that it is possible to distinguish between those who have the disease and those who do not have the disease (through surgery or autopsy, say). Call this the *gold standard*. Then a 2 × 2 table can be set up as in Table 36-2.

Now, based on this table, simple formulas can be given for the sensitivity and specificity of the test:

$$\text{Sensitivity} = a/(a + c); \text{Specificity} = d/(b + d).$$

The *prevalence rate* of the disease is defined as the proportion of persons who have the disease:

$$\text{Prevalence rate} = (a + c)/(a + b + c + d).$$

Note that a and d correspond to the patients whose test result is correct, and that b and c correspond to those whose test result is incorrect.

TABLE 36-2. A 2 × 2 table of the gold standard versus the ultrasound examination result

ULTRASOUND EXAMINATION RESULT	GOLD STANDARD		
	DISEASED	DISEASE-FREE	TOTAL
Positive	a	b	$a + b$
Negative	c	d	$c + d$
Total	$a + c$	$b + d$	$a + b + c + d$

a = Number of patients who are diseased and test positive, b = Number of patients who are disease free and test positive, c = Number of patients who are diseased and test negative, and d = Number of patients who are disease free and test negative.

TABLE 36-3. A 2 × 2 table for a disease with a 50% prevalence rate

ULTRASOUND EXAMINATION RESULT	GOLD STANDARD		
	DISEASED	DISEASE-FREE	TOTAL
Positive	600	75	675
Negative	150	675	825
Total	750	750	1500

More specifically, positive results for persons who are disease free (b) are called *false positives*, and negative results for persons who are diseased (c) are called *false negatives*.

Consider Table 36-3.

According to the above formulas, we have:

$$\text{Sensitivity} = 600/750 = 80\%$$
$$\text{Specificity} = 675/750 = 90\%$$
$$\text{Prevalence rate} = 750/1500 = 50\%$$
$$\text{False positives} = 75$$
$$\text{False negatives} = 150$$

Interpretation. Eighty percent of diseased patients test positive and 90% of disease-free persons test negative. The prevalence rate of the disease is 50%. There are 225 persons for whom the test is inaccurate: 75 false positives and 150 false negatives. A major advantage of sensitivity and specificity as measures of the diagnostic value of a test is that they are independent of the prevalence rate of the disease, so they can be used in cases involving a rare disease, that is, one that has a very low prevalence rate.

Now, suppose it is of interest to predict a person's disease status, given the test result. The two measures of particular interest to clinicians that are used for this purpose are the *positive predictive value (PPV)* of a test and the *negative predictive value (NPV)* of a test. The PPV is defined to be the proportion of those with a positive test result who are diseased, as determined by the gold standard. The NPV is defined to be the proportion of those with a negative test result who are disease free, as determined by the gold standard. From Table 36-2, we have:

$$PPV = a/(a + b); NPV = d/(c + d).$$

Plugging in the values from Table 36-3 we have:

PPV = 600/675 = 88.9%; and NPV = 675/825 = 81.8%.

Interpretation. A person whose test result is positive has an 88.9% chance of being diseased; a person whose test result is negative has an 81.8% chance of being disease free.

One drawback of these two predictive measures is that they are a function of the prevalence rate. So, if the prevalence rate in the above example is 10% instead of 50% (perhaps a more realistic situation), then the predictive values may be very different from the values found above. As an illustration, consider Table 36-4.

The data in Table 36-4 indicate that the sensitivity of the examination is 80% and the specificity 90%, exactly as in Table 36-3; however, the PPV is 47.1% and the NPV is 97.6%. Note that for a test with equal sensitivity and specificity, the reduction in the prevalence rate has the effect of reducing the PPV and increasing the NPV. That is, if fewer diseased persons are tested, fewer diseased persons will have a positive test result so the PPV is lower. Likewise, if more disease-free persons are tested, more disease-free persons will have a negative result, so the NPV is higher.

Whereas the sensitivity and specificity are important indicators of the effectiveness of a diagnostic test, it is the PPV and NPV that are of primary interest to those in clinical obstetrics. They want to know what a given test result means for the patient.

Example 9. In a 1988 article, Townsend and colleagues[20] report on a retrospective review of initial sonograms performed on 65 twin gestations to

TABLE 36-4. A 2 × 2 table for a disease with 10% prevalence rate

ULTRASOUND EXAMINATION RESULT	GOLD STANDARD		
	DISEASED	DISEASE-FREE	TOTAL
Positive	120	135	255
Negative	30	1215	1245
Total	150	1350	1500

TABLE 36-5. Data for Example 9

ULTRASOUND EXAMINATION RESULT	GOLD STANDARD		
	TWO CHORIONS	ONE CHORION	TOTAL
Thick membrane	39	8	47
Thin membrane	3	15	18
Total	42	23	65

evaluate the ability of sonography to distinguish monochorionic from dichorionic gestations based on the thickness of the membrane separating the fetuses. The results are shown in Table 36-5.

For this examination the indicators of diagnostic accuracy are:

Sensitivity = 39/42 = 93%; Specificity = 15/23 = 65%.

The predictive values are:

PPV = 39/47 = 83%; NPV = 15/18 = 83.3%.

The prevalence rate of two chorions is 42/65, or 64.6%. Hence, a thick membrane detected dichorionic gestation with a sensitivity of 93%, and a thin membrane detected monochorionic gestation with a specificity of 65%. The PPV of a thick membrane for two chorions is 83%, and the NPV of a thin membrane for one chorion is 83.3%.

The association of two chorions with a thick membrane and of one chorion to a thin membrane was correct in 54 patients, for an accuracy of 54/65, or 83%. The conclusion of the article is that the

TABLE 36-6. Glossary of statistical terms

TERM	MEANING
Bell-shaped data	Data that cluster about the mean and become less and less frequent as they become more distant from the mean
Correlation coefficient	A measure of the strength of the linear relationship between the x measurements and the y measurements
Hypothesis test	A test procedure used to determine the extent to which data support a claim or hypothesis
Level of significance	The probability of rejecting a true null hypothesis in the hypothesis testing procedure
Mean	Central location of a set of numerical data; sometimes called the average
Median	That value in a data set for which half the measurements are higher and half lower
Negative predictive value	The rate of true negative results; calculated as the proportion of true negative test results over all negative (true negative and false negative) test results
Normal values	Values that fall within two standard deviations of the mean
Null hypothesis	A claim or hypothesis the accuracy of which is to be tested; typically involves a statement of "no change" or "status quo"
Percentile	The proportion (expressed as a percentage) of measurements smaller than the measurement of interest
Population	The set of measurements obtained from all of the people or things that are under study; sometimes called the universe
Positive predictive value	The rate of true positive results; calculated as the proportion of true positive test results over all positive (true positive and false positive) test results
P value	A measure of the extent to which the data in a hypothesis testing procedure contradict the null hypothesis
Range	The largest measurement minus the smallest measurement
Sample	A subset of a population
Sensitivity	Proportion of tests that indicate disease (true positive) over the number of proven diseased patients
Slope	The change in the y measurement for a unit increase in the x measurement
Specificity	Proportion of tests that indicate no disease (true negative) over the number of proven disease-free patients
Standard deviation	The square root of the variance (see variance)
Variance	A measure of the variability in a set of data

appearance of the membrane can be useful in sonographic evaluation of chorionicity and amnionicity in twin gestations.

Further information on diagnostic test evaluation can be found in texts by Riegelman[17] and by Fleiss,[6] and in the article by Stempel.[19]

Conclusion

Often when data analyses are conducted certain of the assumptions necessary for the testing procedures discussed above are invalid. For instance, the sample size may be small ($n < 30$) or the sample mean may not be distributed normally. In these instances, so-called *nonparametric procedures* must be used to make inferences based on the sample data (see, for example, McClave and Dietrich,[15] Chapter 10).

One of the important considerations in planning any experiment involving statistical analysis of data is the sample size. The appropriate sample size for a given experiment depends on the hypotheses being tested, the kind of statistical test being applied, and the degree of accuracy required by the researcher, among other factors. Generally, it is not appropriate to make an intuitive guess as to what the appropriate sample size should be. Further reading on sample size choice is available in Khamis,[12] and Kraemer and Thiemann.[14] For a more detailed presentation of statistical methods in obstetric sonography, see the text by Deter and colleagues.[4] Table 36-6 is a statistics glossary.

If a researcher is ever uncertain about the statistical aspect of a study, it is very important to consult a professional statistician.

References

1. Alverson DC, Aldrich M, Angelus P, et al. Longitudinal trends in left ventricular cardiac output in healthy infants in the first year of life. J Ultrasound Med. 1987; 6:519–524.
2. Brook RJ, Arnold GC, Hassard TH, et al. The Fascination of Statistics. New York: Marcel Dekker; 1986.
3. Chen H-Y, Lu C-C, Cheng Y-T, et al. Antenatal measurement of fetal umbilical venous flow by pulsed Doppler and B-mode ultrasonography. J Ultrasound Med. 1986; 5:319-321.
4. Deter RL, Harrist RB, Birnholz JC, et al. Quantitative Obstetrical Ultrasonography. New York: John Wiley and Sons; 1986.
5. Dunn OJ. Basic Statistics: A Primer for the Biomedical Sciences. ed 2. New York: John Wiley and Sons; 1977.
6. Fleiss JL. Statistical Methods for Rates and Proportions. ed 2. New York: John Wiley and Sons; 1981.
7. Fleiss JL. The Design and Analysis of Clinical Experiments. New York: John Wiley and Sons; 1986.
8. Folks JL. Ideas of Statistics. New York: John Wiley and Sons; 1981.
9. Hooke R. How to Tell the Liars from the Statisticians. New York: Marcel Dekker, 1983.
10. Huff D. How to Lie with Statistics. New York: WW Norton; 1954.
11. Khamis HJ. A statistics refresher: Tests of hypothesis and diagnostic test evaluation. J Diagn Med Sonogr. 1987; 3:123–129.
12. Khamis HJ. Statistics refresher II: Choice of sample size. J Diagn Med Sonogr. 1988; 4:176–183.
13. Khamis HJ, Warner RW. A discussion of the 1986 society of diagnostic medical sonographers professional profile survey. Part II. J Diagn Med Sonogr. 1986; 2:328–333.
14. Kraemer HC, Thiemann S. How Many Subjects? Statistical Power Analysis in Research. Newbury Park, CA: Sage Publications; 1987.
15. McClave JT, Dietrich FH II. Statistics. ed 3. San Francisco: Dellen Publishing Company; 1985.
16. O'Leary DH, Kane RA, Chase BM. A prospective study of the efficacy of B-scan sonography in the detection of deep venous thrombosis in the lower extremities. J Clin Ultrasound. 1988; 16:1–8.
17. Reigelman RK. Studying a Study and Testing a Test: How to Read the Medical Literature. Boston: Little, Brown; 1981.
18. Schefler WC. Statistics for Health Professionals. Reading, MA: Addison-Wesley; 1984.
19. Stempel LE. Einie, meenie, minie, mo . . . What do the data really show? Am J Obstet Gynecol. 1982; 144:745-752.
20. Townsend RR, Simpson GF, Filly RA. Membrane thickness in ultrasound prediction of chorionicity of twin gestations. J Ultrasound Med. 1988; 7:327-332.
21. Zador IE, Sokol RJ, Chik L. Interobserver variability, a source of error in obstetric ultrasound. J Ultrasound Med. 1988; 7:245-249.

CHAPTER **37**

Artifacts in Obstetric and Gynecologic Ultrasound

LINDA J. WADSWORTH, SUSAN E. NEALER, BEVERLY A. SPIRT

Artifacts are an integral part of ultrasound that can both clarify and confuse the diagnostic picture. Sonographers must have a basic understanding of the physics of ultrasound in order to obtain optimal examinations, and to recognize the various artifacts. The reader is referred to one of the many basic texts on ultrasound physics for a more detailed discussion of physical principles.

This chapter describes and explains the artifacts most often encountered in obstetric and gynecologic scanning. Artifacts can be divided into four basic categories of physical principles—*reflection and refraction, reverberation, attenuation, side lobe and slice thickness*—and a fifth category, *operator-dependent* artifacts. For purposes of ultrasound instrumentation, four basic assumptions have been made[6,7]:

1. Transducer acoustic beams travel in a straight line.
2. The returning pulse is received before the next pulse is sent.
3. The round-trip time of the pulse is proportional to the distance it travels.
4. Objects viewed are located in the central portion of the sound beam.

These assumptions are not true in every case, and artifacts are a manifestation of that fact.

Reflection and Refraction

Sound does not always travel in a straight line. When a sound beam travels from one medium to another, it may be transmitted, refracted, and/or reflected, depending on the velocity of sound in the two media, the angle of transmission, and the angle of incidence (Fig. 37-1). This occurs according to Snell's law:

$$\frac{\text{sin angle of transmission}}{\text{sin angle of incidence}} = \frac{\text{velocity of medium 2}}{\text{velocity of medium 1}}$$

Refraction refers to the change in direction of the acoustic beam as it travels from one medium to another. When a sound beam crosses an interface between a low-velocity medium and a high-velocity medium, it is refracted away from the vertical. In the reverse, a beam traveling from a high-velocity to a low-velocity medium is bent toward the vertical. *Reflection* occurs when the sound beam bounces off the interface without entering the second medium (Fig. 37-2).[6,11]

The impact of a beam on a curved specular reflector results in *curved-edge refraction*, which may be of two types. A wide shadow results from the sound beam traveling from a low-velocity to a high-velocity medium when it intersects a curved surface; a narrow shadow results if the beam goes from high-velocity to low-velocity tissue (Fig. 37-3).

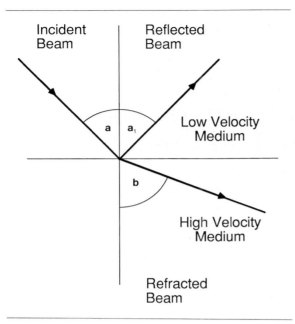

FIGURE 37-1. Reflection and refraction. With oblique incidence, the angle of incidence (a) equals the angle of reflection (a₁). The angle of transmission (b) depends on the incident angle and the velocities of the media.

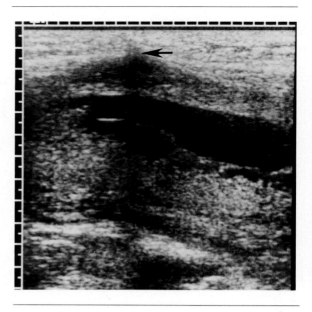

FIGURE 37-2. Reflection. Obstetric sonogram demonstrates total reflection (*arrows*) of the sound beam caused by the transducer-air interface at the umbilicus.

Multiple examples of curved-edge refraction are found in obstetric and gynecologic scanning (Fig. 37-4).

A third type of curved-edge shadowing is *reflective shadowing,* also referred to as *critical angle shadowing.* This is a wide acoustic shadow that is produced when the angle of the incident beam is such that the angle of transmission equals 90 degrees. At this critical angle, the sound beam is completely reflected (see Fig. 37-3).[8,11,12] This artifact is often a source of difficulty in pelvic scanning. When the sound beam intersects the bladder wall at a certain angle it is reflected completely (Fig. 37-5A). This lack of sound transmission should not be misinterpreted as an acoustic shadow caused by calcification as in a myoma or mass. The artifact may be eliminated by changing the angle of the transducer or incident beam (Fig. 37-5B).

A striking example of refraction is the *split-image* or *double-image* artifact. In the pelvis, the sound beam passes through fat and the rectus muscles be-fore reaching the bladder. The beam is refracted away from the perpendicular at the fat-muscle interface and toward the perpendicular when it leaves the muscle. The equipment does not perceive that the beam has been refracted and that the sound is no longer traveling in a straight line. It places the structure in accordance with the time elapsed for the returned signal, causing an extra image to appear. If a structure is located at a particular depth, the image will be totally duplicated (Fig. 37-6).[2,10,13] If the depth is not optimal, partial duplication results. This artifact frequently produces a false double gestational sac, which could be misinterpreted as twins (Fig. 37-7). It may also cause the appearance of a double IUD, an increased crown-rump length (CRL), enlargement of a uterine mass, or a bicornuate uterus. To avoid the split-image artifact the sonographer should scan to the right or left of the midline or have the patient void partially. It has been demonstrated that this artifact appears less frequently when a linear-array transducer is utilized.[13]

Refracted Shadows   ## Reflected Shadow

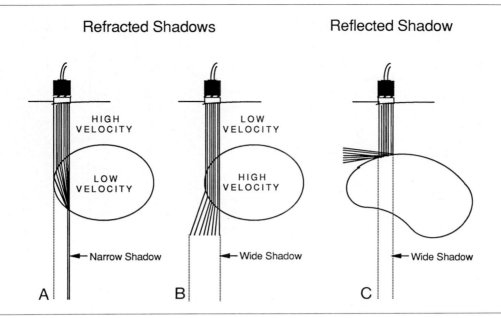

FIGURE 37-3. Curved edge refraction and reflection. (A) High to low velocity. (B) Low to high velocity. (C) Critical angle shadowing.

FIGURE 37-4. Curved edge refraction. Sonogram of fetal skull demonstrates wide edge shadowing (*arrows*) as a result of the sound beam traveling from a low-velocity medium such as amniotic fluid to a high-velocity medium such as bone.

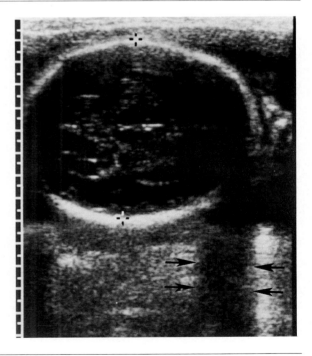

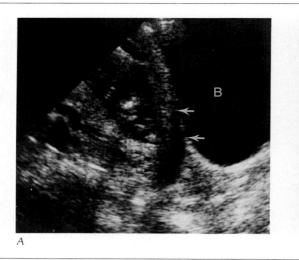
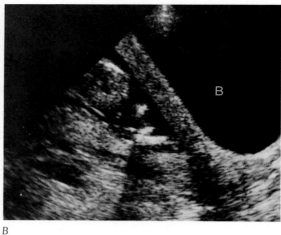

A

B

Figure 37-5. Critical angle shadowing. (A) Sagittal sector scan of the lower uterine segment demonstrates complete reflection of the sound beam (*arrowheads*) at the bladder wall (*arrows*; B, bladder). (B) By changing the transducer angle and further filling the bladder, this artifact is eliminated.

Reverberation

Reverberation is defined as multiple reflections of sound. It occurs when the sound wave strikes an interface with a high degree of acoustic mismatch, such as soft tissue and gas, and most of the sound is reflected back to the transducer. The returning sound is reflected again off the transducer surface, reenters the body, and thus produces more than one reflection from the same surface. Returning echoes are then registered on the monitor at both incorrect and correct locations, equidistant from each other, with decreasing amplitude. The greater the acoustic mismatch, the greater the number of reverberant echos that are produced.

The *pseudomass* is a dramatic example of this phenomenon, wherein a mass effect is created by a combination of reflection and reverberation. This occurs when a highly reflective surface creates strong reverberation echoes that, when mapped into an anechoic or hypoechoic region by the instrument, create the false appearance of a mass (Fig. 37-8).[8,12] Pseudomasses are common artifacts and should be identified promptly by the sonographer. In a thin patient, it should be obvious that the size of the mass visualized cannot possibly exist within

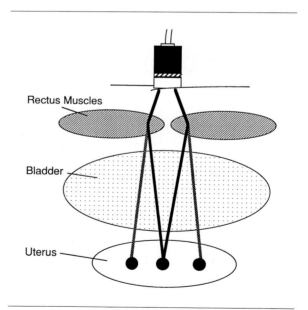

Figure 37-6. Double image artifact. Line representation of acoustic path as it passes through rectus muscles and bladder (see text). The solid line represents the actual sound path and the dotted lines the computer-calculated direction which causes the double image.

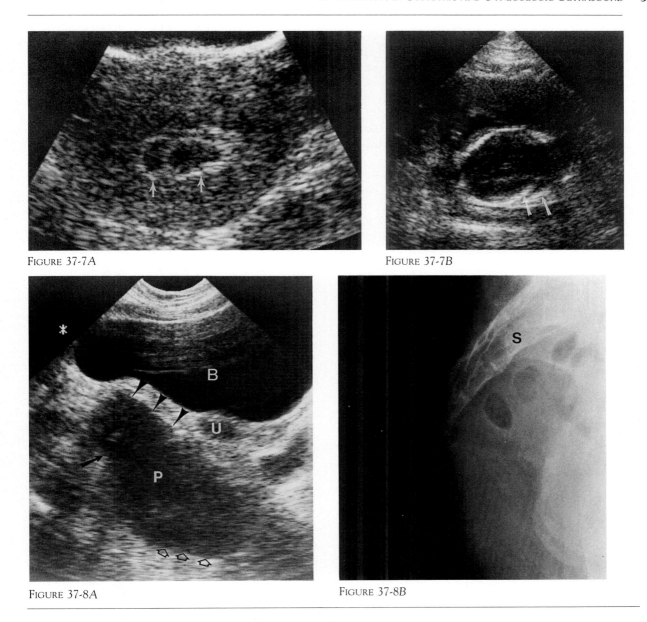

FIGURE 37-7A

FIGURE 37-7B

FIGURE 37-8A

FIGURE 37-8B

FIGURE 37-7. Split image. (A) Transverse sonogram of an early gestation demonstrates artifactual partial duplication of the gestatational sac (*arrows*) due to refraction of the sound beam at the muscle-fat interface. (B) Artifactual double edge of fetal skull (*arrows*) should not be confused with overlapping of fetal skull bones.

FIGURE 37-8. Pseudomass. (A) Longitudinal sonogram of the pelvis demonstrates a pseudomass (P) posterior to the uterus (U). The back wall of the superior aspect of this pseudomass (*arrow*) is created by a reverberation from the highly reflective sacrum (*arrowheads*) in this thin patient. The inferior portion of this pseudomass (*open arrows*) is a duplicated bladder effect secondary to multiple-path reflection (see Fig. 37-9). (B, urinary bladder.) (B) Lateral radiograph confirms the absence of any mass anterior to the sacrum (S).

the patient and that the image must represent artifactual echoes beyond the body cavity. Reducing the gain or changing the direction of the transducer may cause the mass to disappear. If there is doubt, it may help to have the patient void, in order to rearrange the pattern of reflected echoes. If the mass changes or disappears completely, further imaging studies are not necessary. Correlation with physical examination is useful to confirm the presence or absence of a mass.

Multipath reflection or reverberation is a similar artifact. It is caused by the beam striking a curved specular surface, intersecting other curved interfaces, and reflecting in an indirect path back to the transducer. Additional signals are received by the transducer that may be interpreted as part of the primary beam pattern.[6-8] In the pelvis this artifact can duplicate the bladder posteriorly, owing to the increased time required for the reflected beam to return (Figs. 37-8, 37-9). It may be avoided by having the patient void or by repositioning the scanning angle.

Two artifacts that are similar in appearance but are caused by two disparate mechanisms are the

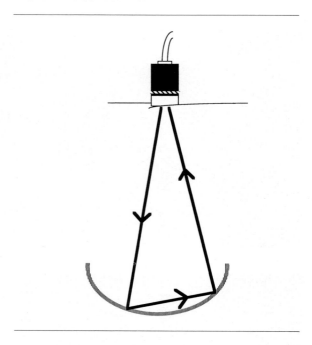

FIGURE 37-9. Multiple-path reflection. The sound beam undergoes multiple reflections as it intersects a curved specular surface.

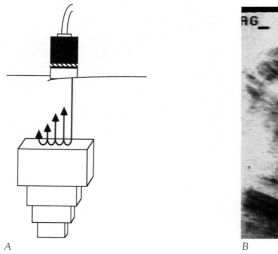

A

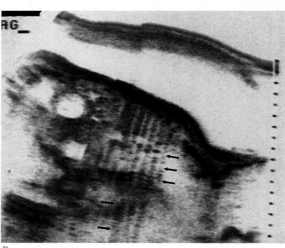

B

FIGURE 37-10. Comet tail. (A) This artifact is characterized by a series of closely spaced reverberations which taper. (B) Coronal section through fetal thorax demonstrates intense comet tail reverberations (*arrows*) from fetal ribs. Polyhydramnios is present.

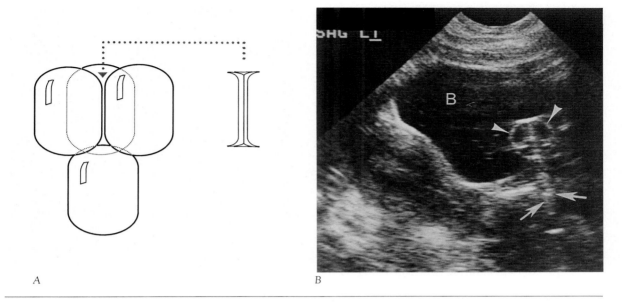

A   B

FIGURE 37-11. Ring down. (*A*) Diagram of bubble-tetrahedron with "fluid bugle" (*arrow*) within (see text). (*B*) Sagittal scan of pelvis shows ring down artifact (*arrows*) from gas in Foley catheter balloon (*arrowheads*; B, bladder).

comet tail and the *ring down* artifacts. In the first, internal reverberations that occur in dense, highly reflective objects such as metal are intense enough and close enough together to produce a distinct and characteristic pattern that appears to merge into a comet tail configuration (Fig. 37-10).[15,17] Reverberations from IUDs, shotgun pellets, and metal surgical clips produce comet tail artifacts.

Ring down is caused by a unique mechanism that is a function of resonance. It is associated with gas collections. We include it here because of its similar sonographic appearance to the comet tail. Ring down appears as a solid line or a series of parallel bands emanating from below a gas pocket. Experiments have shown that it originates from a "fluid bugle," which occurs in the center of a layer of bubbles or a bubble tetrahedron.[1] The fluid bugle acts as an oscillator of the sound beam and causes the liquid in it to vibrate, sending a continuous signal of decreasing amplitude back to the transducer (Fig. 37-11). The fluid bugle resonates at

a frequency determined by its individual size and shape. The frequencies received by the transducer are thus independent of the original frequency.

Reverberations in the fetal head may cause a misleading interpretation of brain anatomy. These reverberations may originate from the highly reflective fetal skull, from the transducer-skin interface, or from maternal tissue layers, particularly in an obese patient. This results in obscuration of the near field, causing a false impression of a unilateral abnormality in a bilateral condition (Fig. 37-12). An arc-shaped structure may appear in the posterior portion of the fetal head. This is referred to as the *pseudoepidural artifact* because of its similarity to epidural collections on computed tomographic scans of the brain. The reverberation echo that produces this artifact originates from the anterior surface of the fetal skull and is placed at twice its depth (Fig. 37-13).[14] With real-time imaging, this artifact may be circumvented by adjusting the angle of the probe while scanning.

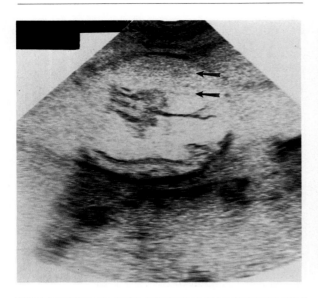

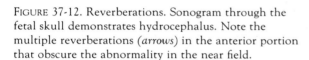

FIGURE 37-12. Reverberations. Sonogram through the fetal skull demonstrates hydrocephalus. Note the multiple reverberations (*arrows*) in the anterior portion that obscure the abnormality in the near field.

FIGURE 37-13. "Pseudoepidural" artifact. Real-time sonogram demonstrates an arc-shaped reverberation (*arrows*) in the posterior aspect of the fetal skull, which should not be confused with an epidural fluid collection.

Attenuation

When a sound wave travels through a medium, its amplitude and intensity decrease. This phenomenon is referred to as *attenuation*. An extremely dense medium such as bone attenuates the sound beam to such an extent that an acoustic shadow is produced. This phenomenon is very useful in diagnostic ultrasound, because an acoustic shadow behind an echogenic focus in an ovarian mass or in the fetal brain or abdomen indicates the presence of calcification (Fig. 37-14A). The degree of shadowing in fetal long bones also provides useful information, since bone absorbs approximately 20 times more sound than soft tissue.[8,16] If the normal degree of shadowing is not seen, an underlying problem of bone mineralization such as osteogenesis imperfecta (Fig. 37-14B) should be considered.[7]

The opposite of shadowing is *enhancement,* an increase in amplitude from reflectors that lie posterior to a weakly attenuating material such as fluid. There is increased transmission of the sound beam through the fluid ("through transmission"), so that

echoes from structures deep to the fluid are of greater amplitude than echoes from tissue adjacent to those structures (Fig. 37-15). The presence of posterior enhancement is the key to whether a mass contains a low attenuating medium such as fluid, hematoma, or abscess (Fig. 37-16). An anechoic mass without posterior enhancement does not represent a simple cyst but rather a complex collection.

Slice Thickness and Side-Lobe Artifacts

Slice-thickness and *side-lobe* artifacts are due to the fact that two of the basic assumptions of ultrasound instrumentation cited above are not always true: (1) The round-trip time of the pulse is proportional to the distance it travels and (2) objects viewed are located in the central portion of the sound beam. Both slice-thickness and side-lobe artifacts may cause a cyst to appear complex.

Side-lobe artifacts result from multiple side beams of lower intensity that emanate from the

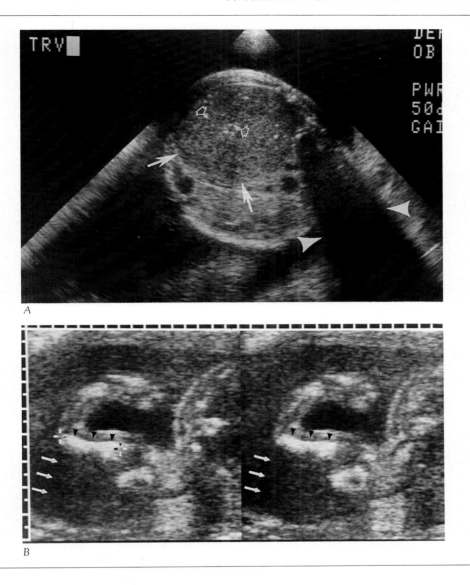

FIGURE 37-14. Acoustic shadow. (A) Transverse scan of fetal abdomen shows prominent acoustic shadow from fetal spine (*arrowheads*). Note acoustic shadows from calcifications (*open arrows*) in abdominal mass (*arrows*), which aided in the diagnosis of fetal neuroblastoma. (Courtesy of Dr. Michael Oliphant, Syracuse, NY.) (B) Note the decreased degree of shadowing (*arrows*) posterior to the humerus (*arrowheads*) of a 17-week fetus with osteogenesis imperfecta.

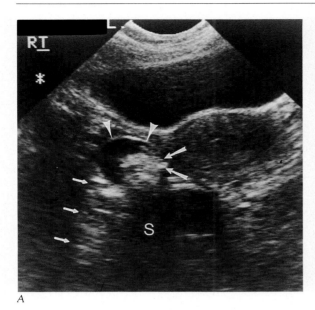

A

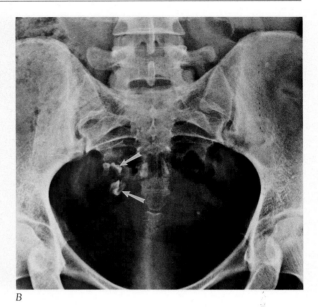

B

FIGURE 37-15. Posterior enhancement. Transverse sonogram (A) and corresponding radiograph (B) of the pelvis in a young woman with dermoid cyst (*arrowheads*) of the right ovary. Both posterior enhancement (*small arrows*) and acoustic shadowing (S) are present on the sonogram. Calcification (*large arrows*) within the dermoid is confirmed on the radiograph.

transducer, surrounding the main beam.[9,12] These lower-intensity lobes radiate to the periphery of the main sound beam, scattering it against specular reflectors such as the bladder or diffuse reflectors like bowel gas. This artifact is frequently seen in the urinary bladder as a debris level or as a line anterior to its floor (Fig. 37-17A). Side-lobe artifacts are dependent on transducer angle and beam intensity but are independent of gravity. They may be eliminated by changing the angle of the transducer and decreasing the gain.

Slice-thickness artifact refutes the assumption that all objects viewed are in a central finite plane. In actuality, a sound beam has width and diverges beyond the focal zone. Despite their true origin, all returning echoes are placed by the equipment on a narrow axis. This produces a "partial volume" effect.[3-6] For example, if a beam is "off axis" to a cyst, an averaging effect of the cyst and surrounding tissue will occur, causing the cyst to fill in with echoes

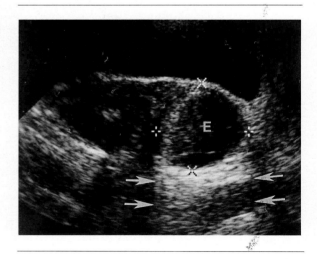

FIGURE 37-16. Posterior enhancement. Transverse sonogram of endometrioma (E) in the left adnexae. Posterior enhancement (*arrows*) is present owing to the weakly attenuating material within the mass.

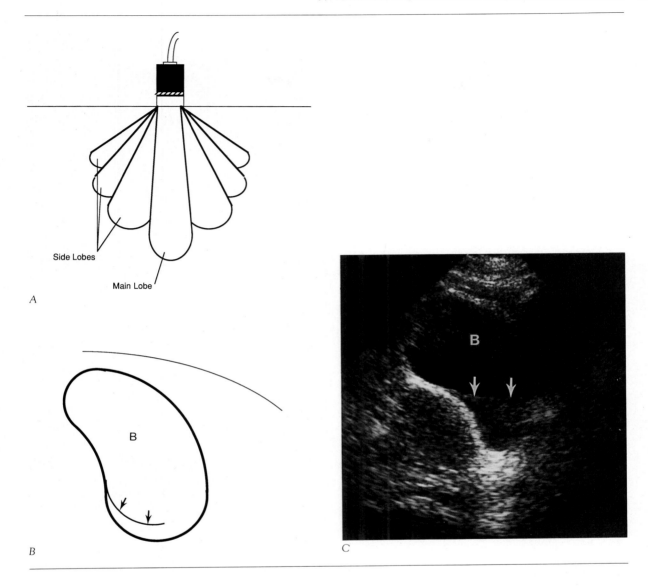

Figure 37-17. Side lobe artifacts. (A) Line representation of main beam with lower-intensity side lobes. (B) Transducer side lobe artifact (*arrows*) located in posterior portion of bladder (B). (C) Sagittal sector scan of pelvis shows low-level echoes (*arrows*) in the dependent portion of the bladder (B) caused by side lobes.

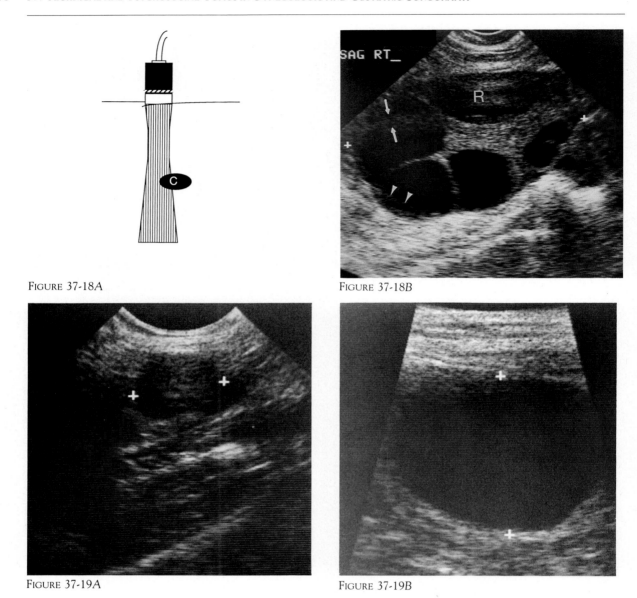

FIGURE 37-18A

FIGURE 37-18B

FIGURE 37-19A

FIGURE 37-19B

FIGURE 37-18. Slice thickness artifact. (A) Sound beam partially intersects tissue adjacent to cyst (C). Echoes from the tissue are misplaced by the equipment into the cyst. (B) Sagittal scan of right ovary in patient with ovarian hyperstimulation syndrome shows spurious band of echoes (arrows) emanating from adjacent soft tissue. Note also reverberations (R) and side lobe artifact (arrowheads).

FIGURE 37-19. Operator-dependent artifacts: transducer selection. (A) Superficial ovarian cyst (cursors) imaged with 5-MHz sector transducer demonstrates no posterior enhancement. Multiple echoes are noted within. (B) The same cyst imaged with 10-MHz transducer shows posterior enhancement and no internal echoes. (Continued on page 607, top)

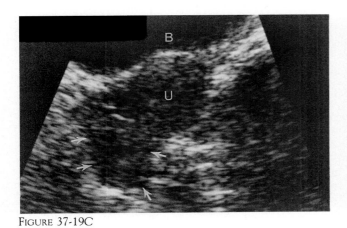

FIGURE 37-19C

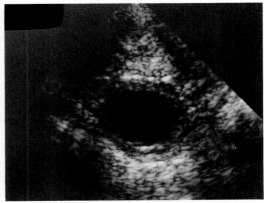

FIGURE 37-19D

FIGURE 37-19. *(continued)* (C) Transabdominal transverse scan through pelvis of obese patient shows uterus (U) and solid-looking right adnexal mass *(arrows;* B, bladder). (D) Transvaginal scan shows that the right adnexal mass actually represents a cyst.

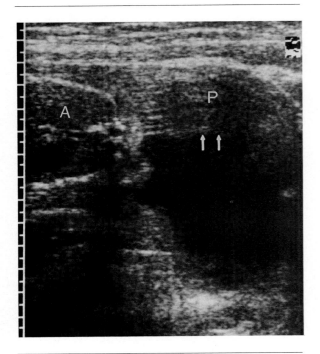

FIGURE 37-20. Operator-dependent artifacts: gain curve selection. Sagittal fetal sonogram shows an apparent anterior placenta (P), which is actually an artifact caused by improper gain curve selection. Note the absence of a chorionic plate *(arrows;* A, fetal abdomen).

from adjacent structures (Fig. 37-18). To minimize this artifact, a narrowly focused beam should be used and the structure should be scanned along its central axis. As with side lobes, the slice-thickness artifact is dependent on equipment output and disappears when the gain setting is lowered.

Operator-Dependent Artifacts

Of all the imaging modalities, ultrasound is the most operator dependent. In ultrasound scanning three variables exist: the sonographer, the instrumentation, and the patient. The unknown variable is the patient. With proper technical and didactic foundation, and appropriate use of equipment, the experienced sonographer can produce anatomically and technically accurate images. The sonographer must select the proper transducer and focal zone and determine machine output and optimal gain curves. Inappropriate transducer and focal zone selection may result in overlooking vital diagnostic information (Fig. 37-19). Improper time gain compensation and output adjustments will lead to a nonuniform display of echoes (Fig. 37-20).

References

1. Avruch L, Cooperberg PL. The ring-down artifact. J Ultrasound Med. 1985; 4:21.

2. Buttery B, Davison G. The ghost artifact. J Ultrasound Med. 1984; 3:49.

3. Fiske CE, Filly RA. Pseudo-sludge. Radiology. 1982; 144:631.

4. Goldstein A, Madrazo BI. Slice-thickness artifacts in gray-scale ultrasound. J Clin Utrasound. 1989; 9:365.

5. Jaffe CC, Rosenfield AT, Sommer G, et al. Technical factors influencing the imaging of small anechoic cysts by B-scan ultrasound. Radiology. 1980; 135:429.

6. Kremkau FW. Diagnostic Ultrasound Principles, Instrumentation, and Exercises. 2nd ed. Orlando, FL: Grune & Stratton; 1984.

7. Kremkau FW, Taylor KJW. Artifacts in ultrasound imaging. J Ultrasound Med. 1985; 5:227–237.

8. Laing FC. Commonly encountered artifacts in clinical ultrasound. Semin Ultrasound. 1983; 4:27.

9. Laing FC, Kurtz AB. The importance of side-lobe artifacts. Radiology. 1982; 145:763.

10. Muller N, Cooperberg PL, Rowley VA, et al. Ultrasonic refraction by the rectus abdominis muscles: The double image artifact. J Ultrasound Med. 1984; 3:515.

11. Robinson DE, Wilson LS, Kossoff G. Shadowing and enhancement in ultrasonic echograms by reflection and refraction. J Clin Ultrasound. 1981; 9:181.

12. Sarti DA. Diagnostic Ultrasound: Text and Cases. Chicago: Year Book Medical Publishers; 1987:54–67.

13. Sauerbrie EE. The split-image artifact in pelvic sonography: The anatomy and the physics. J Ultrasound Med. 1985; 4:29.

14. Stanley JH, Harrell B, Horger EO. Pseudoepidural reverberation artifact: A common ultrasound artifact in the fetal cranium. J Clin Ultrasound. 1986; 14:251–254.

15. Thickman DI, Ziskin MC, Goldenberg NJ, et al. Clinical manifestations of the comet tail artifact. J Ultrasound Med. 1983; 2:225.

16. Ziskin MC. Basic Principles. In: Goldberg BB, Kotler MN, Ziskin MC, et al., eds. Diagnostic Uses of Ultrasound. New York: Grune & Stratton; 1975:1–30.

17. Ziskin MC, Thickman DI, Goldenberg NJ, et al. Clinical manifestations of the comet tail artifact. J Ultrasound Med. 1982; 1:1.

CHAPTER 38

Ethical Issues in Obstetric Sonography

FRANK A. CHERVENAK, LAURENCE B. MCCULLOUGH

Ethical issues frequently arise in the relationships of sonographers with their patients and with physicians who supervise them.[5] After a discussion of ethics in general, medical ethics, and obstetric ethics, we will examine four ethical issues in obstetric ultrasound examinations with special reference to the sonographer's role: competence to perform obstetric ultrasound and referral to specialists; routine screening; disclosure of results; and confidentiality.

The authors understand sonographers to be members of an emerging but not yet fully autonomous profession. This is because sonographers at the present time have no method independent of medicine and physicians for establishing reliable diagnostic categories and nomenclature. This contrasts sharply with, for example, social workers, who have developed autonomous diagnostic categories (e.g., the troubled family or the parent at risk for child abuse). As a consequence of its less than full autonomy, the ethics of sonography are at present most usefully analyzed in terms of the sonographers' role as members of the health care team.

Ethics

Ethics is the disciplined study of morality. Morality concerns right and wrong conduct (what we ought or ought not do) and good and bad character (the kinds of persons we should aspire to be and the virtues we should cultivate). There are many sources of moral beliefs and behavior in our society, including personal experience; the traditions and experiences of families, communities, ethnic and racial groups, and geographic regions; the variety of world religions; and national identity and history, including the laws of the states and of the federal government. These sources of moral beliefs are frequently in conflict. Morality should not be confused with ethics, which seeks to articulate clear, consistent, coherent, and applicable accounts of moral conduct and character.

Historically two academic disciplines have been principally involved in ethics. The first, theological or religious ethics, is based on particular or general religious commitments. There are several problems with this approach. First, religions disagree both intramurally and extramurally about most conduct and character. Second, people of no religious persuasion are excluded from the dialogue. Finally, medical ethics, at least in countries such as the United States, must confront the fact that medicine is a secular profession and that the society that it serves is morally pluralistic.[5]

The second academic discipline involved in ethics is philosophy. To be applicable in a medical context, ethics must transcend moral pluralism by offering an approach without ties to any substantive prior commitment about moral conduct and character. This is what philosophical ethics at-

609

tempts to do. It requires only a commitment to the results of rational discourse, in which all substantive commitments are open to question. Philosophical ethics, therefore, properly serves as the foundation for medical ethics, especially in an international context.[9]

Medical Ethics

Perhaps the most useful beginning point for ethics in sonography is an analysis of the ethical obligation that serves as the foundation of the patient-sonographer relationship: the sonographer's obligation to protect and promote the best interests of the patient. This relationship derives from the patient-physician relationship, because the sonographer's moral authority to care for patients derives from the physician's moral authority as the patient's principal caregiver.

From its beginnings in ancient Greece, Western medicine has made a distinctive claim to know what is in the best interests of the patient. One expression of this claim is *"Primum non nocere,"* which means "First do no harm." In ethics, this is known as the *principle of nonmaleficence.*[1] This principle only partially explains what is in the patient's best interests, however, because medicine, and therefore sonography, seeks to benefit patients, not simply avoid harming them. The use of obstetric ultrasound, like other medical interventions, must be justified by the goal of seeking the greater balance of "good" over "harm,"[1] not simply avoiding harm to the patient at all cost. This ethical principle is called *beneficence,* and is a more adequate basis for ethics in sonography than is nonmaleficence.[1,2]

The principle of beneficence underlies the beneficence model of moral responsibility in medicine[2] and should guide the conduct and character of sonographers.[2] According to the beneficence model, the good ends that sonography should seek for patients are preventing early or premature death (not preventing death itself), preventing and curing disease, injury, and handicapping conditions, or at least alleviating unnecessary pain and suffering.[2] Pain and suffering are unnecessary and therefore represent harms to be avoided when they do not contribute to seeking the goods of the beneficence model.

In the 20th century, first in the United States and more recently in other Western democracies, it has been recognized that patients have their own perspective on their best interests and that that perspective should be on at least an equal footing with medicine's perspective on the patient's best interests. A patient's perspective on his or her best interests is shaped by wide-ranging and sometimes idiosyncratic values and beliefs.[2] *Autonomy* refers to a person's capacity to express and carry out value-based preferences. The ethical principle of respect for autonomy obligates us to acknowledge the integrity of a patient's values and beliefs and of his or her value-based preferences; to avoid interfering with the expression or implementation of these preferences; and when necessary, to assist in their expression and implementation. This principle generates the autonomy model of moral responsibility in medicine.[2] Unlike the beneficence model, no specific goods and harms can be defined because these definitions are left to each individual patient.

Obstetric Ethics

We hold that protecting and promoting the best interests of the pregnant woman and the best interests of the fetus in a pregnancy going to term—and the child the fetus will become—are the basic goals or purposes of obstetric care,[4] and therefore of sonographic examination. These goals form the basis on which the autonomy and beneficence models can be applied in obstetric care. These models generate ethical obligations to the pregnant woman and the fetus.

Maternal best interests are protected and promoted by both autonomy-based and beneficence-based obligations of the sonographer to pregnant women. Fetuses are incapable of having their own perspective on their best interests, because the immaturity of their central nervous system renders them incapable of having the necessary values or beliefs. So, there are no autonomy-based obligations to the fetus.[4] Fetal best interests in sonography are understood exclusively in terms of the beneficence model. This model explains the moral status of the fetus and generates the serious obligations owed to it. The sonographer has beneficence-based obligations to the fetus in a pregnancy going to term, to protect and promote its interests and those of the child it will become, as these are understood from a clinical perspective.[4] The goods to be sought for the child the fetus will become (and, therefore, for the fetus) include prevention of premature death, disease, and handicapping conditions and of unnecessary pain and suffering. It may be appropriate, therefore, to refer to fetuses as patients, with the exception of previable fetuses that are aborted.[4]

The pregnant woman also has beneficence-based obligations to the fetus, because she is its moral fiduciary when the pregnancy will be taken to term. She is expected to protect and promote her fetus's best interests and those of the child it will become.[4] When a pregnant woman elects to have an abortion, however, these fiduciary obligations do not exist. A sonographer with moral objections to abortion should keep two things in mind: First, the moral judgment of the pregnant woman should not be criticized or shortchanged in any way; her autonomy should be respected. Second, the sonographer is free to follow his or her conscience and to withdraw from further involvement with patients who elect abortion. Physicians should respect this important matter of conscience.

Ethical Issues in Obstetric Ultrasound

COMPETENCE AND REFERRAL

The ethical obligation to provide competent obstetric ultrasound examinations is based on the beneficence and autonomy models. Either model alone, and certainly both in combination, require sonographers and physicians to provide patients with accurate and reliable information. To meet this ethical obligation, the clinician must distinguish general from specialized competence both to perform and to interpret the results of obstetric ultrasound examinations.

Ensuring a general level of competence imposes a rigorous standard of training and continuing education. Two problems result when sonographers do not maintain this baseline level of competence. First, they may cause unnecessary harm to the pregnant woman or fetus, thus violating the beneficence model. Second, incomplete or inaccurate reporting of results to the pregnant woman undermines the informed consent process regarding the management of pregnancy, thus violating the autonomy model. Because physicians rely heav-

ily on them, sonographers are in a crucial position to avoid these adverse consequences.

Any sonographer who performs obstetric ultrasound examinations is ethically obligated to assure the pregnant woman that the examinations are performed competently. This obligation also has important implications for physicians who employ a sonographer. Such physicians are ethically obligated to adequately supervise the sonographer's work. The physician must know substantially more than the sonographer, especially about the application of sonographic findings to the diagnosis of anomalies. This more advanced fund of knowledge is essential for the physician to fulfill the additional obligation to regularly review the sonographer's work. In addition, physicians should provide the opportunity for continuing education. In medical care, patients properly rely for their protection on the personal and professional integrity of their clinicians. An important facet of that integrity on the part of physicians is willingness to refer to specialists when the limits of their own knowledge are being approached.

Integrity should also be one of the fundamental virtues of sonographers and, thus, a standard for judging professional character. Like other virtues, such as honesty and compassion, integrity directs sonographers to focus primarily on the patient's best interests, as a way to blunt mere self-interest. As sonography continues to develop as a profession, it will need to identify and address incentives to mere self-interest on the part of sonographers.

Sonographers who work with specialists who receive patients on referral confront two principal ethical concerns. The first is an ethical obligation to ensure that they maintain their standards of general competence. Sonographers as a group have beneficence-based obligations to the patient population. The patient population relies on sonographers' self-regulation as the means to guarantee that these beneficence-based obligations are fulfilled.

The second concern for sonographers involves discovering avoidable errors that a colleague has made. The autonomy model generates an inescapable obligation on the part of the referral specialists to interpret ultrasound examinations made by referring physicians when they are available and to disclose the results of the specialists' examination.

The specialist may sometimes face the obligation to present findings to a pregnant woman that the referring physician should have been competent to detect but did not, due to faulty technique or interpretation. In such an instance, the sonographer's integrity is the only safeguard of the patient's autonomy against the self-interest of the specialist, who may wish to avoid potential loss of income that might result from a conflict with the referring physician. The sonographer should not fail to bring to the attention of the referral specialist (not the patient directly) his or her concern about the inadequacies of the referring physician's sonographic technique. If necessary, the sonographer should become an advocate for disclosure of such information to the pregnant woman.

ROUTINE SCREENING

In many countries routine obstetric ultrasound examination at about 18 weeks has become the standard of care. In others, including the United States, this is not the case. Debate in the United States about routine ultrasound examination has been conducted almost exclusively in terms of the beneficence model applied to both the fetus and the pregnant woman. The result of this ongoing debate seems to be considerable uncertainty about how to balance the goods and harms of routine obstetric ultrasound examinations.[6] The ethical issues concern the physician's responsibilities in informed consent. We include discussion of them because sonographers need to be aware of these issues.

The authors believe that this debate should be expanded to include reference to the autonomy model. In the face of medical uncertainty about the goods and harms of routine ultrasound, it is reasonable to inform patients about that uncertainty and to give them the opportunity to make their own choices about how that uncertainty should be managed. We have argued that prenatal informed consent for sonogram (PICS) should be an indication for the routine use of obstetric ultrasound.[6]

The timing of routine ultrasound is moderated by the autonomy model, because the information obtained is relevant to any woman's decision about whether she will seek an abortion. In pregnancies that will be taken to term, routine ultrasound during the second trimester can enhance a pregnant woman's autonomy. If anomalies are detected, she may begin to prepare herself for the decisions that she will have to confront later about the management of those anomalies in the intrapartum and postpartum periods. Providing this information early in pregnancy permits a pregnant woman ample time to deal with its psychological sequelae before she must confront such decisions.

DISCLOSURE

A number of ethical issues arise about the disclosure of results of ultrasound examinations. First, there must be an adequate informed consent process. This process usually includes disclosure of and discussion about what ultrasound examinations can and cannot detect, the level of sophistication of the ultrasound techniques employed, and the incomplete and sometimes uncertain interpretation of ultrasound images. In routine examinations it may be important for some pregnant women to be aware of the possibility of confronting the unanticipated alternative of terminating a pregnancy in which an anomaly is detected.[8] Sonographers are justified to disclose findings of normal anatomy directly to the pregnant woman. Disclosure of, and discussion about, abnormal findings—if these are to respect and to enhance maternal autonomy and avoid unnecessary psychological harm to the pregnant woman—are the responsibilities of the physician.

The second ethical issue arises in connection with the phenomenon of apparent bonding of pregnant women to their fetuses as a result of the pregnant woman seeing the ultrasound images.[3] Such bonding may benefit pregnancies that will be taken to term but could also complicate decisions to terminate a pregnancy. We recommend that these matters, like abnormal findings, should be discussed with the pregnant woman.

We want to touch on a third issue, which is a matter of ongoing debate: the disclosure of the fetus's gender.[10] We propose that respect for maternal autonomy dictates responding frankly to requests from the pregnant woman for information about the fetus's gender. The pregnant woman should be made aware of the uncertainties of ultrasound gender identification, as part of the disclosure process. The sonographer can use his or her own experience to help the pregnant woman understand those uncertainties.

CONFIDENTIALITY

It should go without saying that the beneficence and autonomy models govern the sonographer's ethical obligations to his or her *patient*. The pregnant woman is indisputably the patient of the sonographer and the physician. Others, including the pregnant woman's spouse, sex partner, and family, should be understood as third parties to the patient-sonographer relationship. Diagnostic information about a woman's pregnancy is confidential. It can be justifiably disclosed to third parties only with the pregnant woman's explicit permission. This is because a potentially acceptable condition for releasing confidential information, avoiding grave harm to others,[1] does not apply in this context. To avoid awkward situations, sonographers and their supervising physicians should establish policies and procedures that reflect this analysis of the ethics of confidentiality.

Conclusion

Because sonographers are sometimes referred to as "technicians," there may be a temptation to be regarded by others, and thus for them a temptation to describe themselves, as mere automatons. The analysis in this chapter of ethical issues in sonography shows why this is a mistake. Sonographers are in an ethically significant relationship with patients and thus are significant members of the health care team. Sonographers have ethical obligations generated by the beneficence and autonomy models. It is important to distinguish, however, limits on those obligations and, therefore, limits on the freedom of sonographers that derive from the patient-physician relationship. Where these limits should be drawn is the fundamental agenda for the future of ethical issues in obstetric sonography. Because sonography is a new and still evolving profession, this distinction is not always easy to make in practice. However, this distinction is crucial for an understanding of the proper role of the sonographer in the health care team.

References

1. Beauchamp TL, Childress JF. Principles of Biomedical Ethics. 3rd ed. New York: Oxford University Press; 1989.
2. Beauchamp TL, McCullough LB. Medical Ethics: The Moral Responsibilities of Physicians. Englewood Cliffs, NJ: Prentice-Hall; 1984.
3. Campbell S, Reading AE, Cox DN, et al. Ultrasound scanning in pregnancy: The short-term psychological effects of early real time scans. J Psychosomat Obstet Gynecol. 1986; 1:57–61.
4. Chervenak FA, McCullough LB. Perinatal ethics: A practical analysis of obligations to mother and fetus. Obstet Gynecol. 1985; 66:442–446.
5. Chervenak FA, McCullough L. Ethics in obstetric ultrasound. J Ultrasound Med. 1989; 8:493–497.
6. Chervenak FA, McCullough LB, Chervenak JL. Prenatal informed consent for sonogram (PICS): An indication for obstetrical ultrasound. Am J Obstet Gynecol. 1989; 161(4):857–860.
7. Engelhardt HT Jr. The Foundations of Bioethics. New York: Oxford University Press; 1986.
8. Faden R, et al. Disclosure of information to patients in medical care. Med Care. 1981; 19:718–733.
9. McCullough LB. Methodological concerns in bioethics. J Med Phil. 1986; 11:17–37.
10. Warren MA. Gendercide. The Implications of Sex Selection. Totowa, NJ: Rowman and Littlefield; 1985.

Appendixes

APPENDIX A. Estimation of gestational age by gestational sac measurement

MEAN PREDICTED GESTATIONAL SAC (MM)	GESTATIONAL AGE (WKS)	MEAN PREDICTED GESTATIONAL SAC (MM)	GESTATIONAL AGE (WKS)
10.0	5.0		
11.0	5.2	36.0	8.8
12.0	5.3	37.0	8.9
13.0	5.5	38.0	9.0
14.0	5.6	39.0	9.2
15.0	5.8	40.0	9.3
16.0	5.9	41.0	9.5
17.0	6.0	42.0	9.6
18.0	6.2	43.0	9.7
19.0	6.3	44.0	9.9
20.0	6.5	45.0	10.0
21.0	6.6	46.0	10.2
22.0	6.8	47.0	10.3
23.0	6.9	48.0	10.5
24.0	7.0	49.0	10.6
25.0	7.2	50.0	10.7
26.0	7.3	51.0	10.9
27.0	7.5	52.0	11.0
28.0	7.6	53.0	11.2
29.0	7.8	54.0	11.3
30.0	7.9	55.0	11.5
31.0	8.0	56.0	11.6
32.0	8.2	57.0	11.7
33.0	8.3	58.0	11.9
34.0	8.5	59.0	12.0
35.0	8.6	60.0	12.2

$$\text{Equation*: Gestational age (wks)} = \frac{\text{Gestational sac (mm)} + 25.43}{7.02}$$

*This formula was expressed in centimeters in its original form.
(From Hellman LM, Kobayashi M, Fillisti L, et al. Growth and development of the human fetus prior to the 20th week of gestation. Am J Obstet Gynecol. 1969;103:784–800.)

Appendix B. Estimation of gestational age by crown-rump length

Crown-rump Length (cm)	Gestational Age (Weeks & Days)	Crown-rump Length (cm)	Gestational Age (Weeks & Days)	Crown-rump Length (cm)	Gestational Age (Weeks & Days)
1.0	7 + 5	2.9	9 + 6	4.8	11 + 5
1.1	7 + 6	3.0	9 + 6	4.9	11 + 5
1.2	8 + 0	3.1	10 + 0	5.0	11 + 6
1.3	8 + 1	3.2	10 + 1	5.1	12 + 0
1.4	8 + 1	3.3	10 + 2	5.2	12 + 0
1.5	8 + 2	3.4	10 + 2	5.3	12 + 1
1.6	8 + 3	3.5	10 + 3	5.4	12 + 1
1.7	8 + 4	3.6	10 + 4	5.5	12 + 2
1.8	8 + 5	3.7	10 + 4	5.6	12 + 3
1.9	8 + 5	3.8	10 + 5	5.7	12 + 3
2.0	8 + 6	3.9	10 + 6	5.8	12 + 4
2.1	9 + 0	4.0	10 + 6	5.9	12 + 4
2.2	9 + 1	4.1	11 + 0	6.0	12 + 5
2.3	9 + 1	4.2	11 + 1	6.1	12 + 6
2.4	9 + 2	4.3	11 + 1	6.2	12 + 6
2.5	9 + 3	4.4	11 + 2	6.3	13 + 0
2.6	9 + 4	4.5	11 + 3	6.4	13 + 0
2.7	9 + 4	4.6	11 + 3	6.5	13 + 1
2.8	9 + 5	4.7	11 + 4	6.6	13 + 2

(Modified from MacGregor SN, Tamura RK, Sabbagha RE, et al. Underestimation of gestational age by conventional crown-rump length dating curves. Obstet Gynecol. 1987;70:347.)

APPENDIX C. Estimation of gestational age by biparietal diameter

BIPARIETAL DIAMETER (MM)	GESTATIONAL AGE (WEEKS)		BIPARIETAL DIAMETER (MM)	GESTATIONAL AGE (WEEKS)	
	MEAN*	90% VARIATION†		MEAN*	90% VARIATION†
20	12.0	12.0	60	23.8	22.3–25.5
21	12.0	12.0	61	24.2	22.6–25.8
22	12.7	12.2–13.2	62	24.6	23.1–26.1
23	13.0	12.4–13.6	63	24.9	23.4–26.4
24	13.2	12.6–13.8	64	25.3	23.8–26.8
25	13.5	12.9–14.1	65	25.6	24.1–27.1
26	13.7	13.1–14.3	66	26.0	24.5–27.5
27	14.0	13.4–14.6	67	26.4	25.0–27.8
28	14.3	13.6–15.0	68	26.7	25.3–28.1
29	14.5	13.9–15.2	69	27.1	25.8–28.4
30	14.8	14.1–15.5	70	27.5	26.3–28.7
31	15.1	14.3–15.9	71	27.9	26.7–29.1
32	15.3	14.5–16.1	72	28.3	27.2–29.4
33	15.6	14.7–16.5	73	28.7	27.6–29.8
34	15.9	15.0–16.8	74	29.1	28.1–30.1
35	16.2	15.2–17.2	75	29.5	28.5–30.5
36	16.4	15.4–17.4	76	30.0	29.0–31.0
37	16.7	15.6–17.8	77	30.3	29.2–31.4
38	17.0	15.9–18.1	78	30.8	29.6–32.0
39	17.3	16.1–18.5	79	31.1	29.9–32.5
40	17.6	16.4–18.8	80	31.6	30.2–33.0
41	17.9	16.5–19.3	81	32.1	30.7–33.5
42	18.1	16.6–19.8	82	32.6	31.2–34.0
43	18.4	16.8–20.2	83	33.0	31.5–34.5
44	18.8	16.9–20.7	84	33.4	31.9–35.1
45	19.1	17.0–21.2	85	34.0	32.3–35.7
46	19.4	17.4–21.4	86	34.3	32.8–36.2
47	19.7	17.8–21.6	87	35.0	33.4–36.6
48	20.0	18.2–21.8	88	35.4	33.9–37.1
49	20.3	18.6–22.0	89	36.1	34.6–37.6
50	20.6	19.0–22.2	90	36.6	35.1–38.1
51	20.9	19.3–22.5	91	37.2	35.9–38.5
52	21.2	19.5–22.9	92	37.8	36.7–38.9
53	21.5	19.8–23.2	93	38.8	37.3–39.3
54	21.9	20.1–23.7	94	39.0	37.9–40.1
55	22.2	20.4–24.0	95	39.7	38.5–40.9
56	22.5	20.7–24.3	96	40.6	39.1–41.5
57	22.8	21.1–24.5	97	41.0	39.9–42.1
58	23.2	21.5–24.9	98	41.8	40.5–43.1
59	23.5	21.9–25.1			

*From weighted least mean square fit equation: $Y = -3.45701 + 0.50157X - 0.00441X^2$
†For each biparietal diameter, 90% of gestational age data points fell within this range.
(From Kurtz AB, et al. Analysis of biparietal diameter as an accurate indicator of gestational age. J Clin Ultrasound. 1980;8:319–326.)

APPENDIX D. Estimation of gestational age by head circumference measurement

HEAD CIRCUMFERENCE (MM)	GESTATIONAL AGE (WEEKS)		HEAD CIRCUMFERENCE (MM)	GESTATIONAL AGE (WEEKS)	
	PREDICTED MEAN VALUES	95% CONFIDENCE LIMITS		PREDICTED MEAN VALUES	95% CONFIDENCE LIMITS
80	13.4	12.1–14.7	220	23.9	22.3–25.5
85	13.7	12.4–15.0	225	24.4	22.1–26.7
90	14.0	12.7–15.3	230	24.9	22.6–27.2
95	14.3	13.0–15.6	235	25.4	23.1–27.7
100	14.6	13.3–15.9	240	25.9	23.6–28.2
105	15.0	13.7–16.3	245	26.4	24.1–28.7
110	15.3	14.0–16.6	250	26.9	24.6–29.2
115	15.6	14.3–16.9	255	27.5	25.2–29.8
120	15.9	14.6–17.2	260	28.0	25.7–30.3
125	16.3	15.0–17.6	265	28.1	25.8–30.4
130	16.6	15.3–17.9	270	29.2	26.9–31.5
135	17.0	15.7–18.3	275	29.8	27.5–32.1
140	17.3	16.0–18.6	280	30.3	27.6–33.0
145	17.7	16.4–19.0	285	31.0	28.3–33.7
150	18.1	16.5–19.7	290	31.6	28.9–34.3
155	18.4	16.8–20.0	295	32.2	29.5–34.8
160	18.8	17.2–20.4	300	32.8	30.1–35.5
165	19.2	17.6–20.8	305	33.5	30.7–36.2
170	19.6	18.0–21.2	310	34.2	31.5–36.9
175	20.0	18.4–21.6	315	34.9	32.2–37.6
180	20.4	18.8–22.0	320	35.5	32.8–38.2
185	20.8	19.2–22.4	325	36.3	32.9–39.7
190	21.2	19.8–22.8	330	37.0	33.6–40.4
195	21.6	20.0–23.2	335	37.7	34.3–41.1
200	22.1	20.5–23.7	340	38.5	35.1–41.9
205	22.5	20.9–24.1	345	39.2	35.8–42.6
210	23.0	21.4–24.6	350	40.0	36.6–43.4
215	23.4	21.8–25.0	355	40.8	37.4–44.2
			360	41.6	38.2–45.0

(Data from Tables 3 and 4 in Handlock FP, Deter RL, Harrist RB, et al. Fetal head circumference: Relation to menstrual age. Am J Roentgenol. 1982;138:649–653.)

APPENDIX E. Lateral ventricular to hemispheric width ratios in fetuses from 15 weeks to term

MENSTRUAL AGE (WEEK)	LATERAL VENTRICULAR WIDTH (2 SD) (MM)	HEMISPHERIC WIDTH (2 SD) (MM)	LATERAL VENTRICULAR WIDTH HEMISPHERIC WIDTH RATIO (LVW/HW) (2 SD) (MM)
15	8 (6–10)	15 (12–18)	56 (38–74)
16	9 (7–11)	15 (13–17)	57 (46–68)
17	9 (8–10)	15 (14–16)	58 (49–67)
18	9 (8–10)	18 (17–19)	51 (41–61)
19	9 (7–11)	20 (19–21)	49 (41–57)
20	9 (7–11)	19 (17–20)	46 (38–54)
21	9 (7–11)	21 (20–22)	42 (31–53)
22	9 (7–11)	23 (21–25)	40 (29–51)
23	8 (7–9)	24 (22–26)	34 (26–42)
24	9 (8–10)	25 (23–27)	35 (27–43)
25	9 (8–10)	28 (25–31)	33 (29–37)
26	9	30	30 (24–36)
27	9	30	28 (23–34)
28	11	33	31 (18–45)
29	10	34	29 (22–37)
30	10	34	30 (26–34)
31	10	34	29 (23–36)
32	11	36	31 (26–36)
33	11	34	31 (25–37)
34	11	38	28 (23–33)
35	11	38	29 (26–31)
36	11	39	28 (23–34)
37	12	41	29 (24–34)
Term	12	43	28 (22–33)

(Data for 15 to 25 gestational weeks from Pretorius DH, Drose JA, Manco-Johnson MI. Fetal lateral ventricular ratio determined during the second trimester. J Ultrasound Med. 1986;5:121–124. Used by permission; for 26 gestational weeks to term: from Johnson ML, Dunne MC, Mack LA, et al. Evaluation of fetal intracranial anatomy by static and realtime ultrasound. J Clin Ultrasound. 1980;8:311–318. Used by permission.)

APPENDIX F. Estimation of gestational age by outer orbital diameter (binocular distance) measurement

Outer Orbital Diameter (MM)	Gestational Age (Weeks)		Outer Orbital Diameter (MM)	Gestational Age (Weeks)	
	Predicted Mean Values	5th–95th Percentiles		Predicted Mean Values	5th–95th Percentiles
15	10.4	7.1–13.9			
16	11.0	7.7–14.4	41	25.9	22.6–29.1
17	11.6	8.3–15.0	42	26.6	23.1–29.9
18	12.1	8.9–15.6	43	27.1	23.9–30.4
19	12.9	9.6–16.1	44	27.7	24.4–31.0
20	13.4	10.1–16.7	45	28.3	25.0–31.6
21	14.0	10.7–17.3	46	28.9	25.6–32.1
22	14.6	11.3–17.9	47	29.6	26.1–32.9
23	15.1	11.9–18.6	48	30.1	26.9–33.4
24	15.9	12.6–19.1	49	30.7	27.3–34.0
25	16.4	13.1–19.7	50	31.3	27.9–34.6
26	17.0	13.7–20.3	51	31.9	28.6–35.1
27	17.6	14.3–20.9	52	32.6	29.1–35.9
28	18.1	14.9–21.6	53	33.0	29.7–36.4
29	18.9	15.6–22.1	54	33.6	30.3–37.0
30	19.4	16.1–22.7	55	34.1	30.9–37.6
31	20.0	16.6–23.3	56	34.9	31.6–38.1
32	20.6	17.1–23.9	57	35.4	32.1–38.7
33	21.1	17.9–24.6	58	36.0	32.7–39.3
34	21.7	18.4–25.1	59	36.6	33.3–39.9
35	22.3	19.0–25.7	60	37.1	33.9–40.6
36	22.9	19.6–26.3	61	37.9	34.6–41.1
37	23.6	20.1–26.9	62	38.4	35.1–41.7
38	24.1	20.6–27.4	63	39.0	35.7–42.3
39	24.7	21.4–28.0	64	39.6	36.3–42.9
40	25.3	22.0–28.6	65	40.1	36.9–43.5

(From Jeanty P, Cantraine F, Cousaert E, et al. The binocular distance: A new way to estimate fetal age. J Ultrasound Med. 1984; 3:241–243. Used by permission.)

APPENDIX G. Estimation of gestational age by abdominal circumference measurement

ABDOMINAL CIRCUMFERENCE (MM)	GESTATIONAL AGE (WEEKS)		ABDOMINAL CIRCUMFERENCE (MM)	GESTATIONAL AGE (WEEKS)	
	PREDICTED MEAN	95% CONFIDENCE LIMITS		PREDICTED MEAN	95% CONFIDENCE LIMITS
100	15.6	13.7–17.5	235	27.7	25.5–29.9
105	16.1	14.2–18.0	240	28.2	26.0–30.4
110	16.5	14.6–18.4	245	28.7	26.5–30.9
115	16.9	15.0–18.8	250	29.2	27.0–31.4
120	17.3	15.4–19.2	255	29.7	27.5–31.9
125	17.8	15.9–19.7	260	30.1	27.1–33.1
130	18.2	16.2–20.2	265	30.6	27.6–33.6
135	18.6	16.6–20.6	270	31.1	28.1–34.1
140	19.1	17.1–21.1	275	31.6	28.6–34.6
145	19.5	17.5–21.5	280	32.1	29.1–35.1
150	20.0	18.0–22.0	285	32.6	29.6–35.6
155	20.4	18.4–22.4	290	33.1	30.1–36.1
160	20.8	18.8–22.8	295	33.6	30.6–36.6
165	21.3	19.3–23.3	300	34.1	31.1–37.1
170	21.7	19.7–23.7	305	34.6	31.6–37.6
175	22.2	20.2–24.2	310	35.1	32.1–38.1
180	22.6	20.6–24.6	315	35.6	32.6–38.6
185	23.1	21.1–25.1	320	36.1	33.6–38.6
190	23.6	21.6–25.6	325	36.6	34.1–39.1
195	24.0	21.8–26.2	330	37.1	34.6–39.6
200	24.5	22.3–26.7	335	37.6	35.1–40.1
205	24.9	22.7–27.1	340	38.1	35.6–40.6
210	25.4	23.2–27.6	345	38.7	36.2–41.2
215	25.9	23.7–28.1	350	39.2	36.7–41.7
220	26.3	24.1–28.5	355	39.7	37.2–42.2
225	26.8	24.6–29.0	360	40.2	37.7–42.7
230	27.3	25.1–29.5	365	40.8	38.3–43.3

(Data from Tables 3 and 4 in Hadlock FP, Deter RL, Harrist RB, et al. Fetal abdominal circumference as a predictor of menstrual age. Am J Roentgenol. 1982;139:367–370.)

Appendix H. Estimation of gestational age by fetal thoracic circumference (in centimeters)

Gestational Age (Week)	Sample Size No.	Predictive Percentiles								
		2.5	5	10	25	50	75	90	95	97.5
16	6	5.9	6.4	7.0	8.0	9.1	10.3	11.3	11.9	12.4
17	22	6.8	7.3	7.9	8.9	10.0	11.2	12.2	12.8	13.3
18	31	7.7	8.2	8.8	9.8	11.0	12.1	13.1	13.7	14.2
19	21	8.6	9.1	9.7	10.7	11.9	13.0	14.0	14.6	15.1
20	20	9.5	10.0	10.6	11.7	12.8	13.9	15.0	15.5	16.0
21	30	10.4	11.0	11.6	12.6	13.7	14.8	15.8	16.4	16.9
22	18	11.3	11.9	12.5	13.5	14.6	15.7	16.7	17.3	17.8
23	21	12.2	12.8	13.4	14.4	15.5	16.6	17.6	18.2	18.8
24	27	13.2	13.7	14.3	15.3	16.4	17.5	18.5	19.1	19.7
25	20	14.1	14.6	15.2	16.2	17.3	18.4	19.4	20.0	20.6
26	25	15.0	15.5	16.1	17.1	18.2	19.3	20.3	21.0	21.5
27	24	15.9	16.4	17.0	18.0	19.1	20.2	21.3	21.9	22.4
28	24	16.8	17.3	17.9	18.9	20.0	21.2	22.2	22.8	23.3
29	24	17.7	18.2	18.8	19.8	21.0	22.1	23.1	23.7	24.2
30	27	18.6	19.1	19.7	20.7	21.9	23.0	24.0	24.6	25.1
31	24	19.5	20.0	20.6	21.6	22.8	23.9	24.9	25.5	26.0
32	28	20.4	20.9	21.5	22.6	23.7	24.8	25.8	26.4	26.9
33	27	21.3	21.8	22.5	23.5	24.6	25.7	26.7	27.3	27.8
34	25	22.2	22.8	23.4	24.4	25.5	26.6	27.6	28.2	28.7
35	20	23.1	23.7	24.3	25.3	26.4	27.5	28.5	29.1	29.6
36	23	24.0	24.6	25.2	26.2	27.3	28.4	29.4	30.0	30.6
37	22	24.9	25.5	26.1	27.1	28.2	29.3	30.3	30.9	31.5
38	21	25.9	26.4	27.0	28.0	29.1	30.2	31.2	31.9	32.4
39	7	26.8	27.3	27.9	28.9	30.0	31.1	32.2	32.8	33.3
40	6	27.7	28.2	28.8	29.8	30.9	32.1	33.1	33.7	34.2

(From Chitkara U, Rosenberg J, Chervenak FA, et al. Prenatal sonographic assessment of the fetal thorax: Normal values. Am J Obstet Gynecol. 1987;156:1071.)

APPENDIX I. Estimation of gestational age by fetal thoracic length (in centimeters)

GESTATIONAL AGE (WEEK)	SAMPLE SIZE NO.	PREDICTIVE PERCENTILES								
		2.5	5	10	25	50	75	90	95	97.5
16	6	0.9	1.1	1.3	1.6	2.0	2.4	2.8	3.0	3.2
17	22	1.1	1.3	1.5	1.8	2.2	2.6	3.0	3.2	3.4
18	31	1.3	1.4	1.7	2.0	2.4	2.8	3.2	3.4	3.6
19	21	1.4	1.6	1.8	2.2	2.7	3.0	3.4	3.6	3.8
20	20	1.6	1.8	2.0	2.4	2.8	3.2	3.6	3.8	4.0
21	30	1.8	2.0	2.2	2.6	3.0	3.4	3.7	4.0	4.1
22	18	2.0	2.2	2.4	2.8	3.2	3.6	3.9	4.1	4.3
23	21	2.2	2.4	2.6	3.0	3.4	3.8	4.1	4.3	4.5
24	27	2.4	2.6	2.8	3.1	3.5	3.9	4.3	4.5	4.7
25	20	2.6	2.8	3.0	3.3	3.7	4.1	4.5	4.7	4.9
26	25	2.8	2.9	3.2	3.5	3.9	4.3	4.7	4.9	5.1
27	24	2.9	3.1	3.3	3.7	4.1	4.5	4.9	5.1	5.3
28	24	3.1	3.3	3.5	3.9	4.3	4.7	5.0	5.4	5.4
29	24	3.3	3.5	3.7	4.1	4.5	4.9	5.2	5.5	5.6
30	27	3.5	3.7	3.9	4.3	4.7	5.1	5.4	5.6	5.8
31	24	3.7	3.9	4.1	4.5	4.9	5.3	5.6	5.8	6.0
32	28	3.9	4.1	4.3	4.6	5.0	5.4	5.8	6.0	6.2
33	27	4.1	4.3	4.5	4.8	5.2	5.6	6.0	6.2	6.4
34	25	4.2	4.4	4.7	5.0	5.4	5.8	6.2	6.4	6.6
35	20	4.4	4.6	4.8	5.2	5.6	6.0	6.4	6.6	6.8
36	23	4.6	4.8	5.0	5.4	5.8	6.2	6.5	6.8	7.0
37	22	4.8	5.0	5.2	5.6	6.0	6.4	6.7	7.0	7.1
38	21	5.0	5.2	5.4	5.8	6.2	6.6	6.9	7.1	7.3
39	7	5.2	5.4	5.6	6.0	6.4	6.8	7.1	7.3	7.5
40	6	5.4	5.6	5.8	6.1	6.5	6.9	7.3	7.5	7.7

(From Chitkara U, Rosenberg J, Chervenak FA, et al. Prenatal sonographic assessment of the fetal thorax: Normal values. Am J Obstet Gynecol. 1987;156:1072.)

APPENDIX J. Estimation of gestational age by femur and humerus measurement

BONE LENGTH (MM)	GESTATIONAL AGE (WEEKS)			
	FEMUR		HUMERUS	
	PREDICTED MEAN	5TH–95TH PERCENTILES	PREDICTED MEAN	5TH–95TH PERCENTILES
10	12.6	10.4–14.9	12.6	9.9–15.3
11	12.9	10.7–15.1	12.9	10.1–15.6
12	13.3	11.1–15.6	13.1	10.4–15.9
13	13.6	11.4–15.9	13.6	10.9–16.1
14	13.9	11.7–16.1	13.9	11.1–16.6
15	14.1	12.0–16.4	14.1	11.4–16.9
16	14.6	12.4–16.9	14.6	11.9–17.3
17	14.9	12.7–17.1	14.9	12.1–17.6
18	15.1	13.0–17.4	15.1	12.6–18.0
19	15.6	13.4–17.9	15.6	12.9–18.3
20	15.9	13.7–18.1	15.9	13.1–18.7
21	16.3	14.1–18.6	16.3	13.6–19.1
22	16.6	14.4–18.9	16.7	13.9–19.4
23	16.9	14.7–19.1	17.1	14.3–19.9
24	17.3	15.1–19.6	17.4	14.7–20.1
25	17.6	15.4–19.9	17.9	15.1–20.6
26	18.0	15.9–20.1	18.1	15.6–21.0
27	18.3	16.1–20.6	18.6	15.9–21.4
28	18.7	16.6–20.9	19.0	16.3–21.9
29	19.0	16.9–21.1	19.4	16.7–22.1
30	19.4	17.1–21.6	19.9	17.1–22.6
31	19.9	17.6–22.0	20.3	17.6–23.0
32	20.1	17.9–22.3	20.7	18.0–23.6
33	20.6	18.3–22.7	21.1	18.4–23.9
34	20.9	18.7–23.1	21.6	18.9–24.3
35	21.1	19.0–23.4	22.0	19.3–24.9
36	21.6	19.4–23.9	22.6	19.7–25.1
37	22.0	19.9–24.1	22.9	20.1–25.7
38	22.4	20.1–24.6	23.4	20.6–26.1
39	22.7	20.6–24.9	23.9	21.1–26.6
40	23.1	20.9–25.3	24.3	21.6–27.1
41	23.6	21.3–25.7	24.9	22.0–27.6
42	23.9	21.7–26.1	25.3	22.6–28.0
43	24.3	22.1–26.6	25.7	23.0–28.6
44	24.7	22.6–26.9	26.1	23.6–29.0
45	25.0	22.9–27.1	26.7	24.0–29.6
46	25.4	23.1–27.6	27.1	24.6–30.0
47	25.9	23.6–28.0	27.7	25.0–30.6
48	26.1	24.0–28.4	28.1	25.6–31.0
49	26.6	24.4–28.9	28.9	26.0–31.6

APPENDIX J. (*continued*)

| BONE LENGTH (MM) | GESTATIONAL AGE (WEEKS) | | | |
| | FEMUR | | HUMERUS | |
	PREDICTED MEAN	5TH–95TH PERCENTILES	PREDICTED MEAN	5TH–95TH PERCENTILES
50	27.0	24.9–29.1	29.3	26.6–32.0
51	27.4	25.1–29.6	29.9	27.1–32.6
52	27.9	25.6–30.0	30.3	27.6–33.1
53	28.1	26.0–30.4	30.9	28.1–33.6
54	28.6	26.4–30.9	31.4	28.7–34.1
55	29.1	26.9–31.3	32.0	29.1–34.7
56	29.6	27.2–31.7	32.6	29.9–35.3
57	29.9	27.7–32.1	33.1	30.3–35.9
58	30.3	28.1–32.6	33.6	30.9–36.4
59	30.7	28.6–32.9	34.1	31.4–36.9
60	31.1	28.9–33.3	34.9	32.0–37.6
61	31.6	29.4–33.9	35.3	32.6–38.1
62	32.0	29.9–34.1	35.9	33.1–38.7
63	32.4	30.1–34.6	36.6	33.9–39.3
64	32.9	30.7–35.1	37.1	34.4–39.9
65	33.4	31.1–35.6	37.7	35.0–40.6
66	33.7	31.6–35.9	38.3	35.6–41.1
67	34.1	32.0–36.4	38.9	36.1–41.7
68	34.6	32.4–36.9	39.6	36.9–42.3
69	35.0	32.6–37.1	40.1	37.4–42.9
70	35.6	33.3–37.7		
71	35.9	33.7–38.1		
72	36.4	34.1–38.6		
73	36.9	34.6–39.0		
74	37.3	35.1–39.6		
75	37.7	35.6–39.9		
76	38.1	36.0–40.4		
77	38.6	36.4–40.9		
78	39.1	36.9–41.3		
79	39.6	37.3–41.7		
80	40.0	37.9–42.1		

(From Jeanty P, Rodesch F, Delbeke D, et al. Estimation of gestational age from measurements of fetal long bones. J Ultrasound Med. 1984;3:75–79.)

Appendix K. Estimation of gestational age by tibia measurement

Tibia Length (mm)	Gestational Age (weeks)		Tibia Length (mm)	Gestational Age (weeks)	
	Predicted Mean	5th–95th Percentiles		Predicted Mean	5th–95th Percentiles
10	13.4	10.6–16.3	40	25.3	22.4–28.1
11	13.7	10.9–16.6	41	25.7	22.9–28.6
12	14.1	11.1–17.0	42	26.1	23.3–29.1
13	14.4	11.6–17.3	43	26.6	23.7–29.6
14	14.9	11.9–17.7	44	27.1	24.1–30.0
15	15.1	12.1–18.0	45	27.6	24.6–30.6
16	15.6	12.6–18.4	46	28.0	25.1–30.9
17	15.9	13.0–18.9	47	28.4	25.6–31.4
18	16.1	13.3–19.1	48	29.0	26.1–31.6
19	16.6	13.7–19.6	49	29.4	26.6–32.3
20	17.0	14.1–19.9	50	29.9	27.0–32.9
21	17.4	14.6–20.3	51	30.4	27.6–33.3
22	17.9	14.9–20.7	52	30.9	28.0–33.9
23	18.1	15.1–21.1	53	31.4	28.6–34.3
24	18.6	15.6–21.4	54	31.9	29.0–34.9
25	18.9	16.0–21.9	55	32.4	29.6–35.3
26	19.3	16.4–22.1	56	32.9	30.0–35.9
27	19.7	16.9–22.6	57	33.4	30.6–36.3
28	20.1	17.1–23.0	58	33.9	31.0–36.9
29	20.6	17.6–23.6	59	34.4	31.6–37.3
30	21.0	18.1–23.9	60	34.9	32.0–37.9
31	21.4	18.6–24.3	61	35.4	32.6–38.3
32	21.9	18.9–24.7	62	35.9	33.0–39.4
33	22.1	19.3–25.1	63	36.6	33.6–39.4
34	22.6	19.7–25.6	64	37.0	34.1–39.9
35	23.1	20.1–26.0	65	37.6	34.6–40.5
36	23.6	20.6–26.4	66	38.0	35.1–41.0
37	23.9	21.0–26.9	67	38.6	35.7–41.6
38	24.4	21.6–27.3	68	39.1	36.1–42.0
39	24.9	21.9–27.7	69	39.7	36.9–42.6

(From Jeanty P, Rodesch F, Delbeke D, et al. Estimation of gestational age from measurements of fetal long bones. J Ultrasound Med. 1984;3:75–79.)

APPENDIX L. Estimation of gestational age by ulna measurement

ULNA LENGTH (MM)	GESTATIONAL AGE (WEEKS)		ULNA LENGTH (MM)	GESTATIONAL AGE (WEEKS)	
	PREDICTED MEAN	5TH–95TH PERCENTILES		PREDICTED MEAN	5TH–95TH PERCENTILES
10	13.1	10.1–16.1	38	25.1	22.1–28.1
11	13.6	10.6–16.4	39	25.6	22.6–28.7
12	13.9	10.9–16.9			
13	14.1	11.1–17.3	40	26.1	23.1–29.1
14	14.6	11.6–17.7	41	26.7	23.6–29.7
15	15.0	11.9–18.0	42	27.1	24.1–30.3
16	15.4	12.3–18.4	43	27.7	24.7–30.9
17	15.7	12.7–18.9	44	28.3	25.1–31.3
18	16.1	13.1–19.1	45	28.9	25.9–31.9
19	16.6	13.6–19.6	46	29.4	26.3–32.4
			47	29.9	26.9–33.0
20	16.9	13.9–20.0	48	30.6	27.4–33.6
21	17.3	14.3–20.6	49	31.1	28.0–34.1
22	17.7	14.7–20.9			
23	18.1	15.1–21.1	50	31.6	28.6–34.7
24	18.6	15.6–21.6	51	32.1	29.1–35.3
25	19.0	16.0–22.1	52	32.9	29.7–35.9
26	19.4	16.4–22.6	53	33.4	30.3–36.4
27	19.9	16.9–22.9	54	34.0	30.9–37.0
28	20.3	17.3–23.4	55	34.6	31.6–37.7
29	20.9	17.7–23.9	56	35.1	32.1–38.3
			57	35.9	32.9–38.9
30	21.1	18.1–24.3	58	36.4	33.4–39.6
31	21.7	18.6–24.9	59	37.1	34.0–40.1
32	22.1	19.1–25.1			
33	22.7	19.6–25.7	60	37.7	34.6–40.9
34	23.1	20.1–26.1	61	38.3	35.3–41.4
35	23.6	20.6–26.7	62	39.0	35.9–42.0
36	24.1	21.1–27.1	63	39.6	36.6–42.7
37	24.6	21.4–27.7	64	40.3	37.1–43.3

(From Jeanty P, Rodesch F, Delbeke D, et al. Estimation of gestational age from measurements of fetal long bones. J Ultrasound Med. 1984;3:75–79.)

APPENDIX M. Estimation of gestational age by femur length (FL) to head circumference (HC) ratio

PREDICTED MEAN GESTATIONAL AGE (WK)	FL/HC RATIO		PREDICTED MEAN GESTATIONAL AGE (WK)	FL/HC RATIO	
	MEAN	RANGE 16–84% (OR 1 SD)		MEAN	RANGE 16–84% (OR 1 SD)
15	16.2	15.3–17.1	30	20.3	19.2–21.4
16	14.9	13.3–16.5	31	20.3	19.3–21.3
17	16.1	14.6–17.6	32	20.2	19.1–21.3
18	16.9	15.8–18.0	33	20.7	19.9–21.5
19	17.2	16.1–18.3	34	20.6	19.4–21.8
20	18.3	16.8–19.8	35	21.2	20.1–22.3
21	18.1	15.9–20.3	36	21.1	20.1–22.1
22	19.3	18.4–20.2	37	21.7	20.8–22.6
23	20.0	19.2–20.8	38	21.8	20.9–22.7
24	19.8	18.7–20.9	39	22.0	20.6–23.4
25	19.5	18.7–20.3	40	21.6	20.7–22.5
26	19.5	18.6–20.4	41	22.4	21.6–23.2
27	19.5	18.6–20.4	42	22.0	20.1–23.9
28	19.7	18.8–20.6			
29	20.2	19.6–20.8			

(From Hadlock FP, Harrist RB, Shah Y, et al. The femur length/head circumference relation in obstetric sonography. J Ultrasound Med. 1984;3:439–442. Used by permission.)

APPENDIX N. Abbreviated fetal weight estimation table

BPD + AD (MM)	EFW (G)	AD + FEM SUM (MM)	EFW (G)
100	490	90	500
110	590	100	620
120	720	110	760
130	870	120	930
140	1050	130	1140
150	1280	140	1400
160	1550	150	1720
170	1880	160	2120
180	2280	170	2600
190	2770	180	3190
200	3350	190	3920
210	4070	200	4810
220	4940		

To use this table, obtain the BPD and/or FEM and two abdominal diameter measurements using standard sonographic methods. Compute the mean (average) AD in millimeters and add to BPD or FEM in millimeters. Look up the estimated fetal weight in the appropriate column.
BPD, biparietal diameter; FEM, femur diaphysis (shaft) length; AD, mean abdominal diameter, i.e., (AD1 + AD2)/2
(Adapted from Rose BI. Abbreviated tables for estimating fetal weight with ultrasound. J Reprod Med. 1988;33:298–300.)

APPENDIX O. Estimation of fetal weight (in grams) by biparietal diameter (BPD) and abdominal circumference (AC)*

BPD (mm)	AC (mm) 155	160	165	170	175	180	185	190	195	200	205	210	215
31	224	234	244	255	267	279	291	304	318	332	346	362	378
32	231	241	251	263	274	286	299	312	326	340	355	371	388
33	237	248	259	270	282	294	307	321	335	349	365	381	397
34	244	255	266	278	290	302	316	329	344	359	374	391	408
35	251	262	274	285	298	311	324	338	353	368	384	401	418
36	259	270	281	294	306	319	333	347	362	378	394	411	429
37	266	278	290	302	315	328	342	357	372	388	404	422	440
38	274	286	298	310	324	337	352	366	382	398	415	432	451
39	282	294	306	319	333	347	361	376	392	409	426	444	462
40	290	303	315	328	342	356	371	386	403	419	437	455	474
41	299	311	324	338	352	366	381	397	413	430	448	467	486
42	308	320	333	347	361	376	392	408	424	442	460	479	498
43	317	330	343	357	371	387	402	419	436	453	472	491	511
44	326	339	353	367	382	397	413	430	447	465	484	504	524
45	335	349	363	377	393	408	425	442	459	478	497	517	538
46	345	359	373	386	404	420	436	454	472	490	510	530	551
47	355	369	384	399	415	431	448	466	484	503	524	544	565
48	366	380	395	410	426	443	460	478	497	517	537	558	580
49	376	391	406	422	438	455	473	491	510	530	551	572	594
50	387	402	418	434	451	468	486	505	524	544	565	587	610
51	399	414	430	446	463	481	499	518	538	559	580	602	625
52	410	426	442	459	476	494	513	532	552	573	595	618	641
53	422	438	455	472	489	508	527	547	567	589	611	634	657
54	435	451	468	485	503	522	541	561	582	604	627	650	674
55	447	464	481	499	517	536	556	577	598	620	643	667	691
56	461	477	495	513	532	551	571	592	614	636	660	684	709
57	474	491	509	527	547	566	587	608	630	653	677	701	727
58	488	505	524	542	562	582	603	625	647	670	695	719	745
59	502	520	539	558	578	598	619	642	664	688	713	738	764
60	517	535	554	573	594	615	636	659	682	706	731	757	784
61	532	550	570	590	610	632	654	677	700	725	750	777	804
62	547	566	586	606	627	649	672	695	719	744	770	797	824
63	563	583	603	624	645	667	690	714	738	764	790	817	845
64	580	600	620	641	663	686	709	733	758	784	811	838	867
65	597	617	638	659	682	705	728	753	778	805	832	860	889
66	614	635	656	678	701	724	748	773	799	826	853	882	911
67	632	653	675	697	720	744	769	794	820	848	876	905	935
68	651	672	694	717	740	765	790	816	842	870	898	928	958
69	670	691	714	737	761	786	811	838	865	893	922	952	983

AC (mm)

BPD (mm)	155	160	165	170	175	180	185	190	195	200	205	210	215
70	689	711	734	758	782	807	833	860	888	916	946	976	1,008
71	709	732	755	779	804	830	856	883	912	941	971	1,002	1,033
72	730	763	777	801	827	853	880	907	936	965	996	1,027	1,060
73	751	775	799	824	850	876	904	932	961	991	1,022	1,054	1,087
74	773	797	822	847	874	901	928	957	987	1,017	1,049	1,081	1,114
75	796	820	845	871	898	925	954	983	1,013	1,044	1,076	1,109	1,143
76	819	844	870	896	923	951	980	1,009	1,040	1,072	1,104	1,137	1,172
77	843	868	894	921	949	977	1,007	1,037	1,068	1,100	1,133	1,167	1,202
78	868	894	920	947	975	1,004	1,034	1,065	1,096	1,129	1,162	1,197	1,232
79	893	919	946	974	1,003	1,032	1,062	1,094	1,126	1,159	1,193	1,228	1,264
80	919	946	973	1,002	1,031	1,061	1,091	1,123	1,156	1,189	1,224	1,259	1,296
81	946	973	1,001	1,030	1,060	1,090	1,121	1,153	1,187	1,221	1,256	1,292	1,329
82	974	1,001	1,030	1,059	1,089	1,120	1,152	1,185	1,218	1,253	1,288	1,325	1,363
83	1,002	1,030	1,059	1,089	1,120	1,151	1,183	1,217	1,251	1,286	1,322	1,359	1,397
84	1,032	1,060	1,090	1,120	1,151	1,183	1,216	1,249	1,284	1,320	1,356	1,394	1,433
85	1,062	1,091	1,121	1,151	1,183	1,216	1,249	1,283	1,318	1,355	1,392	1,430	1,469
86	1,093	1,122	1,153	1,184	1,216	1,249	1,283	1,318	1,354	1,390	1,428	1,467	1,507
87	1,125	1,155	1,186	1,218	1,250	1,284	1,318	1,353	1,390	1,427	1,465	1,505	1,545
88	1,157	1,188	1,220	1,252	1,285	1,319	1,354	1,390	1,427	1,465	1,504	1,543	1,584
89	1,191	1,222	1,254	1,287	1,321	1,356	1,391	1,428	1,465	1,503	1,543	1,583	1,625
90	1,226	1,258	1,290	1,324	1,358	1,393	1,429	1,456	1,504	1,543	1,583	1,624	1,666
91	1,262	1,294	1,327	1,361	1,396	1,432	1,468	1,506	1,544	1,584	1,624	1,666	1,708
92	1,299	1,332	1,365	1,400	1,435	1,471	1,508	1,546	1,586	1,626	1,667	1,709	1,752
93	1,337	1,370	1,404	1,439	1,475	1,512	1,550	1,588	1,628	1,668	1,710	1,753	1,796
94	1,376	1,410	1,444	1,480	1,516	1,554	1,592	1,631	1,671	1,712	1,755	1,798	1,842
95	1,416	1,450	1,486	1,522	1,559	1,597	1,635	1,675	1,716	1,758	1,800	1,844	1,889
96	1,457	1,492	1,528	1,565	1,602	1,641	1,680	1,720	1,762	1,804	1,847	1,892	1,937
97	1,500	1,535	1,572	1,609	1,647	1,686	1,726	1,767	1,809	1,852	1,895	1,940	1,986
98	1,544	1,580	1,617	1,654	1,693	1,733	1,773	1,815	1,857	1,900	1,945	1,990	2,037
99	1,589	1,625	1,663	1,701	1,740	1,781	1,822	1,864	1,907	1,951	1,996	2,042	2,089
100	1,635	1,672	1,710	1,749	1,789	1,830	1,871	1,914	1,958	2,002	2,048	2,094	2,142

(Continues)

Appendix O. Estimation of fetal weight (in grams) by biparietal diameter (BPD) and abdominal circumference (AC)* (Continued)

BPD (mm)	AC (mm)												
	220	225	230	235	240	245	250	255	260	265	270	275	280
31	395	412	431	450	470	491	513	536	559	584	610	638	666
32	405	423	441	461	481	502	525	548	572	597	624	651	680
33	415	433	452	472	493	514	537	560	585	611	638	666	693
34	425	444	463	483	504	526	549	573	598	624	652	680	710
35	436	455	475	495	517	539	562	587	612	638	666	695	725
36	447	466	486	507	529	552	575	600	626	653	681	710	740
37	458	478	498	519	542	565	589	614	640	667	696	725	756
38	470	490	510	532	554	578	602	628	654	682	711	741	772
39	482	502	523	545	568	592	616	642	669	697	727	757	789
40	494	514	536	558	581	606	631	657	684	713	743	773	806
41	506	527	549	572	595	620	645	672	700	729	759	790	828
42	519	540	562	585	609	634	660	688	716	745	776	807	841
43	532	554	576	600	624	649	676	703	732	762	793	825	859
44	545	567	590	614	639	665	692	719	749	779	810	843	877
45	559	581	605	629	654	680	708	736	765	796	828	861	896
46	573	596	620	644	670	696	724	753	783	814	846	880	915
47	588	611	635	660	686	713	741	770	801	832	865	899	934
48	602	626	650	676	702	730	758	788	819	851	884	919	954
49	617	641	666	692	719	747	776	806	837	870	903	938	975
50	633	657	683	709	736	765	794	824	856	889	923	959	996
51	649	674	699	726	754	783	812	843	876	909	944	980	1,017
52	665	690	717	744	772	801	831	863	895	929	964	1,001	1,039
53	682	708	734	762	790	820	851	883	916	950	986	1,023	1,061
54	699	725	752	780	809	839	870	903	936	971	1,007	1,045	1,084
55	717	743	771	799	828	859	891	924	958	993	1,030	1,068	1,107
56	735	762	789	818	848	879	911	945	979	1,015	1,052	1,091	1,131
57	753	780	809	838	869	900	933	966	1,001	1,038	1,075	1,114	1,155
58	772	800	829	858	889	921	954	989	1,024	1,061	1,099	1,139	1,180
59	792	820	849	879	911	943	977	1,011	1,047	1,085	1,123	1,163	1,205
60	811	840	870	900	932	965	999	1,035	1,071	1,109	1,148	1,189	1,231
61	832	861	891	922	955	988	1,023	1,058	1,095	1,134	1,173	1,214	1,257
62	853	882	913	945	977	1,011	1,046	1,083	1,120	1,159	1,199	1,241	1,284
63	874	904	935	967	1,001	1,035	1,071	1,107	1,145	1,185	1,226	1,268	1,311
64	896	927	958	991	1,025	1,059	1,096	1,133	1,171	1,211	1,253	1,295	1,339
65	919	950	982	1,015	1,049	1,084	1,121	1,159	1,198	1,238	1,280	1,323	1,368
66	942	973	1,006	1,039	1,074	1,110	1,147	1,185	1,225	1,266	1,308	1,352	1,397
67	965	997	1,030	1,065	1,100	1,136	1,174	1,213	1,253	1,294	1,337	1,381	1,427
68	990	1,022	1,056	1,090	1,126	1,163	1,201	1,241	1,281	1,323	1,367	1,411	1,458
69	1,015	1,048	1,082	1,117	1,153	1,190	1,229	1,269	1,310	1,353	1,397	1,442	1,489

AC (mm)

BPD (mm)	220	225	230	235	240	245	250	255	260	265	270	275	280
70	1,040	1,074	1,108	1,144	1,181	1,219	1,258	1,298	1,340	1,383	1,427	1,473	1,521
71	1,066	1,100	1,135	1,171	1,209	1,247	1,287	1,328	1,370	1,414	1,459	1,505	1,553
72	1,093	1,128	1,163	1,200	1,238	1,277	1,317	1,358	1,401	1,445	1,491	1,538	1,586
73	1,121	1,156	1,192	1,229	1,267	1,307	1,348	1,390	1,433	1,478	1,524	1,571	1,620
74	1,149	1,184	1,221	1,259	1,297	1,338	1,379	1,421	1,465	1,511	1,557	1,605	1,655
75	1,178	1,214	1,251	1,289	1,328	1,369	1,411	1,454	1,499	1,544	1,592	1,640	1,690
76	1,207	1,244	1,281	1,320	1,360	1,401	1,444	1,487	1,533	1,579	1,627	1,676	1,727
77	1,238	1,275	1,313	1,352	1,393	1,434	1,477	1,522	1,567	1,614	1,663	1,712	1,764
78	1,269	1,306	1,345	1,385	1,426	1,468	1,512	1,557	1,603	1,650	1,699	1,749	1,801
79	1,301	1,339	1,378	1,418	1,460	1,503	1,547	1,592	1,639	1,687	1,737	1,787	1,840
80	1,333	1,372	1,412	1,453	1,495	1,538	1,583	1,629	1,676	1,725	1,775	1,826	1,879
81	1,367	1,406	1,446	1,488	1,531	1,575	1,620	1,666	1,714	1,763	1,814	1,866	1,919
82	1,401	1,441	1,482	1,524	1,567	1,612	1,657	1,704	1,753	1,803	1,854	1,906	1,960
83	1,436	1,477	1,518	1,561	1,605	1,650	1,696	1,744	1,793	1,843	1,895	1,948	2,002
84	1,473	1,513	1,555	1,599	1,643	1,689	1,735	1,784	1,833	1,884	1,936	1,990	2,045
85	1,510	1,551	1,594	1,637	1,682	1,728	1,776	1,825	1,875	1,926	1,979	2,033	2,089
86	1,548	1,589	1,633	1,677	1,722	1,769	1,817	1,866	1,917	1,969	2,022	2,077	2,134
87	1,586	1,629	1,673	1,717	1,764	1,811	1,859	1,909	1,960	2,013	2,067	2,122	2,179
88	1,626	1,669	1,714	1,759	1,806	1,854	1,903	1,953	2,005	2,058	2,113	2,169	2,226
89	1,667	1,711	1,756	1,802	1,849	1,897	1,947	1,998	2,050	2,104	2,159	2,216	2,274
90	1,709	1,753	1,799	1,845	1,893	1,942	1,992	2,044	2,097	2,151	2,207	2,264	2,322
91	1,752	1,797	1,843	1,890	1,938	1,988	2,039	2,091	2,144	2,199	2,255	2,313	2,372
92	1,796	1,841	1,888	1,936	1,984	2,035	2,086	2,139	2,193	2,248	2,305	2,363	2,423
93	1,841	1,887	1,934	1,982	2,032	2,083	2,135	2,188	2,242	2,298	2,356	2,414	2,475
94	1,887	1,934	1,982	2,030	2,080	2,132	2,184	2,238	2,293	2,350	2,407	2,467	2,527
95	1,935	1,982	2,030	2,080	2,130	2,182	2,235	2,289	2,345	2,402	2,460	2,520	2,582
96	1,984	2,031	2,080	2,130	2,181	2,233	2,287	2,342	2,398	2,456	2,515	2,575	2,637
97	2,033	2,082	2,131	2,181	2,233	2,286	2,340	2,396	2,452	2,510	2,570	2,631	2,693
98	2,085	2,133	2,183	2,234	2,286	2,340	2,395	2,451	2,508	2,567	2,627	2,688	2,751
99	2,137	2,186	2,237	2,288	2,341	2,395	2,450	2,507	2,565	2,624	2,684	2,746	2,810
100	2,191	2,241	2,292	2,344	2,397	2,452	2,507	2,564	2,623	2,682	2,743	2,806	2,870

(Continues)

APPENDIX O. Estimation of fetal weight (in grams) by biparietal diameter (BPD) and abdominal circumference (AC)* *(Continued)*

BPD (mm)	AC (mm)												
	285	290	295	300	305	310	315	320	325	330	335	340	345
31	696	726	759	793	828	865	903	943	985	1,029	1,075	1,123	1,173
32	710	742	774	809	844	882	921	961	1,004	1,048	1,094	1,143	1,193
33	725	757	790	825	861	899	938	979	1,022	1,067	1,114	1,163	1,214
34	740	773	806	841	878	916	956	998	1,041	1,087	1,134	1,183	1,235
35	756	789	823	858	896	934	975	1,017	1,061	1,107	1,154	1,204	1,256
36	772	805	840	876	913	953	993	1,036	1,080	1,127	1,175	1,226	1,278
37	788	822	857	893	931	971	1,012	1,056	1,101	1,147	1,196	1,247	1,300
38	805	839	874	911	950	990	1,032	1,076	1,121	1,168	1,218	1,269	1,323
39	822	856	892	930	969	1,009	1,052	1,096	1,142	1,190	1,240	1,292	1,346
40	839	874	911	949	988	1,029	1,072	1,117	1,163	1,212	1,262	1,315	1,369
41	857	892	929	968	1,008	1,049	1,093	1,138	1,185	1,234	1,285	1,338	1,393
42	875	911	948	987	1,028	1,070	1,114	1,159	1,207	1,256	1,308	1,361	1,417
43	893	930	968	1,007	1,048	1,091	1,135	1,181	1,229	1,279	1,331	1,385	1,442
44	912	949	987	1,027	1,069	1,112	1,157	1,204	1,252	1,303	1,355	1,410	1,467
45	932	969	1,008	1,048	1,090	1,134	1,179	1,226	1,275	1,326	1,380	1,435	1,492
46	951	989	1,028	1,069	1,112	1,156	1,202	1,249	1,299	1,351	1,404	1,460	1,518
47	971	1,010	1,049	1,091	1,134	1,178	1,225	1,273	1,323	1,375	1,430	1,486	1,545
48	992	1,031	1,071	1,113	1,156	1,201	1,248	1,297	1,348	1,401	1,455	1,512	1,571
49	1,013	1,052	1,093	1,135	1,179	1,225	1,272	1,322	1,373	1,426	1,482	1,539	1,599
50	1,034	1,074	1,115	1,158	1,203	1,249	1,297	1,347	1,399	1,452	1,508	1,566	1,626
51	1,056	1,096	1,138	1,181	1,226	1,273	1,322	1,372	1,425	1,479	1,535	1,594	1,655
52	1,078	1,119	1,161	1,205	1,251	1,298	1,347	1,398	1,451	1,506	1,563	1,622	1,683
53	1,101	1,142	1,185	1,229	1,276	1,323	1,373	1,425	1,478	1,533	1,591	1,651	1,713
54	1,124	1,166	1,209	1,254	1,301	1,349	1,399	1,452	1,506	1,562	1,620	1,680	1,742
55	1,148	1,190	1,234	1,279	1,327	1,376	1,426	1,479	1,534	1,590	1,649	1,710	1,773
56	1,172	1,215	1,259	1,305	1,353	1,402	1,454	1,507	1,562	1,619	1,678	1,740	1,803
57	1,197	1,240	1,285	1,332	1,380	1,430	1,482	1,535	1,591	1,649	1,709	1,770	1,835
58	1,222	1,266	1,311	1,358	1,407	1,458	1,510	1,564	1,621	1,679	1,739	1,802	1,866
59	1,248	1,292	1,338	1,386	1,435	1,486	1,539	1,594	1,651	1,710	1,770	1,834	1,899
60	1,274	1,319	1,366	1,414	1,464	1,515	1,569	1,624	1,682	1,741	1,802	1,866	1,932
61	1,301	1,346	1,393	1,442	1,493	1,545	1,599	1,655	1,713	1,773	1,835	1,899	1,965
62	1,328	1,374	1,422	1,471	1,522	1,575	1,630	1,686	1,745	1,805	1,868	1,932	1,999
63	1,356	1,403	1,451	1,501	1,552	1,606	1,661	1,718	1,777	1,838	1,901	1,967	2,034
64	1,385	1,432	1,481	1,531	1,583	1,637	1,693	1,751	1,810	1,872	1,935	2,001	2,069
66	1,444	1,492	1,542	1,594	1,647	1,702	1,759	1,817	1,878	1,941	2,006	2,073	2,142
67	1,474	1,523	1,574	1,626	1,679	1,735	1,792	1,852	1,913	1,976	2,042	2,109	2,179
68	1,505	1,555	1,606	1,658	1,713	1,769	1,827	1,887	1,949	2,012	2,078	2,147	2,217
69	1,537	1,587	1,639	1,692	1,747	1,803	1,862	1,922	1,985	2,049	2,116	2,184	2,255

BPD (mm)	AC (mm)												
	285	290	295	300	305	310	315	320	325	330	335	340	345
70	1,570	1,620	1,672	1,726	1,781	1,839	1,898	1,959	2,022	2,087	2,154	2,223	2,295
71	1,603	1,654	1,706	1,761	1,817	1,875	1,934	1,996	2,059	2,125	2,193	2,262	2,334
72	1,636	1,688	1,741	1,796	1,853	1,911	1,971	2,044	2,098	2,164	2,232	2,302	2,375
73	1,671	1,723	1,777	1,832	1,890	1,948	2,009	2,072	2,137	2,203	2,272	2,343	2,416
74	1,706	1,759	1,813	1,869	1,927	1,987	2,048	2,111	2,176	2,244	2,313	2,384	2,458
75	1,742	1,795	1,850	1,907	1,965	2,025	2,087	2,151	2,217	2,285	2,354	2,426	2,501
76	1,779	1,833	1,888	1,945	2,004	2,065	2,127	2,192	2,258	2,326	2,397	2,469	2,544
77	1,816	1,871	1,927	1,985	2,044	2,105	2,168	2,233	2,300	2,369	2,440	2,513	2,588
78	1,855	1,910	1,966	2,025	2,085	2,146	2,210	2,275	2,343	2,412	2,484	2,557	2,633
79	1,894	1,949	2,006	2,065	2,126	2,188	2,252	2,318	2,386	2,456	2,528	2,603	2,679
80	1,934	1,990	2,048	2,107	2,168	2,231	2,296	2,362	2,431	2,501	2,574	2,649	2,725
81	1,975	2,031	2,089	2,149	2,211	2,275	2,340	2,407	2,476	2,547	2,620	2,695	2,773
82	2,016	2,073	2,132	2,193	2,255	2,319	2,385	2,462	2,522	2,594	2,667	2,743	2,821
83	2,059	2,116	2,176	2,237	2,300	2,364	2,431	2,499	2,569	2,641	2,715	2,791	2,870
84	2,102	2,160	2,220	2,282	2,345	2,410	2,477	2,546	2,617	2,689	2,764	2,841	2,920
85	2,146	2,205	2,266	2,328	2,392	2,457	2,525	2,594	2,665	2,739	2,814	2,891	2,970
86	2,192	2,251	2,312	2,375	2,439	2,505	2,573	2,643	2,715	2,789	2,864	2,942	3,022
87	2,238	2,298	2,359	2,423	2,488	2,554	2,623	2,693	2,765	2,840	2,916	2,994	3,074
88	2,285	2,346	2,408	2,472	2,537	2,604	2,673	2,744	2,817	2,892	2,968	3,047	3,128
89	2,333	2,394	2,457	2,521	2,587	2,655	2,725	2,796	2,869	2,944	3,021	3,101	3,182
90	2,382	2,444	2,507	2,572	2,639	2,707	2,777	2,849	2,923	2,998	3,076	3,155	3,237
91	2,433	2,495	2,559	2,624	2,691	2,760	2,830	2,903	2,977	3,053	3,131	3,211	3,293
92	2,484	2,547	2,611	2,677	2,744	2,814	2,885	2,958	3,032	3,109	3,187	3,268	3,350
93	2,536	2,599	2,664	2,731	2,799	2,869	2,940	3,014	3,089	3,166	3,245	3,326	3,409
94	2,590	2,653	2,719	2,786	2,854	2,925	2,997	3,070	3,146	3,224	3,303	3,384	3,468
95	2,644	2,709	2,774	2,842	2,911	2,982	3,054	3,129	3,205	3,283	3,362	3,444	3,528
96	2,700	2,765	2,831	2,899	2,969	3,040	3,113	3,188	3,264	3,343	3,423	3,505	3,589
97	2,757	2,822	2,889	2,958	3,028	3,099	3,173	3,248	3,325	3,404	3,484	3,567	3,651
98	2,815	2,881	2,948	3,017	3,088	3,160	3,234	3,309	3,387	3,466	3,547	3,630	3,715
99	2,874	2,941	3,009	3,078	3,149	3,222	3,296	3,372	3,450	3,529	3,600	3,694	3,779
100	2,935	3,002	3,070	3,140	3,211	3,285	3,359	3,436	3,514	3,594	3,676	3,759	3,845

(Continues)

Appendix O. Estimation of fetal weight (in grams) by biparietal diameter (BPD) and abdominal circumference (AC)* *(Continued)*

BPD (mm)	AC (mm)										
	350	355	360	365	370	375	380	385	390	395	400
31	1,225	1,279	1,336	1,396	1,458	1,523	1,591	1,661	1,735	1,812	1,893
32	1,246	1,301	1,358	1,418	1,481	1,546	1,615	1,686	1,761	1,838	1,920
33	1,267	1,323	1,381	1,441	1,504	1,570	1,639	1,711	1,786	1,865	1,946
34	1,289	1,345	1,403	1,464	1,528	1,595	1,664	1,737	1,812	1,891	1,973
35	1,311	1,367	1,426	1,488	1,552	1,619	1,689	1,762	1,839	1,918	2,001
36	1,333	1,390	1,450	1,512	1,577	1,645	1,715	1,789	1,865	1,945	2,029
37	1,356	1,413	1,474	1,536	1,602	1,670	1,741	1,815	1,893	1,973	2,057
38	1,379	1,437	1,498	1,561	1,627	1,696	1,768	1,842	1,920	2,001	2,086
39	1,402	1,461	1,523	1,586	1,653	1,722	1,794	1,870	1,948	2,030	2,115
40	1,426	1,486	1,548	1,612	1,679	1,749	1,822	1,898	1,977	2,059	2,145
41	1,451	1,511	1,573	1,638	1,706	1,776	1,849	1,926	2,005	2,088	2,174
42	1,475	1,536	1,599	1,664	1,733	1,804	1,878	1,954	2,035	2,118	2,205
43	1,500	1,562	1,625	1,691	1,760	1,832	1,906	1,984	2,064	2,148	2,236
44	1,526	1,588	1,652	1,718	1,788	1,860	1,935	2,013	2,094	2,179	2,267
45	1,552	1,614	1,679	1,746	1,816	1,889	1,964	2,043	2,125	2,210	2,298
46	1,579	1,641	1,706	1,774	1,845	1,918	1,994	2,073	2,156	2,241	2,330
47	1,605	1,669	1,734	1,803	1,874	1,948	2,024	2,104	2,187	2,273	2,363
48	1,633	1,697	1,763	1,832	1,904	1,976	2,055	2,136	2,219	2,306	2,396
49	1,661	1,725	1,792	1,861	1,934	2,009	2,086	2,167	2,251	2,339	2,429
50	1,689	1,754	1,821	1,891	1,964	2,040	2,118	2,200	2,284	2,372	2,463
51	1,718	1,783	1,851	1,922	1,995	2,071	2,150	2,232	2,317	2,406	2,498
52	1,747	1,813	1,882	1,953	2,027	2,103	2,183	2,266	2,351	2,440	2,532
53	1,777	1,843	1,913	1,984	2,059	2,136	2,216	2,299	2,386	2,475	2,568
54	1,807	1,874	1,944	2,016	2,091	2,169	2,250	2,333	2,420	2,510	2,604
55	1,838	1,906	1,976	2,049	2,124	2,203	2,284	2,368	2,456	2,546	2,640
56	1,869	1,938	2,008	2,082	2,158	2,237	2,319	2,403	2,491	2,582	2,677
57	1,901	1,970	2,041	2,115	2,192	2,272	2,354	2,439	2,528	2,619	2,714
58	1,934	2,003	2,075	2,150	2,227	2,307	2,390	2,475	2,564	2,657	2,752
59	1,966	2,037	2,109	2,184	2,262	2,342	2,426	2,512	2,602	2,694	2,790
60	2,000	2,071	2,144	2,219	2,298	2,379	2,463	2,550	2,640	2,733	2,829
61	2,034	2,105	2,179	2,255	2,334	2,416	2,500	2,588	2,678	2,772	2,869
62	2,069	2,140	2,215	2,291	2,371	2,453	2,538	2,626	2,717	2,811	2,909
63	2,104	2,176	2,251	2,328	2,408	2,491	2,577	2,665	2,757	2,851	2,949
64	2,140	2,213	2,288	2,366	2,446	2,530	2,616	2,705	2,797	2,892	2,991
65	2,176	2,250	2,326	2,404	2,485	2,569	2,656	2,745	2,838	2,933	3,032
66	2,213	2,287	2,364	2,443	2,524	2,609	2,696	2,786	2,879	2,975	3,075
67	2,251	2,326	2,403	2,482	2,564	2,649	2,737	2,827	2,921	3,018	3,117
68	2,290	2,365	2,442	2,522	2,605	2,690	2,778	2,869	2,964	3,061	3,161
69	2,329	2,404	2,482	2,563	2,646	2,732	2,821	2,912	3,007	3,104	3,205

BPD (mm)	AC (mm)										
	350	355	360	365	370	375	380	385	390	395	400
70	2,368	2,444	2,523	2,604	2,688	2,774	2,863	2,955	3,050	3,149	3,250
71	2,409	2,485	2,564	2,646	2,730	2,817	2,907	2,999	3,095	3,193	3,295
72	2,450	2,527	2,607	2,689	2,773	2,861	2,951	3,044	3,140	3,239	3,341
73	2,491	2,569	2,649	2,732	2,817	2,905	2,996	3,089	3,186	3,285	3,386
74	2,534	2,612	2,693	2,776	2,862	2,950	3,041	3,135	3,232	3,332	3,435
75	2,577	2,656	2,737	2,821	2,907	2,996	3,088	3,182	3,279	3,380	3,483
76	2,621	2,700	2,782	2,866	2,953	3,042	3,134	3,229	3,327	3,428	3,531
77	2,666	2,746	2,828	2,912	3,000	3,090	3,181	3,277	3,376	3,477	3,581
78	2,711	2,792	2,874	2,959	3,047	3,137	3,230	3,326	3,425	3,526	3,631
79	2,757	2,838	2,921	3,007	3,095	3,186	3,279	3,376	3,475	3,576	3,681
80	2,804	2,886	2,969	3,056	3,144	3,235	3,329	3,426	3,525	3,627	3,733
81	2,852	2,934	3,018	3,105	3,194	3,286	3,380	3,477	3,577	3,679	3,785
82	2,901	2,983	3,068	3,155	3,244	3,336	3,431	3,529	3,629	3,732	3,838
83	2,950	3,033	3,118	3,206	3,296	3,388	3,483	3,581	3,682	3,785	3,891
84	3,001	3,084	3,169	3,257	3,348	3,441	3,536	3,634	3,735	3,839	3,945
85	3,052	3,135	3,221	3,310	3,401	3,494	3,590	3,688	3,790	3,894	4,000
86	3,104	3,188	3,274	3,363	3,454	3,548	3,644	3,743	3,845	3,949	4,056
87	3,157	3,241	3,328	3,417	3,509	3,603	3,700	3,799	3,901	4,005	4,113
88	3,210	3,295	3,383	3,472	3,565	3,659	3,756	3,855	3,958	4,063	4,170
89	3,265	3,351	3,438	3,528	3,621	3,716	3,813	3,913	4,015	4,120	4,228
90	3,321	3,407	3,495	3,585	3,678	3,773	3,871	3,971	4,074	4,179	4,287
91	3,377	3,464	3,552	3,643	3,736	3,832	3,930	4,030	4,133	4,239	4,347
92	3,435	3,522	3,611	3,702	3,795	3,891	3,989	4,090	4,193	4,299	4,408
93	3,494	3,581	3,670	3,761	3,855	3,951	4,050	4,151	4,254	4,361	4,469
94	3,553	3,641	3,738	3,822	3,916	4,013	4,111	4,213	4,316	4,423	4,532
95	3,614	3,701	3,791	3,884	3,978	4,075	4,174	4,275	4,379	4,486	4,595
96	3,675	3,763	3,854	3,946	4,041	4,138	4,237	4,339	4,443	4,550	4,659
97	3,738	3,826	3,917	4,010	4,105	4,202	4,302	4,404	4,508	4,615	4,724
98	3,802	3,890	3,981	4,074	4,170	4,267	4,367	4,469	4,573	4,680	4,790
99	3,866	3,956	4,047	4,140	4,236	4,333	4,433	4,536	4,640	4,747	4,857
100	3,932	4,022	4,113	4,207	4,303	4,400	4,501	4,603	4,708	4,815	4,924

*Antilog 10 (birth weight) = −1.7492 + 0.166 (BPDcm) + 0.046 (ACcm) − 0.00264 (ACcm × BPDcm) will yield estimated weights in kilograms (kg). (Adapted from Shepard MJ, Richards VA, Berkowitz RL, et al. An evaluation of two equations for predicting fetal weight by ultrasound. Am J Obstet Gynecol. 1982;147:47–54. Used by permission.)

APPENDIX P. Estimation of fetal weight (in grams) by abdominal circumference (AC) and femur length (FL)*

FL (mm)	AC (mm)									
	200	205	210	215	220	225	230	235	240	245
40	663	691	720	751	783	816	851	887	925	964
41	680	709	738	769	802	836	871	907	946	986
42	697	726	757	788	821	855	891	928	967	1,007
43	715	745	776	808	841	875	912	949	988	1,029
44	734	764	795	827	861	896	933	971	1,010	1,051
45	753	783	815	847	882	917	954	993	1,033	1,074
46	772	803	835	868	903	939	976	1,015	1,056	1,098
47	792	823	856	889	924	961	999	1,038	1,079	1,122
48	812	844	877	911	947	984	1,022	1,062	1,103	1,146
49	833	865	899	933	969	1,007	1,046	1,086	1,128	1,171
50	855	887	921	956	993	1,031	1,070	1,111	1,153	1,197
51	877	910	944	980	1,016	1,055	1,095	1,136	1,179	1,223
52	899	933	967	1,004	1,041	1,080	1,120	1,162	1,205	1,250
53	922	956	992	1,028	1,066	1,105	1,146	1,188	1,232	1,277
54	946	981	1,016	1,053	1,091	1,131	1,172	1,215	1,259	1,305
55	971	1,005	1,041	1,079	1,118	1,158	1,199	1,242	1,287	1,333
56	995	1,031	1,067	1,105	1,144	1,185	1,227	1,271	1,316	1,362
57	1,021	1,057	1,094	1,132	1,172	1,213	1,255	1,299	1,345	1,392
58	1,047	1,084	1,121	1,160	1,200	1,242	1,285	1,329	1,375	1,422
59	1,074	1,111	1,149	1,188	1,229	1,271	1,314	1,359	1,406	1,454
60	1,102	1,139	1,178	1,217	1,258	1,301	1,345	1,409	1,437	1,485
61	1,130	1,168	1,207	1,247	1,289	1,331	1,376	1,421	1,469	1,518
62	1,160	1,198	1,237	1,278	1,319	1,363	1,408	1,454	1,501	1,551
63	1,189	1,228	1,268	1,309	1,351	1,395	1,440	1,487	1,535	1,585
64	1,220	1,259	1,299	1,341	1,384	1,428	1,473	1,520	1,569	1,619
65	1,251	1,291	1,332	1,373	1,417	1,461	1,507	1,555	1,604	1,655
66	1,284	1,324	1,365	1,407	1,451	1,496	1,542	1,590	1,640	1,691
67	1,317	1,357	1,399	1,441	1,486	1,531	1,578	1,626	1,676	1,728
68	1,351	1,391	1,433	1,477	1,521	1,567	1,615	1,663	1,713	1,765
69	1,385	1,427	1,469	1,513	1,558	1,604	1,652	1,701	1,752	1,804
70	1,421	1,463	1,506	1,550	1,595	1,642	1,690	1,740	1,791	1,843
71	1,458	1,500	1,543	1,588	1,633	1,681	1,729	1,779	1,830	1,883
72	1,495	1,538	1,581	1,626	1,673	1,720	1,769	1,819	1,871	1,924
73	1,534	1,577	1,621	1,666	1,713	1,761	1,810	1,861	1,913	1,966
74	1,573	1,616	1,661	1,707	1,754	1,802	1,852	1,903	1,955	2,009
75	1,614	1,657	1,702	1,749	1,796	1,845	1,895	1,946	1,999	2,053
76	1,655	1,699	1,745	1,791	1,839	1,888	1,939	1,990	2,043	2,098
77	1,698	1,742	1,788	1,835	1,883	1,933	1,983	2,035	2,089	2,144
78	1,741	1,786	1,833	1,880	1,928	1,978	2,029	2,082	2,135	2,191
79	1,786	1,832	1,878	1,926	1,975	2,025	2,076	2,129	2,183	2,238
80	1,832	1,878	1,925	1,973	2,022	2,073	2,124	2,177	2,232	2,287
81	1,879	1,926	1,973	2,021	2,071	2,121	2,173	2,227	2,281	2,337
82	1,928	1,974	2,022	2,070	2,120	2,171	2,224	2,277	2,332	2,388
83	1,978	2,024	2,072	2,121	2,171	2,223	2,275	2,329	2,384	2,440

*Based on regression model: $\log_{10}$ body weight $= 1,3598 + 0.051 \, (AC) + 0.1844 \, (FL) - 0.0037 \, (AC \times FL)$.

APPENDIX P. (*Continued*)

AC (mm)										
250	255	260	265	270	275	280	285	290	295	300
1,006	1,048	1,093	1,139	1,188	1,239	1,291	1,346	1,403	1,463	1,525
1,027	1,070	1,115	1,162	1,211	1,262	1,315	1,371	1,429	1,489	1,551
1,049	1,093	1,138	1,186	1,235	1,287	1,340	1,396	1,454	1,515	1,578
1,071	1,116	1,162	1,209	1,259	1,311	1,365	1,422	1,480	1,541	1,605
1,094	1,139	1,185	1,234	1,284	1,336	1,391	1,448	1,507	1,568	1,632
1,118	1,163	1,210	1,259	1,309	1,362	1,417	1,474	1,534	1,596	1,660
1,142	1,187	1,235	1,284	1,335	1,388	1,444	1,501	1,561	1,623	1,688
1,166	1,212	1,260	1,310	1,316	1,415	1,471	1,529	1,589	1,652	1,717
1,191	1,237	1,286	1,336	1,388	1,442	1,498	1,557	1,618	1,681	1,746
1,216	1,263	1,312	1,363	1,415	1,470	1,527	1,585	1,647	1,710	1,776
1,243	1,290	1,339	1,390	1,443	1,498	1,555	1,615	1,676	1,740	1,806
1,269	1,317	1,367	1,418	1,471	1,527	1,584	1,644	1,706	1,770	1,837
1,296	1,344	1,395	1,447	1,500	1,556	1,614	1,647	1,737	1,801	1,868
1,324	1,373	1,423	1,476	1,530	1,586	1,645	1,705	1,768	1,833	1,900
1,352	1,401	1,452	1,505	1,560	1,617	1,675	1,736	1,799	1,865	1,933
1,418	1,431	1,482	1,535	1,591	1,648	1,707	1,768	1,832	1,897	1,966
1,411	1,461	1,513	1,566	1,622	1,679	1,739	1,801	1,864	1,931	1,999
1,441	1,491	1,544	1,598	1,654	1,712	1,772	1,834	1,898	1,964	2,033
1,472	1,523	1,575	1,630	1,686	1,744	1,805	1,867	1,932	1,999	2,068
1,503	1,555	1,608	1,663	1,719	1,778	1,839	1,902	1,966	2,034	2,103
1,535	1,587	1,641	1,696	1,753	1,812	1,873	1,936	2,002	2,069	2,139
1,568	1,620	1,674	1,730	1,788	1,847	1,908	1,972	2,038	2,105	2,175
1,602	1,654	1,709	1,765	1,823	1,882	1,944	2,008	2,074	2,142	2,212
1,636	1,689	1,744	1,800	1,858	1,919	1,981	2,045	2,111	2,180	2,250
1,671	1,724	1,779	1,836	1,895	1,956	2,018	2,082	2,149	2,218	2,289
1,707	1,760	1,816	1,873	1,932	1,993	2,056	2,121	2,188	2,256	2,328
1,743	1,797	1,853	1,911	1,970	2,031	2,094	2,160	2,227	2,296	2,367
1,780	1,835	1,891	1,949	2,009	2,070	2,134	2,199	2,267	2,336	2,408
1,819	1,873	1,930	1,988	2,048	2,110	2,174	2,240	2,307	2,377	2,449
1,857	1,913	1,970	2,028	2,089	2,151	2,215	2,281	2,348	2,418	2,490
1,897	1,953	2,010	2,069	2,130	2,192	2,256	2,322	2,391	2,461	2,533
1,938	1,994	2,051	2,110	2,171	2,234	2,299	2,365	2,433	2,504	2,576
1,979	2,035	2,093	2,153	2,214	2,277	2,342	2,408	2,477	2,547	2,620
2,021	2,078	2,136	2,196	2,196	2,321	2,386	2,453	2,521	2,592	2,665
2,065	2,122	2,180	2,240	2,302	2,365	2,431	2,498	2,566	2,637	2,710
2,109	2,166	2,225	2,285	2,347	2,411	2,476	2,543	2,612	2,683	2,756
2,154	2,211	2,270	2,331	2,393	2,457	2,523	2,590	2,659	2,730	2,803
2,200	2,258	2,317	2,378	2,440	2,504	2,570	2,638	2,707	2,778	2,851
2,247	2,305	2,365	2,426	2,488	2,553	2,618	2,686	2,755	2,827	2,899
2,295	2,353	2,413	2,474	2,537	2,602	2,668	2,735	2,805	2,876	2,949
2,344	2,403	2,463	2,524	2,587	2,652	2,718	2,785	2,855	2,926	2,999
2,394	2,453	2,513	2,575	2,638	2,702	2,769	2,837	2,906	2,977	3,050
2,446	2,504	2,565	2,626	2,690	2,754	2,821	2,889	2,958	3,029	3,102
2,498	2,557	2,617	2,679	2,743	2,807	2,874	2,942	3,011	3,082	3,155

(From Hadlock FP, Harrist RB, Carpenter RJ, et al. Sonographic estimation of fetal weight: The value of femur length in addition to head and abdomen measurements. Radiology. 1984;150:535–540. Used by permission.)   (*Continued*)

APPENDIX P. Estimation of fetal weight (in grams) by abdominal circumference (AC) and femur length (FL)*
(*Continued*)

FL	AC (mm)									
(mm)	305	310	315	320	325	330	335	340	345	350
40	1,590	1,658	1,729	1,802	1,879	1,959	2,042	2,129	2,220	2,314
41	1,617	1,685	1,756	1,830	1,907	1,987	2,071	2,158	2,249	2,344
42	1,644	1,712	1,783	1,858	1,935	2,016	2,100	2,187	2,279	2,373
43	1,671	1,740	1,812	1,886	1,964	2,054	2,129	2,217	2,308	2,404
44	1,699	1,768	1,840	1,915	1,993	2,075	2,159	2,247	2,339	2,434
45	1,727	1,797	1,869	1,944	2,023	2,105	2,189	2,278	2,370	2,465
46	1,756	1,826	1,898	1,974	2,053	2,135	2,220	2,309	2,401	2,497
47	1,785	1,855	1,928	2,004	2,084	2,166	2,251	2,340	2,432	2,528
48	1,814	1,885	1,959	2,035	2,115	2,197	2,283	2,372	2,464	2,560
49	1,845	1,916	1,990	2,066	2,146	2,229	2,315	2,404	2,497	2,593
50	1,875	1,947	2,021	2,098	2,178	2,261	2,347	2,437	2,530	2,626
51	1,906	1,978	2,053	2,130	2,210	2,294	2,380	2,470	2,563	2,659
52	1,938	2,010	2,085	2,163	2,243	2,327	2,413	2,503	2,597	2,693
53	1,970	2,043	2,118	2,196	2,277	2,360	2,447	2,537	2,631	2,728
54	2,003	2,076	2,151	2,229	2,311	2,395	2,482	2,572	2,665	2,762
55	2,036	2,109	2,185	2,264	2,345	2,429	2,516	2,607	2,700	2,797
56	2,070	2,143	2,220	2,298	2,380	2,464	2,552	2,642	2,736	2,833
57	2,104	2,178	2,254	2,333	2,415	2,500	2,587	2,678	2,772	2,869
58	2,139	2,213	2,290	2,369	2,451	2,536	2,624	2,714	2,808	2,905
59	2,175	2,249	2,326	2,405	2,488	2,573	2,660	2,751	2,845	2,942
60	2,211	2,286	2,363	2,442	2,525	2,610	2,698	2,789	2,883	2,980
61	2,248	2,323	2,400	2,480	2,562	2,647	2,736	2,837	2,921	3,018
62	2,285	2,360	2,438	2,518	2,600	2,686	2,774	2,865	2,959	3,056
63	2,323	2,398	2,476	2,556	2,639	2,725	2,813	2,904	2,998	3,095
64	2,362	2,437	2,515	2,595	2,678	2,764	2,852	2,943	3,037	3,134
65	2,401	2,477	2,555	2,635	2,718	2,804	2,892	2,983	3,077	3,174
66	2,441	2,517	2,595	2,675	2,759	2,844	2,933	3,024	3,118	3,215
67	2,481	2,557	2,636	2,716	2,800	2,885	2,974	3,065	3,159	3,256
68	2,523	2,599	2,677	2,758	2,841	2,927	3,016	3,107	3,200	3,297
69	2,564	2,641	2,719	2,800	2,884	2,969	3,058	3,149	3,242	3,339
70	2,607	2,683	2,762	2,843	2,927	3,012	3,101	3,192	3,285	3,381
71	2,650	2,727	2,806	2,887	2,970	3,056	3,144	3,235	3,328	3,424
72	2,694	2,771	2,850	2,931	3,014	3,100	3,188	3,279	3,372	3,468
73	2,739	2,816	2,895	2,976	3,059	3,145	3,233	3,323	3,416	3,512
74	2,785	2,861	2,940	3,021	3,105	3,190	3,278	3,369	3,461	3,557
75	2,831	2,908	2,987	3,068	3,151	3,236	3,324	3,414	3,507	3,602
76	2,878	2,955	3,034	3,115	3,198	3,283	3,371	3,461	3,553	3,648
77	2,926	3,003	3,081	3,162	3,245	3,331	3,418	3,508	3,600	3,694
78	2,974	3,051	3,130	3,211	3,294	3,379	3,466	3,555	3,647	3,741
79	3,024	3,100	3,179	3,260	3,343	3,427	3,514	3,604	3,695	3,789
80	3,074	3,151	3,229	3,310	3,392	3,477	3,564	3,653	3,744	3,837
81	3,125	3,202	3,280	3,360	3,443	3,527	3,614	3,702	3,793	3,886
82	3,177	3,253	3,332	3,412	3,494	3,578	3,664	3,752	3,843	3,935
83	3,230	3,306	3,384	3,464	3,546	3,630	3,716	3,803	3,893	3,985

*Based on regression model: $\log_{10}$ body weight $= 1.3598 + 0.051 \, (AC) + 0.1844 \, (FL) - 0.0037 \, (AC \times FL)$.

APPENDIX P. *(Continued)*

				AC (mm)					
355	360	365	370	375	380	385	390	395	400
2,413	2,515	2,622	2,734	2,850	2,972	3,098	3,230	3,367	3,511
2,442	2,545	2,652	2,764	2,880	3,002	3,128	3,260	3,397	3,540
2,472	2,575	2,683	2,794	2,911	3,032	3,159	3,290	3,427	3,570
2,503	2,606	2,713	2,825	2,942	3,063	3,189	3,321	3,458	3,600
2,533	2,637	2,744	2,856	2,973	3,094	3,220	3,352	3,488	3,630
2,565	2,668	2,776	2,888	3,004	3,125	3,251	3,383	3,519	3,661
2,596	2,700	2,807	2,919	3,036	3,157	3,283	3,414	3,550	3,692
2,628	2,732	2,840	2,952	3,068	3,189	3,315	3,446	3,582	3,723
2,660	2,764	2,872	2,984	3,100	3,221	3,347	3,478	3,613	3,754
2,693	2,797	2,905	3,017	3,133	3,254	3,380	3,510	3,645	3,786
2,726	2,830	2,938	3,050	3,166	3,287	3,412	3,542	3,677	3,818
2,760	2,864	2,972	3,084	3,200	3,320	3,445	3,575	3,710	3,850
2,794	2,898	3,006	3,117	3,234	3,354	3,479	3,608	3,743	3,882
2,828	2,932	3,040	3,152	3,268	3,388	3,513	3,642	3,776	3,915
2,863	2,967	3,075	3,186	3,302	3,422	3,547	3,676	3,809	3,948
2,898	3,002	3,110	3,221	3,337	3,457	3,581	3,710	3,843	3,981
2,933	3,038	3,145	3,257	3,372	3,492	3,616	3,744	3,877	4,015
2,970	3,074	3,181	3,293	3,408	3,572	3,651	3,779	3,911	4,048
3,006	3,110	3,218	3,329	3,444	3,563	3,686	3,814	3,946	4,082
3,043	3,147	3,254	3,366	3,480	3,599	3,722	3,849	3,981	4,117
3,080	3,184	3,292	3,403	3,517	3,636	3,758	3,885	4,016	4,151
3,118	3,222	3,329	3,440	3,554	3,673	3,795	3,921	4,052	4,186
3,157	3,260	3,367	3,478	3,592	3,710	3,832	3,957	4,087	4,222
3,195	3,299	3,406	3,516	3,630	3,747	3,869	3,994	4,124	4,257
3,235	3,338	3,445	3,555	3,668	3,785	3,906	4,031	4,160	4,293
3,274	3,378	3,484	3,594	3,707	3,824	3,944	4,069	4,197	4,329
3,315	3,418	3,524	3,633	3,746	3,863	3,983	4,106	4,234	4,366
3,355	3,458	3,564	3,673	3,786	3,902	4,021	4,144	4,271	4,402
3,397	3,499	3,605	3,714	3,862	3,941	4,060	4,183	4,309	4,439
3,438	3,541	3,646	3,754	3,866	3,981	4,100	4,222	4,347	4,477
3,481	3,583	3,688	3,796	3,907	4,022	4,140	4,261	4,386	4,514
3,523	3,625	3,730	3,838	3,948	4,062	4,180	4,300	4,425	4,552
3,567	3,668	3,772	3,880	3,990	4,104	4,220	4,340	4,464	4,591
3,610	3,712	3,816	3,922	4,032	4,145	4,261	4,381	4,503	4,629
3,655	3,756	3,859	3,966	4,075	4,187	4,303	4,421	4,543	4,668
3,700	3,800	3,903	4,009	4,118	4,230	4,344	4,462	4,583	4,708
3,745	3,845	3,948	4,053	4,161	4,272	4,387	4,504	4,624	4,747
3,791	3,891	3,993	4,098	4,205	4,316	4,429	4,545	4,665	4,787
3,838	3,937	4,039	4,143	4,250	4,360	4,472	4,588	4,706	4,827
3,885	3,984	4,085	4,188	4,295	4,404	4,515	4,630	4,748	4,868
3,933	4,031	4,131	4,234	4,340	4,448	4,559	4,673	4,790	4,909
3,981	4,079	4,179	4,281	4,386	4,493	4,604	4,716	4,832	4,950
4,030	4,127	4,226	4,328	4,432	4,539	4,648	4,760	4,875	4,992
4,080	4,176	4,275	4,376	4,479	4,585	4,693	4,804	4,918	5,034

(From Hadlock FP, Harrist RB, Carpenter RJ, et al. Sonographic estimation of fetal weight: The value of femur length in addition to head and abdomen measurements. Radiology. 1984;150:535–540. Used by permission.)

Index

ISBN 0-397-50952-9

90000